Handbook of Clinical Infectious Diseases

Handbook of Clinical Infectious Diseases

Editor: Cameron Harris

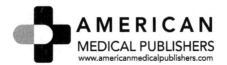

AMERICAN
MEDICAL PUBLISHERS
www.americanmedicalpublishers.com

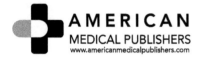

Cataloging-in-Publication Data

Handbook of clinical infectious diseases / edited by Cameron Harris.
    p. cm.
Includes bibliographical references and index.
ISBN 979-8-88740-141-6
1. Communicable diseases. 2. Infection. 3. Communicable diseases--Diagnosis. 4. Communicable diseases--Treatment. 5. Infection--Prevention. I. Harris, Cameron.
RC111 .H36 2023
616.9--dc23

American Medical Publishers,
41 Flatbush Avenue,
1st Floor, New York,
NY 11217, USA

ISBN 979-8-88740-141-6 (Hardback)

Contents

Preface

Infectious diseases are caused by pathogens like fungi, bacteria and viruses. These diseases can spread through direct contact, such as from one person to another, from animal to person, and from mother to an unborn child. They can also be transmitted indirectly through bug bites, contaminated water or food, and exposure to pathogens in the environment. The most common infectious diseases include influenza, hepatitis, common cold, tuberculosis, urinary tract infections (UTIs), strep throat, vaginal candidiasis and clostridioides difficile. The signs of infectious diseases vary based on the pathogens causing the infections, which may include fatigue, fever, congestion, chills, cough, muscle aches and headache, and gastrointestinal symptoms like nausea, vomiting and diarrhea. A weakened immune system as a result of consumption of various medications, or having diseases like HIV and cancer are the risk factors of infectious diseases. The risk of infection can be reduced by washing hands regularly, getting vaccinated, staying back at home during illness, clean and safe preparation of food, and practicing safe sex. This book aims to understand the clinical perspectives of infectious diseases. The readers would gain knowledge that would broaden their perspective in this area of medicine.

This book is a result of research of several months to collate the most relevant data in the field.

When I was approached with the idea of this book and the proposal to edit it, I was overwhelmed. It gave me an opportunity to reach out to all those who share a common interest with me in this field. I had 3 main parameters for editing this text:

1. Accuracy – The data and information provided in this book should be up-to-date and valuable to the readers.

2. Structure – The data must be presented in a structured format for easy understanding and better grasping of the readers.

3. Universal Approach – This book not only targets students but also experts and innovators in the field, thus my aim was to present topics which are of use to all.

Thus, it took me a couple of months to finish the editing of this book.

I would like to make a special mention of my publisher who considered me worthy of this opportunity and also supported me throughout the editing process. I would also like to thank the editing team at the back-end who extended their help whenever required.

Editor

Structural Modeling and Molecular Dynamics of the Immune Checkpoint Molecule HLA-G

Thais Arns[1], Dinler A. Antunes[2], Jayvee R. Abella[2], Maurício M. Rigo[2], Lydia E. Kavraki[2], Silvana Giuliatti[3] and Eduardo A. Donadi[1]*

[1] Department of Basic and Applied Immunology, Ribeirão Preto Medical School, University of São Paulo, Ribeirão Preto, Brazil, [2] Department of Computer Science, Rice University, Houston, TX, United States, [3] Department of Genetics, Ribeirão Preto Medical School, University of São Paulo, Ribeirão Preto, Brazil

***Correspondence:**
Eduardo A. Donadi
eadonadi@usp.br*

HLA-G is considered to be an immune checkpoint molecule, a function that is closely linked to the structure and dynamics of the different HLA-G isoforms. Unfortunately, little is known about the structure and dynamics of these isoforms. For instance, there are only seven crystal structures of HLA-G molecules, being all related to a single isoform, and in some cases lacking important residues associated to the interaction with leukocyte receptors. In addition, they lack information on the dynamics of both membrane-bound HLA-G forms, and soluble forms. We took advantage of *in silico* strategies to disclose the dynamic behavior of selected HLA-G forms, including the membrane-bound HLA-G1 molecule, soluble HLA-G1 dimer, and HLA-G5 isoform. Both the membrane-bound HLA-G1 molecule and the soluble HLA-G1 dimer were quite stable. Residues involved in the interaction with ILT2 and ILT4 receptors (α3 domain) were very close to the lipid bilayer in the complete HLA-G1 molecule, which might limit accessibility. On the other hand, these residues can be completely exposed in the soluble HLA-G1 dimer, due to the free rotation of the disulfide bridge (Cys42/Cys42). In fact, we speculate that this free rotation of each protomer (i.e., the chains composing the dimer) could enable alternative binding modes for ILT2/ILT4 receptors, which in turn could be associated with greater affinity of the soluble HLA-G1 dimer. Structural analysis of the HLA-G5 isoform demonstrated higher stability for the complex containing the peptide and coupled β2-microglobulin, while structures lacking such domains were significantly unstable. This study reports for the first time structural conformations for the HLA-G5 isoform and the dynamic behavior of HLA-G1 molecules under simulated biological conditions. All modeled structures were made available through GitHub (https://github.com/KavrakiLab/), enabling their use as templates for modeling other alleles and isoforms, as well as for other computational analyses to investigate key molecular interactions.

Keywords: HLA-G, HLA-G1 soluble dimer, HLA-G5 isoform, molecular dynamics, structural bioinformatics

INTRODUCTION

The Human Leukocyte Antigen G (HLA-G) is a nonclassical Major Histocompatibility Complex class I (MHC-I) molecule that possesses immunomodulatory properties (1). Its presence is tissue-restricted, being expressed in fetal tissues [trophoblast cells (2)] and constitutively expressed in adult thymic medulla (3), cornea (4), pancreatic islets (5), erythroid, and endothelial cell precursors (6). However, the expression of HLA-G can be induced in several conditions (1), including cancer (7, 8), transplantation (9), viral infections (10, 11), and autoimmune and inflammatory diseases (12, 13).

A well-recognized function of the HLA-G molecule in these pathological and physiological conditions is the inhibition of the cytotoxic activity of Natural Killer (NK) and $CD8^+$ T lymphocytes. This function is mediated by interaction with leukocyte receptors, particularly with the Leukocyte Ig-like Receptors (LILRs), also known as Immunoglobulin-like Transcripts (ILT2, ILT4). ILT2 and ILT4 interact with several classical class I HLA molecules, but have higher affinity for HLA-G (14). ILT2 is expressed by B cells, some subtypes of T cells and NK cells, and all monocytes/dendritic cells (15). It is also described as a receptor for HLA-G associated with β2-microglobulin. On the other hand, ILT4 is myeloid-specific and only expressed by monocytes/dendritic cells (16), being capable of recognizing HLA-G free heavy chains (17, 18). Through these differentially expressed receptors, HLA-G can interact with all these different cell types, primarily inhibiting their functions. In addition, HLA-G may also generate regulatory/suppressor cells. For instance, human tolerogenic dendritic cells (DC-10) express high levels of membrane-bound HLA-G1 and are potent inducers of adaptive allospecific Type 1 regulatory T (Tr1) cells (19). The *HLA-G* gene is located within the MHC region, presenting low polymorphism, in contrast with the highly polymorphic classical class I genes, i.e., *HLA-A, -B, -C* (20). Geragthy et al. (21) first described the *HLA-G* gene in 1987, and its structure is homologous to other HLA class I genes. The *HLA-G* primary transcript may generate at least seven alternative splicing mRNAs that encode membrane-bound (HLA-G1, G2, G3, G4) and soluble (HLA-G5, G6, G7) protein isoforms (22-25). HLA-G1 may also be detected in plasma after proteolytic cleavage by metalloproteases, and presents the same domains (α1, α2, and α3) of classical class I molecules, being also associated with a β2-microglobulin. HLA-G2 is devoid of the α2 domain encoded by exon 3. HLA-G3 does not have the α2 and α3 domains encoded by exons 3 and 4, and HLA-G4 lost the α3 domain. The soluble HLA-G5 and HLA-G6 isoforms have the same extra globular domains as HLA-G1 and HLA-G2, respectively, and are generated by transcripts retaining intron 4, which block translation of the transmembrane domain (exon 5). The 5' region of the intron, in the reading phase with exon 4, is translated into a stop codon and generates the HLA-G5 and HLA-G6 isoforms. These isoforms contain a specific 21 residues long tail involved in molecule solubility. The soluble HLA-G7 isoform is limited to the α1 domain and retains two intron 2

specific amino acids. All alternative transcripts are devoid of exon 7 (26, 27).

Sequence comparison of the HLA-G molecule to other HLA class I proteins reveals some interesting particularities. First, HLA-G has an unusually long half-life on the cell surface, resulting from the absence of an endocytosis motif in its truncated cytoplasmic domain (28). Second, HLA-G sequences have two unique Cysteine residues located at positions 42 and 147. Dimerization of HLA-G occurs through the creation of disulfide bonds between the two unique Cysteine residues at position 42 (Cys42-Cys42 bonds). Since all isoforms carry Cys42, all translated isoforms could potentially form membrane-bound homodimers, soluble homodimers, β2-microglobulin-free homodimers, and possibly homotrimers (associated or not to β2-microglobulin) (29, 30). Noteworthy, HLA-G dimers: i) do not induce significant structural changes to the main backbone of the protomers (i.e., chains forming the dimer) (17); ii) may exhibit distinct inhibitory functions as compared to monomers [e.g., dimers bind to ILT receptors with higher affinity *in vitro* (29) and *in vivo* (31)]; and iii) exhibit slower dissociation rates than monomers (17). ILT recognition of HLA-G dimers has a pivotal role on immune suppression at the maternal-fetal interface, possibly contributing to the prevention of pregnancy complications such as pre-eclampsia and recurrent miscarriages (17, 20).

Since HLA-G5 isoform has the same extra globular domains as HLA-G1, it could potentially be recognized by the same receptors. In fact, it has been reported that ILT2 can interact with β2-microglobulin-associated HLA-G5, while ILT4 could be able to recognize isoforms that are not associated to β2-microglobulin (17, 32). Such β2-microglobulin-free heavy chain has been detected in cell culture supernatants expressing HLA-G5 (33). It has also been shown that the expression of soluble HLA-G5 could inhibit the cytotoxicity of NK cells, and that the degree of inhibition was more evident when induced by HLA-G5, as compared to the membrane-bound HLA-G1. Most importantly, it was shown that the combination of HLA-G1 and HLA-G5 leads to significantly greater suppression than the effects of HLA-G1 or HLA-G5 alone (34). The direct involvement of HLA-G5 in inducing graft acceptance *in vivo* after human transplantation was provided by the observation that HLA-G5 purified from the plasma of transplanted HLA-G-positive patients suppressed alloproliferation of T cells *in vitro* (35).

Considering all the aforementioned structural diversity of known HLA-G isoforms, and the multiple roles of HLA-G in different immunological pathways, it is astonishing how little is known about the structure and dynamics of these molecules. As of today, there are only seven crystal structures of HLA-G receptors in the Protein Data Bank (PDB) (36). Note that these structures are limited to HLA-G1, and that even for this particular isoform they do not capture the full molecule (see **Supplementary Table 1**). In addition, there is only so much that can be understood from a static crystal structure in which relates to the dynamic behavior of these molecules. For instance, previous analysis of the membrane-bound HLA-G1 has indicated an oblique orientation of the protomers. Such orientation makes the ILT2 and ILT4 binding sites slightly more accessible to the interaction with these receptors (17). However, it does not tell us if this oblique orientation is stable in the soluble HLA-G1 dimer, or if other arrangements are possible. Finally, available structural data cannot inform us about the structure and dynamics of all other HLA-G alleles and isoforms.

As a step forward in addressing all these open questions, the present work reports for the first time the complete structure and dynamic behavior of the membrane-bound HLA-G1 model. In addition, it also characterizes the dynamics of the soluble HLA-G1 dimer. These efforts allowed for the first time the observation of a tilting movement of the membrane-bound HLA-G1 monomer, and the total rotational freedom of the HLA-G1 dimer in solution (**Figure 1**). Finally, it investigates the stability of three different proposed structures for the soluble HLA-G5 isoform.

MATERIAL AND METHODS

Molecular Modeling

To obtain the complete HLA-G1 model for the molecule encoded by the *HLA-G*01:01* allele group, homology modeling was performed using Modeller 9.15 software (37) and the PDB_ID: 1YDP structure as a template (38). The selected template structure was obtained by X-ray diffraction crystallography with a 1.9 Å resolution (38), is encoded by the *HLA-G*01:04* allele group, and exhibits 275 resolved residues. It includes the nonapeptide RIIPRHLQL in the binding cleft, and the coupled β2-microglobulin chain. The Rosetta cyclic coordinate descent algorithm (CCD) *ab initio* modeling (39) was applied to unresolved extracellular and intracellular regions in the crystallographic template. Two thousand models were generated in each *ab initio* modeling step. For the transmembrane portion, the GPCR-ITASSER online server was used (40). The complete membrane-bound HLA-G1 model was then applied as template for three possible HLA-G5 isoform structures: monomer, monomer containing the nonapeptide in the cleft, and monomer containing the nonapeptide in the cleft coupled to β2-microglobulin. Isoform residues not included in the membrane-bound HLA-G1 model were resolved using the Rosetta CCD *ab initio* modeling. The

existing structural gaps in the HLA-G1 soluble dimer template (PDB_ID: 2D31) were completed by homology modeling using PDB_ID: 1YDP structure as template. All models were evaluated using several validation software, including QMEAN (41), MODFOLD (42), Verify 3D (43, 44), ERRAT (45), and PROCHECK (46). Images and structure visualization were performed using PyMOL software (47). The BioPython package (48) was applied to identify the interacting residues. The Cα Root Mean Square Deviation (RMSD) and Root Mean Square Fluctuations (RMSF) values were calculated using the initial structures as reference. All structures and simulation movies are available in the **Supplementary Material** and at GitHub (https://github.com/KavrakiLab/).

Lipid Bilayer Insertion

The complete HLA-G1 model was inserted into a phospholipid bilayer (DLPA, *1,2-Dilauroyl-sn-glycero-3-phosphate*). This step was performed with the CHARMM-GUI online server (49, 50).

Molecular Dynamics (MD) Simulations

Three simulations of 100 ns were performed for the complete HLA-G1 inserted into the lipid bilayer, using GROMACS v5.1.4 (51) and CHARMM36m force field (52). MD simulations were also performed in triplicate using GROMACS v4.6.5 package and the G54a7 force field, for a total of 600 ns for the soluble HLA-G1 dimer and a total of 2.1 μs for the HLA-G5 isoform. A cubic box was defined with at least 9 Å of liquid layer around the protein (exact dimensions were different for each protein), using single-point charge water model and periodic boundary conditions. An appropriate number of sodium (Na$^+$) and chloride (Cl$^-$) counter-ions were added to neutralize the system at the final concentration of 0.15 mol/L. Besides the complete membrane-bound HLA-G1, the dynamic system contained 32,560 DLPA molecules, 184,197 water molecules and 380 counter-ions. As for the soluble dimer, it contained 383,325 water molecules and 470 counter-ions. The HLA-G5 monomer dynamic system contained 90,375 water molecules and 187 counter-ions; the monomer containing the nonapeptide in the cleft system had 90,135 water molecules and 185 counter-ions; and the monomer containing the nonapeptide in the cleft coupled to β2-microglobulin had 83,676 water molecules and 179 counter-ions. The algorithms *v-*

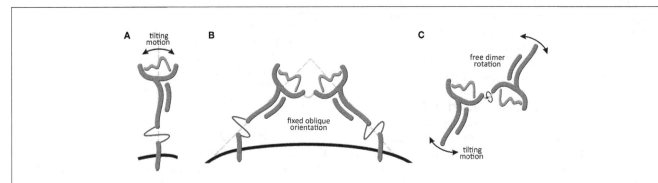

FIGURE 1 | **(A)** Tilting motion of the membrane-bound HLA-G1 structure. **(B)** Membrane-bound HLA-G1 dimer representation, showing the oblique orientation (~45° angle) observed by X-ray crystallography. **(C)** Representation of the complete rotational freedom of the soluble HLA-G1 dimer in solution.

rescale ($\tau t = 0.1$ ps) and *parrinello-rhaman* ($\tau p = 2$ ps) were used for temperature and pressure coupling, respectively. Cutoff values of 1.2 nm were used for both van der Waals and Coulomb interactions, with Fast Particle-Mesh Ewald (PME) electrostatics. For all MD simulations, the production stage was preceded by: *i)* three steps of Energy Minimization (alternating steepest-descent and conjugate gradient algorithms), and *ii)* eight steps of Equilibration as previously described (53). Briefly, the Equilibration stage started with position restraints for all heavy atoms ($5,000$ kJ^{-1}mol^{-1}nm^{-1}) and a temperature of 310 K, for a period of 300 ps, to allow for the formation of solvation layers. The temperature was then reduced to 280 K and the position restraints were gradually reduced. This process was followed by a gradual increase in temperature (up to 300 K). Together, these Equilibration steps represented the first 500 ps of each simulation. During the production stage, the system was held at constant temperature (310 K) without restraints.

Dimensionality Reduction Analysis

Principal component analysis (PCA) was performed using the Python libraries MDTraj (54) and PyEmma (55). PCA is a dimensionality reduction method used to analyze the sampling done by the MDs. PCA maximizes the variance of the transformed coordinates, which is ideal for finding conformations that are geometrically diverse. The residue-residue distances (defined as the distance between the nearest two heavy atoms) between one copy of the dimer and the other were extracted. Only every tenth residue in the system was considered to save memory, resulting in 1,444 features for the dimensionality reduction analysis.

Peptide-Bound Ensemble Modeling and Stability Analysis

A structure-based stability analysis was performed to compare two different HLA-G binders, RIIPRHLQL and RLPKDFRIL. The aforementioned complete model of HLA-G1 (HLA-G*01:01), after removed the bound peptide structure, was used as input to the Anchored Peptide-MHC Ensemble Generator (APE-Gen) (56). Generated ensembles of peptide conformations were later minimized with OpenMM (57), and the lowest energy conformation for each peptide was selected using the Vinardo scoring function (58). All these steps were performed using a customized workflow from the HLA-Arena modeling environment (59). Finally, selected conformations (i.e., lowest energy) were used as input for a structure-based random forest classifier trained on a large dataset of immunopeptidomics experiments (60). This analysis predicted the stability of both complexes, and the individual contribution of each peptide residue toward peptide-MHC complex stability.

Protein-Protein Docking With ILT4

A protein-protein docking study was conducted with the ClusPro webserver (61). A crystal structure of ILT4 was obtained from PDB (PDB_ID: 6AED), and gaps (residues 134 to 143) were filled with loop refinement algorithm from Modeller 9.15 software (37) using UCSF Chimera software (62). This structure was used for protein-protein docking against *(i)* HLA-G monomer and *(ii)* HLA-G dimer structures. The best output structure was chosen considering the frequency of members inside each cluster and the Lowest Energy score.

RESULTS

Membrane-Bound HLA-G1 Molecule Displays Tilting Motion in Solution

A complete model of the mature protein encoded by the *HLA-G*01:01* allele group was generated, containing all 314 residues (**Figure 2A**). The complete modeled system included the HLA-G molecule, sodium (Na$^+$) and chloride (Cl$^-$) counter-ions, and a phospholipid bilayer (**Figure 2B**). During the MD simulations, the average cleft width was 23.2 Å, ranging from 19.4 Å to 25.6 Å (measured at each 10 ns), and the peptide cleft depth was 15.8 Å (**Figure 2A**). The RIIPRHLQL peptide remained stable during the simulations, as observed by the low Root Mean Square Fluctuation (RMSF) (data not shown). The RMSD values for the MD simulations did not exceed 11.46 Å for any of the replicated trajectories, oscillating in the range from 4 Å to 10 Å (**Supplementary Figure 1**). Note that the observed RMSD variation does not reflect unfolding or large conformational changes in the protein, but it relates to oscillations on the angle of the transmembrane region and its impact on the orientation of the extracellular domain (**Figure 2C**). In fact, the RMSD value calculated between the initial and final conformations of the protein is of only 3.13 Å. This conformational stability can also be observed by the PCA analysis, which demonstrates great overlap of sampled conformations among all three simulations. Taken together, these results point to the stability and compactness of the complete membrane-bound HLA-G1 model generated (**Figure 2D**). The transmembrane region extended for 32.7 Å and, alongside the cytoplasmic tail, presented an all direction swinging movement, spanning 22.5 Å.

ILT2 and ILT4 Interacting Residues Are Not Fully Accessible in the Membrane-Bound HLA-G1 Molecule

According to previous studies, ILT2 binds to HLA-G residue F195, while ILT4 binds to F195 and Y197 (17, 38). All these residues are located at the end of the α3 domain, and our model shows that these binding sites are very close to the lipid bilayer (**Figure 3**). Limited access to these residues could explain the lower overall affinity of the HLA-G1 monomer to ILT2/ILT4, when compared to the soluble dimer, as previously demonstrated by *Shiroishi* and collaborators (17). Locations of other potential binding sites are also depicted. CD8α/α contacts the α3 domain of HLA-G1 at residues 223 to 229 (63, 64). Q79 and M76 are candidate interacting residues for KIR2DL4 (26, 65, 66).

Soluble HLA-G1 Dimer Displays Full Rotational Freedom of Protomers

Three simulations of 200 ns were performed for the soluble HLA-G1 dimer, starting from the oblique orientation (~45° angle) observed by X-ray crystallography (**Figure 4A**) for the disulfide-linked HLA-G1 dimer. The RMSD values for the MD simulations

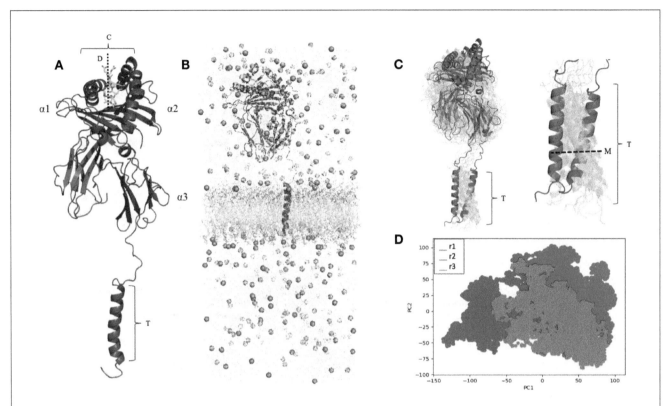

FIGURE 2 | (A) Complete membrane-bound HLA-G1 protein encompassing the α1, α2, α3, transmembrane (T), and intracytoplasmic (I) domains (purple), coupled with β2-microglobulin (pink) and the RIIPRHLQL peptide (green). W (average cleft width) = 23.2 Å, and D (cleft depth) = 15.8 Å; T = 32.7 Å. (B) Complete membrane-bound HLA-G1 molecular dynamics simulation system, including: *i*) water molecules seen in the blue background, *ii*) Na⁺ and Cl⁻ ions (golden spheres), and *iii*) phospholipid bilayer (green). (C) Initial (blue) and final (red) conformations of the 100 ns complete membrane-bound HLA-G1 dynamics (left) and for the transmembrane portion (right). Intermediate conformations obtained at 10ns intervals are displayed in light gray, showing the molecular movement inside the lipid bilayer. M, transmembrane swinging movement over 100 ns. (D) Principal component analysis (PCA) depicting the distribution of conformations extracted from three independent MD trajectories (r1, r2, and r3).

oscillated between 9 Å and 25 Å, depending on the simulation (**Supplementary Figure 2**). Once again, these high RMSD values do not reflect conformational changes of the protomers (**Figures 4B, C**). Instead, they reflect the great conformational freedom of the protomers during the MD simulation, as enabled by the rotation of the disulfide bond (**Figure 4C**). Although the dimer as a whole is very flexible, the folding of the protomers is very stable, and the RIIPRHLQL peptide remained stably bound in the cleft; data consistent with the low Root Mean Square Fluctuation (RMSF) obtained (**Supplementary Figure 3**).

Interestingly, the PCA analysis revealed that each soluble dimer simulation described a different trajectory, exploring different regions of the conformational space (**Figure 4D**). In our PCA analysis, PC1 is most correlated with the distance between LEU81 in one copy and ILE214 in the other copy (**Figure 5A**), while PC2 is most correlated with the distance between GLN141 in one copy and SER91 in the other copy (**Figure 5B**).

HLA-G5 Is More Stable When Associated With β2-Microglobulin and a Peptide Ligand

In this work, we evaluated three HLA-G5 structural possibilities: (*i*) monomer (**Figure 6A**), (*ii*) monomer containing the

nonapeptide in the cleft (**Figure 6B**), and (*iii*) monomer containing the nonapeptide in the cleft coupled to β2-microglobulin (**Figure 6C**). Considering Cα residue fluctuation of all the HLA-G5 structural possibilities, the most stable structure was the monomer containing the nonapeptide in the cleft coupled to β2-microglobulin, which suffered minimal structural deformations during the MD simulation (**Figure 6D**). As seen in (**Supplementary Material—HLA-G5 Monomer, nonapeptide, and coupled β2-microglobulin Simulation Video; Supplementary Figure 4**), the stability is mainly due to the interaction of the tail from intron 4 and the coupled β2-microglobulin, which prevents the tail from reaching up and destabilizing the peptide cleft. In fact, this disruptive behavior was observed in the absence of β2-microglobulin, leading to complete dissociation of the nonapeptide from the HLA-G5 cleft (**Figure 6D** and **Supplementary Material—HLA-G5 Monomer and nonapeptide Simulation Video**). Specifically, the interaction with the tail from intron 4 (last 21 residues) resulted in an increase of the cleft's width, causing the peptide's anchor residues to lose important interactions with residues in the cleft's β-sheet floor and surrounding α-helices (**Supplementary Figure 4**). At the beginning of the simulation

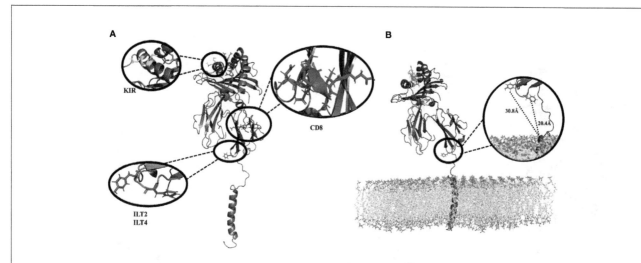

FIGURE 3 | **(A)** Complete membrane-bound HLA-G1 protein (without lipid bilayer), indicating the interacting residues for CD8 receptor (blue: residues D223, Q224, T225, Q226, D 227, V228, E229), ILT2 receptor (red: residues F195), and ILT4 receptor (red: residues F195, Y197). Residues suggested to interact with KIR2DL are also depicted (green: residues Q79, M76) **(B)** Complete membrane bound HLA-G1 protein (including the lipid bilayer), emphasizing the localization and distance of the ILT2 (red: residues F195, 20.4 Å to the membrane) and ILT4 receptors (red: residues F195, Y197, 30.8 Å to the membrane), both of which are close to the lipid bilayer. (D, Aspartic acid; E, Glutamic acid; F, Phenylalanine; M, Methionine; Q, Glutamine; T, Threonine; and V, Valine).

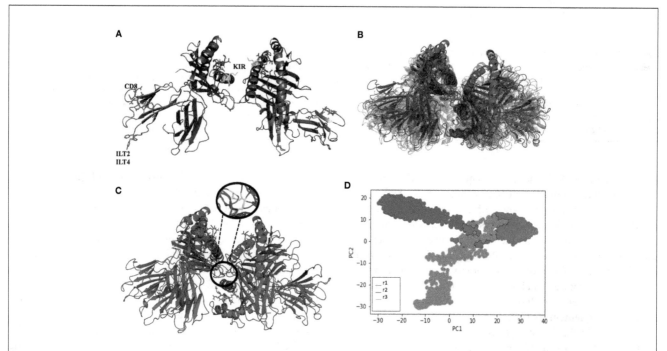

FIGURE 4 | **(A)** Soluble HLA-G1 protein indicating the interacting for CD8 receptor (blue: residues D223, Q224, T225, Q226, D 227, V228, E229), ILT2 receptor (red: residue F195) and ILT4 receptor (red: residues F195, Y197). Residues suggested to interact with KIR2DL are also depicted (green: residues Q79, M76) **(B)** Initial (blue) and final (red) conformations of the 200 ns soluble HLA-G1 dimer dynamics. Twenty-nanosecond intervals (light gray) showing the significant dimer rotation. **(C)** Initial (blue) and final (red) conformations of the 200-ns soluble HLA-G1 dimer dynamics, depicting the zoomed area showing the disulfide bridge. **(D)** Principal component analysis (PCA) depicting the distribution of conformations extracted from three independent MD trajectories (r1, r2, and r3).

the cleft width measured 15.6 Å (**Figure 7A**), increasing its size up to 17.4 Å around 200 ns of the simulation, when the peptide escapes the cleft (**Figure 7B**). The cleft width reduces to about 14.6 Å after the unbinding of the peptide (**Figure 7C**). The superimposed images reveal the variation in cleft's width during the simulated time (**Figure 7D**).

Some structural instability was also observed for the soluble HLA-G5 monomer alone (**Figure 6D**). Both monomer and

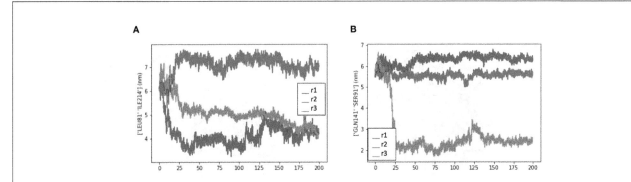

FIGURE 5 | Measurement of the distance between residues to evaluate the dimer flexibility at the disulfide bridge. Measurement data extracted from three dimer simulations (r1, r2, and r3) showed that the residues exhibited similar spatial behavior in all simulations, depending on the residue-residue distance that is observed. **(A)** Measurement data from LEU81 and SER91, **(B)** Measurement data from LEU81 and ILE214. (LEU, Leucine; ILE, Isoleucine; GLN, Glutamine; SER, Serine).

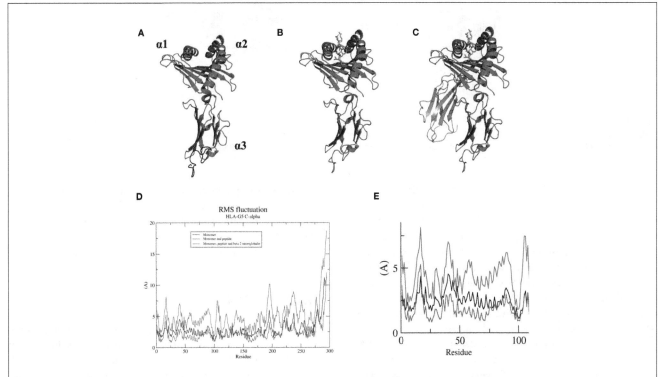

FIGURE 6 | **(A)** Soluble HLA-G5 isoform (pink) and 21 amino acid tail from intron 4 (black, but represented in the following figures in pink). Domain location (α1, α2, and α3) shown. **(B)** Soluble HLA-G5 isoform (pink) and nonapeptide RIIPRHLQL (green). **(C)** Soluble HLA-G5 isoform (pink), nonapeptide RIIPRHLQL (green) and β2-microglobulin (lavender). **(D)** RMSF of all three HLA-G5 structural possibilities: monomer (black), monomer containing the nonapeptide in the cleft (red), and monomer containing the nonapeptide in the cleft coupled to β2-microglobulin (blue). **(E)** Zoomed α-1 domain residues (residue number 1–100), taken from RMSF plot **(D)**, showing HLA-G5 monomer (black), monomer containing the nonapeptide in the cleft (red), and monomer containing the nonapeptide in the cleft coupled to β2-microglobulin (blue).

monomer containing the nonapeptide in the cleft showed much higher RMSF values for the α1-domain region, which constitutes residues 1 to 100. Such residues were extremely important in order to keep the peptide cleft folded, and suffered the majority of the destabilizing interactions induced by the movement of the portion relative to the tail from intron 4 (**Figure 6E** and **Supplementary Material**—HLA-G5 Monomer Simulation Video, **Supplementary Material**—HLA-G5 Monomer and nonapeptide Simulation Video).

Produced Models Can Be Used for Additional Structural Analysis

All produced 3D models were made available through GitHub (github.com/KavrakiLab/hla-g-models) and can now be used as input for additional structural analysis. To demonstrate this point, we conducted a *(i)* peptide-docking analysis comparing two different HLA-G peptide-binders, and a *(ii)* protein-protein docking analysis of binding modes for ILT4.

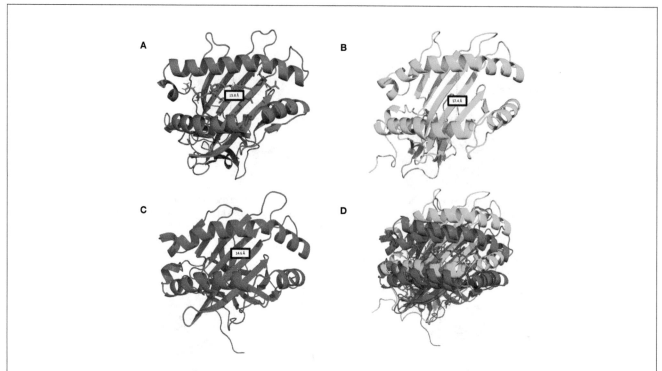

FIGURE 7 | **(A)** HLA-G5 cleft in the absence of the β2-microglobulin, demonstrating the nonapeptide RIIPRHLQL in the initial moments of the simulations. **(B)** Around 200 ns of simulation, due to structural instability, the cleft widens and the nonapeptide RIIPRHLQL loses all interactions with the surrounding structures, escaping the cleft. **(C)** As there is no peptide left in the cleft, its width is diminished. **(D)** Superimposition of **Figures 6A–C**.

Our structural analysis of the peptide-ligands indicated a similar overall contribution to complex stability. A structure-based machine learning method predicted a ~70% probability of stable binding for both peptides (**Supplementary Figure 5**). Moreover, the decomposition of the individual contributions of peptide residues indicated the dominant role of the conserved Leucine in p9 toward complex stability in both systems. As expected, there were differences in secondary interactions with other peptide's residues, with a slight advantage toward RLPKDFRIL. Therefore, our analysis suggests that RLPKDFRIL would provide similar or slightly better stability to the tested HLA-G systems. This prediction is in agreement with recent experimental data showing no significant differences between these peptides regarding the binding of HLA-G1 to ILT2/ILT4 (67).

Our protein-protein docking analysis further corroborated the findings that better interaction with ILT4 is possible when using conformations of the soluble HLA-G1 dimer, as compared to the the membrane-bound HLA-G1 monomer. The putative ILT4-binding site is formed by a relatively hydrophobic patch formed by F195/Y197 residues. This is conserved in HLA-G molecules, but not in other classical HLAs (30). Indeed, our best HLA-G1 dimer/ILT4 interaction models are represented by hydrophobic-favored interactions involving these two HLA residues. Moreover, the ILT4 domains involved in this interaction were domains 1 and 2, which is in accordance to previous binding experiments (30) (**Supplementary Figure 6**). The best interaction model between the monomer of HLA-G and ILT4 was favored by electrostatic interactions and it is depicted in **Supplementary Figure 6A**. Note that the best results indicated a binding mode in which ILT4 approaches HLA-G1 from the "bottom" (**Supplementary Figure 6C**). This binding mode is different from that previously described by Wang et al. (67), and might only be possible for the soluble forms of HLA-G.

DISCUSSION

HLA-G plays an important role on the suppression of immune responses, and both membrane-bound and soluble isoforms may exert this function. As of September 2020, the IMGT-HLA database includes 80 *HLA-G* alleles, encoding 21 complete and 4 truncated proteins (*HLA-G1**01:05N, G*01:13N, G*01:21N and G*01:25N) (68, 69). All alleles encoding the complete protein have the potential to *i)* form dimers through the conserved Cysteine at position 42, *ii)* form the seven commonly described HLA-G isoforms (HLA-G1 to HLA-G7), and *iii)* interact with the leukocyte receptors (26). This remarkable structural diversity must be studied in detail in order to clarify the diverse roles played by HLA-G molecules in both physiological and pathological conditions. Unfortunately, many questions remain unanswered about the structure, dynamics, expression and interaction patterns of different HLA-G alleles and isoforms. For instance, previous experimental studies have provided structures for the membrane-bound HLA-G1, and HLA-G1 dimer, either alone or interacting with other receptors. However, even in these cases the structures were incomplete. In addition, there was no available information on the dynamics of membrane-bound and soluble isoforms. Our goal was to conduct accurate structural modeling and molecular dynamics analysis of *i)* the complete membrane bound HLA-G1, *ii)* the soluble HLA-G1 dimer, and the soluble HLA-G5 monomer. This work moves the field forward, providing both insights on the dynamics of these complexes and complete 3D models that can now be used by other groups for further analysis.

Our complete model of HLA-G1 encompasses the heavy-chain (α1, α2, and α3 domains), connecting peptide, transmembrane portion and cytoplasmic tail of the most frequently observed *HLA-G*01:01* molecule. The *HLA-G*01:01* allele group encompasses 25 synonymous substitutions, as reported for the *HLA-G*01:01:01:01* to *HLA-G*01:01:25* alleles (68, 69). The associated light-chain (β2-microglobulin) was also included in our complete model. Finally, the RIIPRHLQL peptide, derived from histone H2A, was selected to be used in this study since (*i*) it is known to confer stability to the HLA-G molecule (64), (*ii*) is one of the most abundant peptides displayed by HLA-G (70), and (*iii*) was present in the cell cultures used for previous HLA-G X-ray diffraction studies (70). Note that an additional structural analysis comparing the binding of RIIPRHLQL with another HLA-G-binder, RLPKDFRIL, suggested that both peptides should provide similar level of stability to HLA-G complexes.

As expected, the MD simulations (**Figure 2B**) showed a stable membrane-bound HLA-G1 molecule, without evidence of unfolding of secondary structures (i.e., α-helices and β-sheets) (**Figure 2D**). In addition, both the β2-microglobulin and the coupled peptide ligand remained stably-bound during all simulations. Interestingly, we observed for the first time the natural "tilting" movement of the membrane-bound HLA-G1 in solution (**Supplementary Figure 1**). This motion, in addition to the lateral swinging movement of the transmembrane portion in the lipid bilayer (spanning 22.5 Å), is reflected on the observed RMSD values. However, the PCA analysis shows great agreement between simulations in terms of sampled conformations. The superposition of frames from the beginning and end of the simulation (**Figure 2D**) also shows that all secondary and tertiary structures were preserved during MD. These results confirms the stability and compactness of the complete membrane-bound HLA-G1 model generated (**Figure 2C**), which could now be used for additional structural analyses.

We also report for the first time the complete model of the soluble HLA-G1 dimer (**Figure 4A**), and the great conformational flexibility of this molecule in solution (**Figure 4B**). While the disulfide-linked dimer is locked into a 45° angle between the protomers (**Figure 1**), our simulations demonstrate that the soluble dimer is able to explore the full rotational flexibility enabled by the disulfide bridge (**Figure 4C**). Note that the secondary and tertiary structures of each protomer were very stable in solution (**Figure 4D**), despite overall dimer flexibility. The peptide-ligands also remained stably-bound to the respective clefts (**Figures 4A, B**). The PCA analysis of the three independent simulations of the soluble HLA-G1 dimer (**Figure**

4B) demonstrated that every dimer explored a different region of the conformational space, while still presenting similar collective motions, as demonstrated by the residue-residue distance comparisons (**Figures 5A, B**). A direct comparison between the PCAs for the membrane-bound HLA-G1 monomer and soluble HLA-G1 dimer is not possible, since the principal components used in each case reflect features that better capture the movements observed in each system. However, it is possible to observe that the soluble HLA-G1 dimer PCA captures a much greater conformational freedom.

Our HLA-G1 dimer model includes residues located at positions 195, 196, 197, 266, and 267, which were missing in the available crystal structure of the disulfide-linked dimer (17). All these residues are located in the α3 domain, where major leukocyte receptor binding sites are located. For instance, they include the putative binding sites for ILTs (residues 195 and 197) and CD8 (residues 223-229 residues). Note that these sites are very close to membrane in the membrane-bound HLA-G1 monomer (**Figure 3B**), which might limit interaction with these protein-ligands. It has indeed been observed that HLA-G1 dimers display higher affinity for leukocyte receptors than monomers (17, 20). This advantage has been associated with the 45° angle of the protomers in the disulfide-linked dimer, which can help exposing these sites for interaction (17, 67). Note that the free rotation of the protomers in the HLA-G1 soluble dimer, as observed in our simulations, would enable even greater exposure of these biding sites. In order to further explore our models and investigate the interaction with ILT4, we decided to conduct a protein-protein docking experiment with ClusPro. As expected, ClusPro successfully identified binding modes in which the D1 domain of ILT4 interacts with the α3 domain of HLA-G1, specifically involving F195 and Y197. Some of the predicted binding modes displayed ILT4 approaching HLA-G from the "top," as previously described by Wang et al. (67). The authors of that study discuss the limited flexibility of ILT4 in terms of bending between Ig-like domains, and describe this "top-down" binding mode as the only interaction possible for membrane-bound forms of HLA-G1. Interestingly, in the absence of the membrane, ClusPro predicted better binding modes in which ILT4 approaches HLA-G1 from the "bottom," while still preserving interactions between D1 and F195/Y197. Based on these results, we can speculate that higher affinity of soluble HLA-G1 dimer for ILT2/ILT4 ligands could be explained by the possibility of using this alternative "bottom-up" binding mode. Further computational and experimental studies would be necessary to investigate the occurrence and stability of alternative binding modes involving ILT2 and ITL4.

The interaction of HLA-G with T CD8[+] cells may induce FasL up-regulation, soluble FasL secretion and CD8[+] cell apoptosis by Fas-FasL interaction, whose binding sites have not been determined yet (71). Compared to classical class I molecules (e.g., HLA-A, -B, -C), HLA-G binds to CD8α/α loop (residues 223-229) with medium affinity (63, 64), thus inhibiting the T CD8[+] cytotoxic function. Although little is known regarding the HLA-G dimer interaction with CD8, it is possible that the interaction confers increased avidity in a proper structural orientation, permitting an efficient signaling to CD8 as well as it does for ILT2/ILT4 (17, 38). The freedom of rotation reported in this study for the soluble HLA-G1 dimer, exposing two easily accessible binding sites for ILTs/CD8 receptors, corroborates the potential for multiple orientations of the dimer. Considering that these major leukocyte receptors are adjacent to each other, it is possible the formation of complexes containing multiple combinations of one HLA-G dimer and two leukocyte receptors (ILT2/ILT2, ILT4/ILT4; ILT2/ILT4, ILT2/CD8, ILT4/ CD8, CD8/CD8).

It has been proposed that HLA-G could interact with the killer cell immunoglobulin-like receptor KIR2DL4 (25), and that such interaction could induce both inhibitory as well as activating signals (28, 72, 73). Although the inhibition of the innate and adaptive immune response is the most accepted role of HLA-G, activating responses have also been reported (74). The soluble form of HLA-G could be the natural KIR2DL4 ligand, since it accumulates in KIR2DL4$^+$ endosomes and induces endosome signaling (75). In fact, structural representations (17) indicate that steric constraints would prevent KIR2DL4 from interacting with HLA-G dimers (65, 66, 75). Considering that KIR2DL binding residues are located in the α1 domain of the HLA-G molecule, and considering the HLA-G1 dimer rotation presented here, it is possible that the KIR2DL4 binding area would be more accessible in the soluble HLA-G1 dimer as opposed to the membrane-bound HLA-G1 dimer. However, it is important to stress that we have not tested this interaction in our study, and that recent studies have not found evidence of HLA-G/KIR2DL4 interaction. Once again, the models produced in this work can now be used to further investigate this potential interaction.

Contrary to what was observed for the aforementioned systems, greater instability was observed in two of our HLA-G5 models. Specifically, the only stable system was the one containing both the nonapeptide RIIPRHLQL and ß2-microglobulin (**Figure 6** and **Supplementary Material** – HLA-G5 Monomer, nonapeptide, and coupled β2-microglobulin Simulation Video). Previous studies have reported HLA-G5 isoforms both with and without β2-microglobulin (33, 76). However, our results suggest that the monomeric form of HLA-G5 would not be stable without these other chains (**Supplementary Material** – HLA-G5 Monomer Simulation Video). On the other hand, it is possible that HLA-G5 dimers could be stable in the β2-microglobulin-free form, which was not tested here. For instance, the intronic tails of both protomers could interact with each other, not causing the effect of cleft deformation observed in our simulations (**Supplementary Material** – HLA-G5 Monomer and nonapeptide Simulation Video). Such dimeric structures for HLA-G5 without β2-

microglobulin could be similar to the dimers composed by the α1–α3: α1–α3 domains, as in the work published by Kuroki et al., in which HLA-G2 isoform (membrane bound α1–α3) naturally formed a β2-microglobulin-free homodimer which did not have disulfide bridges keeping the structures in place (77). Electron microscopy revealed that the general structure and domain organization of such HLA-G2 homodimers resembled those of class II HLA heterodimers (α1–α2: β1–β2) (20). Published data (77) described the binding of β2-microglobulin and β2-microglobulin-free forms of HLA molecules to members of ILT receptor family and demonstrated that, in addition to ILT4, β2-microglobulin-free structures are recognized by several other members of this receptor family. In fact, the "activating" members of the ILT family showed a preference for such structures. Therefore, it is possible that this could also be the case for HLA-G. This would support the notion that structural variations of HLA-G may be relevant in the modulation of biological function (32). It's also intriguing to consider that, similar to classic class I HLA molecules, HLA-G may have activating receptors. In fact, it is possible that there are other receptors for HLA-G, specific for isoforms or not, and the study of HLA-G structures other than HLA-G1 and HLA-G5 may allow us to identify them (32).

In conclusion, the present study describes for the first time the complete membrane-bound HLA-G1 3D structure and its dynamic behavior in solution. Our study also described the dynamics of the soluble HLA-G1 dimer. Our simulations highlighted the great flexibility enabled by the disulfide bridge, which could even promote alternative binding modes with ILT2/ ILT4 receptors. Our study of the HLA-G5 isoform and its structural alternatives demonstrated greater structural instability when the peptide or β2-microglobulin were absent. More comprehensive structural studies will be necessary to verify the existence of other structural conformations for HLA-G5. This work produced insights on the structure, dynamics, and interaction patterns of important HLA-G variants. It also produced 3D models that can now be used to further investigate these and other HLA-G molecules, to identify new HLA-G ligands, and to design potential pharmacological interventions.

AUTHOR CONTRIBUTIONS

TA, DA and ED contributed to the conception and design of the study. TA generated all structural models. TA and DA performed simulations. TA, DA, MR and JA performed the analysis. SG and LK supervised the analysis. TA, DA and ED wrote the article. All authors contributed to the article and approved the submitted version.

REFERENCES

Carosella ED, Favier B, Rouas-Freiss N, Moreau P, Lemaoult J. Beyond the Increasing Complexity of the Immunomodulatory HLA-G Molecule. *Blood* (2008) 111(10):4862–70. doi: 10.1182/blood-2007-12-127662

Kovats S, Main EK, Librach C, Stubblebine M, Fisher SJ, DeMars R. A Class I Antigen, HLA-G, Expressed in Human Trophoblasts. *Sci (N Y NY)* (1990) 248 (4952):220–23. doi: 10.1126/science.2326636

Mallet V, Blaschitz A, Crisa L, Schmitt C, Fournel S, King A, et al. HLA-G in the Human Thymus: A Subpopulation of Medullary Epithelial but Not CD83 (+)

Dendritic Cells Expresses HLA-G as a Membrane-Bound and Soluble Protein. *Int Immunol* (1999) 11(6):889–98. doi: 10.1093/intimm/11.6.889

Le Discorde M, Moreau P, Sabatier P, Legeais J-M, Carosella ED. Expression of HLA-G in Human Cornea, an Immune-Privileged Tissue. *Hum Immunol* (2003) 64(11):1039–44. doi: 10.1016/j.humimm.2003.08.346

Cirulli V, Zalatan J, McMaster M, Prinsen R, Salomon DR, Ricordi C, et al. The Class I HLA Repertoire of Pancreatic Islets Comprises the Nonclassical Class Ib Antigen HLA-G. *Diabetes* (2006) 55(5):1214–22. doi: 10.2337/db05-0731

Menier C, Rabreau Michèle, Challier J-C, Le Discorde M, Carosella ED, Rouas-Freiss N. Erythroblasts Secrete the Nonclassical HLA-G Molecule from Primitive to Definitive Hematopoiesis. Blood (2004) 104(10):3153–60. doi: 10.1182/blood-2004-03-0809

Paul P, Rouas-Freiss N, Khalil-Daher I, Moreau P, Riteau B, Le Gal FA, et al. HLA-G Expression in Melanoma: A Way for Tumor Cells to Escape from Immunosurveillance. Proc Natl Acad Sci U States America (1998) 95(8):4510–15. doi: 10.1073/pnas.95.8.4510

Rouas-Freiss N, Moreau P, Ferrone S, Carosella ED. HLA-G Proteins in Cancer: Do They Provide Tumor Cells with an Escape Mechanism? Cancer Res (2005) 65(22):10139–44. doi: 10.1158/0008-5472.CAN-05-0097

Lila N, Carpentier A, Amrein C, Khalil-Daher I, Dausset J, Carosella ED. Implication of HLA-G Molecule in Heart-Graft Acceptance. Lancet (London England) (2000) 355(9221):2138. doi: 10.1016/S0140-6736(00)02386-2

Lozano JM, González R, Kindelán JM, Rouas-Freiss N, Caballos R, Dausset J, et al. Monocytes and T Lymphocytes in HIV-1-Positive Patients Express HLA-G Molecule. AIDS (London England) (2002) 16(3):347–51. doi: 10.1097/00002030-200202150-00005

Lafon M, Prehaud C, Megret F, Lafage M, Mouillot G, Roa M, et al. Modulation of HLA-G Expression in Human Neural Cells after Neurotropic Viral Infections. J Virol (2005) 79(24):15226–37. doi: 10.1128/JVI.79.24.15226-15237.2005

Wiendl H, Feger U, Mittelbronn M, Jack C, Schreiner B, Stadelmann C, et al. Expression of the Immune-Tolerogenic Major Histocompatibility Molecule HLA-G in Multiple Sclerosis: Implications for CNS Immunity. Brain: A J Neurol (2005) 128(Pt 11):2689–704. doi: 10.1093/brain/awh609

Khosrotehrani K, Le Danff C, Reynaud-Mendel B, Dubertret L, Carosella ED, Aractingi S. HLA-G Expression in Atopic Dermatitis. J Invest Dermatol (2001) 117(3):750–52. doi: 10.1046/j.0022-202x.2001.01487.x

Boyson JE, Erskine R, Whitman MC, Chiu M, Lau JM, Koopman LA, et al. Disulfide Bond-Mediated Dimerization of HLA-G on the Cell Surface. Proc Natl Acad Sci U States America (2002) 99(25):16180–85. doi: 10.1073/pnas.212643199

Colonna M, Navarro F, Bellón T, Llano M, Garcıa P, Samaridis J, et al. A Common Inhibitory Receptor for Major Histocompatibility Complex Class I Molecules on Human Lymphoid and Myelomonocytic Cells. J Exp Med (1997) 186(11):1809–18. doi: 10.1084/jem.186.11.1809

Colonna M, Samaridis J, Cella M, Angman L, Allen RL, O'Callaghan CA, et al. Human Myelomonocytic Cells Express an Inhibitory Receptor for Classical and Nonclassical MHC Class I Molecules. J Immunol (Baltimore Md: 1950) (1998) 160(7):3096–100.

Shiroishi M, Kuroki K, Ose T, Rasubala L, Shiratori I, Arase H, et al. Efficient Leukocyte Ig-like Receptor Signaling and Crystal Structure of Disulfide-Linked HLA-G Dimer. J Biol Chem (2006) 281(15):10439–47. doi: 10.1074/jbc.M512305200

Gonen-Gross T, Achdout H, Arnon TII, Gazit R, Stern N, HorejsıV, et al. The CD85J/Leukocyte Inhibitory Receptor-1 Distinguishes between Conformed and Beta 2-Microglobulin-Free HLA-G Molecules. J Immunol (Baltimore Md: 1950) (2005) 175(8):4866–74. doi: 10.4049/jimmunol.175.8.4866

Amodio G, Comi M, Tomasoni D, Emma Gianolini M, Rizzo R, LeMaoult J, et al. HLA-G Expression Levels Influence the Tolerogenic Activity of Human DC-10. Haematologica (2015) 100(4):548–57. doi: 10.3324/haematol.2014.113803

Kuroki K, Maenaka K. Immune Modulation of HLA-G Dimer in Maternal- Fetal Interface. Eur J Immunol (2007) 37(7):1727–29. doi: 10.1002/eji.200737515

Geraghty DE, Koller BH, Orr HT. A Human Major Histocompatibility Complex Class I Gene That Encodes a Protein with a Shortened Cytoplasmic Segment. Proc Natl Acad Sci U States America (1987) 84 (24):9145–49. doi: 10.1073/pnas.84.24.9145

Fujii T, Ishitani A, Geraghty DE. A Soluble Form of the HLA-G Antigen Is Encoded by a Messenger Ribonucleic Acid Containing Intron 4. J Immunol (Baltimore Md: 1950) (1994) 153(12):5516–24.

Ishitani A, Geraghty DE. Alternative Splicing of HLA-G Transcripts Yields Proteins with Primary Structures Resembling Both Class I and Class II Antigens. Proc Natl Acad Sci U States America (1992) 89(9):3947–51. doi: 10.1073/pnas.89.9.3947

Paul P, Cabestre FA, Ibrahim EC, Lefebvre S, Khalil-Daher I, Vazeux G, et al. Identification of HLA-G7 as a New Splice Variant of the HLA-G MRNA and Expression of Soluble HLA-G5, -G6, and -G7 Transcripts in Human Transfected Cells. Hum Immunol (2000) 61(11):1138–49. doi: 10.1016/s0198-8859(00)00197-x

Carosella ED, Moreau P, Le Maoult J, Le Discorde M, Dausset J, Rouas-Freiss N. HLA-G Molecules: From Maternal-Fetal Tolerance to Tissue Acceptance. Adv Immunol (2003) 81:199–252. doi: 10.1016/s0065-2776(03)81006-4

Donadi EA, Castelli EC, Arnaiz-Villena A, Roger M, Rey D, Moreau P. Implications of the Polymorphism of HLA-G on Its Function, Regulation, Evolution and Disease Association. Cell Mol Life Sci: CMLS (2011) 68(3):369–95. doi:10.1007/s00018-010-0580-7

Carosella ED, Moreau P, Lemaoult J, Rouas-Freiss N. HLA-G: From Biology to Clinical Benefits. Trends Immunol (2008) 29(3):125–32. doi: 10.1016/j.it.2007.11.005

Diehl M, Münz C, Keilholz W, Stevanović S, Holmes N, Loke YW, et al. Nonclassical HLA-G Molecules Are Classical Peptide Presenters. Curr Biol: CB (1996) 6(3):305–14. doi: 10.1016/s0960-9822(02)00481-5

Gonen-Gross T, Achdout H, Gazit R, Hanna J, Mizrahi Sa'ar, Markel G, et al. Complexes of HLA-G Protein on the Cell Surface Are Important for Leukocyte Ig-like Receptor-1 Function. J Immunol (Baltimore Md: 1950) (2003) 171(3):1343–51. doi:10.4049/jimmunol.171.3.1343

Shiroishi M, Tsumoto K, Amano K, Shirakihara Y, Colonna M, Braud VM, et al. Human Inhibitory Receptors Ig-like Transcript 2 (ILT2) and ILT4 Compete with CD8 for MHC Class I Binding and Bind Preferentially to HLA-G. Proc Natl Acad Sci U States America (2003) 100(15):8856–61. doi: 10.1073/pnas.1431057100

Apps R, Gardner L, Sharkey AM, Holmes N, Moffett A. A Homodimeric Complex of HLA-G on Normal Trophoblast Cells Modulates Antigen-Presenting Cells via LILRB1. Eur J Immunol (2007) 37(7):1924–37. doi: 10.1002/eji.200737089

HoWangYin K-Y, Loustau M, Wu J, Alegre E, Daouya M, Caumartin J, et al. Multimeric Structures of HLA-G Isoforms Function through Differential Binding to LILRB Receptors. Cell Mol Life Sci: CMLS (2012) 69(23):4041–49. doi: 10.1007/s00018-012-1069-3

Juch H, Blaschitz A, Daxböck C, Rueckert C, Kofler K, Dohr G. A Novel Sandwich ELISA for Alpha1 Domain Based Detection of Soluble HLA-G Heavy Chains. J Immunol Methods (2005) 307(1–2):96–106. doi: 10.1016/j.jim.2005.09.016

Zhang W-Q, Xu D-P, Liu D, Li Y-Y, Ruan Y-Y, Lin A, et al. HLA-G1 and HLA-G5 Isoforms Have an Additive Effect on NK Cytolysis. Hum Immunol (2014) 75(2):182–89. doi: 10.1016/j.humimm.2013.11.001

Le Rond S, Azéma C, Krawice-Radanne I, Durrbach A, Guettier C, Carosella ED, et al. Evidence to Support the Role of HLA-G5 in Allograft Acceptance through Induction of Immunosuppressive/Regulatory T Cells. J Immunol (Baltimore Md: 1950) (2006) 176(5):3266–76. doi: 10.4049/jimmunol.176.5.3266

Berman HM, Westbrook J, Feng Z, Gilliland G, Bhat TN, Weissig H, et al. The Protein Data Bank. Nucleic Acids Res (2000) 28(1):235–42. doi: 10.1093/nar/28.1.235

Webb B, Sali A. Comparative Protein Structure Modeling Using MODELLER. Curr Protoc Bioinf (2016) 54(20 2016):5.6.1–5.6.37. doi: 10.1002/cpbi.3

Clements CS, Kjer-Nielsen L, Kostenko L, Hoare HL, Dunstone MA, Moses E, et al. Crystal Structure of HLA-G: A Nonclassical MHC Class I Molecule Expressed at the Fetal-Maternal Interface. Proc Natl Acad Sci U States America (2005) 102(9):3360–65. doi: 10.1073/pnas.0409676102

Wang C, Bradley P, Baker D. Protein-Protein Docking with Backbone Flexibility. J Mol Biol (2007) 373(2):503–19. doi: 10.1016/j.jmb.2007.07.050

Yang J, Zhang Y. I-TASSER Server: New Development for Protein Structure and Function Predictions. Nucleic Acids Res (2015) 43(W1):W174–181. doi: 10.1093/nar/gkv342

Benkert P, Biasini M, Schwede T. Toward the Estimation of the Absolute Quality of Individual Protein Structure Models. Bioinf (Oxford England) (2011) 27(3):343–50. doi: 10.1093/bioinformatics/btq662

Maghrabi AHA, McGuffin LJ. ModFOLD6: An Accurate Web Server for the Global and Local Quality Estimation of 3D Protein Models. Nucleic Acids Res (2017) 45(W1):W416–21. doi: 10.1093/nar/gkx332

Bowie JU, Lüthy R, Eisenberg D. A Method to Identify Protein Sequences That Fold into a Known Three-Dimensional Structure. Sci (N Y NY) (1991) 253 (5016):164–70. doi: 10.1126/science.1853201

Lüthy R, Bowie JU, Eisenberg D. Assessment of Protein Models with Three-Dimensional Profiles. Nature (1992) 356(6364):83–5. doi: 10.1038/356083a0

Colovos C, Yeates TO. Verification of Protein Structures: Patterns of Nonbonded Atomic Interactions. Protein Sci: A Publ Protein Soc (1993) 2 (9):1511–19. doi: 10.1002/pro.5560020916

Laskowski RA. PDBsum: Summaries and Analyses of PDB Structures. Nucleic Acids Res (2001) 29(1):221–22. doi: 10.1093/nar/29.1.221

Holec PV, Hackel BJ. PyMOL360: Multi-User Gamepad Control of Molecular Visualization Software. J Comput Chem (2016) 37(30):2667–69. doi: 10.1002/jcc.24489

Biopython: Freely Available Python Tools for Computational Molecular Biology and Bioinformatics. Available at: https://www.ncbi.nlm.nih.] +computational+molecular+biology+and+bioinformatics (Accessed January 29, 2020).

Wu EL, Cheng X, Jo S, Rui H, Song KC, Dávila-Contreras EM, et al. CHARMM-GUI Membrane Builder toward Realistic Biological Membrane Simulations. J Comput Chem (2014) 35(27):1997–2004. doi: 10.1002/jcc.23702

Lee J, Patel DS, Ståhle J, Park S-J, Kern NR, Kim S, et al. CHARMM-GUI Membrane Builder for Complex Biological Membrane Simulations with Glycolipids and Lipoglycans. *J Chem Theory Comput* (2019) 15(1):775–86. doi: 10.1021/acs.jctc.8b01066

Abraham MJ, Murtola T, Schulz R, Páll S, Smith JC, Hess B, et al. GROMACS: High Performance Molecular Simulations through Multi-Level Parallelism from Laptops to Supercomputers. *SoftwareX* (2015) 1–2:19–25. doi: 10.1016/j.softx.2015.06.001

Huang J, Rauscher S, Nawrocki G, Ran T, Feig M, de Groot BL, et al. CHARMM36m: An Improved Force Field for Folded and Intrinsically Disordered Proteins. *Nat Methods* (2017) 14(1):71–3. doi: 10.1038/nmeth.4067

Devaurs D, Antunes DA, Papanastasiou M, Moll M, Ricklin D, Lambris JD, et al. Coarse-Grained Conformational Sampling of Protein Structure Improves the Fit to Experimental Hydrogen-Exchange Data. *Front Mol Biosci* (2017) 4:13:13. doi: 10.3389/fmolb.2017.00013

McGibbon RT, Kyle A. B, Harrigan MP, Klein C, Swails JM, Hernández CX, et al. MDTraj: A Modern Open Library for the Analysis of Molecular Dynamics Trajectories. *Biophys J* (2015) 109(8):1528–32. doi: 10.1016/j.bpj.2015.08.015

Scherer MK, Trendelkamp-Schroer B, Paul F, Pérez-Hernández G, Hoffmann M, Plattner N, et al. PyEMMA 2: A Software Package for Estimation, Validation, and Analysis of Markov Models. *J Chem Theory Comput* (2015) 11(11):5525–42. doi: 10.1021/acs.jctc.5b00743

Abella JR, Dinler A.A, Clementi C, Kavraki LE. APE-Gen: A Fast Method for Generating Ensembles of Bound Peptide-MHC Conformations. *Mol (Basel Switzerland)* (2019) 24(5):881–94. doi: 10.3390/molecules24050881

Eastman P, Swails J, Chodera JD, McGibbon RT, Zhao Y, Beauchamp KA, et al. OpenMM 7: Rapid Development of High Performance Algorithms for Molecular Dynamics. *PloS Comput Biol* (2017) 13(7):e1005659. doi: 10.1371/journal.pcbi.1005659

Quiroga R, Villarreal MA. Vinardo: A Scoring Function Based on Autodock Vina Improves Scoring, Docking, and Virtual Screening. *PloS One* (2016) 11 (5):e0155183. doi: 10.1371/journal.pone.0155183

Antunes DA, Abella JR, Hall-Swan S, Devaurs D, Conev A, Moll M, et al. HLA-Arena: A Customizable Environment for the Structural Modeling and Analysis of Peptide-HLA Complexes for Cancer Immunotherapy. *JCO Clin Cancer Inf* (2020) 4:623–36. doi: 10.1200/CCI.19.00123

Abella JR, Antunes DA, Clementi C, Kavraki LE. Large-Scale Structure-Based Prediction of Stable Peptide Binding to Class I HLAs Using Random Forests. *Front Immunol* (2020) 11:1583:1583. doi: 10.3389/fimmu.2020.01583

Kozakov D, Hall DR, Xia B, Porter KA, Padhorny D, Yueh C, et al. The ClusPro Web Server for Protein-Protein Docking. *Nat Protoc* (2017) 12 (2):255–78. doi: 10.1038/nprot.2016.169

Pettersen EF, Goddard TD, Huang CC, Couch GS, Greenblatt DM, Meng EC, et al. UCSF Chimera–a Visualization System for Exploratory Research and Analysis. *J Comput Chem* (2004) 25(13):1605–12. doi: 10.1002/jcc.20084

Gao GF, Willcox BE, Wyer JR, Boulter JM, O'Callaghan CA, Maenaka K, et al. Classical and Nonclassical Class I Major Histocompatibility Complex Molecules Exhibit Subtle Conformational Differences That Affect Binding to CD8alphaalpha. *J Biol Chem* (2000) 275(20):15232–38. doi: 10.1074/jbc.275.20.15232

Estibaliz A, Rizzo R, Bortolotti D, Fernandez-Landázuri S, Fainardi E, González A. Some Basic Aspects of HLA-G Biology. *J Immunol Res* (2014) 2014:657625. doi: 10.1155/2014/657625

Hsu KC, Chida S, Geraghty DE, Dupont B. The Killer Cell Immunoglobulin-like Receptor (KIR) Genomic Region: Gene-Order, Haplotypes and Allelic Polymorphism. *Immunol Rev* (2002) 190:40–52. doi: 10.1034/j.1600-065x.2002.19004.x

Apps R, Gardner L, Moffett A. A Critical Look at HLA-G. *Trends Immunol* (2008) 29(7):313–21. doi: 10.1016/j.it.2008.02.012

Wang Q, Song H, Cheng H, Qi J, Nam G, Tan S, et al. Structures of the Four Ig-like Domain LILRB2 and the Four-Domain LILRB1 and HLA-G1 Complex. *Cell Mol Immunol* (2020) 17(9):966–75. doi: 10.1038/s41423-019-0258-5

Robinson J, Barker DJ, Georgiou X, Cooper MA, Flicek P, Marsh SGE. IPD-IMGT/HLA Database. *Nucleic Acids Res* (2020) 48(D1):D948–55. doi: 10.1093/nar/gkz950

Robinson J, Soormally AR, Hayhurst JD, Marsh SGE. The IPD-IMGT/HLA Database - New Developments in Reporting HLA Variation. *Hum Immunol* (2016) 77(3):233–37. doi: 10.1016/j.humimm.2016.01.020

Ishitani A, Sageshima N, Lee N, Dorofeeva N, Hatake K, Marquardt H, et al. Protein Expression and Peptide Binding Suggest Unique and Interacting Functional Roles for HLA-E, F, and G in Maternal-Placental Immune Recognition. *J Immunol (Baltimore Md: 1950)* (2003) 171(3):1376–84. doi: 10.4049/jimmunol.171.3.1376

Contini P, Ghio M, Poggi A, Filaci G, Indiveri F, Ferrone S, et al. Soluble HLA- A,-B,-C and -G Molecules Induce Apoptosis in T and NK CD8+ Cells and Inhibit Cytotoxic T Cell Activity through CD8 Ligation. *Eur J Immunol* (2003) 33(1):125–34. doi: 10.1002/immu.200390015

Selvakumar A, Steffens U, Dupont B. NK Cell Receptor Gene of the KIR Family with Two IG Domains but Highest Homology to KIR Receptors with Three IG Domains. *Tissue Antigens* (1996) 48(4 Pt 1):285–94. doi: 10.1111/j.1399-0039.1996.tb02647.x

Faure M, Long EO. KIR2DL4 (CD158d), an NK Cell-Activating Receptor with Inhibitory Potential. *J Immunol (Baltimore Md: 1950)* (2002) 168(12):6208–14. doi: 10.4049/jimmunol.168.12.6208

Fu B, Zhou Y, Ni X, Tong X, Xu X, Dong Z, et al. Natural Killer Cells Promote Fetal Development through the Secretion of Growth-Promoting Factors. *Immunity* (2017) 47(6):1100–13.e6. doi: 10.1016/j.immuni.2017.11.018

Rajagopalan S, Long EO. KIR2DL4 (CD158d): An Activation Receptor for HLA-G. *Front Immunol* (2012) 3:258. doi: 10.3389/fimmu.2012.00258

Morales PJ, Pace JL, Platt JS, Langat DK, Hunt JS. Synthesis of b2- Microglobulin-Free, Disulphide-Linked HLA-G5 Homodimers in Human Placental Villous Cytotrophoblast Cells. *Immunology* (2007) 122(2):179. doi: 10.1111/j.1365-2567.2007.02623.x

Kimiko K, Mio K, Takahashi A, Matsubara H, Kasai Y, Manaka S, et al. Cutting Edge: Class II–like Structural Features and Strong Receptor Binding of the Nonclassical HLA-G2 Isoform Homodimer. *J Immunol (Baltimore Md: 1950)* (2017) 198(9):3399–403. doi: 10.4049/jimmunol.1601296

2

B Cell-Based Vaccine Transduced with ESAT6-Expressing Vaccinia Virus and Presenting α-Galactosylceramide is a Novel Vaccine Candidate Against ESAT6-Expressing Mycobacterial Diseases

Bo-Eun Kwon[1], Jae-Hee Ahn[1], Eun-Kyoung Park[1], Hyunjin Jeong[1], Hyo-Ji Lee[2], Yu-Jin Jung[2], Sung Jae Shin[3], Hye-Sook Jeong[4], Jung Sik Yoo[4], EunKyoung Shin[4], Sang-Gu Yeo[5], Sun-Young Chang[6] and Hyun-Jeong Ko[1]*

[1] *Laboratory of Microbiology and Immunology, College of Pharmacy, Kangwon National University, Chuncheon, South Korea,*
[2] *Department of Biological Sciences, Kangwon National University, Chuncheon, South Korea,* [3] *Department of Microbiology, Institute for Immunology and Immunological Disease, Brain Korea 21 PLUS Project for Medical Science, Yonsei University College of Medicine, Seoul, South Korea,* [4] *Division of Vaccine Research, Center for Infectious Disease Research, Korea National Institute of Health (KNIH), Korea Centers for Disease Control and Prevention (KCDC), Cheongju, South Korea,* [5] *Sejong Institute of Health and Environment, Sejong, South Korea,* [6] *Laboratory of Microbiology, College of Pharmacy and Research Institute of Pharmaceutical Science and Technology (RIPST), Ajou University, Suwon, South Korea*

*Correspondence:
Hyun-Jeong Ko
hjko@kangwon.ac.kr

Early secretory antigenic target-6 (ESAT6) is a potent immunogenic antigen expressed in *Mycobacterium tuberculosis* as well as in some non-tuberculous mycobacteria (NTM), such as *M. kansasii*. *M. kansasii* is one of the most clinically relevant species of NTM that causes mycobacterial lung disease, which is clinically indistinguishable from tuberculosis. In the current study, we designed a novel cell-based vaccine using B cells that were transduced with vaccinia virus expressing ESAT6 (vacESAT6), and presenting α-galactosylceramide (αGC), a ligand of invariant NKT cells. We found that B cells loaded with αGC had increased levels of CD80 and CD86 after *in vitro* stimulation with NKT cells. Immunization of mice with B/αGC/vacESAT6 induced CD4$^+$ T cells producing TNF-α and IFN-γ in response to heat-killed *M. tuberculosis*. Immunization of mice with B/αGC/vacESAT6 ameliorated severe lung inflammation caused by *M. kansasii* infection. We also confirmed that immunization with B/αGC/vacESAT6 reduced *M. kansasii* bacterial burden in the lungs. In addition, therapeutic administration of B/αGC/vacESAT6 increased IFN-γ$^+$ CD4$^+$ T cells and inhibited the progression of lung pathology caused by *M. kansasii* infection. Thus, B/αGC/vacESAT6 could be a potent vaccine candidate for the prevention and treatment of ESAT6-expressing mycobacterial infection caused by *M. kansasii*.

Keywords: *Mycobacterium kansasii*, *Mycobacterium tuberculosis*, non-tuberculous mycobacteria, **ESAT6, vaccine**, α-galactosylceramide

INTRODUCTION

Non-tuberculous mycobacteria (NTM) are one of the mycobacteria species which cause pulmonary disease as a common manifestation (1). *Mycobacterium kansasii* belongs to NTM species and is one of the major causative agent of NTM lung disease (2). Symptoms of *M. kansasii* are mild under single infection, but it is known that more severe symptoms occur when contracted along with other illnesses such as inflammatory pseudotumor (3), sarcoidosis (4), and HIV (5). Especially, it has been reported that in Brazil, most patients who acquire lung disease caused by NTM had previously received tuberculosis treatment (6). These reports implied that NTM was closely associated with other diseases, and therefore is one of the important factors in pulmonary infection.

Bacillus Calmette-Guerin (BCG) is the only approved live attenuated vaccine strain induced from *M. bovis* through multiple sub-culturing for a long period of time (7). The protective efficacy of BCG against tuberculous meningitis and tuberculosis (TB) is well-known in children, however, protection for primary infection or latent infection in adults seems poor (8). Also, BCG vaccination did not provide protection against NTM infection (9). Due to this limitation of BCG, more persistent research is needed to identify novel vaccine candidates.

Early secretory antigenic target-6 (ESAT6) is a protein encoded by a gene located in the region of difference 1, which is expressed in *M. tuberculosis* but not in BCG (10). ESAT6 has sufficient immunogenicity in both humans and mice post *M. tuberculosis* infection (11). Interestingly, some NTM species, including *M. kansasii* also contain genes for ESAT6 homolog. In the present study, we expressed ESAT6 in B cells using ESAT6-expressing vaccinia virus to deliver ESAT6 antigen to B cells, and presented α-galactosylceramide (αGC), an invariant natural killer cell (iNKT) ligand, on CD1d molecule of B cells. Previous studies have suggested that a B cell vaccine which expressed tumor antigen showed potent anti-tumor effect facilitated by activated NKT cells (12, 13).

In the current study, we developed an ESAT6-expressing B cell-based vaccine which was loaded with αGC (B/αGC/vacESAT6) and assessed its preventive and therapeutic effect in a murine model of *M. kansasii* infection.

MATERIALS AND METHODS

Construction of Vaccinia Virus Vector Expressing ESAT6

ESAT6 gene of *M. tuberculosis* strain H37Rv with human optimized codon was synthesized and cloned into vaccinia virus delivery vector PVVT1-C7L (PVVT1-C7L-Tpa-esat6) which contains *tPA* gene for secretion of intracellular signal peptide. Sfi1 restriction enzyme was used for cloning. PVVT1-C7L-Tpa-esat6 was transformed to *E. coli* DH5 competent cells for amplification. The expression of *ESAT6* gene was confirmed by PCR using the following primers; 5′-TTT GAA GCA TTG GAA GCA ACT-3′ (VVTK-F) and 5′-ACGTTGAAATGTCCCATCGACT-3′ (VVTK-R).

Preparation of Recombinant Vaccinia Virus Expressing ESAT6

Vero cells in 12-well plates were infected with vaccinia virus (KCCM11574P) at a multiplicity of infection (MOI) of 0.02 for 2 h, and the infected Vero cells were transfected with PVVT1-C7L-Tpa-esat6 plasmid using Lipofectamine 2000 (Thermo Fisher Scientific, Waltham, MA, USA) transfection reagent for 4 h. Vero cells were incubated for 3–4 days to observe the cytopathic effects, and recombinant viruses were obtained by plaque isolation. For high efficacy and purity, recombinant vaccinia virus expressing ESAT6 (vacESAT6) was concentrated by ultracentrifugation. The expression of ESAT6 protein by Vero cells and isolated B cells after transduction with vacESAT6 was confirmed by confocal microscopy (**Figures 1A,B, Supplementary Figure 1**).

Preparation of B Cell-Based Vaccine and Immunization of BCG

B220$^+$ cells were magnetically purified from splenocytes of naïve C57BL/6 mice using CD45R/B220 biotin (BD biosciences, California, USA) and anti-biotin microbeads (Miltenyi Biotec, Bergisch Gladbach, Germany) according to the manufacturer's instructions. Labeled cells were purified through LS column (Miltenyi Biotec, Bergisch Gladbach, Germany). Isolated B220$^+$ cells (2×10^7 cells seeded) were transduced with vacESAT6 (MOI of 1) for 2 h and then loaded with αGC (Enzo life sciences, New York, USA) (1 μg/ml) for 22 h and incubated in a CO_2 incubator. After washing three times with PBS, mice were immunized with cultured cells (B cell-based vaccine) by tail vein injection. As for the comparison group, mice were intramuscularly immunized with BCG (10^5 CFU/mouse).

To confirm preventive effect of Bvac, mice were either immunized with BCG by intramuscular injection at a 10^5 CFU/mouse or administered with Bvac by tail vein injection at day 0 for the priming and day 7 for the boost. At day 14, mice were challenged with 10^7 CFU/mouse of *M. kansasii*. To confirm the therapeutic effect of Bvac, mice were infected with 10^7 CFU of *M. kansasii* per mouse at Day 0, and were administrated with BCG or Bvac at 3 days post-infection. The mice were boosted with Bvac at 7 days post-infection. We analyzed histology, protein levels and bacterial loads from lung and liver after 14 days following *M. kansasii* infection.

Murine Infection Model of *M. kansasii*

C57BL/6 mice were purchased at 6–7 weeks of age from Charles River Laboratories (Orient Bio Inc., Seongnam, Korea). All animal experiments, including the *M. kansasii* challenge experiment, were approved by the Institutional Animal Care and Use Committee of Kangwon National University (Permit Number: KW-160201-4). A hypervirulent *M. kansasii* SM#1 clinical isolate was used for challenge *in vivo* (14). To induce infection, mice were intravenously injected with *M. kansasii* (10^7 CFU/mouse). We checked the bodyweight and survival rate of mice every day following *M. kansasii* infection.

The lungs and liver of infected mice were isolated for determining the bacterial count in these organs at 2 weeks

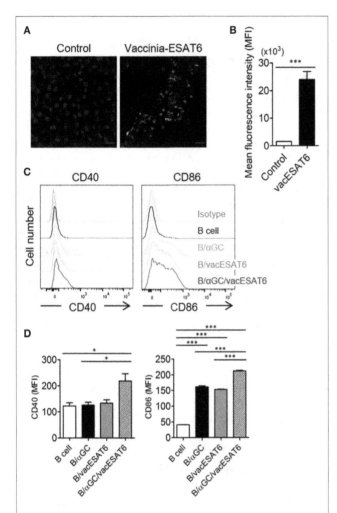

FIGURE 1 | B/αGC/vacESAT6 up-regulates co-stimulatory molecules on B cells. **(A,B)** Vero cells were transduced with vaccinia-ESAT6 (vacESAT6) at a multiplicity of infection (MOI) of 1. Transduced cells were fluorescently stained for ESAT6 (green) and counterstained with DAPI (blue) for nuclei which were analyzed by confocal microscopy to detect the expression of ESAT6 (scale bar = 20 μm). **(A)** Representative confocal images and **(B)** Representation of the evaluation of green fluorescent area. **(C,D)** B220⁺ cells were isolated from splenocytes of naïve C57BL/6 mice. Isolated B220⁺ cells were transduced with vacESAT6 at a MOI of 1 and/or loaded with 1 μg/ml of αGC and then co-cultured with naïve splenocytes for 24 h. Incubated cells were stained to examine the expression of B220, CD40, and CD86. Expression levels of CD40 and CD86 in B220⁺ cells were analyzed by flow cytometry. **(C)** Representative flow cytometry histogram and **(D)** summary of mean fluorescence intensity of CD40 and CD86 expression in B cells. ANOVA. *$p < 0.05$, ***$p < 0.001$.

post *M. kansasii* infection. Lungs were homogenized in 1X PBS containing 0.04% tween 80 and liver was homogenized in 1X PBS containing 1 mM EDTA (125 mg of tissues/ml). The homogenized supernatants were 10-fold serial diluted in Difco™ Middlebrook 7H9 Broth (BD biosciences, California, USA) containing ADC [Sodium Chloride (Duchefa, BH Haarlem, The Nederlands), Dextrose (SHOWA, Gyoda, Japan), Bovine Albumin Fraction V (MPBio, Santa Ana, USA), Catalase (Sigma-Aldrich, St. Louis, USA)] and each diluent

was drop cultured in Difco™ Middlebrook 7H10 Agar (BD biosciences, California, USA) containing OADC [Sodium Chloride, Dextrose, Bovine Albumin Fraction V, Catalase, Oleic acid (Sigma-Aldrich, St. Louis, USA)]. Smear plates were cultured in a 37°C incubator and colonies were counted after 2–3 weeks.

Isolation of Cells and Measurement of Co-stimulatory Molecules in B Cells

For the isolation of T cells, splenocytes were labeled with CD8α-PE and anti-PE microbeads (Miltenyi Biotec, Bergisch Gladbach, Germany) according to the manufacturer's instructions. The labeled cells were then purified through LS column (Miltenyi Biotec, Bergisch Gladbach, Germany). CD4⁺ T cells were isolated by using the mouse CD4⁺ T cell isolation kit (Miltenyi Biotec, Bergisch Gladbach, Germany). CD11c⁺ DCs were purified by using CD11c⁺ microbeads (Miltenyi Biotec, Bergisch Gladbach, Germany). B220⁺ cells were purified by using CD45R/B220 biotin (BD biosciences, California, USA) and anti-Biotin microbeads (Miltenyi Biotec, Bergisch Gladbach, Germany) from splenocytes of naïve C57BL/6 mice. Purified B cells were transduced with vacESAT6 at a MOI of 1 and/or loaded with 1 μg/ml of αGC and then co-cultured with naïve splenocytes for 24 h. Incubated cells were stained to examine the expression of B220, CD40, and CD86 using antibodies such as APC-conjugated anti-B220 (BD biosciences, California, USA), PE-conjugated isotype control (eBioscience, San Diego, USA), anti-CD40 (Biolegend, San Diego, USA), and anti-CD86 Ab (BD biosciences, California, USA). Cells were analyzed by flow cytometry.

Measurement of Intracellular Cytokines in CD4⁺ T Cells

For measurement of intracellular cytokines, dendritic cells and CD4⁺ T cells were co-cultured and stimulated for 3 days with heat-killed H37Rv at 0.1 MOI or overnight with anti-CD3 and anti-CD28 antibody in culture media. H37Rv strain was generously provided by Sang-Nae Cho (Yonsei University). Brefeldin A Solution (1000 x) Thermo Fisher Scientific, Waltham, MA, USA) was added for 4 h before harvest and then harvested cells were stained with PerCP-Cy™5.5 rat anti-mouse CD4 (BD biosciences, California, USA) or PE rat anti-mouse CD8α (BD biosciences, California, USA). Stained cells were permeabilized with IC Fixation Buffer (Thermo Fisher Scientific, Waltham, MA, USA) according to the manufacturer's recommendations. Next, permeabilized cells were stained with TNF-α mAb, APC (Thermo Fisher Scientific, Waltham, MA, USA) and IFN-γ mAb (XMG1.2) PE (Thermo Fisher Scientific, Waltham, MA, USA).

The supernatants of homogenized tissues were analyzed for cytokine production using BD™ Cytometric Bead Array (CBA) Mouse Inflammation kit (BD biosciences, California, USA) according to the manufacturer's instructions.

Western Blotting

Total protein lysates of *M. kansasii* were sonicated with PRO-PREP™ protein extraction solution (iNtRON

Biotechnology, Daejeon, Korea). Lysates were boiled at 100°C and proteins were separated by performing SDS-PAGE. Proteins were transferred onto PVDF membranes (Millipore, Burlington, USA) and then blocked with 5% skim milk in TBS with tween 20. Next, the membranes were incubated with anti-ESAT6 primary antibody [11G4] (Abcam, Cambridge, USA) and proteins were detected using HRP conjugated goat anti-mouse polyclonal antibody (Enzo life sciences, New York, USA). Membranes were developed using femtoLUCENT™ PLUS-HRP chemiluminescence detection system (G-Biosciences, St. Louis, USA).

Flow Cytometry

Cells were collected from spleen and stained with markers such as APC-conjugated anti-B220 (BD biosciences, California, USA) and anti-Ly6C (BD biosciences, California, USA) Ab, FITC-conjugated anti-CD11b Ab (BD biosciences, California, USA), PE-conjugated isotype control (eBioscience, San Diego, USA), anti-CD40 Ab (Biolegend, San Diego, USA), and anti-CD86 (BD biosciences, California, USA) Ab. Flow cytometry was performed on a FACSVerse instrument (BD biosciences, California, USA) and data were analyzed using FlowJo software (Flowjo, San Carlos, USA).

Histology

Mice were sacrificed and lungs were isolated from each group. They were fixed with 4% formalin overnight. Lung tissues were processed using a tissue processor (Leica, Wetzlar, Germany) and then embedded in paraffin. Paraffin-embedded tissue blocks were cut into 5 μm thick sections and stained with hematoxylin and eosin.

Confocal Microscopy

Uninfected or vaccinia virus-infected Vero cells and B cells were cultured in a 37°C incubator for 24 h. Cells were fixed with 4% paraformaldehyde and stained with anti-ESAT6 Ab (Abcam, Cambridge, USA), and further stained with anti-mouse IgG (H+L), F(ab')$_2$ Fragment (Alexa Fluor® 488-conjugated) (Cell signaling, Danvers, USA) or DyLight™ 405 affinipure donkey anti-mouse IgG (H+L) (DyLight™ 405-conjugated). Cells were visualized by confocal microscopy (Carl Zeiss, LSM880 with Airyscan, Zena, Germany).

Statistics

Statistical analysis was conducted with GraphPad Prism 5.0 (GraphPad Software, La Jolla, USA). Differences between groups were assessed by the Student's t-test. Comparisons between multiple-groups were carried out by one-way ANOVA analysis of variance followed by the Bonferroni's multiple comparison test. P values < 0.05 were considered as significant at a 95% confidence interval for all analyses.

RESULTS

B/αGC/vacESAT6 Upregulated the Expression of Co-stimulatory Molecules on B Cells

It has been previously reported that αGC-loaded B cell-based vaccines expressing tumor antigens showed significant antitumor effects *in vivo* (15, 16). Thus, we decided to adopt this vaccine strategy for the development of preventive and therapeutic anti-mycobacterial vaccine. B cells were transduced with recombinant vaccinia virus expressing ESAT6 (vacESAT6), and the transduced B cells were loaded with αGC. We found that B cells loaded with αGC/vacESAT6 (B/αGC/vacESAT6) (Bvac) increased the expression of co-stimulatory molecules including CD40 and CD86 when they were co-cultured with splenocytes from naïve C57BL/6 mice for 24 h (**Figures 1C,D**). B cells loaded with αGC or B cells transduced with vacESAT6 increased the expression of CD86, which further increased in B/αGC/vacESAT6 (**Figures 1C,D**). B cells transduced with vacGFP control virus also increased the expression of CD86 (**Supplementary Figure 2**) suggesting that infection of vaccinia virus alone could be stimulatory for B cells. These results suggested that activated NKT cells by αGC on B cells as well as vaccinia virus infection activated the B cells to increase the expression of co-stimulatory molecules including CD40 and CD86, which help B cells to function as professional antigen presenting cells to induce effective T cells.

B/αGC/vacESAT6 Induced CD4$^+$ T Cell Responses Against H37Rv

We next determined whether B/αGC/vacESAT6 induced CD4$^+$ T cell response *in vivo*. Groups of mice were immunized with either saline, BCG or B/αGC/vacESAT6, and mice were sacrificed to obtain splenocytes. We analyzed TNF-α- and IFN-γ-producing CD4$^+$ T cells after 3 days of co-culturing the splenocytes with dendritic cells pulsed with heat-killed H37Rv. As a result, we found that the percentage of CD4$^+$ T cells producing TNF-α$^+$ and IFN-γ$^+$ was higher in mice vaccinated with B/αGC/vacESAT6 as compared to control and BCG-immunized mice (**Figures 2A,B**). In addition, IFN-γ production was also increased in the culture supernatant of splenocytes from B/αGC/vacESAT6 group compared to control and BCG group (**Figure 2C**). These results show that B/αGC/vacESAT6 induced the H37Rv-specific CD4$^+$ T cell-mediated cellular immunity which might be critical for the regulation of mycobacterial infection.

Mice Infected With *M. kansasii* Showed Severe Lung Inflammation

M. kansasii is one of the NTM which expresses ESAT6 homolog as a major antigen. We confirmed the expression of ESAT6 in *M. kansasii* by western blotting analysis (**Figure 3A**). We found that the bodyweight of mice significantly decreased with intravenous (i.v) injection of *M. kansasii* (10^7 CFU/mouse). For humane reasons, mice were monitored two times every

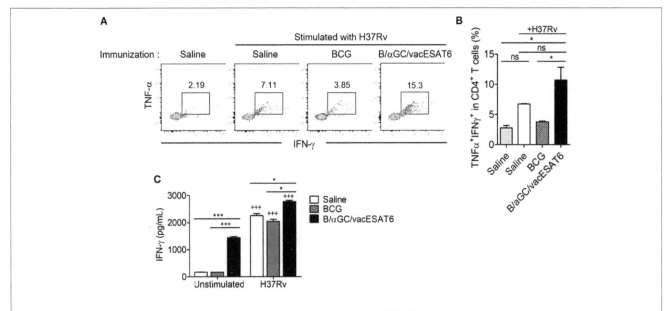

FIGURE 2 | B/αGC/vacESAT6 induced *M. tuberculosis* specific CD4+ T cell response. Splenic CD4+ T cells were isolated from mice which were immunized with BCG (10^5 CFU/mouse) or with B/αGC/vacESAT6 (Bvac), and they were co-cultured with CD11c+ dendritic cells which were stimulated with heat-killed *M. tuberculosis* H37Rv at 0.1 MOI. After 72 h co-culture, CD4+ T cells were analyzed by flow cytometry to detect intracellular TNF-α and IFN-γ production. **(A)** Representative intracellular staining of TNF-α and IFN-γ. **(B)** Summary of TNF-α and IFN-γ secreting CD4+ T cells. **(C)** Secreted IFN-γ levels were measured in culture supernatant by ELISA. ANOVA. *$p < 0.05$, ***$p < 0.001$, +++$p < 0.001$ compared to unstimulated counterpart.

day and sacrificed when they weighed <80% of their initial bodyweight. In addition, there was significant lung injury including infiltration of immune cells around bronchial tubes as well as formation of granuloma-like lesions. We also confirmed the presence of bacteria in lungs of *M. kansasii*-infected mice at 2 weeks after infection. On the contrary, immunization of mice with Bvac ameliorated loss of bodyweight and increased survival rate following *M. kansasii* infection (**Figures 3B,C**). In addition, lungs of mice immunized with Bvac had moderate injury with reduced cell infiltration as compared with non-vaccinated mice after *M. kansasii* infection (**Figures 3D,E**). Bvac also decreased the bacterial burden in the lungs of *M. kansasii*-infected mice (**Figure 3F**). We also analyzed the proportion of NK cells and NKT cells in splenocytes by flow cytometry. We confirmed that Bvac immunization increased the percentage of NKT cells as compared with that of non-vaccinated mice as assessed after *M. kansasii* infection (**Supplementary Figure 3**). We also compared the therapeutic effects of Bvac and BCG vaccine in *M. kansasii*-infected mice. As a result, mice therapeutically treated with BCG and Bvac showed moderate levels of inflammation with reduced cell infiltration and decreased the bacterial burden in the lungs of *M. kansasii*-infected mice (**Supplementary Figures 4A,B**). Intriguingly, however, immunization of mice with Bvac significantly decreased the bacterial burden in the liver than BCG immunization after *M. kansasii* infection (**Supplementary Figures 4C,D**). Collectively, we established a murine model of infection of *M. kansasii* and showed that Bvac had preventive effect against *M. kansasii* expressing ESAT6.

B/αGC/vacESAT6 Had Therapeutic Effects Against *M. kansasii* Infection

We speculated whether B/αGC/vacESAT6 (Bvac) had therapeutic effects against mice infected with *M. kansasii*. To evaluate therapeutic efficacy of Bvac, mice were i.v. challenged with 10^7 CFU/mouse of *M. kansasii*, and 14 days later, they were injected with Bvac at day 3 and 7 post-infection. When we checked the bodyweight, mice administered with Bvac showed alleviation in loss of body weight as compared to mice infected with *M. kansasii* (**Figure 4A**). Further, survival rate increased in mice treated with Bvac (**Figure 4B**). Histological analysis of lungs of infected mice confirmed the therapeutic effects of Bvac against *M. kansasii* infection (**Figures 4C,D**). Bacterial load in the lungs was significantly reduced in mice administered with Bvac as compared to *M. kansasii* infected mice (**Figure 4E**). Also, administered with BCG did not show the therapeutic effect, while Bvac administration reduced bacterial loads in lungs of the infected mice (**Supplementary Figure 5**). Furthermore, production of TNF and IL-6, which were increased in lungs of infected mice following *M. kansasii* infection, were significantly decreased when administered with Bvac (**Figure 5A**). Collectively these results suggested that Bvac had a therapeutic effect in mice infected with *M. kansasii*.

Bvac Increased the Production of IFN-γ in CD4+ T Cells in a Therapeutic Mouse Model

Finally, we assessed the production of intracellular cytokines in CD4+ T cells after therapeutic treatment with Bvac in *M.*

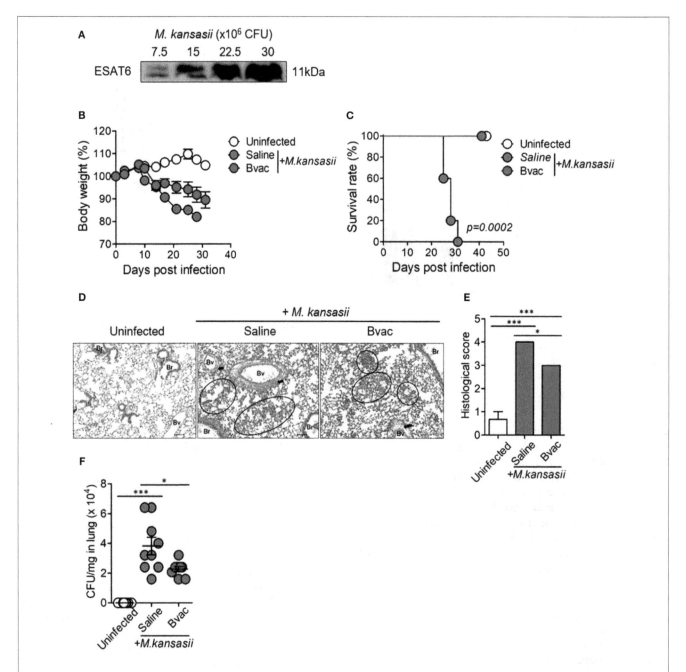

FIGURE 3 | Immunization of mice with Bvac prevented *M. kansasii* infection. **(A)** Expression of 11 kDa ESAT6 obtained from lysates of various CFU of *M. kansasii* by western blotting. **(B–F)** Mice were intravenously immunized with Bvac via tail vein. After 14 days of immunization mice were challenged with *M. kansasii* (10^7 CFU/mouse) ($n = 5$ for uninfected, $n = 6$ for saline and Bvac group). After 14 days following *M. kansasii* infection, histology and bacterial CFU were determined from lungs. **(B)** Bodyweight. ANOVA. $*p < 0.05$, *M. kansasii* vs. Bvac+ *M. kansasii*. **(C)** Survival rate. Log-rank test. **(D)** Representative hematoxylin and eosin staining of lung sections from each group of mice (scale bar = 100 μm). Bv (Blood vessel), Br (Bronchus), circle indicates interstitial necrotizing inflammatory foci, and arrow is perivascular inflammatory cell infiltration. **(E)** Histological scores of the lung sections. **(F)** CFU of *M. kansasii* from lung homogenates. ANOVA. $*p < 0.05$, $***p < 0.001$.

kansasii infected mice. IFN-γ-producing T cells are known to play a key role in resistance against various pathogens including *M. tuberculosis* (17). Mice were infected with *M. kansasii* (10^7 CFU/mouse), and i.v. injected with Bvac at day 3 and 7 post infection. After 14 days following *M. kansasii* infection, lung homogenates were analyzed for the production of TNF, IFN-γ,

and IL-6. Interestingly, although the levels of TNF, IFN-γ and IL-6, were highly increased in mice infected with *M. kansasii*, the levels of TNF and IL-6 were significantly reduced. When CD4$^+$ T cells obtained from the spleen of the treated mice were analyzed for IFN-γ production, we found that splenocytes of mice administered with Bvac showed increased production of

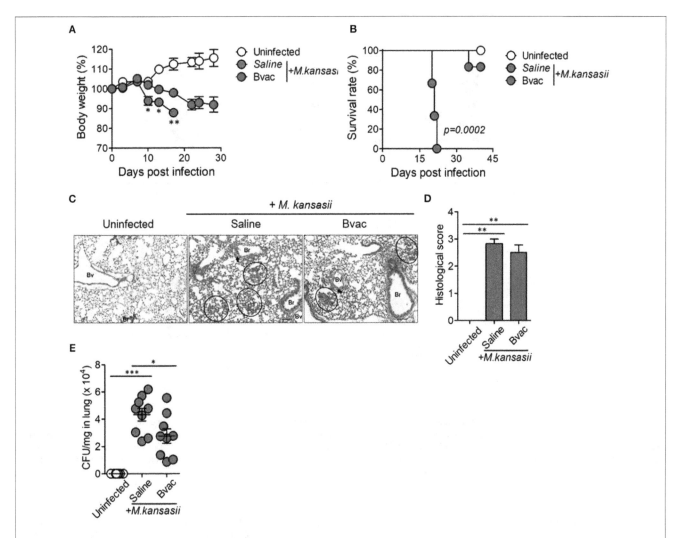

FIGURE 4 | Bvac has therapeutic effect on mice infected with *M. kansasii*. To evaluate therapeutic efficacy of Bvac, mice were infected with 10^7 CFU of *M. kansasii* per mouse, and Bvac was administered via tail vein injection at day 3 and 7 post infection ($n = 5$ for uninfected, $n = 6$ for saline and Bvac group). After 14 days following *M. kansasii* infection, histology and bacterial CFU were determined from lung. **(A)** Body weights of mice are shown, ANOVA. $^*p < 0.05$, $^{**}p < 0.01$, *M. kansasii* vs. Bvac + *M. kansasii*. **(B)** Survival rate. Log-rank test. **(C)** Representative hematoxylin and eosin staining of lung sections from each group of mice (scale bar = $100\,\mu$m). Bv (Blood vessel), Br (Bronchus), circle indicates interstitial necrotizing inflammatory foci, and arrow is perivascular inflammatory cell infiltration. **(D)** Histological scores of the lung sections. **(E)** CFU of *M. kansasii* from lung homogenates. ANOVA. $^*p < 0.05$, $^{***}p < 0.001$.

IFN-γ in CD4$^+$ T cells compared to *M. kansasii*-infected mice (**Figure 5B**). Consequently, these results suggest that Bvac could induce IFN-γ-producing CD4$^+$ T cell response, resulting in preventive and therapeutic effects against *M. kansasii* expressing ESAT6 (**Supplementary Figure 6**).

DISCUSSION

Tuberculosis is the most dangerous and incurable disease in the world (18–20). Although most patients with *M. tuberculosis* infection can be cured with appropriate treatment with anti-tuberculosis drugs such as isoniazid, rifampin, pyrazinamide, and ethambutol, it is difficult to treat multidrug resistant tuberculosis (MDR-TB) and extensively drug-resistant tuberculosis (XDR-TB) (21). Novel drugs including bedaquiline and delamanid

have been introduced to deal with MDR-TB (22). In addition, drug repositioning approaches have provided linezolid, imatinib, and metformin for the treatment of TB patients (23–27). However, since treatment of MDR-TB requires at least 4 months, studies on the development of new anti-tuberculosis drugs are still needed. In this study, we suggest a novel approach to treat mycobacterial infection including *M. tuberculosis* using a therapeutic vaccine.

Currently, the only licensed vaccine for TB is BCG. BCG is made by attenuating *M. bovis*. However, there are several limitations of BCG as TB vaccine since it cannot prevent the development of primary infection and reactivation of latent pulmonary infection. Besides, the efficacy of BCG vaccine has a broad range and limited efficacy in adults. Due to the limitation of BCG vaccine, there is

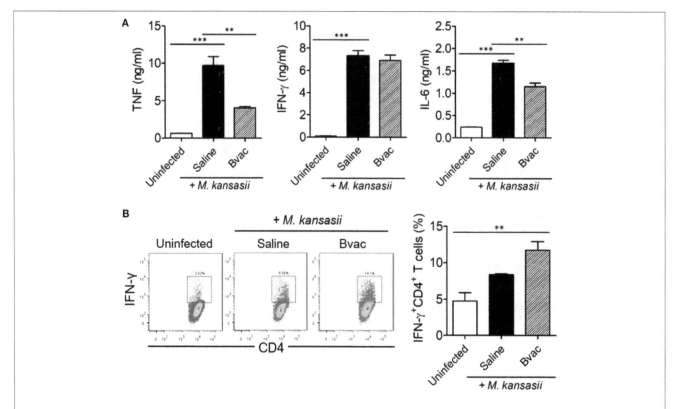

FIGURE 5 | Therapeutic administration of Bvac increased the production of IFN-γ in CD4+ T cells in *M. kansasii*-infected mice. Mice were infected with 10^7 CFU/mouse of *M. kansasii*, and then they were intravenously injected with Bvac at day 3 and 7 post infection. After 14 days following *M. kansasii* infection, lung and spleen were isolated to analyze cytokine production. **(A)** The levels of TNF, IFN-γ, and IL-6 from lung homogenates. **(B)** Splenic CD4+ T cells were analyzed for IFN-γ production after *in vitro* stimulation with plate-coated anti-CD3 and anti-CD28 antibodies. Representative histogram (left) and summary (right) for the percentages of IFN-γ producing CD4+ T cells. ANOVA. **p < 0.01, ***p < 0.001.

an immediate need for further research to develop a novel mycobacterial vaccine.

NTM is another contagious disease-causing pathogen in humans (17). It has been reported that the incidence of multiple NTM infections and NTM-associated mortality rates have dramatically increased in recent times (28, 29). Non-tuberculous mycobacterial pulmonary disease (NTM-PD) is one of the main conditions caused by NTM (30, 31) and the radiological manifestation of NTM-PD is classified as fibrocavitary form (similar to pulmonary tuberculosis) and nodular bronchiectatic form (similar to MAC pulmonary disease) (32, 33). It has been reported that NTM-PD infection increases with age (34), co-infection with chronic obstructive pulmonary disease (COPD) and asthma, in patients (35).

M. kansasii is known as one of the main pathogens causing NTM-PD (36). It has been reported that *M. kansasii*-infected patients are mostly infected with other disorders such as tuberculosis, other types of NTM, and HIV, which are resulting in exacerbated symptoms and weakened immune system (2). Treatment of *M. kansasii* infection is typically by administering rifampin, but sometimes fails due to resistance to rifampin. Ethambutol and isoniazid are also used, but drug resistance against these drugs have also been reported (37, 38). Since NTM-PD is accompanied by other diseases, we presumed that a novel

approach using an immunotherapeutic agent or vaccine could be used to treat NTM infection as well as *M. tuberculosis*, which essentially increases host immunity.

To control *M. tuberculosis* or NTM infection, it has been recognized that Th1 response is important. IFN-γ, which is mainly expressed by Th1, supports to activate macrophages and empowers it to successfully degrade invaded bacteria. Additionally, activation of Th1 cells helps B cells to produce antibodies which suppress free bacteria by inducing the formation of immune complexes. However, a recent study reported anomalies of CD4+ T cell physiology in NTM-infected host. NTM infected patients, especially when infected with *M. intracellulare* or *M. avium*, showed reduced CD4+ T cells in PBMC (39). In addition, the importance of IFN-γ production seems controversial in a mouse infection model. A systemic infection model induced by intravenous injection of *M. kansasii* showed CD4+ T cell-dependent reduction of mycobacterial burden in multiple organs. However, intranasal infection revealed no significant alteration of severity between WT and IL-12p40-, CD4-, or IFN-γ- deficient mice, triggered by *M. kansasii* infection (40, 41). These data suggested the restricted contribution of CD4+ T cell function in suppressing *M. kansasii* in intranasally-induced lung infection model. Collectively, these reports imply that the generation of IFN-γ producing CD4$^+$ T cell response is crucial to control systemic *M. kansasii* infection similar to other species of mycobacterium.

Recently, vaccines using antigen-presenting cells including dendritic cells and B cells have been suggested to induce strong T cell-mediated immunity (11, 15). B cell vaccine is one of the cell-based vaccine approaches developed by using pathogen-specific antigens to induce diverse immune responses including Th1, cytotoxic T cell, and pathogenic antigen-specific antibody response. To augment CD4$^+$ T cell response, αGC, a ligand of NKT cell receptor, was used to load into the CD1d molecules on B cell surface (11).

In the current study, we designed a B cell-based vaccine (B/αGC/vacESAT6), which was transduced by vaccinia virus expressing ESAT6 and loaded with αGC. ESAT6 is a 6 kDa secretory protein and is one of the critical antigens, widely used as a candidate antigen for the development of new TB vaccine. ESAT6 has been shown to have sufficient immunogenicity such as CD4$^+$ T cell and CTL responses in both rodents and humans (42). Although ESAT6 is one of the promising antigen candidates, it might inhibit innate immunity by TLR2 binding, and can also inhibit the function of MHC molecules by the phagosomal rupture. However, we could not find any significant adverse effect after the administration of B/αGC/vacESAT6.

The ESAT6 of *M. bovis* and *M. tuberculosis* is identical (43, 44) and the amino acid sequence of ESAT6 homolog of *M. kansasii* is highly similar to that of *M. bovis*. Thus, we presumed that ESAT6 of *M. tuberculosis* could protect *M. kansasii* infection. In the current study, we confirmed that immunization with B/αGC/vacESAT6 ameliorated pulmonary inflammation caused by *M. kansasii* infection. Especially, therapeutic treatment of B/αGC/vacESAT6 decreased bodyweight loss and bacterial load in the lungs following *M.*

kansasii infection, as well as increased the survival rate of *M. kansasii*-infected mice. The therapeutic administration of B/αGC/vacESAT6 increased IFN-γ production by CD4$^+$ T cells. In addition, B/αGC/vacESAT6 altered the composition of other immune cells in lungs such as CD8 T cells and myeloid cells.

Collectively, we developed a αGC-loaded, ESAT6 expressing B-cell based vaccine (B/αGC/vacESAT6) and confirmed the preventive and therapeutic effect of B/αGC/vacESAT6 vaccine in a murine model of *M. kansasii* infection.

ETHICS STATEMENT

The animal study was reviewed and approved by Institutional Animal Care and Use Committee of Kangwon National University, Kangwon National University, Chuncheon Gangwon-do 24341, South Korea (Permit Number: KW-160201-4).

AUTHOR CONTRIBUTIONS

B-EK and H-JK designed this study. H-SJ, JY, ES, S-GY, SS, H-JL, and Y-JJ contributed with materials and analysis tools. B-EK performed and analyzed *in vivo* animal experiments together with E-KP and HJ. B-EK and J-HA performed data interpretation and discussion. B-EK, J-HA, S-YC, and H-JK wrote the manuscript. All authors reviewed the manuscript.

ACKNOWLEDGMENTS

We thank Byung-Il Yoon, College of Veterinary Medicine and Institute of Veterinary Science at Kangwon National University for providing technical assistance for histopathological examinations.

REFERENCES

Kim YJ, Han SH, Kang HW, Lee JM, Kim YS, Seo JH, et al. NKT ligand-loaded, antigen-expressing B cells function as long-lasting antigen presenting cells *in vivo*. Cell Immunol. (2011) 270:135–44. doi: 10.1016/j.cellimm.2011.04.006

Johnston JC, Chiang L, Elwood K. *Mycobacterium kansasii*. Microbiol Spectr. (2017) 5:TNMI7-0011-2016. doi: 10.1128/microbiolspec.TNMI7-0011-2016

Marras TK, Daley CL. Epidemiology of human pulmonary infection with nontuberculous mycobacteria. Clin Chest Med. (2002) 23:553–67. doi: 10.1016/S0272-5231(02)00019-9

Kwon BE, Ahn JH, Min S, Kim H, Seo J, Yeo SG, et al. Development of new preventive and therapeutic vaccines for tuberculosis. Immune Netw. (2018) 18:e17. doi: 10.4110/in.2018.18.e17

Vynnycky E, Fine PE. The natural history of tuberculosis: the implications of age-dependent risks of disease and the role of reinfection. Epidemiol Infect. (1997) 119:183–201. doi: 10.1017/S0950268897007917

Al-Zahid S, Wright T, Reece P. Laryngeal inflammatory pseudotumour secondary to *Mycobacterium kansasii*. Case Rep Pathol. (2018) 2018:9356243. doi: 10.1155/2018/9356243

van Herwaarden N, Bavelaar H, Janssen R, Werre A, Dofferhoff A. Osteomyelitis due to *Mycobacterium kansasii* in a patient with sarcoidosis. IDCases. (2017) 9:1–3. doi: 10.1016/j.idcr.2017.04.001

Procop GW. HIV and mycobacteria. Semin Diagn Pathol. (2017) 34:332–9. doi: 10.1053/j.semdp.2017.04.006

Carneiro MDS, Nunes LS, David SMM, Dias CF, Barth AL, Unis G. Nontuberculous mycobacterial lung disease in a high tuberculosis incidence setting in Brazil. J Bras Pneumol. (2018) 44:106–11. doi: 10.1590/s1806-37562017000000213

Kendall EA, Azman AS, Clobelens FG, Dowdy DW. MDR-TB treatment as prevention: the projected population-level impact of expanded treatment for multidrug-resistant tuberculosis. PLoS ONE. (2017) 12:e0172748. doi: 10.1371/journal.pone.0172748

Seo H, Jeon I, Kim BS, Park M, Bae EA, Song B, et al. IL-21-mediated reversal of NK cell exhaustion facilitates anti-tumour immunity in MHC class I- deficient tumours. Nat Commun. (2017) 8:15776. doi: 10.1038/ncomms15776

Mangtani P, Abubakar I, Ariti C, Beynon R, Pimpin L, Fine PE, et al. Protection by BCG vaccine against tuberculosis: a systematic review of randomized controlled trials. Clin Infect Dis. (2014) 58:470–80. doi: 10.1093/cid/cit790

Zimmermann P, Finn A, Curtis N. Does BCG vaccination protect against nontuberculous mycobacterial infection? A systematic review and meta-analysis. J Infect Dis. (2018) 218:679–87. doi: 10.1093/infdis/jiy207

Lim YJ, Choi HH, Choi JA, Jeong JA, Cho SN, Lee JH, et al. *Mycobacterium kansasii*-induced death of murine macrophages involves endoplasmic reticulum stress responses mediated by reactive oxygen species generation or calpain activation. Apoptosis. (2013) 18:150–9. doi: 10.1007/s10495-012-0792-4

Chung Y, Kim BS, Kim YJ, Ko HJ, Ko SY, Kim DH, et al. CD1d-restricted T cells license B cells to generate long-lasting cytotoxic antitumor immunity *in vivo*. Cancer Res. (2006) 66:6843–50. doi: 10.1158/0008-5472.CAN-06-0889

Kim YJ, Ko HJ, Kim YS, Kim DH, Kang S, Kim JM, et al. alpha-Galactosylceramide-loaded, antigen-expressing B cells prime a wide spectrum of antitumor immunity. Int J Cancer. (2008) 122:2774–83. doi: 10.1002/ijc.23444

Griffith DE. Nontuberculous mycobacterial lung disease. Curr Opin Infect Dis. (2010) 23:185–90. doi: 10.1097/QCO.0b013e328336ead6

Havlir DV, Getahun H, Sanne I, Nunn P. Opportunities and challenges for HIV care in overlapping HIV and TB epidemics. JAMA. (2008) 300:423–30. doi: 10.1001/jama.300.4.423

Lonnroth K, Castro KG, Chakaya JM, Chauhan LS, Floyd K, Glaziou P, et al. Tuberculosis control and elimination 2010-50: cure, care, and social development. *Lancet.* (2010) 375:1814– 29. doi: 10.1016/S0140-6736(10)60483-7

Rehm J, Samokhvalov AV, Neuman MG, Room R, Parry C, Lonnroth K, et al. The association between alcohol use, alcohol use disorders and tuberculosis (TB). A systematic review. *BMC Public Health.* (2009) 9:450. doi: 10.1186/1471-2458-9-450

CDC. Emergence of *Mycobacterium tuberculosis* with extensive resistance to second-line drugs–worldwide, 2000-2004. *MMWR Morb Mortal Wkly Rep.* (2006) 55:301–5.

Pontali E, Sotgiu G, D'Ambrosio L, Centis R, Migliori GB. Bedaquiline and multidrug-resistant tuberculosis: a systematic and critical analysis of the evidence. *Eur Respir J.* (2016) 47:394–402. doi: 10.1183/13993003.01891-2015

Agyeman AA, Ofori-Asenso R. Efficacy and safety profile of linezolid in the treatment of multidrug-resistant (MDR) and extensively drug-resistant (XDR) tuberculosis: a systematic review and meta-analysis. *Ann Clin Microbiol Antimicrob.* (2016) 15:41. doi: 10.1186/s12941-016-0156-y

Bruns H, Stegelmann F, Fabri M, Dohner K, van Zandbergen G, Wagner M, et al. Abelson tyrosine kinase controls phagosomal acidification required for killing of *Mycobacterium tuberculosis* in human macrophages. *J Immunol.* (2012) 189:4069–78. doi: 10.4049/jimmunol.1201538

Napier RJ, Norris BA, Swimm A, Giver CR, Harris WA, Laval J, et al. Low doses of imatinib induce myelopoiesis and enhance host anti-microbial immunity. *PLoS Pathog.* (2015) 11:e1004770. doi: 10.1371/journal.ppat.1004770

Napier RJ, Rafi W, Cheruvu M, Powell KR, Zaunbrecher MA, Bornmann W, et al. Imatinib-sensitive tyrosine kinases regulate mycobacterial pathogenesis and represent therapeutic targets against tuberculosis. *Cell Host Microbe.* (2011) 10:475–85. doi: 10.1016/j.chom.2011.09.010

Singhal A, Jie L, Kumar P, Hong GS, Leow MK, Paleja B, et al. Metformin as adjunct antituberculosis therapy. *Sci Transl Med.* (2014) 6:263ra159. doi: 10.1126/scitranslmed.3009885

Cassidy PM, Hedberg K, Saulson A, McNelly E, Winthrop KL. Nontuberculous mycobacterial disease prevalence and risk factors: a changing epidemiology. *Clin Infect Dis.* (2009) 49:e124–9. doi: 10.1086/648443

Mirsaeidi M, Machado RF, Garcia JG, Schraufnagel DE. Nontuberculous mycobacterial disease mortality in the United States, 1999- 2010: a population-based comparative study. *PLoS ONE.* (2014) 9:e91879. doi: 10.1371/journal.pone.0091879

Marras TK, Mendelson D, Marchand-Austin A, May K, Jamieson FB. Pulmonary nontuberculous mycobacterial disease, Ontario, Canada, 1998- 2010. *Emerg Infect Dis.* (2013) 19:1889–91. doi: 10.3201/eid1911.130737

Strollo SE, Adjemian J, Adjemian MK, Prevots DR. The burden of pulmonary nontuberculous mycobacterial disease in the United States. *Ann Am Thorac Soc.* (2015) 12:1458–64. doi: 10.1513/AnnalsATS.201503-173OC

Kwon YS, Koh WJ. Diagnosis and treatment of nontuberculous mycobacterial lung disease. *J Korean Med Sci.* (2016) 31:649– 59. doi: 10.3346/jkms.2016.31.5.649

Christensen EE, Dietz GW, Ahn CH, Chapman JS, Murry RC, Anderson J, et al. Initial roentgenographic manifestations of pulmonary *Mycobacterium tuberculosis*, *M. kansasii*, and *M. intracellularis* infections. *Chest.* (1981) 80:132–6. doi: 10.1378/chest.80.2.132

Marras TK, Mehta M, Chedore P, May K, Al Houqani M, Jamieson F. Nontuberculous mycobacterial lung infections in Ontario, Canada: clinical and microbiological characteristics. *Lung.* (2010) 188:289–99. doi: 10.1007/s00408-010-9241-8

Usemann J, Fuchs O, Anagnostopoulou P, Korten I, Gorlanova O, Roosli M, et al. Predictive value of exhaled nitric oxide in healthy infants for asthma at school age. *Eur Respir J.* (2016) 48:925–8. doi: 10.1183/13993003.00439-2016

Moon SM, Choe J, Jhun BW, Jeon K, Kwon OJ, Huh HJ, et al. Treatment with a macrolide-containing regimen for *Mycobacterium kansasii* pulmonary disease. *Respir Med.* (2019) 148:37–42. doi: 10.1016/j.rmed.2019.01.012

Abate G, Hamzabegovic F, Eickhoff CS, Hoft DF. BCG vaccination induces *M. avium* and *M. abscessus* cross-protective immunity. *Front Immunol.* (2019) 10:234. doi: 10.3389/fimmu.2019.00234

Ahn CH, Wallace RJ Jr, Steele LC, Murphy DT. Sulfonamide-containing regimens for disease caused by rifampin-resistant *Mycobacterium kansasii*. *Am Rev Respir Dis.* (1987) 135:10–6.

Lim A, Allison C, Tan DB, Oliver B, Price P, Waterer G. Immunological markers of lung disease due to non-tuberculous mycobacteria. *Dis Markers.* (2010) 29:103–9. doi: 10.1155/2010/347142

Wieland CW, Florquin S, Pater JM, Weijer S, van der Poll T. CD4 + cells play a limited role in murine lung infection with *Mycobacterium kansasii*. *Am J Respir Cell Mol Biol.* (2006) 34:167–73. doi: 10.1165/rcmb.2005- 0198OC

Hepper KP, Collins FM. Immune responsiveness in mice heavily infected with *Mycobacterium kansasii*. *Immunology.* (1984) 53:357–64.

Pathak SK, Basu S, Basu KK, Banerjee A, Pathak S, Bhattacharyya A, et al. Direct extracellular interaction between the early secreted antigen ESAT-6 of *Mycobacterium tuberculosis* and TLR2 inhibits TLR signaling in macrophages. *Nat Immunol.* (2007) 8:610–8. doi: 10.1038/ni1468

Cole ST, Brosch R, Parkhill J, Garnier T, Churcher C, Harris D, et al. Deciphering the biology of *Mycobacterium tuberculosis* from the complete genome sequence. *Nature.* (1998) 393:537–44. doi: 10.1038/24206

Garnier T, Eiglmeier K, Camus JC, Medina N, Mansoor H, Pryor M, et al. The complete genome sequence of *Mycobacterium bovis*. *Proc Natl Acad Sci USA.* (2003) 100:7877–82. doi: 10.1073/pnas.1130426100

3

A Ligation/Recombinase Polymerase Amplification Assay for Rapid Detection of SARS-CoV–2

Pei Wang[1†], Chao Ma[2†], Xue Zhang[2†], Lizhan Chen[2], Longyu Yi[1], Xin Liu[1], Qunwei Lu[1*], Yang Cao[2*] and Song Gao[2*]

[1] Key Laboratory of Molecular Biophysics of Ministry of Education, Department of Biomedical Engineering, College of Life Science and Technology, Center for Human Genome Research, Huazhong University of Science and Technology, Wuhan, China, [2] Jiangsu Key Laboratory of Marine Pharmaceutical Compound Screening, Jiangsu Key Laboratory of Marine Biological Resources and Environment, Co-Innovation Center of Jiangsu Marine Bio-industry Technology, School of Pharmacy, Jiangsu Ocean University, Lianyungang, China

*Correspondence:
Qunwei Lu
luqw@hust.edu.cn
Yang Cao
2020000088@jou.edu.cn
Song Gao
gaos@jou.edu.cn

[†]These authors have contributed equally to this work

The pandemic of COVID-19 caused by severe acute respiratory syndrome coronavirus-2 (SARS-CoV-2) has led to more than 117 million reported cases and 2.6 million deaths. Accurate diagnosis technologies are vital for controlling this pandemic. Reverse transcription (RT)-based nucleic acid detection assays have been developed, but the strict sample processing requirement of RT has posed obstacles on wider applications. This study established a ligation and recombinase polymerase amplification (L/RPA) combined assay for rapid detection of SARS-CoV–2 on genes N and ORF1ab targeting the specific biomarkers recommended by the China CDC. Ligase-based strategies usually have a low-efficiency problem on RNA templates. This study has addressed this problem by using a high concentration of the T4 DNA ligase and exploiting the high sensitivity of RPA. Through selection of the ligation probes and optimization of the RPA primers, the assay achieved a satisfactory sensitivity of 10^1 viral RNA copies per reaction, which was comparable to RT-quantitative polymerase chain reaction (RT-qPCR) and other nucleic acid detection assays for SARS-CoV–2. The assay could be finished in less than 30 min with a simple procedure, in which the requirement for sophisticated thermocycling equipment had been avoided. In addition, it avoided the RT procedure and could potentially ease the requirement for sample processing. Once validated with clinical samples, the L/RPA assay would increase the practical testing availability of SARS-CoV-2. Moreover, the principle of L/RPA has an application potential to the identification of concerned mutations of the virus.

Keywords: SARS-CoV-2, T4 DNA ligase, ligation, recombinase polymerase amplification, nucleic acid detection

INTRODUCTION

The pandemic of COVID-19 caused by severe acute respiratory syndrome coronavirus-2 (SARS-CoV-2) has led to more than 117 million reported cases and 2.6 million deaths globally, and the numbers are still increasing (https://www.who.int/). Specific therapeutics, effective vaccines, and accurate diagnosis are vital for control of the pandemic (Jindal and Gopinath, 2020; Liu et al., 2020).

Determination of the 29,903-nucleotide (nt), single-stranded RNA (ssRNA) genome sequence of SARS-CoV-2 had made nucleic acid detection of the virus possible (Wu et al., 2020). Based on the sequence information, reverse transcription-quantitative polymerase chain reaction (RT-qPCR) assays were rapidly developed and had become the primary means for detection and diagnosis (Chan et al., 2020; Udugama et al., 2020). The procedure of a typical RT-qPCR assay included converting the viral RNA to complementary DNA (cDNA) and exponential amplification of the detection biomarker with thermal cycling (Feng et al., 2020). Obvious limitations of the RT-qPCR assays were the dependence on sophisticated thermocycling equipment and well-trained personnel. For the diagnosis needs of COVID-19 in resource-limited areas, family self-testing or mass screening, assays based on isothermal amplification technologies like loop-mediated isothermal amplification (LAMP) and recombinase polymerase amplification (RPA) had been developed to reduce the thermocycler dependence (Notomi et al., 2000; Piepenburg et al., 2006; Rabe and Cepko, 2020). Some assays incorporated the clustered regularly interspaced short palindromic repeats (CRISPR) technology to increase the specificity and sensitivity (Broughton et al., 2020; Huang et al., 2020; Zhang et al., 2020). Visualization technologies were applied to read the amplification signals with simple devices or the naked eye, such as portable fluorescence readers or lateral flow strips (LFS) (Behrmann et al., 2020; Zhang C. et al., 2021). These assays provided more choices for practical testing needs of SARS-CoV-2.

Reverse transcription (RT) that converts the viral RNA to cDNA is the fundamental first step of these assays before the nucleic acid amplification, because PCR, LAMP and RPA technologies can only amplify DNA templates. The RT procedure requires high quality of the template RNA as it involves sequential covalent bonding events along the continuous RNA strand. Because RNA is vulnerable to degradation by environmental ribonucleases (RNases), a strict sample processing requirement must be complied with to avoid RNase contamination, which poses obstacles on wide application of the RT-based assays. False negative risk exists when conditions cannot meet the requirement of preparation of RT templates. In this study, we established a ligation and RPA (L/RPA) combined assay for rapid detection of SARS-CoV-2 (Figure 1). The L/RPA assay avoided the RT procedure and had a potentially lower operating requirement as compared to RT-based assays. The DNA ligase of bacteriophage T4, an important tool enzyme widely used in molecular cloning and next-generation sequencing (NGS), was the key factor of the assay. The detection biomarkers of the L/RPA assay were RNA fragments on ORF1ab gene and N gene, as recommended by China CDC. For each biomarker, a set of ligation probes (Probe A and Probe B) were designed. Each probe had a portion complementary to the RNA biomarker, and an "amplification arm" to facilitate the RPA amplification. With the presence of viral RNA, the probe set would anneal to the biomarker and be ligated into a single-stranded DNA (ssDNA) fragment by the T4 DNA ligase. The ssDNA fragment would be exponentially

amplified in the subsequent isothermal RPA reaction, and the amplification signal could be read in real-time using the SYBR Green I fluorescence dye (Figure 1).

Ligase-based strategies had been used for gene rearrangement and single nucleotide polymorphism (SNP) detections (Albrecht et al., 2013; Ruiz et al., 2020), but there had been no report of applications to nucleic acid detection of RNA virus. This was because DNA ligases (e.g., T4 DNA ligase) were not efficient on RNA templates, which could affect sensitivity of the detection (Nilsson et al., 2001; Bullard and Bowater, 2006; Lohman et al., 2014; Wee and Trau, 2016). In this study, we addressed this problem by optimizing the ligation protocol and exploiting the high sensitivity of RPA (Euler et al., 2013; Mayboroda et al., 2018). A satisfactory sensitivity of 10^1 viral RNA copies per reaction was achieved, which was comparable to that of RT-qPCR. The assay could finish in less than 30 min with a simple procedure. The requirement for sophisticated thermocycling equipment had been avoided. The requirement for sample processing could potentially be eased because the RT procedure had been avoided. Once validated with clinical samples, the L/RPA assay would increase the practical testing availability of SARS-CoV-2. Moreover, the principle of L/RPA has an application potential to the identification of concerned mutations of the virus, which now mainly depends on sequencing.

METHODS

Design of Probes and Primers
The ligation probes targeted the N gene and the ORF1ab gene of the SARS-CoV-2 genome (GenBank accession no. NC_045512.2). The RNA fragments matching the forward primer, probe, and reverse primer sequences of the RT-qPCR (TaqMan) assay that recommended by the China CDC were selected as the potential detection biomarkers (http://ivdc.chinacdc.cn/kyjz/202001/t20200121_211337.html). Exact complementary sequences of these potential biomarkers were used to design the "annealing portion" of the ligation probes. The "amplification arms" of the probes were artificial sequences that had considered to avoid similarity to nucleic acid sequences of any microorganisms or human by using the NCBI-BLAST. The amplification primers for RPA were determined by the "amplification arm" sequences of the corresponding probes. The general requirements for designing RPA primers were also considered. The Primer Premier 5.0 software was used to analyze the cross-dimerization possibilities between the amplification primers and corresponding ligation probes. The primer and probe sequences are listed in Supplementary Table 1. The probes and primers were synthesized by General Biosystems Co Ltd, Anhui, China.

SARS-CoV-2 Pseudovirus and RNA Extraction
The SARS-CoV-2 pseudovirus (Fubio Biological Technology Co Ltd, Shanghai, China) was composed of a retrovirus capsid with

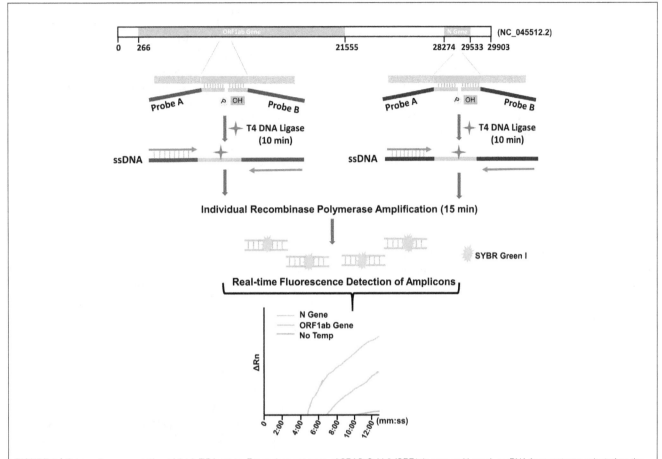

FIGURE 1 | Schematic representation of the L/RPA assay. For each target gene of SRAS-CoV-2 (ORF1ab gene or N gene), an RNA fragment was selected as the detection biomarker. A probe pair (Probe A and Probe B) was designed with the "annealing portions" exactly complementary to the targeted biomarker sequence (indicated with color blue or yellow) and the "amplification arms" completely artificial (indicated with color purple or dark blue). With the presence of the viral RNA, the probe set would anneal to the targeted biomarker and be ligated into one ssDNA fragment with the T4 DNA ligase. The ligation product for each biomarker was individually amplified by RPA with the forward and reverse primers matching the "amplification arm" sequences. With the fluorescence dye SYBR Green I, the amplification signals were detected in real-time. No Temp: the control with no viral RNA template.

RNA fragments containing the ORF1ab gene, E gene and N gene sequences of SARS-CoV-2. The pseudovirus at a concentration of 10^8 particles/ml was stored in nuclease-free water under -20°C. RNA in the pseudovirus was extracted with the TIANamp Virus RNA Kit (Tiangen Biotech Co Ltd, Beijing, China) and served as the template.

RNA Standards of ORF1ab Gene and N Gene Fragments

The pseudovirus RNA was used as the reverse transcription template to synthesize cDNA with the HiScript 1st Strand cDNA Synthesis Kit (Vazyme Biotech Co Ltd, Nanjing, China), and the cDNA was used for PCR amplification to produce DNA fragments of the N gene and the ORF1ab gene. The N gene fragment contained the entire gene sequence, while the ORF1ab gene fragment contained nucleotides from position 13237 to position 13560 of the SARS-CoV-2 genome sequence (GenBank accession no. NC_045512.2), which covered the three potential detection biomarkers on the ORF1ab gene. The PCR products

were inserted into pET-28b(+) vector between the T7 promotor and T7 terminator (restriction sites: BamHI/XhoI) to produce the two constructs for transcription of N gene and ORF1ab gene fragments *in vitro*. The two constructs were confirmed by sequencing (General Biosystems Co Ltd). *In vitro* transcription was conducted according to the manufacturer's instructions of the T7 High Efficiency Transcription Kit (TransGen Biotech Co Ltd, Beijing, China). The transcription products were quantified with a Qubit 4 fluorometer (Thermo Fisher Scientific Inc, Wilmington, DE, USA) and served as the RNA standards. The RNA copy number was calculated based on the transcription size.

L/RPA Procedure

A 4-µl annealing mixture containing the RNA template and 0.5 µl of each ligation probe (1 µM) was heated to 85°C for 2 min and cooled on ice to anneal the probes to the template. Then 0.5 µl of the 10X T4 DNA ligase buffer and 0.5 µl (equal to 40-500 cohesive end units according to the enzyme concentration) of the T4 DNA ligase (Thermo Fisher Scientific Inc) were added to the mixture. Ligation was done in 8-10 min at 37°C and inactivated at 95°C for 2 min. The whole ligation mixture was added to the RPA mixture of the RAA-Basic Nucleic Acid Amplification Reagent (Hangzhou ZC Bio-Sci & Tech Co Ltd, Hangzhou, China) containing 2 μl of each primer (10 μM), 36 μl of A Buffer and 2.5 μl of B Buffer (Hangzhou ZC Bio-Sci & Tech Co Ltd). SYBR Green I fluorescent dye (10,000X) (Beijing Solarbio Science & Technology Co Ltd, Beijing, China) was diluted to 15X by A Buffer and 2.5 μl was used in each RPA reaction (total volume 50 μl). The reaction was conducted on an Applied Biosystems 7900HT Fast Real-Time PCR System at 37°C with signal reads at 20-sec intervals for 15 min.

RT-qPCR

The RT-qPCR reactions were performed according to the manufacturer's instructions of the Novel Coronavirus (2019-nCoV) Dual Probes qRT-PCR Kit (Beyotime Biotechnology Inc, Shanghai, China). The primer and probe sequences were designed according to the China CDC's recommendation (**Supplementary Table 1**). A total of 5 μl of the RNA template was added to the reaction premix to make the total reaction volume to 25 μl. Reactions were conducted on an Applied Biosystems 7900HT Fast Real-Time PCR System. The cycle setting was 20 min at 50°C for reverse transcription, 2 min at 95°C for denaturation, followed by 45 cycles of 15 sec at 95°C and 20 sec at 60°C. The fluorescence channels were VIC for ORF1ab gene and FAM for N gene.

RESULTS

Selection of the Detection Biomarkers

For this study, potential detection markers were the RNA fragments of the virus genome matching the forward primer, probe, and reverse primer sequences of RT-qPCR (TaqMan) that recommended by the China CDC for detection of SARS-CoV–2 (**Supplementary Table 1**). Thus, there were three potential detection biomarkers on the N gene, and another three on the ORF1ab gene. For each potential biomarker, a set of two ligation probes (Probe A and Probe B) was designed (**Figure 1**). More specifically, for N gene, N-Probe 1A and 1B targeted the fragment matching the qPCR forward primer sequence; N-Probe 2A and 2B targeted the fragment matching the qPCR probe sequence; and N-Probe 3A and 3B targeted the fragment matching the qPCR reverse primer sequence. Similarly, a series of O-Probes were designed for the potential biomarkers on the ORF1ab gene (**Supplementary Table 1**).

The ligation efficiency of the L/RPA procedure was fundamental for the overall performance of the detection. A series of preliminary experiments were conducted to increase the ligation efficiency and found that the concentration of T4 ligase in the ligation system was a key factor. It was determined to use 500 U (cohesive end units) of T4 ligase in the 5-μl ligation mixture (**Supplementary Table 2**). Briefly, 40 U, 200 U and 500 U of T4 ligase per reaction were tested for both N gene and ORF1ab gene. For N gene, we used N-Probe 2A and 2B for ligation and the amplification primer set N-Primer 1F and 1R for RPA. For ORF1ab gene, we used O-Probe 1A and 1B and O-Primer 1F and 1/2R. According to the principle, the ligation probes shared the same sequences of the "amplification arms" that matched the amplification primer set (**Supplementary Table 1**). Different template amounts (10^7, 10^3 and 10^1 copies) were tested and the Threshold time (Tt) of the fluorescent signals were compared with the reactions with no template (No Temp). The differences of Tt (ΔTt) between the reaction with no template and the reactions with various amounts of template reflected the performance of the assay. For both genes, acceptable ΔTt were obtained for the various template amounts when 500 U/reaction of T4 ligase was used. Poor ΔTt were observed for 10^3 or 10^1 copies of template when 200 U or 40 U of T4 ligase per reaction was used (**Supplementary Table 2**). Thus, it was determined to use 500 U/reaction of T4 ligase in this assay.

To select the biomarker for the N gene, probe pairs 1 (N-Probe 1A and 1B), 2 (N-Probe 2A and 2B), and 3 (N-Probe 3A and 3B) were tried in the L/RPA reactions using the same amplification primer set (N-Primer 1F and 1R) (**Supplementary Table 1**). The amplification signals of reactions with 10^7 N gene copies and reactions with no template were compared for each probe pair. The probe pair 2 produced the most distinct signals (the most different Tt values) between reactions with 10^7 N gene copies and reactions with no template, suggesting that the RNA fragment on the N gene matching the qPCR probe sequence should be selected as the biomarker for the N gene (**Figure 2A** and **Supplementary Table 3**).

Similarly, to select the biomarker for the ORF1ab gene, O-Probe 1A and 1B, 2A and 2B, and 3A and 3B were tried in the L/RPA reactions using O-Primer 1F and 1/2R (**Supplementary Table 1**). The probe pair 1 produced the most distinct signals and the most different Tt values between reactions with 10^7 ORF1ab gene copies and reactions with no template, suggesting that the RNA fragment on the ORF1ab gene matching the qPCR forward primer sequence should be selected as the biomarker for the ORF1ab gene (**Figure 2B** and **Supplementary Table 3**).

Screening for Optimal RPA Primer Sets

The limit of detection (LOD) of the L/RPA assay for the N gene using the probe pair 2 (N-Probe 2A and 2B) and primer set 1 (N-Primer 1F and 1R) was tested with series dilutions of the N gene RNA fragments. The results showed close signal curves and Tt values of reactions with 10^3 copies, 10^1 copies, and no template (**Figure 3A** and **Supplementary Table 4**). Similar results were obtained from the L/RPA assay for the ORF1ab gene detection using the probe pair 1 (O-Probe 1A and 2B) and primer set 1 (O-Primer 1F and 1/2R) (**Figure 3B** and **Supplementary Table 4**).

For better LOD, signals of reactions with no template should appear later and distinct from reactions with 10^1 copies of template. Possible cross-dimerization between the amplification primers and ligation probes were analyzed with the Primer Premier 5.0 software and additional probe and primer sets were designed (**Supplementary Table 1**). For the N gene, one

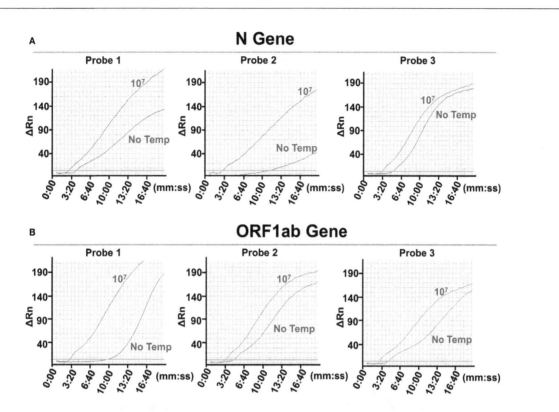

FIGURE 2 | Selection of the detection biomarkers. The images were the fluorescence history diagrams of RPA amplifications of the ligation products from the N gene RNA standard template **(A)** and the ORF1ab gene RNA standard template **(B)**. The diagrams showed the fluorescence signal (ΔRn) *vs*. time (mm:ss). For each target gene, 3 potential detection biomarkers were targeted by ligation probe pairs 1, 2, and 3 that were indicated at the top of the respective diagrams. The curves indicated with "10⁷" represented amplification signals from ligations with 10⁷ the RNA templates. The curves indicated with "No Temp" represented amplification signals from the ligation controls with no RNA template. Every diagram was one typical outcome of three independent experiments.

additional forward primer (N-Primer 2/3F) and two additional reverse primer (N-Primer 2R and 3R) were designed and used as Primer-Set 2 (N-Primer 2/3F and 2R) and Primer-Set 3 (N-Primer 2/3F and 3R). Because the "amplification arm" sequences of the ligation probes should match the amplification primer sequences, N-Probe 2A-2/3, N-Probe 2B-2, and N-Probe 2B-3 were designed and used together with N-Primer 2/3F, N-Primer 2R, and N-Primer 3R, respectively. For the ORF1ab gene, one additional forward primer (O-Primer 2F) was designed and used in Primer-Set 2 (O-Primer 2F and 1/2R). O-Probe 1A-2 was designed and used together with O-Primer 2F.

These newly designed primer sets showed later signals and bigger *Tt* values of the no template reactions that led to better LOD. For the N gene, Primer-Set 2 showed close signal curves of reactions with 10³ and 10¹ copies of template, and Primer-Set 3 was selected (**Figure 3A** and **Supplementary Table 4**). For the ORF1ab gene, Primer-Set 2 was selected (**Figure 3B** and **Supplementary Table 4**). For both the N gene and the ORF1ab gene, the L/RPA assay exhibited a LOD of 10¹ copies per reaction.

The finally selected probes and primers in the L/RPA assay were listed in **Supplementary Table 1** with the primer/probe names indicated in red. The sequences were as follows (5'-3', the complementary portions of the probes were italicized):

N-Probe 2A-2/3, ***GCAGCAGCAA***GACGAGGGAAAGAG CAGTACCTAA;

N-Probe 2B-3, TGTGTACGAATCCCACTAATTCG CC***AATCTGTCAA***;

N-Primer 2/3F, TTAGGTACTGCTCTTTCCCTCGTC;

N-Primer 3R, TGTGTACGAATCCCACTAATTCGCC;

O-Probe 1A-2, ***AACCCACAGGG***CAATAGGGAGATCAT AGGAGTTGGCT;

O-Probe 1B, TAACTCATATTGTAGAAGAGTAGAAG ***TTAAGTGTAA***;

O-Primer 2F, AGCCAACTCCTATGATCTCCCTATTG;

O-Primer 1/2R, TAACTCATATTGTAGAAGAGTAGAAG.

Validation With SARS-CoV-2 Pseudovirus

The L/RPA assay was validated with SARS-CoV-2 pseudovirus. RNA extracted from the SARS-CoV-2 pseudovirus was 10-fold serially diluted and detected by the L/RPA assay for both the N gene and the ORF1ab gene. The results were compared with the RT-qPCR method (**Figure 4** and **Supplementary Table 5**). For both genes, up to dilution multiple of 10⁵, the L/RPA assay could give positive signals. At this dilution multiple, the RT-qPCR detection gave a non-linear signal for the N gene, and gave a

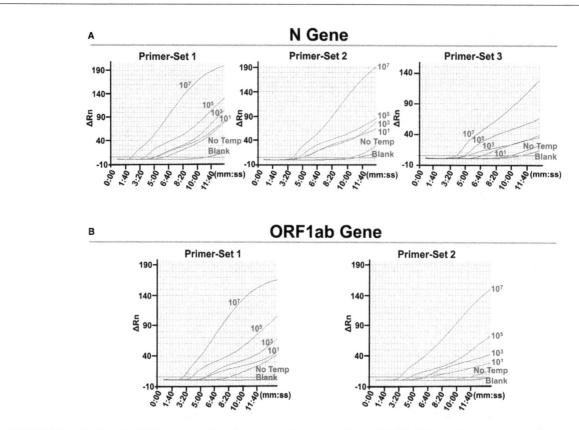

FIGURE 3 | Screening for optimal RPA primer sets. The images were the fluorescence history diagrams of RPA amplifications with different primer sets for the detection of N gene **(A)** and ORF1ab gene **(B)**. For RPA reactions using each primer set, the corresponding probe pairs were used for the preceding ligation reactions. The diagrams showed the fluorescence signal (ΔRn) *vs.* time (mm:ss). The blue numbers beside the curves indicated the amount of RNA standard templates (in copies) used in the corresponding L/RPA assays. No Temp: the control with no RNA template. Blank: the control RPA reactions without the ligation reaction components and the RNA template. Every diagram was one typical outcome of three independent experiments.

signal in the range of "suspected" for the ORF1ab gene, which suggested that the template amount was close to the detection limit. Thus, the sensitivity of L/RPA assay was at the same level as RT-qPCR.

DISCUSSION

Rapid and simple SARS-CoV-2 detection methods that are not limited by sophisticated thermocycling equipment are valuable for diagnosis needs in resource-limited areas, family self-testing or mass screening. For this purpose, assays based on LAMP, RPA and CRISPR technologies have been developed (Rabe and Cepko, 2020; Haq et al., 2021; Zhang W. S. et al., 2021). These assays are generally faster and simpler than RT-qPCR, providing more choices for the testing needs of SARS-CoV-2 under different situations. Reverse transcription (RT) is the fundamental first step of these assays that converts the viral RNA to cDNA, the initial material for nucleic acid amplification. Because of the ubiquitous environmental RNase, the RT procedure has strict operating requirements for RNase-free environment, containers, and reagents, which complicate the application of RT-based assays. The L/RPA assay established in

this study avoided the RT procedure. Instead, two ligation probes were annealed to adjacency on the RNA template and ligated into a ssDNA fragment for subsequent amplification. This strategy used the RNA template only for the ligation, a "one covalent bonding" event that was quicker and much simpler than RT. The fewer RNA involvement should potentially ease the operating requirement of the whole assay.

This is the first application of ligase-based strategies to the detection of RNA virus. Because the T4 DNA ligase is inefficient on RNA templates (Nilsson et al., 2001; Bullard and Bowater, 2006), it is important to bring up the ligation efficiency to the level that exponential amplification of the ligation product can occur. During the optimization of the ligation protocol, we found that using small reaction volume and keeping high concentration of the T4 DNA ligase were the key factors. It was determined that using 500 U of the T4 ligase in a 5-μl reaction mixture could achieve sufficient ligation efficiency. On the other hand, the highly sensitive RPA technology had to be used, while PCR was not sensitive enough to guarantee a satisfactory sensitivity of the assay.

The detection biomarkers of the L/RPA assay were selected from the viral RNA fragments matching the forward primer, probe, and reverse primer sequences of RT-qPCR (TaqMan) that

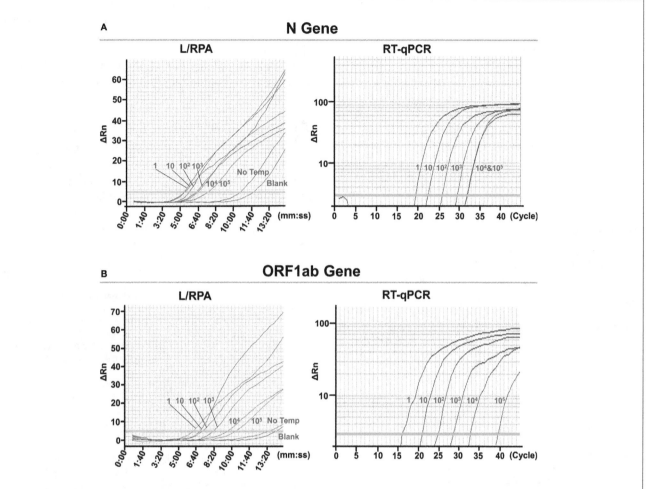

FIGURE 4 | Validation with SARS-CoV-2 pseudovirus. The images were the fluorescence history diagrams of the detection results of the N gene **(A)** and the ORF1ab gene **(B)** of SARS-CoV-2 pseudovirus using the L/RPA assay and RT-qPCR. The diagrams of L/RPA showed the fluorescence signal (ΔRn) *vs.* time (mm: ss). The diagrams of RT-qPCR showed the fluorescence signal (ΔRn) *vs. Ct* (cycle). The blue numbers beside the curves indicated the dilution multiple of the RNA extracted from the pseudovirus used in the corresponding assays. No Temp: the control with no RNA template. Blank: the control reactions without the ligation reaction components and the RNA template. Every diagram was one typical outcome of three independent experiments.

recommended by the China CDC. One biomarker was selected for each of the target genes, N and ORF1ab. This ensured the good specificity of the selected biomarkers towards SARS-CoV-2, because the sequences had been used in hundreds of millions of clinical detections worldwide in RT-qPCR assays. For each biomarker, sequence optimizations were carefully conducted for the L/RPA assay. The sequence optimization process of this study suggested that the sequences of the "amplification arms" of the probes were important. Inappropriate sequences could possibly form cross-dimers between the amplification primers and ligation probes and produce noise fluorescence signals, affecting the sensitivity.

The L/RPA assay showed a sensitivity of 10^1 viral RNA copies per reaction, which was comparable to that of RT-qPCR and other nucleic acid detection assays for SARS-CoV-2 (Behrmann et al., 2020; Zhang C. et al., 2021; Zhang W. S. et al., 2021). The assay could be finished in less than 30 min with simple operation and without dependence on sophisticated thermocycling

equipment. Because of the enzyme characteristics, both the ligation and the RPA reactions does not demand strict temperature control, and the set temperature of 37°C can even be provided by the body heat. Although a qPCR machine was used in this study to read the fluorescence signal, the thermocycling function had been avoided. Fluorescent signal detection of SYBR Green I DNA staining is a mature technology, and battery-powered portable tube scanners are commercially available and ready to be applied to the fluorescence detection of the L/RPA assay (Mondal et al., 2016).

Though the sensitivity of 10^1 viral RNA copies per reaction was comparable to RT-qPCR, our results did not show a good relationship between the *Tt* value and the template amount. This means quantitative detection of SARS-CoV-2 could not be achieved by the L/RPA assay. One possible reason was that the amplification substrate was the ligation product of the two ligation probes, and the ligation efficiency was not linearly related to the template amount. Considering the major need of practical SARS-CoV-2 tests was to give an answer of positive or negative, the L/RPA assay without the capacity of quantification was still a competent detection choice. Based on the results of this study, a tentative evaluation standard for both N gene and ORF1ab gene could be: $\Delta Tt \geq 2.0$ min, positive; 2.0 min > $\Delta Tt \geq 0.5$ min, suspected; $\Delta Tt < 0.5$ min, negative; where $\Delta Tt = Tt_{\text{No Temp}} - Tt_{\text{Sample}}$. As a future direction, validation of the L/RPA assay with clinical samples should be a requirement before it can be applied to practical testing, and a more accurate evaluation standard should be determined based on the detection of adequate clinical samples.

In conclusion, this study established a ligation-based L/RPA assay for rapid detection of SARS-CoV-2. The assay is more easily operated than the RT-based assays because the RNA involvement has been reduced. Not limited by sophisticated thermocycling equipment, the assay provides more choice for the detection of SARS-CoV-2 at point of need. Furthermore, the principle of the assay is readily applicable to the identification of concerned mutations of the virus, which now mainly depends on sequencing.

AUTHOR CONTRIBUTIONS

QL, YC, and SG designed the research. PW, CM, XZ, LC, and LY conducted the research. PW, CM, XZ, and XL analyzed the data. PW and SG wrote the manuscript. All authors contributed to the article and approved the submitted version.

REFERENCES

Albrecht, J. C., Kotani, A., Lin, J. S., Soper, S. A., and Barron, A. E. (2013). Simultaneous Detection of 19 K-ras Mutations by Free-Solution Conjugate Electrophoresis of Ligase Detection Reaction Products on Glass Microchips. *Electrophoresis* 34, 590–597. doi: 10.1002/elps.201200462

Behrmann, O., Bachmann, I., Spiegel, M., Schramm, M., Abd El Wahed, A., Dobler, G., et al. (2020). Rapid Detection of SARS-CoV-2 by Low Volume Real-Time Single Tube Reverse Transcription Recombinase Polymerase Amplification Using an Exo Probe With an Internally Linked Quencher (Exo-Iq). *Clin. Chem.* 66, 1047–1054. doi: 10.1093/clinchem/hvaa116

Broughton, J. P., Deng, X., Yu, G., Fasching, C. L., Servellita, V., Singh, J., et al. (2020). Crispr-Cas12-based Detection of SARS-Cov-2. *Nat. Biotechnol.* 38, 870–874. doi: 10.1038/s41587-020-0513-4

Bullard, D. R., and Bowater, R. P. (2006). Direct Comparison of Nick-Joining Activity of the Nucleic Acid Ligases From Bacteriophage T4. *Biochem. J.* 398, 135–144. doi: 10.1042/bj20060313

Chan, J. F.-W., Yip, C. C.-Y., To, K. K.-W., Tang, T. H.-C., Wong, S. C.-Y., Leung, K.-H., et al. (2020). Improved Molecular Diagnosis of COVID-19 by the Novel, Highly Sensitive and Specific COVID-19-Rdrp/Hel Real-Time Reverse Transcription-PCR Assay Validated in Vitro and With Clinical Specimens. *J. Clin. Microbiol.* 58, e00310–e00320. doi: 10.1128/jcm.00310-20

Euler, M., Wang, Y., Heidenreich, D., Patel, P., Strohmeier, O., Hakenberg, S., et al. (2013). Development of a Panel of Recombinase Polymerase Amplification Assays for Detection of Biothreat Agents. *J. Clin. Microbiol.* 51, 1110–1117. doi: 10.1128/jcm.02704-12

Feng, W., Newbigging, A. M., Le, C., Pang, B., Peng, H., Cao, Y., et al. (2020). Molecular Diagnosis of COVID-19: Challenges and Research Needs. *Anal. Chem.* 92, 10196–10209. doi: 10.1021/acs.analchem.0c02060

Haq, F., Sharif, S., Khurshid, A., Ikram, A., Shabbir, I., Salman, M., et al. (2021). Reverse Transcriptase Loop-Mediated Isothermal Amplification (RT-LAMP)-based Diagnosis: A Potential Alternative to Quantitative Real-Time PCR Based Detection of the Novel SARS-COV-2 Virus. *Saudi. J. Bio. Sci.* 28, 942–947. doi: 10.1016/j.sjbs.2020.10.064

Huang, Z., Tian, D., Liu, Y., Lin, Z., Lyon, C. J., Lai, W., et al. (2020). Ultra-Sensitive and High-Throughput CRISPR-p Owered COVID-19 Diagnosis. *Biosens. Bioelectron.* 164:112316. doi: 10.1016/j.bios.2020.112316

Jindal, S., and Gopinath, P. (2020). Nanotechnology Based Approaches for Combatting COVID-19 Viral Infection. *Nano Express.* 1, 022003. doi: 10.1088/2632-959x/abb714

Liu, Y., Gayle, A. A., Wilder-Smith, A., and Rocklöv, J. (2020). The Reproductive Number of COVID-19 is Higher Compared to SARS Coronavirus. *J. Travel. Med.* 27, taaa021. doi: 10.1093/jtm/taaa021

Lohman, G. J., Zhang, Y., Zhelkovsky, A. M., Cantor, E. J., and Evans, T. C.Jr. (2014). Efficient DNA Ligation in DNA-RNA Hybrid Helices by Chlorella Virus DNA Ligase. *Nucleic Acids Res.* 42, 11846–11846. doi: 10.1093/nar/gku792

Mayboroda, O., Katakis, I., and O'Sullivan, C. K. (2018). Multiplexed Isothermal Nucleic Acid Amplification. *Anal. Biochem.* 545, 20–30. doi: 10.1016/j.ab.2018.01.005

Mondal, D., Ghosh, P., Khan, M. A. A., Hossain, F., Böhlken-Fascher, S., Matlashewski, G., et al. (2016). Mobile Suitcase Laboratory for Rapid Detection of Leishmania Donovani Using Recombinase Polymerase Amplification Assay. *Parasit. Vectors.* 9, 281. doi: 10.1186/s13071-016-1572-8

Nilsson, M., Antson, D.-O., Barbany, G., and Landegren, U. (2001). RNA-Templated DNA Ligation for Transcript Analysis. *Nucleic Acids Res.* 29, 578–581. doi: 10.1093/nar/29.2.578

Notomi, T., Okayama, H., Masubuchi, H., Yonekawa, T., Watanabe, K., Amino, N., et al. (2000). Loop-Mediated Isothermal Amplification of DNA. *Nucleic Acids Res.* 28, e63–e63. doi: 10.1093/nar/28.12.e63

Piepenburg, O., Williams, C. H., Stemple, D. L., and Armes, N. A. (2006). DNA Detection Using Recombination Proteins. *PLoS Biol.* 4, e204. doi: 10.1371/journal.pbio.0040204

Rabe, B. A., and Cepko, C. (2020). Sars-CoV-2 Detection Using Isothermal Amplification and a Rapid, Inexpensive Protocol for Sample Inactivation and Purification. *PNAS* 117, 24450–24458. doi: 10.1073/pnas.2011221117

Ruiz, C., Huang, J., Giardina, S. F., Feinberg, P. B., Mirza, A. H., Bacolod, M. D., et al. (2020). Single-Molecule Detection of Cancer Mutations Using a Novel PCR-LDR-qPCR Assay. *Hum. Mutat.* 41, 1051–1068. doi: 10.1002/humu.23987

Udugama, B., Kadhiresan, P., Kozlowski, H. N., Malekjahani, A., Osborne, M., Li, V. Y. C., et al. (2020). Diagnosing COVID-19: The Disease and Tools for Detection. *ACS Nano.* 14, 3822–3835. doi: 10.1021/acsnano.0c02624

Wee, E. J. H., and Trau, M. (2016). Simple Isothermal Strategy for Multiplexed, Rapid, Sensitive, and Accurate miRNA Detection. *ACS Sens.* 1, 670–675. doi: 10.1021/acssensors.6b00105

Wu, F., Zhao, S., Yu, B., Chen, Y.-M., Wang, W., Song, Z.-G., et al. (2020). A New Coronavirus Associated With Human Respiratory Disease in China. *Nature* 579, 265–269. doi: 10.1038/s41586-020-2008-3

Zhang, F., Abudayyeh, O. O., and Gootenberg, J. S. (2020) *A Protocol for Detection of COVID-19 Using CRISPR Diagnostics*. Available at: https://www.broadinstitute.org/files/publications/special/COVID-19%20detection%20(updated).pdf (Accessed 2021-03-13).

Zhang, W. S., Pan, J., Li, F., Zhu, M., Xu, M., Zhu, H., et al. (2021). Reverse Transcription Recombinase Polymerase Amplification Coupled With CRISPR-Cas12a for Facile and Highly Sensitive Colorimetric Sars-CoV-2 Detection. *Anal. Chem.* 93, 4126–4133. doi: 10.1021/acs.analchem.1c00013

Zhang, C., Zheng, T., Wang, H., Chen, W., Huang, X., Liang, J., et al. (2021). Rapid One-Pot Detection of SARS-CoV-2 Based on a Lateral Flow Assay in Clinical Samples. *Anal. Chem.* 93, 3325–3330. doi: 10.1021/acs.analchem.0c05059

4

Phenotypic and Genotypic Characterization of Novel Polyvalent Bacteriophages with Potent *In Vitro* Activity Against an International Collection of Genetically Diverse *Staphylococcus aureus*

Elliot Whittard[1], James Redfern[1], Guoqing Xia[2], Andrew Millard[3], Roobinidevi Ragupathy[1], Sladjana Malic[1] and Mark C. Enright[1*]

[1] Department of Life Sciences, Manchester Metropolitan University, Manchester, United Kingdom, [2] Lydia Becker Institute of Immunology and Inflammation, University of Manchester, Manchester, United Kingdom, [3] Department of Genetics and Genome Biology, University of Leicester, Leicester, United Kingdom

Correspondence:
Mark C. Enright
m.enright@mmu.ac.uk

Phage therapy recently passed a key milestone with success of the first regulated clinical trial using systemic administration. In this single-arm non-comparative safety study, phages were administered intravenously to patients with invasive *Staphylococcus aureus* infections with no adverse reactions reported. Here, we examined features of 78 lytic *S. aureus* phages, most of which were propagated using a *S. carnosus* host modified to be broadly susceptible to staphylococcal phage infection. Use of this host eliminates the threat of contamination with staphylococcal prophage — the main vector of *S. aureus* horizontal gene transfer. We determined the host range of these phages against an international collection of 185 *S. aureus* isolates with 56 different multilocus sequence types that included multiple representatives of all epidemic MRSA and MSSA clonal complexes. Forty of our 78 phages were able to infect > 90% of study isolates, 15 were able to infect > 95%, and two could infect all 184 clinical isolates, but not a phage-resistant mutant generated in a previous study. We selected the 10 phages with the widest host range for *in vitro* characterization by planktonic culture time-kill analysis against four isolates:- modified *S. carnosus* strain TM300H, methicillin-sensitive isolates D329 and 15981, and MRSA isolate 252. Six of these 10 phages were able to rapidly kill, reducing cell numbers of at least three isolates. The four best-performing phages, in this assay, were further shown to be highly effective in reducing 48 h biofilms on polystyrene formed by eight ST22 and eight ST36 MRSA isolates. Genomes of 22 of the widest host-range phages showed they belonged to the *Twortvirinae* subfamily of the order *Caudovirales* in three main groups corresponding to *Silviavirus*, and two distinct groups of *Kayvirus*. These genomes assembled as single-linear dsDNAs with an average length of 140 kb and a GC content of *c.* 30%. Phages that could infect > 96% of *S. aureus* isolates were found in all three groups, and these have great potential as therapeutic candidates if, in future studies, they can be formulated to maximize their efficacy and eliminate emergence of phage resistance by using appropriate combinations.

Keywords: *Staphylococcus aureus*, bacteriophage, biofilm, methicillin-resistant *Staphylococcus aureus*, genomics

INTRODUCTION

Staphylococcus aureus is one of the major causes of both hospital- and community-acquired infections globally. It is an extremely versatile pathogen, causing a broad spectrum of diseases ranging in severity from minor skin and soft-tissue infections to life-threatening invasive infections (Lowy, 1998). Hospitalized patients are particularly prone to *S. aureus* infections because of the presence of compromised immune systems and surgical site infections caused by the implantation of indwelling medical devices (Brandt et al., 1999). *S. aureus* is commonly resistant to penicillin and methicillin-resistant *S. aureus* (MRSA) infections, resistant to all beta-lactam antibiotics, are most frequently treated with intravenous vancomycin, the antibiotic of "last resort" for resistant staphylococcal infections. However, resistance to this antibiotic (Centers for Disease Control and Prevention, 2002) and newer agent, such as linezolid (Tsiodras et al., 2001) and daptomycin (Skiest, 2006), have emerged, and there is a great and ever-increasing need for novel antibiotics and other therapeutic strategies for treating this pathogen.

Phage therapy exploits the natural ability of lytic bacteriophages (phages) to invade, multiply intracellularly, and then kill their host. Obligately, lytic phage are regarded as the most appropriate candidates in human health because they are capable of rapidly killing their host, greatly reducing the chances of bacteria developing phage resistance (Skurnik et al., 2007; Cui et al., 2017b). They also lack the required genetic factors for genome incorporation found in temperate phages. Despite widespread use in the 1930s, phage therapeutics were largely eclipsed by the discovery and clinical development of broad-spectrum antibiotics in western countries. However, phage therapy continues to be used at The G. Eliava Institute of Bacteriophage, Microbiology, and Virology in Tbilisi, Georgia and the Institute of Immunology and Experimental Therapy in Wroclaw, Poland, and these have become major centers for the development and application of phage therapy (Summers, 2001; Kutter et al., 2010). Success rates exceeding 85% have been reported in treating antibiotic-resistant infections caused by pathogens, including *S. aureus*, *Pseudomonas aeruginosa*, *Klebsiella pneumoniae*, and *Escherichia coli* in Poland (O'Flaherty et al., 2009) in studies involving large patient numbers. To date, there have been three early-stage clinical trials of phages for the treatment of *S. aureus* infections. In 2009, Rhoads et al. reported safety in a trial of phages against venous leg ulcers (Rhoads et al., 2009) and more recently McCallin et al. (2018) demonstrated the safety of a broad-spectrum phage cocktail in a placebo-controlled study, including nasal and oral administration. A recent study in Australia demonstrated safety of a good manufacturing practice — quality three-phage cocktail administered intravenously to 13 patients with invasive *S. aureus* infections (Petrovic Fabijan et al., 2020). This study marked a milestone in phage therapy, the first regulated clinical trial of systemically administered phages.

Most reports in the literature regarding lytic staphylococcal phages show that these are typically members of the *Twortvirinae* subfamily, which currently comprises five genera representing distinct lineages — *Kayvirus, Sepunavirus, Silviavirus, Twortvirus*, and unclassified *Twortvirinae*. These phages display a broad host range, infecting most *S. aureus* isolates and even those of other staphylococcal species (Lobocka et al., 2012). Studies on these group of phages and also their lytic enzymes hold promise for future clinical development alone or in combination with antibiotics (Berryhill et al., 2021) especially as comparative genomic analysis show little similarity between phages from different lineages in gene complement or in their lytic gene sequences (O'Flaherty et al., 2005a; Synnott et al., 2009; Lobocka et al., 2012). These may therefore represent an important and diverse source of phages for traditional therapy or development of treatments based on novel antimicrobial enzymes.

Here, we report on the isolation and characterization of 78 lytic phages with broad host range against a diverse collection of *S. aureus*. These 185 isolates include members of all globally disseminated MRSA and methicillin-sensitive lineages, including multiple isolates of clonal complexes (CCs) 1, 5, 8, 22, 30, 45, 59, and CC80 containing the main MRSA lineages (Chatterjee and Otto, 2013). Wherever possible, we isolated and propagated phages on a modified *S. carnosus* isolate that is avirulent (Rosenstein et al., 2009), containing none of the virulence genes associated with *S. aureus* prophages that could potentially compromise the safe production of phages for therapeutic use. We examined the *in vitro* characteristics of selected phages in planktonic and biofilm culture and characterized the genomic similarity and taxonomy of 22 phages with some of the broadest host ranges.

MATERIALS AND METHODS

Bacterial Strains

A modified *S. carnosus* strain, TM300H, a hybrid strain derived from TM300H expressing both its native glycerol-phosphate (GroP)- and *S. aureus* ribitol-phosphate (RboP)-type wall teichoic acids, was used for phage isolation and propagation. *S. carnosus* is a non-virulent staphylococcal species used in meat production, and as such, we considered it a benign propagating host for phage production. TM300H was transformed with a chloramphenicol resistance plasmid encoding polyribitol-phosphate (RboP) repeating units of *S. aureus* wall teichoic acid to promote phage adsorption (Winstel et al., 2013). This required supplementation of growth medium with 10 μg/ml chloramphenicol. The methicillin-sensitive isolate D329 was used as an alternative host for phage propagation where this was not possible using TM300H. *S. aureus* isolate 15981 (obtained from Prof ATA Jenkins, University of Bath, UK) was also included in this study as it is a very strong biofilm producer and has been used in several studies of *S. aureus* virulence and biofilm regulation including those by Valles et al. (2003) and Toledo-Arana et al. (2005). All bacterial isolates were cultured in tryptone soy broth (TSB) or agar (TSA) and stored at −80°C in TSB containing 25% (v/v) glycerol. One hundred eighty-five genetically diverse isolates of *S. aureus* from our collection, including isolates from 13 published studies of human and animal carriage and disease, were used in this study (**Table 1**). They comprised 126 MRSA and 59 MSSA isolates from 14 different countries with 58 different multilocus sequence types (Enright et al., 2000). This collection contains multiple representative isolates of all major MRSA and MSSA lineages (Enright et al., 2002; Feil et al., 2003; Holden et al., 2013), including those associated with community-onset (Vandenesch et al., 2003) and livestock-associated (van Belkum et al., 2008) MRSA infections. **Table 1** shows the MLST sequence type and clonal complex of each isolate, as well as a reference to the original study where the isolate was first characterized using MLST, and for MRSA isolates — SCC*mec* typing. Further information on study isolates are available from the cited source and, in most cases, from the PubMLST website at https://pubmlst.org/organisms/staphylococcus-aureus.

Phage Isolation, Propagation, and Host Range Determination

Sewage effluent samples were collected from various process tanks at Davyhulme and Eccles wastewater treatment works, Manchester, England. Organic matter was removed from samples by centrifugation at 3,000*g* for 30 min. 10-ml aliquots of supernatant were filtered (0.22 μm pore size), before being combined with 10 ml of double-strength TSB and 100 μl of exponentially growing bacterial cultures, followed by incubation at 37°C, in an orbital incubator at 150 rpm for 24 h. Bacterial debris were removed by centrifugation (3,000*g*, 30 min), and supernatants were filtered (0.22 μm) and stored at 4°C. This supernatant was used to check the presence of lytic phages using the double-agar overlay method (Kropinski et al., 2009). Isolated single plaques were picked into SM buffer (50 mM Tris-HCl, 8 mM MgSO₄, 100 mM NaCl, and 0.01% gelatin, pH 7.5) in sterile distilled water, and successive rounds of single plaque purification were carried out until purified plaques were obtained. Purified phage suspensions were maintained at 4°C. *S. carnosus* strain TM300H was used for phage propagation whenever possible; however, for some phages, the methicillin-sensitive *S. aureus* isolate D329 was used (**Table 1**).

Phage host range was determined by spot test, 100 μl of log phase bacterial culture was mixed with 10 ml soft agar, the mixture poured onto 10 ml TSA plates and 10 μl phage lysate (~10⁶ pfu/ml) spotted onto the plate prior to overnight incubation at 37°C. Bacterial strains were classed as wholly sensitive to a particular phage if spot test resulted in a clear plaque, intermediately sensitive if plaques showed evidence of clearing but were hazy or turbid and resistant if no clearing was present. All host range assays were performed in triplicate.

A collection of 32 uncharacterized *S. aureus* phages collected in previous studies was also included in this study.

In Vitro Growth Experiments
Growth Kinetics in Planktonic Culture

The growth rate of each bacterial isolate in liquid culture was studied in 96-well flat-bottomed microtiter plates by measuring absorbance of each well using the method of Alves et al. (2014). Briefly, bacterial growth was measured by absorbance (600 nm) over 19 h at 37°C, with shaking, using a microplate reader (FLUOstar Omega, BMG LABTECH). The plate reader provided absorbance data points every 180 s following a 10-s agitation at 200 rpm. Data points after every 30 min were used for analysis.

Time-Kill Assays

Time-kill assays were performed to determine the sensitivity of planktonic bacterial cells to phage infection and to investigate the frequency of phage-resistant bacterial mutants using the method described in Alves et al. (2014). Briefly, 200 μl of 1:100 dilutions of overnight bacterial cultures were added to wells of 96-well microtiter plates. Dilutions were made using TSB. After 2 h of incubation at 37°C, phage lysate, at an MOI of 0.1, was added, and the microplates were incubated for a further 17 h. Experiments were performed in triplicate.

Formation and Treatment of *S. aureus* Biofilms

Biofilm assays followed a standard 96-well plate method as described previously (Alves et al., 2014). Briefly, 200 μl of 1:100 dilutions of overnight bacterial culture, made using TSB supplemented with 1% D-(+)-glucose (TSBg), were added to microtiter plates. Microtiter plates with lids were sealed with Parafilm were wrapped in moistened paper towel, then placed in a sealed plastic box to maintain humidity. Plates were incubated at 37°C for 48 h without agitation to allow biofilm formation. After 24 h, 50 μl of spent medium was withdrawn and replaced with 50 μl of fresh TSBg. Plates were then incubated for a further 24 h at 37°C. Biofilms were washed three times with PBS before air drying and staining with 0.1% (w/v) crystal violet (CV). Stained biofilms were rinsed with PBS, air dried then solubilized in 200 μl of 30% (v/v) glacial acetic acid. Biofilm mass was measured spectrophotometrically using a FLUOstar plate reader at absorbance of 590 nm. Enumeration of *S. aureus* cells recovered from 48-h biofilms was performed by washing with PBS to remove non-adherent bacteria and residual media. Biofilms were then resuspended in 200-μl PBS and serially diluted, with 100 μl spread on TSA plates to determine the CFU for each isolate.

48-h biofilms were treated with 200 μl of diluted phage lysate at two different MOIs, of 1.0 and 0.1. Quantification of biofilm biomass and viable cell counts following exposure to phage for 6 and 24 h was performed as described above.

Phage Genome Sequencing
Isolation of Phage Genomic DNA

Phage genomic DNA was extracted by a phenol/chloroform/isoamyl alcohol (25:24:1 [v/v]) method using 1.5 ml of lysate (10⁷ to 10⁹ pfu/ml). Lysates were centrifuged at 10,000*g* for 10 min at 4°C, and 1-ml supernatant was transferred into a fresh microfuge tube and treated with DNase I (10 μl of 1 mg/ml DNase I) and RNase A (4 μl of 12.5 mg/ml RNase A). 1 ml of phenol (pH 10) was added to each tube, before vortexing for 30 s, and centrifugation at 10,000*g* for 10 min at 4°C. The aqueous layer was removed to a fresh tube and 1 ml phenol/

TABLE 1 | Details of *Staphylococcus aureus* isolates used in this study.

Isolate	ST	CC	MRSA	Country	Year	Reference
H462	1	1	N	UK	1997	(Avrani and Lindell, 2015)
NL0118512	1	1	N	Netherlands	1999	(Bankevich et al., 2012)
BTN2164	1	1	N	UK	1999	(Cui et al., 2017a)
HT2001-254	1	1	Y	USA	2001	(Dickey and Perrot, 2019)
A93-0066	5	5	Y	France	1993	(Adriaenssens and Brister, 2017)
FIN61974	5	5	Y	Finland	2002	(Adriaenssens and Brister, 2017)
H157	5	5	N	UK	1997	(Avrani and Lindell, 2015)
AR110735	5	5	Y	Ireland	1993	(Avrani and Lindell, 2012)
BK519	5	5	Y	USA	1991	(Bankevich et al., 2012)
NJ992	5	5	Y	USA	2002	(Bankevich et al., 2012)
D10	5	5	N	UK	1997	(Beeton et al., 2015)
CDC-USA800	5	5	Y	USA	1998	(Chatterjee and Otto, 2013)
BTN2242	5	5	N	UK	2002	(Cui et al., 2017a)
C56	6	5	N	UK	1997	(Avrani and Lindell, 2015)
E228	8	8	N	Denmark	1957	(Alves et al., 2014)
99ST22111	8	8	Y	Australia	1997	(Bankevich et al., 2012)
EMRSA13	8	8	Y	UK	1999	(Bankevich et al., 2012)
EMRSA2	8	8	Y	UK	1999	(Brandt et al., 1999)
EMRSA6	8	8	Y	UK	1999	(Avrani and Lindell, 2015)
EMRSA7	8	8	Y	UK	1999	(Avrani and Lindell, 2012)
NL010548-1	31	30	N	Netherlands	1999	(Bankevich et al., 2012)
D137	8	8	N	UK	1997	(Beeton et al., 2015)
NOT110	34	30	N	UK	2000	(Brandt et al., 1999)
CDC-USA300	8	8	Y	USA	1998	(Chatterjee and Otto, 2013)
15981	8	1	N	Spain	2003	(Abedon, 1992)
H169	36	30	Y	Finland	1996	(Adriaenssens and Brister, 2017)
D295	36	30	N	UK	1997	(Avrani and Lindell, 2015)
D316	36	30	N	UK	1997	(Beeton et al., 2015)
H117	36	30	N	UK	1997	(Avrani and Lindell, 2015)
D329	36	30	Y	UK	1997	(Beeton et al., 2015)
H402	13	30	N	UK	1997	(Avrani and Lindell, 2015)
C154	14	15	N	UK	1997	(Avrani and Lindell, 2015)
C357	15	15	Y	UK	1997	(Avrani and Lindell, 2015)
H291	18	15	N	UK	1997	(Beeton et al., 2015)
D17	20	15	N	UK	1997	(Avrani and Lindell, 2015)
98/10618	36	22	Y	UK	1998	(Adriaenssens and Brister, 2017)
SwedenAO9973	22	22	Y	Sweden	1999	(Avrani and Lindell, 2015)
WW1678/96	22	22	Y	Germany	1996	(Adriaenssens and Brister, 2017)
C101	22	22	N	UK	1997	(Avrani and Lindell, 2015)
C720	22	22	Y	UK	1998	(Avrani and Lindell, 2015)
H182MRSA	22	22	Y	UK	1997	(Avrani and Lindell, 2015)
H65	22	22	N	UK	1998	(Avrani and Lindell, 2015)
EMRSA15-90	22	22	Y	UK	1990	(Bankevich et al., 2012)
NL011399-5	22	22	N	Netherlands	1999	(Bankevich et al., 2012)
403.02	22	22	N	UK	2002	(Berryhill et al., 2021)
434.07	22	22	Y	UK	2007	(Berryhill et al., 2021)
723.07	22	22	N	UK	2007	(Berryhill et al., 2021)
921.07	22	22	Y	UK	2007	(Berryhill et al., 2021)
930.02	22	22	Y	UK	2002	(Berryhill et al., 2021)
1018.07	22	22	Y	UK	2007	(Berryhill et al., 2021)
1091	22	22	Y	UK	2008	(Berryhill et al., 2021)
729192	22	22	Y	UK	2007	(Berryhill et al., 2021)
98.4823.X	38	30	N	UK	1998	(Berryhill et al., 2021)
AR0650784	42	22	N	Ireland	1993	(Berryhill et al., 2021)
ARI10	45	45	Y	UK	2007	(Berryhill et al., 2021)
ARI11	45	45	Y	UK	2007	(Cui et al., 2017a)

Isolate	ST	CC	MRSA	Country	Year	Reference
ARI7	22	22	Y	UK	1997	(Avrani and Lindell, 2015)
F86956	22	22	Y	Netherlands	1999	(Bankevich et al., 2012)
H43162	22	22	N	UK	1999	(Cui et al., 2017a)
H91491	22	22	Y	USA	2001	(Dickey and Perrot, 2019)
H05060412	22	22	Y	France	1993	(Adriaenssens and Brister, 2017)
H05322054809	22	22	Y	Finland	2002	(Adriaenssens and Brister, 2017)
H07230040705	22	22	Y	UK	1997	(Avrani and Lindell, 2015)
H07374046805	22	22	Y	Ireland	1993	(Avrani and Lindell, 2012)
M81008	22	22	Y	USA	1991	(Bankevich et al., 2012)
T27706	22	22	Y	USA	2002	(Bankevich et al., 2012)
T50530	22	22	N	UK	1997	(Beeton et al., 2015)
W44936	22	22	Y	USA	1998	(Chatterjee and Otto, 2013)
370.07	22	22	N	UK	2002	(Cui et al., 2017a)
RH06000061/09	22	22	Y	Australia	1999	(Avrani and Lindell, 2015)
BTN1626	22	22	N	UK	2002	(Cui et al., 2017a)
C49	23	22	N	UK	1997	(Beeton et al., 2015)
D279	25		N	UK	1997	(Beeton et al., 2015)
H118	28		N	UK	1997	(Beeton et al., 2015)
CUBA4030	30	30	N	Cuba	1999	(Beeton et al., 2015)
C390	31	30	N	UK	1999	(Bankevich et al., 2012)
H399	33	30	N	UK	1997	(Beeton et al., 2015)
C160	34	30	N	UK	2000	(Brandt et al., 1999)
MRSA252-0Knut	36	30	Y	USA	1998	(Chatterjee and Otto, 2013)
FIN75916	36	30	Y	Spain	2003	(Adriaenssens and Brister, 2017)
UK96/22010	36	30	N	UK	1997	(Adriaenssens and Brister, 2017)
H119MRSA	36	30	Y	UK	1996	(Avrani and Lindell, 2015)
H325	36	30	N	UK	1997	(Beeton et al., 2015)
MRSA252	36	30	N	UK	1997	(Beeton et al., 2015)
EMRSA16	36	30	N	UK	1997	(Beeton et al., 2015)
NottmA	13	30	Y	UK	1997	(Avrani and Lindell, 2015)
NottmA2	36	30	N	UK	2000	(Brandt et al., 1999)
03.1791.F	36	30	Y	UK	2003	(Centers for Disease Control and Prevention, 2002)
06.9570.L	36	30	N	UK	2006	(Centers for Disease Control and Prevention, 2002)
07.1227.Z	36	30	N	UK	2007	(Centers for Disease Control and Prevention, 2002)
07.1696.F	36	30	Y	UK	2007	(Centers for Disease Control and Prevention, 2002)
07.2449.K	36	30	Y	UK	2007	(Centers for Disease Control and Prevention, 2002)
07.2496.L	36	30	Y	UK	2007	(Centers for Disease Control and Prevention, 2002)
07.2589.M	36	30	N	UK	2007	(Centers for Disease Control and Prevention, 2002)
07.2880.V	36	30	Y	UK	2007	(Centers for Disease Control and Prevention, 2002)
07.3841.N	36	30	Y	UK	2007	(Centers for Disease Control and Prevention, 2002)
07.6636.Y	36	30	N	UK	2007	(Centers for Disease Control and Prevention, 2002)
07.6659.K	36	30	Y	UK	2007	(Centers for Disease Control and Prevention, 2002)
07.7206.Y	36	30	N	UK	2007	(Centers for Disease Control and Prevention, 2002)
97.2483.Hb	36	30	Y	USA	1997	(Chatterjee and Otto, 2013)
98.5806.F	36	30	Y	UK	1998	(Berryhill et al., 2021)
USA300	36	30	Y	USA	1998	(Berryhill et al., 2021)
BTN1429	36	30	Y	UK	2002	(Berryhill et al., 2021)
BTN2172	36	30	Y	UK	2002	(Berryhill et al., 2021)
BTN2292	36	30	Y	UK	2002	(Berryhill et al., 2021)
BTN766	36	30	N	UK	2008	(Berryhill et al., 2021)
H137	38	30	N	UK	1997	(Berryhill et al., 2021)
C253	40	30	N	UK	1998	(Berryhill et al., 2021)
C427	42	22	N	UK	1997	(Berryhill et al., 2021)
FIN76167	45	45	Y	Finland	1996	(Berryhill et al., 2021)
BTN2299	45	45	Y	UK	2007	(Cui et al., 2017a)

Isolate	ST	CC	MRSA	Country	Year	Reference
D97	55	30	N	UK	1997	(Beeton et al., 2015)
D318	57	15	N	UK	1997	(Beeton et al., 2015)
D508	58		N	UK	1997	(Beeton et al., 2015)
D535	59		N	UK	1997	(Beeton et al., 2015)
D551	59		N	UK	1997	(Beeton et al., 2015)
D473	69	1	N	UK	1997	(Beeton et al., 2015)
CDCUSA700	72	8	Y	USA	1998	(Chatterjee and Otto, 2013)
SWEDEN8980/99	80	80	Y	Sweden	1999	(Adriaenssens and Brister, 2017)
HT2002-0664	80	80	Y	France	2002	(Dickey and Perrot, 2019)
HT200040991	80	80	Y	France	2004	(Dickey and Perrot, 2019)
BK1563	88		Y	USA	1991	(Bankevich et al., 2012)
HT2001-0634	93	93	Y	Australia	2001	(Dickey and Perrot, 2019)
HT2002-0635	93	93	Y	Australia	2002	(Dickey and Perrot, 2019)
H560	121		N	UK	1998	(Avrani and Lindell, 2015)
D139	145		N	UK	1997	(Beeton et al., 2015)
FIN62305	156		Y	Finland	1990	(Adriaenssens and Brister, 2017)
D22	182		N	UK	1997	(Beeton et al., 2015)
CAN6428-011	188	1	N	Canada	2002	(Bankevich et al., 2012)
D470	207		N	UK	1997	(Beeton et al., 2015)
NOT116	227		N	UK	2000	(Brandt et al., 1999)
WW2594/97-2	228	5	Y	Germany	1997	(Adriaenssens and Brister, 2017)
GERMANY131/98	228	5	Y	Germany	1998	(Bankevich et al., 2012)
CDC16	231	5	Y	USA	1998	(Chatterjee and Otto, 2013)
93.3759.V	235	5	Y	UK	2002	(Bankevich et al., 2012)
91-4990	239	8	Y	Netherlands	1991	(Adriaenssens and Brister, 2017)
EMRSA11	239	8	Y	UK	1999	(Bankevich et al., 2012)
EMRSA4	239	8	Y	UK	1999	(Bankevich et al., 2012)
FFP200	239	8	Y	Portugal	1996	(Bankevich et al., 2012)
EMRSA9	240	8	Y	UK	1999	(Bankevich et al., 2012)
SWEDEN408/99	246	8	Y	Sweden	1999	(Adriaenssens and Brister, 2017)
FRA97393	247	8	Y	France	2002	(Adriaenssens and Brister, 2017)
82MRSA	247	8	Y	UK	1997	(Avrani and Lindell, 2015)
EMRSA5	247	8	Y	UK	1999	(Bankevich et al., 2012)
EMRSA8	250	8	Y	UK	1999	(Bankevich et al., 2012)
KD12168	250	8	Y	UK	1965	(Bankevich et al., 2012)
27969	398	398	Y	UK	2012	N/A
09.4620.V	398	398	Y	UK	2012	N/A
09.6440.M	398	398	Y	UK	2012	N/A
11.1299.J	398	398	Y	UK	2012	N/A
11.2530.K	398	398	Y	UK	2012	N/A
11.3281.H	398	398	Y	UK	2012	N/A
11.4910.K	398	398	Y	UK	2012	N/A
11.5252.H	398	398	Y	UK	2012	N/A
11.5654.T	398	398	Y	UK	2012	N/A
12.2167.C	398	398	Y	UK	2012	N/A
12.2539.L	398	398	Y	UK	2012	N/A
12.2732.H	398	398	Y	UK	2012	N/A
42-57	398	398	Y	UK	2012	N/A
BVCA92	398	398	Y	UK	2012	N/A
C7-4011	398	398	Y	UK	2007	N/A
C7(P11)	398	398	Y	UK	2007	N/A
C7(P4)	398	398	Y	UK	2007	N/A
GKP136-53	398	398	Y	UK	2012	N/A
h-RVC57276	398	398	Y	UK	2012	N/A
m-38-53	398	398	Y	UK	2012	N/A
m-mecA-17-57	398	398	Y	UK	2012	N/A

(Continued)

TABLE 1 | Continued

Isolate	ST	CC	MRSA	Country	Year	Reference	Isolate	ST	CC	MRSA	Country	Year	Reference	Isolate	ST	CC	MRSA	Country	Year	Reference
ARI2	22	22	Y	UK	2007	(Berryhill et al., 2021)	BTN2306	45	45	Y	UK	1999	(Cui et al., 2017a)	RV2007-06745-3'A'	398	398	Y	UK	2007	N/A
ARI15	22	22	Y	UK	2007	(Berryhill et al., 2021)	C316	49		N	UK	1997	(Avrani and Lindell, 2015)	RV2007-13689-13	398	398	Y	UK	2007	N/A
ARI26	22	22	Y	UK	2007	(Berryhill et al., 2021)	H417	50		N	UK	1997	(Avrani and Lindell, 2015)	NOT161	843	97	N	UK	2000	(Brandt et al., 1999)
ARI31	22	22	Y	UK	2007	(Berryhill et al., 2021)	C3	51		N	UK	1997	(Avrani and Lindell, 2015)	NOT290	848	1	N	UK	2000	(Brandt et al., 1999)
ARI4	22	22	Y	UK	2007	(Berryhill et al., 2021)	D49	53	45	N	UK	1997	(Beeton et al., 2015)	BTN2289	868	5	N	UK	1999	(Cui et al., 2017a)
ARI5	22	22	Y	UK	2007	(Berryhill et al., 2021)	D98	54	45	N	UK	1997	(Beeton et al., 2015)							

chloroform/isoamylalcohol (25:24:1) was added, vortexed for 30 s, and centrifuged at 10,000g for a further 10 min at 4°C. The phenol/chloroform/isoamylalcohol step was then repeated before DNA was precipitated with two volumes of ice-cold absolute ethanol and 1/10 volume of 7.5 M ammonium acetate, and stored at −20°C overnight. Samples were centrifuged at 10,000g for 20 min at 4°C, and DNA pellets were washed twice with 1 ml 70% ethanol (v/v), then resuspended in 100 µl nuclease-free water.

Whole-Genome Sequencing

Libraries of the selected phage DNA samples (input DNA 0.2 ng/µl) were prepared using the Illumina NexteraXT DNA Sample Preparation Kit following manufacturer's instructions. Sequencing of phage DNA (paired-end 2 × 150 high output) was carried out using the Illumina NextSeq500 platform at Manchester Metropolitan University, UK.

Genome Assembly, Annotation, and Comparison

Sequence reads were assembled using SPAdes v3.11 (Bankevich et al., 2012). All phage assemblies resulted in a single large contig plus a number of small repeats. The largest contig and their coverage were assessed and visualized using Bandage (Wick et al., 2015), individual genome assemblies were analyzed using Artemis (Rutherford et al., 2000), and the largest scaffolds were compared to the similarity of previously sequenced genomes using BLASTN. Based on the similarity between our query sequences and the top hits (closely related genomes) identified using BLASTn, genome assemblies of all related phage infecting *S. aureus* were retrieved from GenBank (https://www.ncbi.nlm.nih.gov/nuccore) and the European Nucleotide Archive (ENA) databases in April 2021 to achieve a final collection of 122 phage genomes.

Genomes were annotated with PROKKA v1.14.6 (Seemann, 2014) using a custom *Caudovirales* gene database (Michniewski et al., 2019). Neighbor-joining trees were constructed using min-hash distances implemented in Mashtree (Katz et al., 2019). Genome comparisons were made using min-hash implemented in MASH (Ondov et al., 2016), and the pan-genome analysis tool Roary v3.13.0 (Page et al., 2015) was used to assess the number of genes shared by each genome (Page et al., 2015). Phylogenetic trees were constructed using Archaeopteryx v0.9929 (https://sites.google.com/site/cmzmasek/home/software/archaeopteryx).

Statistical Analysis

Planktonic and biofilm experiments were performed with a minimum of three replicates, and these values were used to plot mean ± standard deviation. Statistical analysis was performed using GraphPad Prism Version 7.0 software package, data were analyzed as an ordinary one-way analysis of variance (ANOVA) and Sidak's multiple comparison test to determine significance of results. Results were taken as significantly different by a p value of < 0.05 unless otherwise stated.

RESULTS

Phage Isolation

The modified *S. carnosus* strain TM300H and *S. aureus* strain D329 were used to isolate and propagate 46 phages from 150 filtered sewage samples over a period of several months. Plaques were all small in size with most being <1 mm in diameter (*n*=39) and the largest being 2 mm. 39 of 46 phages were propagated on TM300H; however, the remainder (EW20, EW29, EW30, EW41, and EW44-46) could not reliably infect this strain and were propagated on *S. aureus* D239 instead. Phages were named in accordance with recent guidance on nomenclature with the designations vB_SauM_EW1 to vB_SauM_EW46 (Adriaenssens and Brister, 2017) and are henceforth referred to as EW1, EW2 …

EW46. The 32 phages isolated previously were propagated on modified TM300H and were named EW47 to EW78.

Host Range

The host range of the 78 phages was determined by spot test of lysates against 185 *S. aureus* isolates (**Table 2**) in agar overlays. Bacterial strains were classified as sensitive, intermediately sensitive, or resistant, depending on plaque morphology — examples of these are shown in **Figure 1**. The majority

TABLE 2 | Percentage coverage of EW phage against 185 *S. aureus* isolates.

Phage	Isolates Resistant	Isolates Intermediate	Isolates Sensitive	Coverage	Phage	Isolates Resistant	Isolates Intermediate	Isolates Sensitive	Coverage
EW1	80	104	1	56.76%	EW40	17	158	10	90.81%
EW2	80	104	1	56.76%	EW41	6	124	54	96.76%
EW3	27	149	9	85.41%	EW42	6	163	16	96.76%
EW4	59	124	2	68.11%	EW43	11	159	15	94.05%
EW5	26	153	6	85.95%	EW44	44	112	29	76.22%
EW6	42	137	6	77.30%	EW45	36	147	2	80.54%
EW7	48	117	20	74.05%	EW46	65	116	4	64.86%
EW8	163	21	1	11.89%	EW47	123	62	0	33.51%
EW9	70	110	5	62.16%	EW48	60	122	3	67.57%
EW10	59	117	9	68.11%	EW49	14	147	24	92.43%
EW11	97	83	5	47.57%	EW50	139	41	5	24.86%
EW12	71	112	2	61.62%	EW51	15	151	19	91.89%
EW13	82	100	3	55.68%	EW52	6	152	27	96.76%
EW14	80	101	4	56.76%	EW53	27	149	9	85.41%
EW15	7	119	59	96.22%	EW54	16	94	75	91.35%
EW16	69	57	59	62.70%	EW55	76	96	13	58.92%
EW17	76	52	57	58.92%	EW56	19	119	47	89.73%
EW18	3	98	84	98.38%	EW57	16	116	53	91.35%
EW19	70	59	56	62.16%	EW58	14	107	64	92.43%
EW20	71	60	54	61.62%	EW59	13	101	71	92.97%
EW21	18	109	58	90.27%	EW60	12	84	89	93.51%
EW22	26	102	57	85.95%	EW61	13	99	73	92.97%
EW23	37	119	29	80.00%	EW62	12	94	79	93.51%
EW24	30	139	16	83.78%	EW63	12	99	74	93.51%
EW25	46	130	9	75.14%	EW64	11	97	77	94.05%
EW26	7	116	62	96.22%	EW65	13	107	65	92.97%
EW27	5	126	54	97.30%	EW66	12	96	77	93.51%
EW28	19	146	20	89.73%	EW67	11	94	80	94.05%
EW29	6	142	37	96.76%	EW68	11	97	77	94.05%
EW30	16	158	11	91.35%	EW69	10	103	72	94.59%
EW31	19	154	12	89.73%	EW70	1	88	96	99.46%
EW32	54	122	9	70.81%	EW71	1	83	101	99.46%
EW33	19	160	6	89.73%	EW72	5	91	89	97.30%
EW34	36	138	11	80.54%	EW73	13	95	77	92.97%
EW35	4	169	12	97.84%	EW74	2	76	107	98.92%
EW36	7	164	14	96.22%	EW75	8	81	96	95.68%
EW37	14	167	4	92.43%	EW76	10	83	92	94.59%
EW38	36	148	1	80.54%	EW77	13	89	83	92.97%
EW39	142	41	2	23.24%	EW78	10	85	90	94.59%

The phage host range is scored as resistant, intermediate, and susceptible based on the level of clearing on host overlays. Percentage coverage is the cumulative number of isolates that displayed intermediate and sensitive susceptibility to phage.

Coloured shading has been used to indicate level of resistance (red), intermediate-sensitivity (orange), and sensitivity of the isolate collection to phage infection.

exhibited a broad host range phenotype with 40 of our 78 phage capable of infecting over 90% of isolates as determined by their sensitivity or intermediate-sensitivity to phages in this assay (**Table 2**). Fifteen of these were capable of disrupting the growth of over 95% (178/185) of isolates. Phages EW70 and EW71 had the broadest host range and were capable of infecting 184 of the 185 isolates. Of the 184 isolates, they could infect 96 (53%), and 101 (55%) were fully susceptible, respectively, that is, they produced distinct clear plaques. The only phage they could not infect was a mutant of isolate MRSA252 generated in a previous study during growth of the isolate in liquid culture with phage K (Alves et al., 2014).

Time Kill Assays in Planktonic Culture

To investigate the dynamics of phages and their hosts in liquid culture, we quantified the ability of phages to reduce bacterial numbers in broth cultures and observed any phage-resistant mutant emergence. We selected ten of the fourteen phages that were able to infect > 96% of isolates tested, for time kill experiments (from **Table 2**). These were phages EW15, EW18, EW27, EW29, EW36, EW41, EW52, EW71, EW72, and EW74. Suspensions of these ten phages were tested against TM300H, D329, MRSA252, and 15981. These isolates were chosen as they include the two propagating bacteria used, MRSA252,

a representative of a major MRSA lineage (CC30) and the first genome sequenced MRSA isolate (Holden et al., 2004) and the well-studied abundant biofilm producing isolate 15981. Phages were introduced to growing cultures to achieve a multiplicity of infection (MOI) of 0.1, and incubated for 19 h with OD_{600} readings taken every 3 min.

Both EW41 and EW52, propagated on D329 were the only phage ineffective against TM300H in this planktonic culture assay. The remaining eight phages were successful in reducing the growth of TM300H within 4 h following their introduction and they prevented any observable growth of phage-resistant mutants after 19 h (**Figure 2A**). With isolate D329, phages EW27 and EW29 initially took an hour longer than other phage before having any effect on the host as seen in **Figure 2B**. However, both EW27 and EW29 effectively reduced the growth of D329 after 4 and 6 h, respectively, while preventing the emergence of phage-resistant mutants. As for phage EW72, it was unsuccessful at depleting bacterial numbers before phage-resistant mutants emerged after 5 h, although this had an effect on the growth rate of D329 when compared with controls. Interestingly, an increase in bacterial density compared with the control was observed in D329 following addition of EW36. Individual growth phases appear less clearly defined with MRSA252 when challenged with phage (**Figure 2C**), which is also observed with strain 15981 (**Figure 2D**).

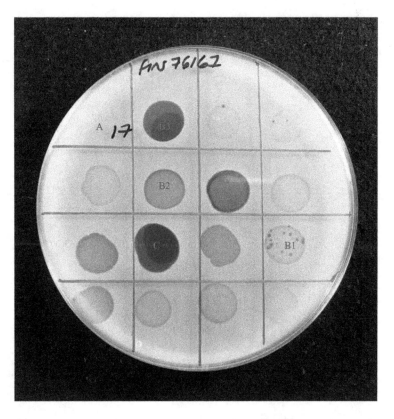

FIGURE 1 | Host range assay showing effect of 16 phages against *S. aureus* strain Fin76167. Plaque formation was scored based on the level of clearing, **(A)** Resistant with no disturbance to lawn, **(B)** Intermediate-sensitivity varied from, B1 Few plaques with slight disturbance to lawn, B2 Substantial turbidity throughout clear zone, B3 High degree of clearing of with numerous mutant colonies present, to **(C)** Sensitive with complete clearing of bacterial lawn.

It is clear that a number of phages could not effectively reduce bacterial numbers before resistant mutants emerge. A reduced rate of killing was observed among phage when challenged against other strains compared with their propagating hosts, decreasing bacterial numbers at a much more gradual rate, with some phage such as EW15 taking several hours. Interestingly, phage EW71 and EW74 appeared to have a bacteriostatic effect on strain 15981 with no change in absorbance observed for c. 14 h before slowly increasing (**Figure 2D**).

As observed in D329, EW36 seemed to have a positive effect on the growth of MRSA252 when compared with the control, as a significant increase in OD_{600} with time was observed. The same trend was also observed with EW72 on the growth of 15981, however, only slightly more than the control. Interestingly, EW52 appeared to have a brief positive effect on the growth rate of MRSA252 for a period of 2 h when initially introduced to the wells, followed by a prolonged infection period in which MRSA252 appeared to increase in concentration momentarily, before eventually decreasing in bacterial density below the initial concentration after 15 h. For all three S. aureus isolates used, phages that were able to successfully reduce the optical density and prevent bacterial regrowth were able to achieve it within 8 h relative to controls. Nevertheless, there were a number of phages including EW15, EW27, EW29, and EW52 that exhibited a lower degree of bacteriolytic ability against their hosts, taking up to ~13 h

to have any inhibitory and bactericidal effect on the bacteria. Isolate 15981 rapidly evolved resistance to phages EW18 and EW52. However, phage EW52 was successful in reducing bacterial density eventually, whereas phage EW18, moderately reduced growth of 15981 but elicited resistant mutants. Strain 15981 was found to be the most resistant to phage infection killing in this assay. Reductions to growth were at a much lower rate compared to other hosts and the appearance of phage-resistance was observed in each experiment. Phage EW41 was the most effective at inhibiting the growth of all three S. aureus isolates, decreasing cell densities rapidly, within 2 h following phage application. However, as EW41 was isolated and propagated on D329 because it could not be propagated on TM300H, it is not surprising that it had little or no effect on TM300H in this assay.

S. aureus Biofilms

The two most common MRSA lineages in the UK have MLST sequence types (ST) 22 and 36 and these currently have global distributions (Holden et al., 2004; Holden et al., 2013). We selected isolates from these lineages to examine their biofilm forming properties and susceptibility to phages as these genotypes are the most common in our collection. We compared the biofilm densities produced by 43 ST22, and 27 ST36 isolates after 48 h by measurement of absorbance at OD_{590}

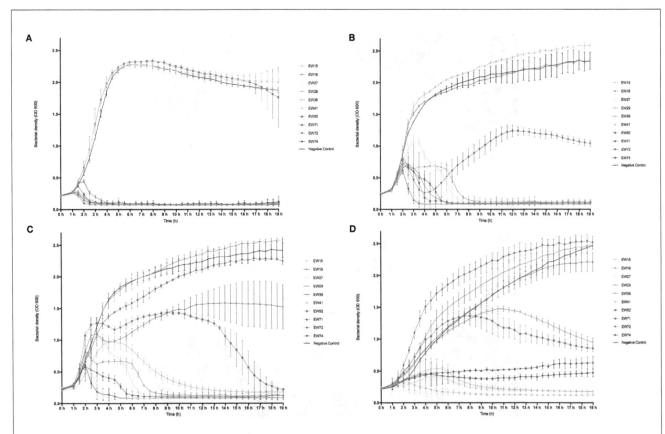

FIGURE 2 | Time-kill curve of four mid-exponential phase planktonic S. aureus strains by ten different phages at a multiplicity of infection (MOI) of 0.1. Absorbance readings at 600 nm were taken using a plate reader every 30 min for 19 h while shaking at 37°C, three independent experiments were performed in total. **(A)** Modified S. carnosus isolate TM300H; **(B)** S. aureus isolate D329, **(C)** S. aureus isolate MRSA252, and **(D)** S. aureus isolate 15981.

following CV staining. We found considerable variation within isolates of these genotypes (**Supplementary Figure 1**) with an obvious dichotomy between relatively little biofilm produced by most ST22 isolates compared to those of ST36. This can be seen by visual inspection of stained biofilms from the four most proficient biofilm producing isolates from each ST with ST36 isolate biofilms being generally darker stained than those of ST22 (**Supplementary Figure 2**).

We used the same ST22 isolates; ARI10, WW44936, 1018.07, and HO5322054809 and ST36 isolates; 07.1696.F, 06.9570.L, 07.1227.Z, and 07.2880.V (see **Table 1** for details on isolates) to examine the relationship between biofilm biomass and viable cell count. We compared OD_{590} readings of CV-stained 48 h mature biofilms for these eight isolates and compared these to viable cell counts. **Supplementary Figure 3** shows that the variation in biofilm biomass between strongest and weakest biofilm formers does not necessarily correlate to the number of viable cells present. All isolates had approximately similar numbers of cells in their biofilms but there was markedly greater variation within OD_{590} readings for some isolates. ST22 isolates ARI10 and WW936 produced significantly more CV-stained biofilm than 1018.07 and 370.07 and similarly for ST36 isolates 07.1696.F and 06.9570.L produced much more CV-stained biofilm than the other two isolates of this genotype.

ST22 strains displayed a propensity to form moderately adhered biofilms that had significantly lower ODs than the best ST36 biofilm formers, yet they had consistently higher cell counts — similar to those values observed from ST36 isolates. The biofilms produced by *S. aureus* were found at the air-biofilm interface and as large aggregates at the solid-liquid interface at the base of microtiter plate wells.

Effect of Phages on 48 h Biofilms

We selected four phages (EW27, EW36, EW41, and EW71) for analysis of biofilm reduction on the basis of; i) their broad host range against study isolates (**Table 2**) and ii) rapidly lytic characteristics in planktonic culture and observed lack of resistant-mutant selection (**Figure 2**). Each of these four phages was added to 48 h biofilms at an MOI of 0.1 or 1.0 and viable cell counts and OD_{600} readings of CV-stained biofilms were performed after 6 and 24 h following phage application. Biofilm readings for each phage and corresponding viable cell counts are presented in **Supplementary Figures 4–7** and biofilm readings summarized in **Table 3**.

EW27

Viable cell counts recovered from each EW27 phage-treated biofilm for all ST22 and ST36 isolates except for isolate 07.2496.L, were significantly reduced ($p < 0.001$) following a 6-h exposure to EW27 when compared to untreated biofilm controls (**Table 3** and **Supplementary Figure 4**). However, following an initial decrease in CFU/ml after 6 h, an increase in bacterial concentration can be seen across all phage-treated ST22 isolates after 24 h, suggesting that resistance to phage had occurred within that time. There was no significant difference

between CFU counts from wells treated with phage for 6 and 24 h ($p < 0.05$). When considering the overall biofilm biomass following phage exposure and CV staining, results revealed phage EW27 was highly effective at reducing the biofilms produced by all ST22 and ST36 strains. For EW27 treated ST36 isolates, biofilm biomass significantly increased in isolates 07.1696.F, 06.9570.L, and BTN 2172 using both MOI 1 and 0.1 ($p < 0.05$), despite a minor reduction in bacterial numbers after 24-h treatments compared to 6 h. Following treatment of EW27 after both timepoints, EW27 at a MOI of 0.1 proved to be the most effective at both reducing bacterial cells and biofilm biomass for almost all ST22 and ST36 strains.

EW36

Phage EW36 produced significant reductions in biofilm biomass for all study isolates except for 07.2496.L at both MOIs ($p < 0.01$), with MOI 0.1 proving to be most effective (**Table 3** and **Supplementary Figure 5**). For both ST22 and ST36, no increase to biofilm density was observed from 6 to 24 h, suggesting that phage EW36 successfully disrupted biofilms preventing regrowth. This is further supported by the greater reduction in viable cell counts when biofilms were treated for 24 h. Interestingly, the populations of viable bacteria recovered from each biofilm produced by the four ST22 and ST36 isolates were found to be higher in wells treated by phage EW36 at MOI 0.1, despite producing lower absorbance readings than biofilms treated with a higher titer of phage at a MOI 1. EW36 was able to reduce viable cell numbers for both ST22 and ST36 isolates by at least one-log after 6 h and two-logs after 24 h at an MOI 0.1. With biofilms treated at an MOI 1, two-log reductions were observed after 6 h and three-log reductions after 24 h.

EW41

Significant reductions ($p < 0.01$) in biofilm biomass were observed for all ST22 and ST36 isolates tested with phage EW41 except for isolate 370.07 where two-log reductions in cells recovered and 60% to 93% reductions in biofilm biomass were observed after 6 h treatment (**Table 3** and **Supplementary Figure 6**). Interestingly, phage EW41 had the least effect in reducing biofilm biomass of isolate W449 36 after 6 h — reducing it by roughly 22% at an MOI 1 and 19% at an MOI 0.1; however, viable cell counts were relative to all other isolates and two-log reductions were observed across both time points. Furthermore, biofilm biomass and viable cell counts recovered from the biofilms challenged with EW41 after 24 h produced levels similar to 6 h exposure. Phage EW41 was able to further reduce biofilm levels of W449 36 by ~85% when exposed for 24 h. ST36 biofilms challenged with phage EW41 for 24 h produced higher levels of biofilm biomass and increase in cells recovered by up to one-log when compared to 6 h exposure, suggesting regrowth had occurred within that time. Across all ST22 and ST36 isolates, both biofilm biomass and viable cells recovered were consistently lower in wells challenged with EW41 at an MOI 0.1 when compared with MOI 1, although this was not significant.

TABLE 3 | Summary table showing the relative difference in biofilm reduction of study phage at two multiplicities of infection (MOI) against four ST22 and four ST36 isolates.

	ST22	OD590	MOI 1	EW27MOI 0.1	MOI 1	EW36MOI 0.1	MOI 1	EW41MOI 0.1	MOI 1	EW71MOI 0.1
	ARI 10	1.2034	-44%	-61%	-47%	-63%	-80%	-85%	-84%	-87%
6 h	W449 36	1.1929	-71%	-78%	-77%	-78%	-22%	-19%	-75%	-68%
	1018.07	0.5941	-59%	-74%	-58%	-72%	-59%	-70%	-67%	-73%
	370.07	0.4381	-43%	-68%	-52%	-63%	-43%	-69%	-63%	-76%
	ARI 10	1.2034	-58%	-55%	-81%	-82%	-82%	-83%	-87%	-86%
24 h	W449 36	1.1929	-68%	-77%	-82%	-85%	-85%	-86%	-84%	-84%
	1018.07	0.5941	-20%	-49%	-68%	-69%	-69%	-70%	-76%	-74%
	370.07	0.4381	-25%	-43%	-59%	-68%	-63%	-66%	-78%	-75%
	ST36	OD590	MOI 1	EW27MOI 0.1	MOI 1	EW36MOI 0.1	MOI 1	EW41MOI 0.1	MOI 1	EW71MOI 0.1
	07.1696.F	3.0191	-89%	-89%	-79%	-79%	-90%	-86%	-95%	-95%
6 h	06.9570.L	2.7274	-75%	-60%	-81%	-80%	-71%	-74%	-91%	-92%
	BTN 2172	1.0997	-74%	-72%	-76%	-73%	-86%	-85%	-83%	-83%
	07.2496.L	0.7536	-64%	-69%	-20%	-29%	-70%	-70%	-81%	-79%
	07.1696.F	3.0191	-77%	-80%	-88%	-90%	-86%	-89%	-89%	-95%
24 h	06.9570.L	2.7274	-25%	-51%	-89%	-90%	-59%	-84%	-90%	-92%
	BTN 2172	1.0997	-30%	-57%	-73%	-78%	-83%	-68%	-77%	-83%
	07.2496.L	0.7536	-40%	-66%	-56%	-60%	-36%	-66%	-59%	-79%

48 h biofilms were challenged with phage for 6 and 24 h, percentages are based on control values.
Colour used to indicate different treatments.

EW71

Phage EW71 was the most effective of the four in reducing biofilm density and viable cell numbers (**Table 3** and **Supplementary Figure 7**). Phage EW71 was effective at reducing ($p < 0.01$) biofilm biomass after 6 h treatment while greatly limiting the amount of regrowth after 24 h. Furthermore, phage EW71 was successful in reducing the number of viable cells by up to three-logs after 6 h, and continued to reduce after 24 h treatment by up to four logs versus controls. Biofilm densities of ST22 following treatment of EW71 after 6 h ranged from 63% to 87% while consequently preventing the regrowth of all four ST22 hosts after 24 h, further reducing biofilm densities. Greater reductions in biofilm densities were also observed when ST36 isolates were challenged with phage EW71 with OD_{590} values reduced by 59 95% after 6 h. Interestingly, a marginal increase in absorbance was observed in across all four ST36 biofilms when exposed to phage for 24 h. However, increases to viable cell counts were only observed for 07.1696.F and 07.2496.L suggesting phage resistance and regrowth had occurred within the two sampling periods. Phage applied to biofilms at an MOI 1 were found to be the most effective at reducing viable cell counts within the biofilm after 6 and 24 h exposures; however, biofilm densities were somewhat higher with this MOI. Even so, biofilm biomasses were approximately similar across the majority of hosts for both 6- and 24-h treatments, except for isolate W449 36; however, this difference was not significant.

Evaluation of Phage Biofilm Assays

Table 3 and **Supplementary Figures 4–7** show the percentage reduction of *S. aureus* ST22 and ST36 isolate biofilms when challenged by EW27, EW36, EW41, and EW71 at MOIs of 1 and 0.1 after 6 and 24 h. For all ST22 isolates the median reduction in biofilm biomass for MOI 1 and MOI 0.1 after 6 h was 59% and

71% respectively, whereas the median reduction for MOI 1 and MOI 0.1 after 24 h exposure was 72% and 75%, respectively. Whereas, for ST36 isolates, the median biofilm biomass reduction for MOI 1 and MOI 0.1 after 6 h was 80% and 79%, respectively. After 24 h treatment, the median reduction for MOI 1 and MOI 0.1 for ST36 isolates was 75% and 80%, respectively.

Overall, the highest biofilm biomass reductions after 6 and 24 h phage treatments was observed with phages EW41 and EW71 respectively, with an MOI of 0.1. Although significant reductions in biofilm biomass was observed when treated with both MOIs of phage, the greatest reductions across all ST22 and ST36 isolates after 6 and 24 h exposure was achieved when biofilms were treated at an MOI 0.1. Although each phage was able to disperse the biofilms of all study isolates, complete elimination of cells was not observed across any of the hosts at either MOI as cells were recoverable when treated with phages for 6 h and 24 h.

Phage-Resistant Mutants

The morphology of colonies recovered from phage-treated biofilms were heterogeneous and this was most marked for isolates treated with phage EW71 as shown in **Figure 3**. Phage-resistant mutant isolates recovered from each phage experiment were found to be resistant to all phage upon spot testing on agar overlays.

Genomics

We sequenced the genomes of 22 phages with broad host range based upon spot testing results (**Table 2**). All are *Myoviruses* and members of the *Twortvirinae* sub-family of the family *Herelleviridae* based on BLASTN similarity. To further investigate the relatedness and taxonomy of our phages we compared their genomes to the 100 publicly available *Twortvirinae* genomes in Genbank (as of April 2021) using the min-hash algorithm implemented in MASH (Ondov et al., 2016) to generate distance matrices that were used to construct the neighbor-joining dendrograms shown in **Figure 4**. The 22-phage genomes segregated into three main groups, designated 1 3.

Group 1

This group contains five phages EW15, EW20, EW22, EW27, and EW41 (shown in red in **Figure 4**). They share very high similarity (MASH distances < 1%) with each other, except for phage EW41 that differs by 1.6% (**Supplementary Table 1**). It also has a slightly smaller genome of 132,999 bp compared to the others which are c.135,800 bp in size. These phages are very similar to, and cluster with 11 staphylococcal phages of the genus *Silviavirus* (**Figure 4B**). They include the broad host-range phages Romulus and Remus, proposed as an ideal candidate phages for human therapy due to their broad host-range and virulence (Vandersteegen et al., 2013).

Group 2

The largest group in this study contains 11 phages of the genus *Kayvirus* based on genomic sequence similarity, with genomes that share >95% similarity (*i.e.* < 5% MASH distance) with each other (**Figure 4** and **Supplementary Table 1**). It contains three subgroups A, B, and C, and these are colored green in **Figure 4**. Group 2A contains phages EW36 and EW42 that are 139,881 and 139,874 bp in length, respectively. Group 2B is made up of phages EW1, EW2, EW4 that are very similar (>99%) to each other and EW13 that differs from these by about 1.8% of bases The first three phages have genomes that are 140,906 bp long, about 4 kb shorter than that of EW13 at 145,736 bp. Group 2C comprises phages EW3, EW5, EW6, EW7, and EW9 with genomes of between 141,953 and 143,288 bp. Their genomes are >99.5% similarity to each other. Group 2 phages form a distinct clade on their own in the dendrogram in **Figure 4B** and are most closely related to genomes belonging to phages of the

genus *Kayvirus* that include the species "Staphylococcus phage MCE-2014" (Alves et al., 2014) and several unclassified Kayviruses, sharing c.90% sequence similarity. Phage MCE-2014 (also known as DRA88) was first reported in a study where it was used in combination with phage K to treat experimental *S. aureus* biofilms. The phage K mutant of strain MRSA252 used here was derived from this study (**Table 1**).

Group 3

This group contains two closely related subgroups pf phages whose genomes differ by c.3%. The four group 3A phages in this group are EW18, EW26, EW29, and EW72 with genomes of 143, 240 to 143,287 bp that are > 99.5% similar to each other. These cluster most closely with database isolates of the genus *Kayvirus* that include the species phiPLA-Rodi whose reference phage, phiPLA-RODI, has been used in several studies, including those involving *S. aureus* biofilms (Gutierrez et al., 2015; Gonzalez et al., 2017). The genomes of group 3B phages EW71 and EW74 are 139,939 and 139,896 bp in length respectively, and they share >99% sequence similarity with each other and with the genomes of three phages in Genbank from the genus *Kayvirus*. These include phage K (Gill, 2014), the most well known of the staphylococcal phages (**Figure 4B**) that is commonly included in staphylococcal phage preparations (O'Flaherty et al., 2005b).

Overall, the genomes of *Silviavirus* phages of group 1 share about 25% to 26% DNA sequence similarity to those of group 2 and group 3 *Kayvirus* phages. Groups 2 and 3 are more similar with approximately 90% DNA similarity using min-hash distances (**Supplementary Table 1**). **Supplementary Table 2** lists all annotated genes in the 122 *Twortvirinae* studied and shows their presence absence (BLASTP identity > 95%). Group 1 phages had no genes in common with those of groups 2 and 3 using Roary with default parameters. Groups 2 and 3 shared 38 genes common at BLASTP identity > 95% (18% of the 202 genes in the EW1 genome). No known function could be assigned to 33

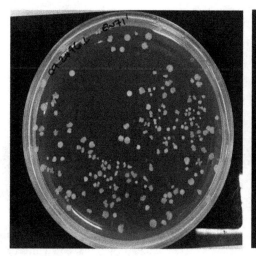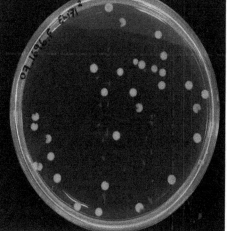

FIGURE 3 | Heterogeneous colony phenotypes produced by *S. aureus* phage-resistant mutants of 07.2496.L and 07.1696.F following exposure to EW71.

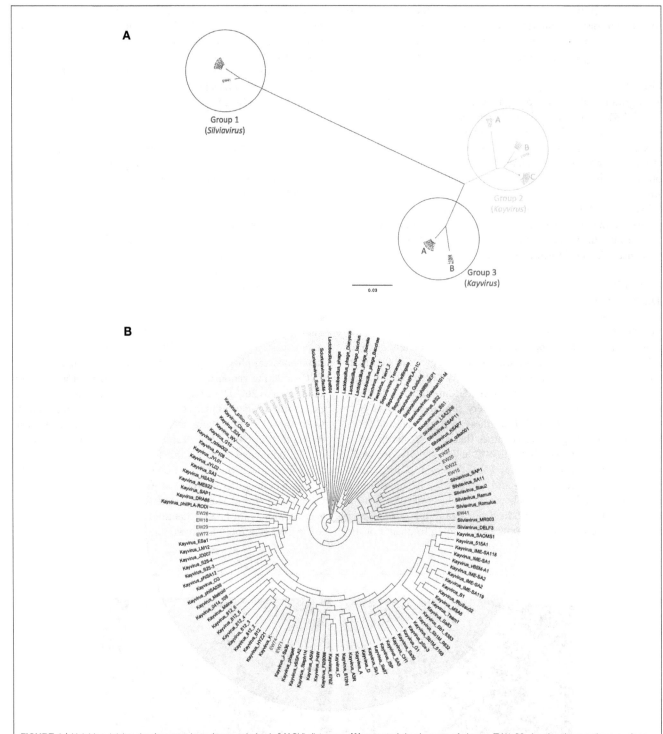

FIGURE 4 | Neighbor-joining dendrograms based upon min-hash (MASH) distances. **(A)** unrooted dendrogram of phages EW1-22 showing three major groupings and subgroupings. **(B)** Circular dendrogram showing the relatedness of the same phages in relation to 100 *Twortvirinae* genome assemblies and the phage genera they represent. Dendrogram is rooted at the midpoint of the longest branch.

but the core genes comprised a terminase gene, an intron-encoded endonuclease, a LysM domain-containing protein, a putative DNA repair protein, and a virion component protein.

The host range of group 1 phages as measured by percentage of strains able to be infected (coverage) varied from 61.62%

to 97.3%. In group 2 this coverage varied from 56.76% to 96.76% and in group 3 from 96.22% to 99.46% (**Table 2**). All three groups therefore had phages that could infect the great majority, if not all 184 clinical isolates, but not the phage K mutant MRSA252 strain.

DISCUSSION

Phage therapy has potential for the treatment of many bacterial diseases, but for most bacterial pathogens, the limited host range of lytic phages means that empiric use requires the use of cocktails of different phage strains with varying host ranges and virulence characteristics. Broad host range, highly virulent S. aureus phages are relatively easy to isolate, and their use in phage therapy, especially in Georgia and Poland, has been associated with a high degree of success. This study confirms reports of the extremely broad host range of some Myoviridae, especially some of the Kayviruses and Silviaviruses characterized here. Two of these Kayviruses, EW70 and EW71, were able to infect the complete panel of our genetically diverse 185 S. aureus isolates in agar overlays that included a very wide range of MRSA and MSSA genotypes. Nine other phages could infect >96% of isolates, and these comprised three Silviaviruses, two Kayviruses of a different clade from EW70 and EW71, as well as four others that are closely related to EW70 and EW71. The broad host range of S. aureus Myoviruses is in part explained by their sharing a common receptor that has been found to be the backbone of cell wall teichoic acids (Xia et al., 2011; Winstel et al., 2013).

In our planktonic assays, all 10 phages were able to infect at least one of the four S. aureus isolates tested, and five were able to infect and significantly reduce the growth of two. EW41 was found to be the most effective under planktonic conditions, as it immediately reduced bacterial cell numbers preventing the regrowth of all three S. aureus isolates, yet it had no effect on the modified S. carnosus isolate. As it was propagated on S. aureus strain D239 host, its specificity may be more limited compared to other phages in infecting coagulase-negative staphylococci. Four phages had no effect on the growth of at least one of the three S. aureus hosts in liquid culture. However, phages that were effective were able to prevent the appearance of resistant mutants throughout the duration of the experiment. When resistance mutants were observed, the growth rate and presumably, fitness of these phage-resistant cells was clearly affected and did not recover to the levels achieved by uninfected controls. This suggests that resistance to phage infection was at the expense of growth capacity (Middelboe, 2000; Avrani and Lindell, 2015). Emergence of spontaneous phage resistance can involve selection of sub-populations with altered receptor structures that in S. aureus includes wall techoic acid (Hall et al., 2011; Xia et al., 2011; Avrani and Lindell, 2015). Fitness costs associated when acquiring phage-resistance, can cause a variety of structural and morphological changes (Inal, 2003; Ormala and Jalasvuori, 2013). One approach is concealing surface receptors that phages used as docking sites to adsorb to their hosts; however, these sites are often used for the uptake of nutrients (Mizoguchi et al., 2003), thus possibly limiting their growth and virulence which may be why cell numbers were able to recover after 24 h treatment compared with 6 h, yet biofilm densities remained considerably low.

When applied at low concentrations (MOI 0.1), phage must infect and replicate enough to increase their number to surpass the rate of replication for the bacterial host. This would explain why most host isolates continued to grow for at least 1 h following introduction. In similar studies comparing phage infection at various MOIs (Abedon, 1992; Beeton et al., 2015; Cui et al., 2017a), the greater the MOI the more effective the phage was in the study, which presumably is largely because of the increased rate of phage collisions and infections, thus leading to higher densities in viral progeny in a shorter time frame.

The four S. aureus phages used in biofilm studies were selected based on their lytic potential in spot plate assays and in liquid culture. All four exhibited generally high efficacy in effectively reducing biofilm biomass and cell numbers of each S. aureus isolate after 6 and 24 h. Cell regrowth was detected following 24 h infection with phage compared to 6 h by at least one of the hosts suggesting growth of phage-resistant mutants had occurred, however this was at the expense of biofilm regrowth. These observations were similar to those reported in a previous study of S. aureus biofilm (Melo et al., 2018). The observation of biofilm regrowth and phage resistance still remains a major issue and is something regularly observed in biofilms when challenged by single lytic phage that promotes mutant selection (Drilling et al., 2014). This necessitates a phage combination approach using phage cocktails or co-administration with antibiotics to prevent the emergence of phage-resistant mutant bacteria. Previous studies have made use of the disruptive ability of phage to reduce biofilm structures produced by S. aureus and reduce bacterial populations enough to facilitate the penetration of antibiotics and eradicate infection (Tkhilaishvili et al., 2018; Dickey and Perrot, 2019). Previous evidence suggests that the phage resistance phenotype increases sensitivity to antibiotics and also results in a loss of fitness (Leon and Bastias, 2015). Additionally, the application of phage cocktails consisting of multiple polyvalent phage that target different receptor proteins to prevent multi-resistance, but also increase the rate of killing, thus greatly reducing the probability of hosts acquiring resistance to phage (Gu et al., 2012). The anti-biofilm capabilities and broad host range demonstrated by the four study phage make them promising candidates for possible future combination studies.

Previous phage/host studies have demonstrated that by increasing the concentration of phage-to-bacteria (MOI), which, essentially increases the rate of collisions between phage and biofilm cells leads to increased rate of bacterial killing (Gupta and Prasad, 2011; Lopes et al., 2018). Additionally, greater reductions could have been facilitated by direct bacterial lysis the lysis from without effect. However there was no significant difference between MOI values, suggesting that an increased phage-to-bacteria ratio offered no advantages in reducing biofilm biomass, as described previously (Lopes et al., 2018). Overall, reductions in biofilm biomass (OD_{590}) were generally higher in biofilms treated at an MOI 0.1 (compared to 1) using any of the four phage after both 6 and 24 h treatments. The effectiveness of the low MOI demonstrates the self-perpetuating nature of lytic phage to proliferate in number, therefore only requiring small initial dosing.

Compared to the characteristic smooth, round colonies phenotypes typically produced by S. aureus, the recovery of heterogenous morphotypes produced by phage-resistant derivatives following phage exposure were regularly detected during this study, although most commonly observed in biofilms treated with EW71. Similar irregular-shaped colonies have been reported in previous studies and are thought to be caused by a subpopulation within a colony that has reverted back to a phage-sensitive phenotype, subsequently leading to cell death as the colony forms (Mizoguchi et al., 2003; O'Flynn et al., 2007; Kocharunchitt et al., 2009). However, the observation of "pacman"-like colonies, as seen here, has not been as well documented and warrants further investigation.

A major consideration in producing phages for human therapy is the possible presence of induced prophage from propagating host bacteria. *S. aureus* isolates typically harbor several prophages in their genomes and these mediate horizontal gene transfer and contain virulence genes such as toxins (Xia and Wolz, 2014). In this study, we found that most phages could be propagated on an avirulent *S. carnosus* strain that could be used to increase the safety of staphylococcal phage therapeutics in future GMP manufacturing if used in place of potentially virulent *S. aureus* hosts.

AUTHOR CONTRIBUTIONS

ME conceived this study. ME, EW, JR, GX, AM, RR, and SM designed experimental procedures. EW, ME, JR, SM, and RR performed the experiments, analyzed and curated the data. EW and ME assembled the phage collection. ME, EW, JR, AM, and GX wrote the manuscript. All authors contributed to the article and approved the submitted version.

ACKNOWLEDGMENTS

We acknowledge expert microbiology support from the 4th floor technical team at Manchester Metropolitan University. We thank Phil Jones at United Utilities for his invaluable help.

SUPPLEMENTARY MATERIAL

Supplementary Figure 1 | Biofilm formation of **(A)** 43 *S. aureus* ST22; and **(B)** 27 ST36 isolates grown in tissue culture microtiter plates over 48 h at 37°C. Biofilms densities produced were assessed following crystal violet staining, dissolved in 30% acetic acid, and measured at an OD590. Each assay was performed in triplicate, data presented as mean values (± standard deviation).

Supplementary Figure 2 | Variation in biofilm production by ST22 **(A)** and ST36 **(B)** isolates after 48 h incubation in TSB supplemented with 1% D-(+)-glucose. Biofilms were visualized following staining with 0.1% crystal violet.

Supplementary Figure 3 | Comparison of biofilm densities of eight *S. aureus* isolates assessed by CV staining **(A)** and corresponding viable cell counts **(B)**.

Supplementary Figure 4 | Effect of phage EW27 on mature biofilms of S. aureus ST22 **(A)** and ST36 isolates **(B)**. Static biofilms were initially grown in tissue-culture microtiter plates for 48 hand challenged with EW36 at a multiplicity of infection of 1 and 0.1 for a period of 6 and 24 h. **(A)** Biofilms initially stained with crystal violet and optical density was measured at an absorbance of 590 nm. **(B)** Viable cells were recovered from phage treated wells by scratching and dislodging the biofilms from the surface plate wells and plated out in triplicate. Each assay was performed in triplicate, data presented as mean values (± standard deviation).

Supplementary Figure 5 | Effect of phage EW36 on mature biofilms of *S. aureus* ST22 **(A)** and ST36 isolates **(B)**. Static biofilms were initially grown in tissue-culture microtiter plates for 48 h and challenged with EW36 at a multiplicity of infection of 1 and 0.1 for a period of 6 and 24 h. Top Biofilms initially stained with crystal violet and optical density was measured at an absorbance of 590 nm. Bottom Viable cells were recovered from phage treated wells by scratching and dislodging the biofilms from the surface plate wells and plated out in triplicate. Each assay was performed in triplicate, data presented as mean values (± standard deviation).

Supplementary Figure 6 | Effect of phage EW41 on mature biofilms of *S. aureus* ST22 **(A)** and ST36 isolates **(B)**. Static biofilms were initially grown in tissue-culture microtiter plates for 48 h and challenged with EW36 at a multiplicity of infection of 1 and 0.1 for a period of 6 and 24 h. Top Biofilms initially stained with crystal violet and optical density was measured at an absorbance of 590 nm. Bottom Viable cells were recovered from phage treated wells by scratching and dislodging the biofilms from the surface plate wells and plated out in triplicate. Each assay was performed in triplicate, data presented as mean values (± standard deviation).

Supplementary Figure 7 | Effect of phage EW71 on mature biofilms of *S. aureus* ST22 **(A)** and ST36 isolates **(B)**. Static biofilms were initially grown in tissue-culture microtiter plates for 48 h and challenged with EW36 at a multiplicity of infection of 1 and 0.1 for a period of 6 and 24 h. Top Biofilms initially stained with crystal violet and optical density was measured at an absorbance of 590 nm. Bottom Viable cells were recovered from phage treated wells by scratching and dislodging the biofilms from the surface plate wells and plated out in triplicate. Each assay was performed in triplicate, data presented as mean values (± standard deviation).

Supplementary Table 1 | Min-hash distances of study phage genomes expressed as percent.

Supplementary Table 2 | Gene presence or absence in 122 study phage genomes (BLASTP>95%).4L2_Filename: fcimb.2021.698909_styled.docx

REFERENCES

Abedon, S. T. (1992). Lysis of Lysis-Inhibited Bacteriophage T4-Infected Cells. *J. Bacteriol.* 174 (24), 8073–8080. doi: 10.1128/jb.174.24.8073-8080.1992

Adriaenssens, E., and Brister, J. R. (2017). How to Name and Classify Your Phage: An Informal Guid. *Viruses* 9 (4), 1–9. doi: 10.3390/v9040070

Alves, D. R., Gaudion, A., Bean, J. E., Perez Esteban, P., Arnot, T. C., Harper, D. R., et al. (2014). Combined Use of Bacteriophage K and a Novel Bacteriophage to Reduce Staphylococcus Aureus Biofilm Formation. *Appl. Environ. Microbiol.* 80 (21), 6694–6703. doi: 10.1128/AEM.01789-14

Avrani, S., and Lindell, D. (2015). Convergent Evolution Toward an Improved Growth Rate and a Reduced Resistance Range in Prochlorococcus Strains Resistant to Phage. *Proc. Natl. Acad. Sci. U. S. A.* 112 (17), E2191–E2200. doi: 10.1073/pnas.1420347112

Bankevich, A., Nurk, S., Antipov, D., Gurevich, A. A., Dvorkin, M., Kulikov, A. S., et al. (2012). SPAdes: A New Genome Assembly Algorithm and Its Applications to Single-Cell Sequencing. *J. Comput. Biol.* 19 (5), 455–477. doi: 10.1089/cmb.2012.0021

Beeton, M. L., Alves, D. R., Enright, M. C., and Jenkins, A. T. (2015). Assessing Phage Therapy Against Pseudomonas Aeruginosa Using a Galleria Mellonella Infection Model. *Int. J. Antimicrob. Agents* 46 (2), 196–200. doi: 10.1016/j.ijantimicag.2015.04.005

Berryhill, B. A., Huseby, D. L., McCall, I. C., Hughes, D., and Levin, B. R. (2021). Evaluating the Potential Efficacy and Limitations of a Phage for Joint Antibiotic and Phage Therapy of Staphylococcus Aureus Infections. *Proc. Natl. Acad. Sci. U. S. A.* 118 (10), 1–8. doi: 10.1073/pnas.2008007118

Brandt, C. M., Duffy, M. C., Berbari, E. F., Hanssen, A. D., Steckelberg, J. M., and Osmon, D. R. (1999). Staphylococcus Aureus Prosthetic Joint Infection Treated With Prosthesis Removal and Delayed Reimplantation Arthroplasty. *Mayo. Clin. Proc.* 74 (6), 553–558. doi: 10.4065/74.6.553

Centers for Disease Control and Prevention (2002). Staphylococcus Aureus Resistant to Vancomycin–United States 2002. *MMWR Morb. Mortal. Wkly. Rep.* 51 (26), 565–567.

Chatterjee, S. S., and Otto, M. (2013). Improved Understanding of Factors Driving Methicillin-Resistant Staphylococcus Aureus Epidemic Waves. *Clin. Epidemiol.* 5, 205–217. doi: 10.2147/CLEP.S37071

Cui, Z., Feng, T., Gu, F., Li, Q., Dong, K., Zhang, Y., et al. (2017a). Characterization and Complete Genome of the Virulent Myoviridae Phage JD007 Active Against a Variety of Staphylococcus Aureus Isolates From Different Hospitals in Shanghai, Chin. Virol. J. 14 (1), 26. doi: 10.1186/s12985-017-0701-0

Cui, Z., Guo, X., Dong, K., Zhang, Y., Li, Q., Zhu, Y., et al. (2017b). Safety Assessment of Staphylococcus Phages of the Family Myoviridae Based on Complete Genome Sequences. Sci. Rep. 7, 41259. doi: 10.1038/srep41259

Dickey, J., and Perrot, V. (2019). Adjunct Phage Treatment Enhances the Effectiveness of Low Antibiotic Concentration Against Staphylococcus Aureus Biofilms In Vitro. PLoS One 14 (1), e0209390. doi: 10.1371/journal.pone.0209390

Drilling, A., Morales, S., Jardeleza, C., Vreugde, S., Speck, P., and Wormald, P. J. (2014). Bacteriophage Reduces Biofilm of Staphylococcus Aureus Ex Vivo Isolates From Chronic Rhinosinusitis Patients. Am. J. Rhinol. Allergy 28 (1), 3-11. doi: 10.2500/ajra.2014.28.4001

Enright, M. C., Day, N. P., Davies, C. E., Peacock, S. J., and Spratt, B. G. (2000). Multilocus Sequence Typing for Characterization of Methicillin-Resistant and Methicillin-Susceptible Clones of Staphylococcus Aureus. J. Clin. Microbiol. 38 (3), 1008-1015. doi: 10.1128/JCM.38.3.1008-1015.2000

Enright, M. C., Robinson, D. A., Randle, G., Feil, E. J., Grundmann, H., and Spratt, B. G. (2002). The Evolutionary History of Methicillin-Resistant Staphylococcus Aureus (MRS). Proc. Natl. Acad. Sci. U. S. A. 99 (11), 7687-7692. doi: 10.1073/pnas.122108599

Feil, E. J., Cooper, J. E., Grundmann, H., Robinson, D. A., Enright, M. C., Berendt, T., et al. (2003). How Clonal Is Staphylococcus Aureus? J. Bacteriol. 185 (11), 3307-3316. doi: 10.1128/JB.185.11.3307-3316.2003

Gill, J. J. (2014). Revised Genome Sequence of Staphylococcus Aureus Bacteriophage K. Genome Announc. 2 (1), e01173-13. doi: 10.1128/genomeA.01173-13

Gonzalez, S., Fernandez, L., Campelo, A. B., Gutierrez, D., Martinez, B., Rodriguez, A., et al. (2017). The Behavior of Staphylococcus Aureus Dual-Species Biofilms Treated With Bacteriophage phiIPLA-RODI Depends on the Accompanying Microorganis. Appl. Environ. Microbiol. 83 (3), e02821-16. doi: 10.1128/AEM.02821-16

Gu, J., Liu, X., Li, Y., Han, W., Lei, L., Yang, Y., et al. (2012). A Method for Generation Phage Cocktail With Great Therapeutic Potential. PLoS One 7 (3), e31698. doi: 10.1371/journal.pone.0031698

Gupta, R., and Prasad, Y. (2011). Efficacy of Polyvalent Bacteriophage P-27/HP to Control Multidrug Resistant Staphylococcus Aureus Associated With Human Infections. Curr. Microbiol. 62 (1), 255-260. doi: 10.1007/s00284-010-9699-x

Gutierrez, D., Vandenheuvel, D., Martinez, B., Rodriguez, A., Lavigne, R., and Garcia, P. (2015). Two Phages, phiIPLA-RODI and phiIPLA-C1C, Lyse Mono- and Dual-Species Staphylococcal Biofilm. Appl. Environ. Microbiol. 81 (10), 3336-3348. doi: 10.1128/AEM.03560-14

Hall, A. R., Scanlan, P. D., and Buckling, A. (2011). Bacteria-Phage Coevolution and the Emergence of Generalist Pathogens. Am. Nat. 177 (1), 44-53. doi: 10.1086/657441

Holden, M. T., Feil, E. J., Lindsay, J. A., Peacock, S. J., Day, N. P., Enright, M. C., et al. (2004). Complete Genomes of Two Clinical Staphylococcus Aureus Strains: Evidence for the Rapid Evolution of Virulence and Drug Resistance. Proc. Natl. Acad. Sci. U. S. A. 101 (26), 9786-9791. doi: 10.1073/pnas.0402521101

Holden, M. T., Hsu, L. Y., Kurt, K., Weinert, L. A., Mather, A. E., Harris, S. R., et al. (2013). A Genomic Portrait of the Emergence, Evolution, and Global Spread of a Methicillin-Resistant Staphylococcus Aureus Pandemic. Genome Res. 23 (4), 653-664. doi: 10.1101/gr.147710.112

Inal, J. M. (2003). Phage Therapy: A Reappraisal of Bacteriophages as Antibiotics. Arch. Immunol. Ther. Exp. (Warsz). 51 (4), 237-244.

Katz, L. S., Griswold, T., Morrison, S. S., Caravas, J. A., Zhang, S., den Bakker, H., et al. (2019). Mashtree: A Rapid Comparison of Whole Genome Sequence Files. J. Open Source Softw. 4 (44), 1-6. doi: 10.21105/joss.01762

Kocharunchitt, C., Ross, T., and McNeil, D. L. (2009). Use of Bacteriophages as Biocontrol Agents to Control Salmonella Associated With Seed Sprouts. Int. J. Food Microbiol. 128 (3), 453-459. doi: 10.1016/j.ijfoodmicro.2008.10.014

Kropinski, A. M., Mazzocco, A., Waddell, T. E., Lingohr, E., and Johnson, R. P. (2009). Enumeration of Bacteriophages by Double Agar Overlay Plaque Assay. Methods Mol. Biol. 501, 69-76. doi: 10.1007/978-1-60327-164-6_7

Kutter, E., De Vos, D., Gvasalia, G., Alavidze, Z., Gogokhia, L., Kuhl, S., et al. (2010). Phage Therapy in Clinical Practice: Treatment of Human Infections. Curr. Pharm. Biotechnol. 11 (1), 69-86. doi: 10.2174/138920110790725401

Leon, M., and Bastias, R. (2015). Virulence Reduction in Bacteriophage Resistant Bacteria. Front. Microbiol. 6, 343. doi: 10.3389/fmicb.2015.00343

Lobocka, M., Hejnowicz, M. S., Dabrowski, K., Gozdek, A., Kosakowski, J., Witkowska, M., et al. (2012). Genomics of Staphylococcal Twort-Like Phages–Potential Therapeutics of the Post-Antibiotic Era. Adv. Virus Res. 83, 143-216. doi: 10.1016/B978-0-12-394438-2.00005-0

Lopes, A., Pereira, C., and Almeida, A. (2018). Sequential Combined Effect of Phages and Antibiotics on the Inactivation of Escherichia Coli. Microorganisms 6 (4), 1-20. doi: 10.3390/microorganisms6040125

Lowy, F. D. (1998). Staphylococcus Aureus Infections. N. Engl. J. Med. 339 (8), 520-532. doi: 10.1056/NEJM199808203390806

McCallin, S., Sarker, S. A., Sultana, S., Oechslin, F., and Brussow, H. (2018). Metagenome Analysis of Russian and Georgian Pyophage Cocktails and a Placebo-Controlled Safety Trial of Single Phage Versus Phage Cocktail in Healthy Staphylococcus Aureus Carriers. Environ. Microbiol. 20 (9), 3278-3293. doi: 10.1111/1462-2920.14310

Melo, L. D. R., Brandao, A., Akturk, E., Santos, S. B., and Azeredo, J. (2018). Characterization of a New Staphylococcus Aureus Kayvirus Harboring a Lysin Active Against Biofilm. Viruses 10 (4), 1-16. doi: 10.3390/v10040182

Michniewski, S., Redgwell, T., Grigonyte, A., Rihtman, B., Aguilo-Ferretjans, M., Christie-Oleza, J., et al. (2019). Riding the Wave of Genomics to Investigate Aquatic Coliphage Diversity and Activity. Environ. Microbiol. 21 (6), 2112-2128. doi: 10.1111/1462-2920.14590

Middelboe, M. (2000). Bacterial Growth Rate and Marine Virus-Host Dynamic. Microb. Ecol. 40 (2), 114-124. doi: 10.1007/s002480000050

Mizoguchi, K., Morita, M., Fischer, C. R., Yoichi, M., Tanji, Y., and Unno, H. (2003). Coevolution of Bacteriophage PP01 and Escherichia Coli O157:H7 in Continuous Culture. Appl. Environ. Microbiol. 69 (1), 170-176. doi: 10.1128/AEM.69.1.170-176.2003

O'Flaherty, S., Coffey, A., Meaney, W., Fitzgerald, G. F., and Ross, R. P. (2005a). The Recombinant Phage Lysin LysK has a Broad Spectrum of Lytic Activity Against Clinically Relevant Staphylococci, Including Methicillin-Resistant Staphylococcus Aureus. J. Bacteriol. 187 (20), 7161-7164. doi: 10.1128/JB.187.20.7161-7164.2005

O'Flaherty, S., Ross, R. P., and Coffey, A. (2009). Bacteriophage and Their Lysins for Elimination of Infectious Bacteria. FEMS Microbiol. Rev. 33 (4), 801-819. doi: 10.1111/j.1574-6976.2009.00176.x

O'Flaherty, S., Ross, R. P., Meaney, W., Fitzgerald, G. F., Elbreki, M. F., and Coffey, A. (2005b). Potential of the Polyvalent Anti-Staphylococcus Bacteriophage K for Control of Antibiotic-Resistant Staphylococci From Hospitals. Appl. Environ. Microbiol. 71 (4), 1836-1842. doi: 10.1128/AEM.71.4.1836-1842.2005

O'Flynn, G., Coffey, A., Fitzgerald, G., and Ross, R. P. (2007). Salmonella Enterica Phage-Resistant Mutant Colonies Display an Unusual Phenotype in the Presence of Phage Felix 01. Lett. Appl. Microbiol. 45 (6), 581-585. doi: 10.1111/j.1472-765X.2007.02242.x

Ondov, B. D., Treangen, T. J., Melsted, P., Mallonee, A. B., Bergman, N. H., Koren, S., et al. (2016). Mash: Fast Genome and Metagenome Distance Estimation Using MinHas. Genome Biol. 17 (1), 132. doi: 10.1186/s13059-016-0997-x

Ormala, A. M., and Jalasvuori, M. (2013). Phage Therapy: Should Bacterial Resistance to Phages Be a Concern, Even in the Long Run? Bacteriophage 3 (1), e24219. doi: 10.4161/bact.24219

Page, A. J., Cummins, C. A., Hunt, M., Wong, V. K., Reuter, S., Holden, M. T. G., et al. (2015). Roary: Rapid Large-Scale Prokaryote Pan Genome Analysis. Bioinformatics 31 (22), 3691-3693. doi: 10.1093/bioinformatics/btv421

Petrovic Fabijan, A., Lin, R. C. Y., Ho, J., Maddocks, S., Ben Zakour, N. L., Iredell, J. R., et al. (2020). Safety of Bacteriophage Therapy in Severe Staphylococcus Aureus Infection. Nat. Microbiol. 5 (3), 465-472. doi: 10.1038/s41564-019-0634-z

Rhoads, D. D., Wolcott, R. D., Kuskowski, M. A., Wolcott, B. M., Ward, L. S., and Sulakvelidze, A. (2009). Bacteriophage Therapy of Venous Leg Ulcers in Humans: Results of a Phase I Safety Trial. J. Wound Care 18 (6), 237-238, 240-233. doi: 10.12968/jowc.2009.18.6.42801

Rosenstein, R., Nerz, C., Biswas, L., Resch, A., Raddatz, G., Schuster, S. C., et al. (2009). Genome Analysis of the Meat Starter Culture Bacterium Staphylococcus Carnosus TM300. Appl. Environ. Microbiol. 75 (3), 811-822. doi: 10.1128/AEM.01982-08

Rutherford, K., Parkhill, J., Crook, J., Horsnell, T., Rice, P., Rajandream, M. A., et al. (2000). Artemis: Sequence Visualization and Annotation. *Bioinformatics* 16 (10), 944–945. doi: 10.1093/bioinformatics/16.10.944

Seemann, T. (2014). Prokka: Rapid Prokaryotic Genome Annotation. *Bioinformatics* 30 (14), 2068–2069. doi: 10.1093/bioinformatics/btu153

Skiest, D. J. (2006). Treatment Failure Resulting From Resistance of Staphylococcus Aureus to Daptomycin. *J. Clin. Microbiol.* 44 (2), 655–656. doi: 10.1128/JCM.44.2.655-656.2006

Skurnik, M., Pajunen, M., and Kiljunen, S. (2007). Biotechnological Challenges of Phage Therapy. *Biotechnol. Lett.* 29 (7), 995–1003. doi: 10.1007/s10529-007-9346-1

Summers, W. C. (2001). Bacteriophage Therapy. *Annu. Rev. Microbiol.* 55, 437–451. doi: 10.1146/annurev.micro.55.1.437

Synnott, A. J., Kuang, Y., Kurimoto, M., Yamamichi, K., Iwano, H., and Tanji, Y. (2009). Isolation From Sewage Influent and Characterization of Novel Staphylococcus Aureus Bacteriophages With Wide Host Ranges and Potent Lytic Capabilities. *Appl. Environ. Microbiol.* 75 (13), 4483–4490. doi: 10.1128/AEM.02641-08

Tkhilaishvili, T., Lombardi, L., Klatt, A. B., Trampuz, A., and Di Luca, M. (2018). Bacteriophage Sb-1 Enhances Antibiotic Activity Against Biofilm, Degrades Exopolysaccharide Matrix and Targets Persisters of Staphylococcus Aureus. *Int. J. Antimicrob. Agents* 52 (6), 842–853. doi: 10.1016/j.ijantimicag.2018.09.006

Toledo-Arana, A., Merino, N., Vergara-Irigaray, M., Debarbouille, M., Penades, J. R., and Lasa, I. (2005). Staphylococcus Aureus Develops an Alternative, Ica-Independent Biofilm in the Absence of the arlRS Two-Component System. *J. Bacteriol.* 187 (15), 5318–5329. doi: 10.1128/JB.187.15.5318-5329.2005

Tsiodras, S., Gold, H. S., Sakoulas, G., Eliopoulos, G. M., Wennersten, C., Venkataraman, L., et al. (2001). Linezolid Resistance in a Clinical Isolate of Staphylococcus Aureus. *Lancet* 358 (9277), 207–208. doi: 10.1016/S0140-6736(01)05410-1

Valles, J., Rello, J., Ochagavia, A., Garnacho, J., and Alcala, M. A. (2003). Community-Acquired Bloodstream Infection in Critically Ill Adult Patients: Impact of Shock and Inappropriate Antibiotic Therapy on Survival. *Chest* 123 (5), 1615–1624. doi: 10.1378/chest.123.5.1615

van Belkum, A., Melles, D. C., Peeters, J. K., van Leeuwen, W. B., van Duijkeren, E., Huijsdens, X. W., et al. (2008). Methicillin-Resistant and -Susceptible Staphylococcus Aureus Sequence Type 398 in Pigs and Humans. *Emerg. Infect. Dis.* 14 (3), 479–483. doi: 10.3201/eid1403.070760

Vandenesch, F., Naimi, T., Enright, M. C., Lina, G., Nimmo, G. R., Heffernan, H., et al. (2003). Community-Acquired Methicillin-Resistant Staphylococcus Aureus Carrying Panton-Valentine Leukocidin Genes: Worldwide Emergence. *Emerg. Infect. Dis.* 9 (8), 978–984. doi: 10.3201/eid0908.030089

Vandersteegen, K., Kropinski, A. M., Nash, J. H., Noben, J. P., Hermans, K., and Lavigne, R. (2013). Romulus and Remus, Two Phage Isolates Representing a Distinct Clade Within the Twortlikevirus Genus, Display Suitable Properties for Phage Therapy Applications. *J. Virol.* 87 (6), 3237–3247. doi: 10.1128/JVI.02763-12

Wick, R. R., Schultz, M. B., Zobel, J., and Holt, K. E. (2015). Bandage: Interactive Visualization of De Novo Genome Assemblies. *Bioinformatics* 31 (20), 3350–3352. doi: 10.1093/bioinformatics/btv383

Winstel, V., Liang, C., Sanchez-Carballo, P., Steglich, M., Munar, M., Broker, B. M., et al. (2013). Wall Teichoic Acid Structure Governs Horizontal Gene Transfer Between Major Bacterial Pathogens. *Nat. Commun.* 4, 2345. doi: 10.1038/ncomms3345

Xia, G., Corrigan, R. M., Winstel, V., Goerke, C., Grundling, A., and Peschel, A. (2011). Wall Teichoic Acid-Dependent Adsorption of Staphylococcal Siphovirus and Myovirus. *J. Bacteriol.* 193 (15), 4006–4009. doi: 10.1128/JB.01412-10

Xia, G., and Wolz, C. (2014). Phages of Staphylococcus Aureus and Their Impact on Host Evolution. *Infect. Genet. Evol.* 21, 593–601. doi: 10.1016/j.meegid.2013.04.022

5

Increased PD-1 Level in Severe Cervical Injury is Associated with the Rare Programmed Cell Death 1 (*PDCD1*) rs36084323 A Allele in a Dominant Model

Mauro César da Silva[1], Fernanda Silva Medeiros[1], Neila Caroline Henrique da Silva[1], Larissa Albuquerque Paiva[2], Fabiana Oliveira dos Santos Gomes[1], Matheus Costa e Silva[3], Thailany Thays Gomes[1], Christina Alves Peixoto[1], Maria Carolina Valença Rygaard[4], Maria Luiza Bezerra Menezes[5], Stefan Welkovic[6], Eduardo Antônio Donadi[3] and Norma Lucena-Silva[1,4]*

[1] Laboratory of Immunogenetics, Department of Immunology, Aggeu Magalhães Institute, Oswaldo Cruz Foundation, Recife, Brazil, [2] Getúlio Vargas Hospital, Pernambuco Health Department, Recife, Brazil, [3] Clinical Immunology Division, Department of Medicine, School of Medicine of Ribeirão Preto, University of São Paulo (USP), Ribeirão Preto, Brazil, [4] Laboratory of Molecular Biology, IMIP Hospital, Pediatric Oncology Service, Recife, Brazil, [5] Department of Maternal and Child, Faculty of Medical Sciences, University of Pernambuco, Recife, Brazil, [6] Integrated Health Center Amaury de Medeiros (CISAM), University of Pernambuco, Recife, Brazil

Correspondence:
Norma Lucena-Silva
norma.lucena@hotmail.com

The high-risk oncogenic human papillomavirus (HPV) has developed mechanisms for evasion of the immune system, favoring the persistence of the infection. The chronic inflammation further contributes to the progression of tissue injury to cervical cancer. The programmed cell death protein (PD-1) after contacting with its ligands (PD-L1 and PD-L2) exerts an inhibitory effect on the cellular immune response, maintaining the balance between activation, tolerance, and immune cell-dependent lesion. We evaluated 295 patients exhibiting or not HPV infection, stratified according to the location (injured and adjacent non-injured areas) and severity of the lesion (benign, pre-malignant lesions). Additionally, we investigated the role of the promoter region *PDCD1* -606G>A polymorphism (rs36084323) on the studied variables. PD-1 and *PDCD1* expression were evaluated by immunohistochemistry and qPCR, respectively, and the *PDCD1* polymorphism was evaluated by nucleotide sequencing. Irrespective of the severity of the lesion, PD-1 levels were increased compared to adjacent uninjured areas. Additionally, in cervical intraepithelial neoplasia (CIN) I, the presence of HPV was associated with increased ($P = 0.0649$), whereas in CIN III was associated with decreased ($P = 0.0148$) PD-1 levels, compared to the uninjured area in absence of HPV infection. The *PDCD1* -606A allele was rare in our population (8.7%) and was not associated with the risk for development of HPV infection, cytological and histological features, and aneuploidy. In contrast, irrespective of the severity of the lesion, patients exhibiting the mutant *PDCD1* -606A allele at single or double doses exhibited increased protein and gene expression when compared to the *PDCD1* -606GG wild type genotype. Besides, the presence of

HPV was associated with the decrease in *PDCD1* expression and PD-1 levels in carriers of the -606 A allele presenting severe lesions, suggesting that other mediators induced during the HPV infection progression may play an additional role. This study showed that increased PD-1 levels are influenced by the -606G>A nucleotide variation, particularly in low-grade lesions, in which the A allele favors increased *PDCD1* expression, contributing to HPV immune system evasion, and in the high-grade lesion, by decreasing tissue PD-1 levels.

Keywords: PD-1, CIN, HPV, polymorphism, inflammation, cancer

INTRODUCTION

Human papillomavirus (HPV) is the most common sexually transmitted biological agent, responsible for causing several types of cancer, particularly in the anogenital region, accounting for about 85% of the cervical tumors (World Health Organization, 2017; De Oliveira et al., 2019). The high-risk oncogenic HPVs have developed immune system evasion mechanisms, favoring viral persistence and chronic inflammation, which play an important role in the progression from cervical injury to cancer (Aggarwal et al., 2006; Grivennikov et al., 2010; Senba and Mori, 2012; Marinelli et al., 2019).

The programmed cell death protein (PD-1), together with its ligands PD-L1 or PD-L2, exerts an inhibitory effect on the cellular immune response, maintaining the balance between activation and tolerance of the immune cell function. The PD-1/PD-L1 signaling pathway has been used by microorganisms and tumor cells to decrease host immune system activity, permitting chronic infection, cell transformation into the tumor, and tumor cell survival (Ishida et al., 1992; Keir et al., 2008). PD-1 protein is mainly expressed on the membrane of T- and B- lymphocytes, NK cells, dendritic cells, activated monocytes, and immature Langerhans cells (Boussiotis, 2016).

Belonging to the immunoglobulin superfamily, PD-1 is a type I transmembrane monomeric protein, which has a cytoplasmic tyrosine-based inhibitory motif (ITIM) and a tyrosine-based switch motif (ITSM) that transmit inhibitory signals to the

immune system cells. Once the peptide-MHC complex on the surface of the antigen-presenting cell (APC) binds to the T-cell receptor (TCR), the PD-L1 expressed on APC binds to the PD-1 receptor on T-cells and induces the phosphorylation of ITIM and ITSM motifs. The recruitment of the SHP-1 and SHP-2 phosphatases causes dephosphorylation of other signaling molecules of the cascade, inhibiting phosphatidylinositol 3-kinase (PI3K) and protein kinase B (Akt). These events culminate in immune response inhibition, reflected by i) decreased production of cytokines, such as IFN-γ, IL-2, and TNF-α, ii) inhibition of proliferation and survival of T cells, and iii) re-establishment of the immunological homeostasis, decreasing the expression of co-stimulatory molecules at the immunological synapse (Muenst et al., 2016; Salmaninejad et al., 2018). Nevertheless, the PD-1/PD-L1 signaling pathway may be used by tumor cells to attenuate or escape anti-tumor immunity, facilitating tumor progression. In human malignancies, high T-cell PD-1 expression has been reported in Hodgkin's lymphoma, chronic lymphocytic leukemia, and breast, bladder, and ovarian cancers, suggesting a state of functional exhaustion of T cells (Muenst et al., 2016; Hollander et al., 2018; Kawahara et al., 2018; Lewinsky et al., 2018; Wieser et al., 2018; Jiang et al., 2019).

The *PDCD1* gene is located at chromosome 2 (2q37.3), presents 5 exons, and encodes a 288 amino acid PD-1 protein. Alternative splicing can generate different isoforms that are expressed at similar levels after T cell activation (Shinohara et al., 1994; Keir et al., 2008); however, genetic variants at *PDCD1* coding and regulatory 5' and 3' untranslated regions (UTR) may influence protein levels and the natural history of cancer development (Tao et al., 2017; Wang et al., 2018). Several *PDCD1* polymorphic sites have been described, including i) 298 single nucleotide polymorphisms (SNPs) at the coding region, of which 213 missense, 112 synonymous, 7 nonsense, and 4 frameshift mutations; ii) 512 SNPs at the extended 5'UTR, iii) 490 SNPs at the extended 3'UTR, and iv) 1,791 intronic sequence mutations. Among these SNPs, 36 at the coding region, 57 at 5'UTR, 56 at 3'UTR and 283 intronic ones have clinical importance (https://www.ncbi.nlm.nih.gov/SNP/). Among all these polymorphic sites, the *PDCD1* promoter region -606G>A polymorphism (rs36084323) has been associated with the oncogenic p53 protein in breast cancer (Hua et al., 2011), in measles-induced autoimmune neurological manifestations (Ishizaki et al., 2010), and the susceptibility to hepatitis B infection (Hou et al., 2017).

Abbreviations: Akt, Protein kinase B; ASC – H, Atypical squamous cells-cannot exclude high-grade squamous intraepithelial lesion; ASC-US, Atypical squamous cells of undetermined significance; CI, Confidence interval; CIN, Cervical intraepithelial neoplasia (I-III); CISAM, Integrated Health Center Amaury de Medeiros; DNA, Deoxyribonucleic acid; DMSO, Dimethyl sulfoxide; GAPDH, Glyceraldehyde phosphate dehydrogenase; HE, Hematoxylin-eosin; HBV, Hepatitis B virus; HIV, Human immunodeficiency virus; *HLA-G*, Human leukocyte antigen G; HPV, Human papillomavirus; HSIL, High-grade squamous intraepithelial lesion; IMIP, Professor Fernando Figueira Institute of Integral Medicine; IHC, Immunohistochemistry; ITIM, Immunoreceptor tyrosine-based inhibitory motif; ITSM, Immunoreceptor tyrosine-based switch motif; LGSIL, Low-grade squamous intraepithelial lesion; NSCLC, Non-small cell lung cancer; OEGE, Online Encyclopedia for Genetic Epidemiology; OR, Odds ratio; *P*, *P*-value; PBMC, Peripheral blood mononucleated cells; PCR, Polymerase chain reaction; PI3K, Phosphatidylinositol 3-kinase; PD-1/*PDCD1*, Programmed cell death 1; PD-L1/PD-L2, Programmed cell death ligand 1 or 2; SNP, Single nucleotide polymorphisms; SSPE, Subacute sclerosing panencephalitis; TAE, Tris-acetate-EDTA buffer; TCR, T-cell receptor; UTR, Untranslated regions.

To study the role of PD-1 on the progression of cervical lesions, we evaluated PD-1 tissue and *PDCD1* gene expression in women infected or not by HPV. To understand the contribution of genetic factors on PD-1 and *PDCD1* expression, we evaluated the *PDCD1* promoter region -606G>A polymorphism (rs36084323) in these patients.

MATERIALS AND METHODS

Study Population and Ethical Consideration

The study population encompassed 295 women, aged 18-71 years (median=37 years). Among the 107 HPV-infected women, 90 were infected by high-risk, 11 by low-risk HPV, and in 6 samples the HPV viral genotype was not identified. Patients attending the Integrated Health Center Amaury de Medeiros (CISAM) and in the Professor Fernando Figueira Institute of Integral Medicine (IMIP), in Pernambuco, Brazil, between April 2016 to October 2018, were invited to participate in this study during the routine gynecological consultations for evaluation of the Papanicolaou smears, which are performed annually in asymptomatic and symptomatic women. This study was approved by the Ethics Committee of the Aggeu Magalhães Institute (CAAE: 51111115.9.0000.5190), and all participants signed an informed consent form after receiving a detailed explanation about the research. HIV-positive patients were not included in this study.

Clinical and laboratory data were obtained from medical records and interviews, using a standard questionnaire (**Table 1**). Venous blood and cervical exfoliative cells and biopsies were obtained during routine colposcopy analysis and evaluated by experienced gynecologists.

For the *PDCD1* gene expression analysis, the reference group was women presenting no atypia in the cytopathological Papanicolaou smear, who were not eligible to be subjected to biopsy due to ethical restriction. Abnormal cytology was classified using the Bethesda system. Cervical abnormalities were stratified as the low-grade squamous intraepithelial lesion (LGSIL) and high-grade squamous intraepithelial lesion (HGSIL). Women presenting abnormal cytology were subjected to cervical biopsies for histological stratification into the benign lesions, low-grade cervical intraepithelial neoplasia (CIN) I, and high-grade CIN II and CIN III. For the immunohistochemistry evaluation of PD-1 protein levels, the reference controls were specimens from the uninjured area adjacent to the lesion.

Histopathology

Biopsies of the cervical lesion and the adjacent area were fixed in formalin (10%) and embedded in paraffin. Four µm tissue sections were cut using a manual microtome (American Optical, Rotary, Leica, Buffalo Grove, IL), placed on silanized glass slides (Agilent-Dako, Santa Clara, CA), stained with hematoxylin-eosin (HE) and mounted with the medium

TABLE 1 | Demographic, clinical, and laboratory features of women exhibiting cervical lesion associated with the HPV-infections [low-grade squamous intraepithelial lesion (LGSIL), the high-grade squamous intraepithelial lesion (HGSIL) and cervical intraepithelial neoplasia (CIN)] or non-associated with the HPV infection [atypical squamous cells of undifferentiated (ASC-US), atypical squamous cells not excluding high-grade squamous intraepithelial lesion (ASC-H)].

Patients characteristics	TOTAL		HPV +		HPV -		
	N = 295	%	N = 107	36.3%	N = 188	63.7%	
Age - years							
Median (minimum - maximum)	37.8 (18-70)		36 (18-66)		38 (19-72)		P= 0.3066
Use of oral contraceptives	293		107		188		
Yes	68	23.2	19	17.9	49	26.2	P= 0.1152
No	225	76.8	87	82.1	138	73.8	
Data missing	2		1		1		
Cytological alterations	255		107		188		
No atypias	104	40.8	24	25.5	80	49.6	P< 0.0001
ASC-US and ASC-H	26	10.2	6	6.4	20	12.4	
LGSIL	51	20.0	22	23.4	29	18.0	
HGSIL	74	29.0	42	44.7	32	19.9	
Data missing	40		13		27		
Histological alterations	267		107		188		
Uninjured (not submitted to biopsy)*	74	27.7	11	11.7	63	36.4	P< 0.0001
Benign injury	41	15.4	9	9.6	32	18.5	
CIN I	23	8.6	8	8.5	15	8.7	
CIN II	67	25.1	33	35.1	34	19.6	
CIN III	62	23.2	33	35.1	29	16.8	
Data missing	24		13		15		
Cellular ploidy	122		107		188		
Aneuploidy	27	22.1	10	23.8	63	78.8	P< 0.0001
Diploidy	95	77.9	32	76.2	17	21.2	
Data missing	173		65		108		

To evaluate possible differences between the groups of infected and uninfected by HPV, Mann-Whitney test (age-years), Chi-square test (cytological and histological alterations), and Fisher test (Use of oral contraceptives and Cellular ploidy) were performed. *According to the Brazilian Ministry of Health's screening policy for cervical cancer, there is no indication for colposcopy for these patients, due to the absence of changes in the cytological examination.

Entellan® (MERCK, Burlington, MA). The sections were visualized with 400x magnification in an inverted microscope (Zeiss, Göttingen, Germany) equipped with a camera and with a 4.7.4 Image Analysis Program (AxionCam MRm Zeiss). HE-stained slides were blindly evaluated by a cervical pathologist.

HPV Detection and Typing

Genomic DNA was extracted from 500µL of a cervical cell suspension, using the Illustra Blood kit (Healthcare®, Little Chalfont, Buckinghamshire, UK), according to the manufacturer's instructions, and quantified using the NanoDrop 2000 spectrophotometer (ThermoScientific, Waltham, MA). The quality of the extracted DNA was also assessed by PCR-amplification using the human constitutive glyceraldehyde phosphate dehydrogenase (*GAPDH*) gene (Martins et al., 2014). HPV infection in cervical samples was diagnosed by amplifying a fragment of the viral *L1* gene with the degenerate MY09 and MY11 primers (Manos et al., 1989), using the L1-fragment encoded plasmid as the positive control. A reaction without adding any sample was used as a negative control. The presence of a band of approximately 450 base pairs (bp) in the 2% agarose gel confirmed the presence of the viral infection. Each amplification product was directly sequenced with the MY11 primer in the Genetic AnalyzerABI 3500 (Applied Biosystems, Foster City, CA) sequencer, using the BigDye terminator v3.1 cycle sequencing kit (Applied Biosystems). The chromatograms were visualized in the Mega 6.0 program (Tamura et al., 2011) to assess the quality of the sequence. Samples with defined peaks and low background in the chromatogram were submitted to Papillomavirus Episteme (https://pave.niaid.nih.gov/) to HPV genotyping.

Determination of Cellular Ploidy

Cervical cells of the uterine cervix (150µL) were ruptured using 2mL of Pharm Lyse lysis buffer (Becton Dickinson, Franklin Lakes, NJ), vigorously homogenized, and incubated in the dark for 10 minutes, and centrifuged for 120 seconds at 1,000 x g. The supernatant was discarded and the pellet resuspended in 2mL of FACs flow buffer, gently homogenized, and recentrifuged for 120 seconds at 1,000 x g. After discarding the supernatant, the pellet was resuspended in 500 µL of propidium iodide plus 10 µL of RNase (100 µg/mL), and incubated at room temperature for 30 minutes at 4°C and then for 10 minutes at 8°C. DNA fluorescence was measured by laser excitation at 488 nm and emission above 600 nm. The DNA index was estimated by comparing the proportion of DNA from the cervical cells analyzed with the diploid blood cells, using the software ModFitLT V3.0 (Verity Software House Inc., Topsham, ME). Aneuploidy was defined by a deviation in the DNA histogram in more than 10% of the cell population analyzed in the area corresponding to G0- G1 of the cell cycle in the sample (Martins et al., 2014).

Cervical Cell PD-1 Levels

Immunohistochemistry (IHC) analysis for cervical biopsies was manually performed using the DAKO EnVision ™ FLEX kit (Agilent-DAKO, Santa Clara, CA). For antigenic recovery, tissue was pretreated with citrate buffer, pH 6.1 (Agilent-DAKO), and heated for 30 minutes. After blocking with endogenous peroxidase, the tissue sample was incubated with the primary monoclonal anti-PD-1 mouse antibody (ABCAM, Cambridge, UK) diluted (1:100) with DAKO antibody diluent for 1h. After washing, the sections were incubated with secondary antibody for 20 minutes and then visualized with the DAB reagent (3,3'-diaminobenzidine tetrahydrochloride, DAKO). After labeling, tissue sections were counterstained with Harris' hematoxylin and assembled with Entellan® (MERCK).

The IHC slides of the cervical lesion and the adjacent uninjured area were independently analyzed by two specialist pathologists. Cell areas showing brown staining were considered to be positive for the expression of PD-1 and quantified in three fields showing the highest labeling per slide, using the Gimp 2.10.18 software (GNU Image Manipulation Program, UNIX platforms, www.gimp.org). To minimize possible reading errors, we measured pixels in areas with an intense and less intense stained area in the same picture; and combined both readings to generate the final PD-1 expression value.

Cervical Cell *PDCD1* Gene Expression

Total RNA was extracted from a 1000 µL of cervical cell suspension, using Trizol® reagent (Invitrogen), and submitted to cDNA synthesis using the MLLV reverse transcriptase (Invitrogen), accordingly to the manufacturer's instructions. For *PDCD1* expression, the qPCR was prepared with 1µL cDNA and 10 pmoles of each PD1F: 5' GAT GGT TCT TAG ACT CCC CAG ACA G 3', and PD1R: 5' GGC TCA TGC GGT ACC AGT TTA GCA C 3' primers, in Power SYBR™ Green PCR Master Mix (Applied Biosystems, Foster City, CA). For the expression of the *GAPDH* constitutive gene, we used also 1 µL cDNA and 10 pmoles of GAPDH2F: 5' AGA AGG CTG GGG CTC ATT TG 3' and GAPDH2R: 5' GTG GTC ATG AGT CCT TCC AC 3' primers in Power SYBR™ Green PCR Master Mix. All primers were designed nearby the exon-intron junction to amplify a fragment that covers two exons, assuring amplification of the cDNA target. The qPCR was performed in a final volume of 20 µL containing 10 µL of 2× Power SYBR® Green PCR Master Mix, 1 µl forward and 1 µl reverse PCR primers (500nM), 1µL cDNA and 7 µL nuclease-free water. The reaction mixtures were processed with an initial holding period at 95°C for 10 min, followed by a two-step PCR program for 40 cycles that consisted of 95°C for 15 sec and 60°C for 1 min. The *PDCD1* and *GAPDH* calibration curves showed similar amplification efficiency, and samples were evaluated in duplicate in Quant Studio 5 (Applied Biosystem). Only samples showing a melting curve with single and specific peaks, and only duplicates showing standard deviation less than 0.5 were considered for analyses. A unique threshold was settled for each gene amplification in all plates, and the sample CTs were annotated. *PDCD1* relative expression was determined by ΔCT-comparative quantification, in which *PDCD1* expression was normalized by the endogenous gene expression (ΔCT $=$CT$_{PDCD1}$ − CT$_{GAPDH}$) for each sample, and the final results were expressed in fold-change, using the equation (Fold-change=$2^{-\Delta CT}$).

PDCD1 Promoter Region Polymorphism

DNA from peripheral blood mononuclear cells, extracted using DNAzol® Reagent (Invitrogen, Carlsbad, CA) was used for the detection of the -606G>A (rs36084323) SNP. Briefly, DNA was amplified using the *PD-1* PROMO F (5 'GAA AGA TCT GGA ACT GTG GC 3') and PD-1 PROMO R (5 'TGA GAG TGA AAG GTC CCT CC 3') primers. The amplification reaction was performed in a final volume of 20 μL containing 1x of polymerase buffer (Applied Biosystems), 0.5 mM MgCl$_2$, 2% DMSO, 200 μM dNTP's, 1.0 μM of each primer, 1.0 unit of Ampli-Taq Gold (Applied Biosystems) and 80-200 ng of genomic DNA for the amplification of a 962 bp-PD1 fragment. The cycling conditions included an initial stage at 94°C for 10 min; 40 cycles of denaturation at 94°C for 1 min, annealing at 62 °C for 1 min and extension at 72 °C for 1.2 min, and final extension for 7 min at 72°C. The PCR product was visualized using a 1.5% agarose gel and, subsequently, sequenced by the SANGER method, following the BigDye protocol on ABI 3500 sequencer (Applied Biosystems). Polymorphic sites were determined using the Seqman® program (Roche 454, Life ScienceTM, Branford, CT) and individually annotated in an Excel 2016 spreadsheet.

Bioinformatics Analysis

To propose a list of possible microRNAs (miRNA) associated with the *PDCD1* rs36084323 SNP, we took advantage of two separated approaches using: i) the mirDIP Version 4.1.11.1 (Tokar et al., 2018), which integrates 30 different databases of miRNA target prediction, together with a unidirectional search query with *PDCD1* (PD-1 alias), to search for all predicted miRNAs without filtering any specific 'Score class'; ii) the sequence of 100 base pairs that surrounds the SNP, as retrieved from Genome Browser Gateway (http://genome.ucsc.edu/), and blasted using miRBase Release 22.1 (Kozomara et al., 2019). Then, we selected the miRNAs that annealed with the SNP site taking into account the two possible alleles.

Statistical Analysis

Association analyses of allele and genotype frequencies with clinical variables were performed using the two-tailed Fisher's exact and chi-square tests, considering a significance level of $P < 0.05$. The Hardy-Weinberg Equilibrium was assessed by the Online Encyclopedia for Genetic Epidemiology (OEGE). The D'Agostino-Pearson test was used to assess the homogeneity of the PD-1 expression in pixels and fold-change. The central tendency was expressed as a median and the Kruskal-Wallis and Mann-Whitney tests were used to compare numeric variables. The graphics were prepared using GraphPad Prism Software version 5.0 for windows (www.graphpad.com, La Jolla, CA).

RESULTS

PD-1 Detection in Cervical Samples

PD-1 expression was evaluated in samples exhibiting HPV infection and in samples without HPV infection. Irrespective of lesion severity, we observed three patterns of PD-1 staining in cervical samples: i) exclusive labeling of the stratified squamous epithelium, ii) exclusive labeling of stromal cells, and iii) labeling of epithelium and stroma. Considering the uninjured adjacent areas, the expression of PD-1 in epithelium and stroma (n = 50, median = 4,313 pixels) was higher when compared to sections that labeled only the epithelium (n = 48, median = 2,810 pixels, $P = 0.0302$). Considering the injured areas (cervical lesions), the expression of PD-1 in epithelium and stroma (n = 32, median = 21,184 pixels) was also significantly higher when compared to specimens that exclusively labeled the epithelium area (n = 20, median = 6,339 pixels, $P < 0.0001$) (**Figure 1A**).

The evaluation of PD-1 protein level according to the severity of the lesion revealed the following results: i) PD-1 expression in benign lesions, and cervical intraepithelial neoplasia (CIN I, CIN II, and CIN III) was significantly higher when compared to uninjured adjacent tissue ($P<0.0001$, for each comparison, **Figure 1B**); ii) the PD-1 expression in benign lesions did not differ from CIN II ($P = 0.7431$) and CIN III ($P = 0.5854$) and, similarly, CIN II did not differ from CIN III ($P = 0.5122$); and iii) the PD-1 levels in low-grade lesions (CIN I) (n = 12, median = 44,215 pixels) were higher than in those presenting high-grade (CIN II and CIN III) lesions (n = 54, median = 18,942 pixels, $P = 0.0046$); however, the pattern of expression was different. PD-1 labeling in low-grade lesions was higher in infiltrating immune cells of the stroma compared to the epithelium, whereas in high-grade lesions PD-1 expression was observed primarily in the epithelium (**Figure 2**). Additionally, irrespective of the severity of the lesion, PD-1 levels were increased compared to adjacent uninjured areas. Also, in CIN I the presence of HPV was associated with increased PD-1 protein levels ($P = 0.0649$), whereas in CIN III was associated with decreased levels ($P = 0.0148$) compared to correspondent tissue lesion in absence of HPV infection (**Figures 1C, D**).

Polymorphism of the *PDCD1* Promoter Region

Irrespective of the severity of the cervical lesion, the frequency of the wild -606G allele was 91.3%, and the distribution of the GG (83.7%), GA (15.2%), and AA (1.1%) genotypes adhered to the Hardy-Weinberg equilibrium ($\chi^2 = 0.48$). Taking into account the low frequency of the AA genotype, we lumped together the AA and GA genotypes to allow statistical analysis. Women carrying the -606A allele were not at increased risk for i) development of HPV infection, ii) exhibiting cytological and histological HPV and non-HPV changes, and ii) presenting aneuploidy (**Table 2**).

Considering the differential exposure of HPV according to age and the risk for developing cervical lesions, we evaluated the influence of the patient age on the studied variables. Age did not influence the *PDCD1* genotype frequency among patients presenting or not HPV ($P = 0.3066$), and among patients exhibiting benign injury ($P = 0.1692$), CIN I ($P = 0.5698$), CIN II ($P = 0.0746$) or CIN III ($P = 0.7366$) compared to women with normal cytomorphological results.

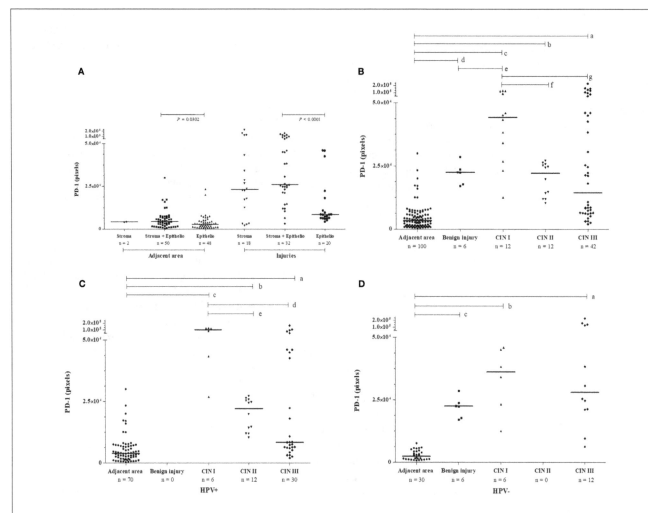

FIGURE 1 | Pattern of PD-1 immunochemistry labeling observed in cervical samples, according to **(A)** the tissue location in injured and uninjured adjacent areas, **(B)** the severity of lesion irrespective to HPV infection, **(C)** in the presence of HPV infection, and **(D)** the absence of HPV infection. PD-1 labeling was analyzed by two independent pathologists, and the intensity of the labeling (pixels) was quantified in three fields per slide. Data were presented as medians, and the comparisons were performed using the Kruskal-Wallis test followed by Mann Whitney U test. In graph B, PD-1 levels were high irrespective of the severity of cervical lesions, CIN III (in a, $P<0.0001$); CIN II (in b, $P<0.0001$); CIN I (in c, $P<0.0001$); and benign lesions (in d, $P<0.0001$) compared to the uninjured adjacent area; and between benign lesion vs. CIN I (in e, $P = 0.0131$); however, CIN I lesions showed the highest PD-1 level compared to the CIN II (in f, $P = 0.0014$) and CIN III (in g, $P = 0.0172$). In graph C, in presence of HPV the PD-1 levels were high in CIN III (in a, $P<0.0001$), CIN II (in b, $P<0.0001$), and CIN I (in c, $P<0.0001$) compared to uninjured tissue, and lower PD-1 levels were observed in CIN III (in d, $P = 0.0048$) and CIN II (in e, $P = 0.0012$) compared to the levels in low-grade lesion CIN I. In graph D, in women non-infected by HPV, high PD-1 levels were also observed in CIN III (in a, $P<0.0001$), CIN I (in b, $P = 0.0001$), and benign injury (in c $P = 0.0001$) compared to the uninjured adjacent area.

Association of the *PDCD1* Gene Expression in the Cervical Lesion With *PDCD1* Polymorphism

The presence of cervical injury was not associated with a greater *PDCD1* expression by exfoliative cervical cells when compared to cervical samples from women with a normal cytomorphological smear (**Figure 3A**). However, considering samples altogether, the mutant -606A allele in single or double dose was associated with higher *PDCD1* gene expression in cervical cells compared to the wild type -606GG genotype (**Figure 3B**). There was no statistical difference ($P = 0.4692$) between *PDCD1* expression levels in lesions of different severities in carriers of the -606GG genotype (**Figure 3C**). However, among carriers of the -606A allele in homo or heterozygosis, the expression of *PDCD1* was

higher in exfoliative cells of patients exhibiting high-grade CIN III lesions compared to those presenting benign ($P = 0.0453$) or CIN II ($P = 0.0233$) lesions (**Figure 3D**). Moreover, despite no association of HPV-infection with *PDCD1* expression (P=0.8329) was observed (**Figure 3E**), the presence of HPV increased *PDCD1* expression, particularly in women presenting CIN I lesion (**Figures 3F, G**), a finding that may have been influenced by the -606A allele (**Figure 3H**).

Association Between PD-1 Protein Levels and *PDCD1* Polymorphism

We also evaluated whether the PD-1 tissue levels were associated with the presence of the rare *PDCD1* -606G>A polymorphic sites. Considering the dominant model for the rare allele, women

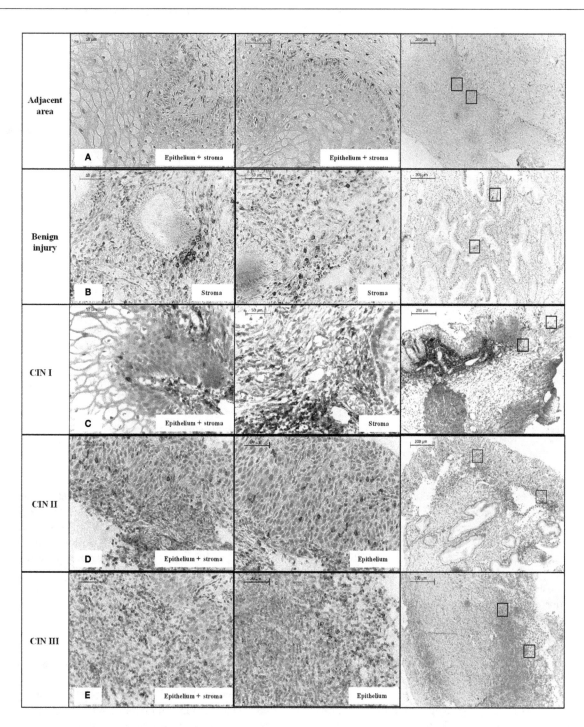

FIGURE 2 | Immunohistochemistry labeling of PD-1 level observed in specimens obtained from the mucosa of the uterine cervix, stratified according to the presence or not of the lesion, and according to the severity of the cervical lesion. **(A)** cervix without lesion, **(B)** benign injury, **(C)** CIN I, **(D)** CIN II, **(E)** CIN III, at 100X and 400X magnifications. PD-1 protein was primarily detected in the stratified epithelium and stroma of the cervical mucosa.

carrying the A allele in homozygosis or heterozygosis (n = 46, median = 7,381 pixels) exhibited increased PD-1 levels in cervical samples when compared to those homozygous for the *G* allele (n = 126, median = 5,697 pixels, *P* = 0.0234) (**Figure 4A**). Besides, the association of *PDCD1* -606A allele with the PD-1

expression was strengthened when we specifically evaluated women with high-grade cervical lesions (CIN III); i.e., women carrying the -606A allele at homo- or heterozygosis exhibited higher PD-1 levels in the cervical lesions when compared to women carrying the homozygous -606G allele (GA + AA with

TABLE 2 | Allelic and genotypic frequency of the promoter region *PDCD1*-606 G>A (rs36084323) polymorphism observed in women exhibiting grades of cervical lesions, stratified according to i) presence or not of the HPV infection, ii) cytological/histological alterations, and iii) cellular ploidy.

Patients characteristics	PDCD1 (rs36084323)										
	GG		GA+AA		P	OR (CI-95%)	G		A		P	OR (CI-95%)
	N= 231	83.7%	N=45	16.3%			N= 504	91.3%	N=48	8.7%		
HPV Infection												
Yes	83	35.9	17	37.8	0.8659	0.92 (0.48-1.79)	182	36.1	18	37.5	0.8757	0.94 (0.51-1.74)
No	148	64.1	28	62.2			322	63.9	30	62.5		
Total	231	100.0	45	100.0			504	100.0	48	100.0		
Cytological alterations												
HGSIL	55	27.8	16	40.0	0.3018	n/a	125	28.8	17	40.5	0.2864	n/a
ASC-US, ASC-H and LGSIL	62	31.3	10	25.0			133	30.6	11	26.2		
No atypias	81	40.9	14	35.0			176	40.6	14	33.3		
Total	198	100.0	40	100.0			434	100.0	42	100.0		
Presence of histological alterations												
Presence of CIN	118	56.5	23	56.1	1.0000	1.01 (0.52-1.99)	259	56.8	23	52.3	0.6337	1.20 (0.64-2.23)
Absence of CIN	91	43.5	18	43.9			197	43.2	21	47.7		
Total	209	100.0	41	100.0			456	100.0	44	100.0		
Histological alterations												
CIN III	48	23.0	10	24.4	0.8669	n/a	106	23.2	10	22.7	0.7133	n/a
CIN II	51	24.4	11	26.8			113	24.8	11	25.0		
CIN I	19	9.1	2	4.9			40	8.8	2	4.5		
Benign injury	33	15.8	8	19.5			72	15.8	10	22.7		
Uninjured	58	27.8	10	24.4			125	27.4	11	25.0		
Total	209	100.0	41	100.0			456	100.0	44	100.0		
Cellular ploidy												
Aneuploidy	22	24.2	3	12.0	0.2737	2.34 (0.64-8.57)	47	22.8	3	11.5	0.3092	2.27 (0.65-7.88)
Diploidy	69	75.8	22	88.0			159	77.2	23	88.5		
Total	91	100.0	25	100.0			206	100.0	26	100.0		

Atypical squamous cells of undetermined significance (ASC-US), atypical squamous cells-not excluding high-grade squamous intraepithelial lesion (ASC-H), the low-grade squamous intraepithelial lesion (LGSIL), the high-grade squamous intraepithelial lesion (HGSIL), cervical intraepithelial neoplasia (CIN). N, sample number; P, P-value; G, wild allele; A, variant allele; OR, odds ratio and 95%CI, confidence interval. The frequencies of alleles and genotypes were compared using the two-tailed Fisher's exact and Chi-square tests.

the median of 48,117 pixels *vs.* GG with the median of 8,539 pixels, $P = 0.0010$ (**Figure 4B**). However, PD-1 levels in uninjured adjacent tissue were not associated with the -606G>A variation site (GA + AA with the median of 3,358 pixels *vs. GG* with the median of 3,409 pixels, $P = 0.8646$) (**Figure 4C**). In the presence of HPV infection, the high PD-1 levels previously associated with the presence of the -606A allele was not observed anymore (**Figures 4D, E**); however, the influence of HPV infection on PD-1 levels continue to be observed for high-grade CIN III lesions even being in less magnitude (**Figure 4F**).

Predicted miRNA and *PDCD1* rs36084323 SNP Association

Considering the discrepancy regarding the results of the protein (**Figure 4F**) and gene expression (**Figure 3H**) levels, we further evaluated the differential targeting of miRNAs at the *PDCD1* -606 variation site. An in-silico study showed that the hsa-miR-204-3p binds exclusively to the *G* allele, whereas the hsa-miR-6798-5p, hsa-miR-6775-5p, and hsa-miR-4776-5p bind only to the A allele, and the hsa-miR-6771-5p targeted both alleles. Notably, the miRNAs that targeted the -606G>A variation site were included among the 2,586 miRNAs that have been predicted to target the *PDCD1* gene, according to the mirDIP analysis (**Figure 5**).

In summary, our results showed that the -606A allele is rare in our population and, considering the dominant model, women carrying the -606 AX genotype (X= A or G) are more likely to respond to HPV-induced cervical lesions with decreased production of PD-1, and the intensity and pattern of labeling is related to the degree of the cervical injury.

DISCUSSION

Since healthy cervical specimens are not easily available due to ethical reasons, in this study we evaluated PD-1 expression in cervical biopsies obtained from patients presenting several stages of the cervical lesion (injured areas) and used, as controls, the adjacent uninjured cervical areas. Irrespective of the severity of the lesion, injured cervical specimens overexpressed PD-1 when compared to the adjacent uninjured area, and particularly observed in the stromal layer (**Figure 1A**). Notably, samples presenting high-grade (CIN II-III) lesions expressed less PD-1 when compared to low-grade (CIN I) lesions (**Figure 1B**). PD-1 expression predominated in the stroma in low-grade lesions, and the epithelium in high-grade lesions (**Figure 2**). The stroma-rich T cell-infiltrate in low-grade cervical lesions associated with the increased tissue PD-1 (Hemmat and Bannazadeh Baghi, 2019)

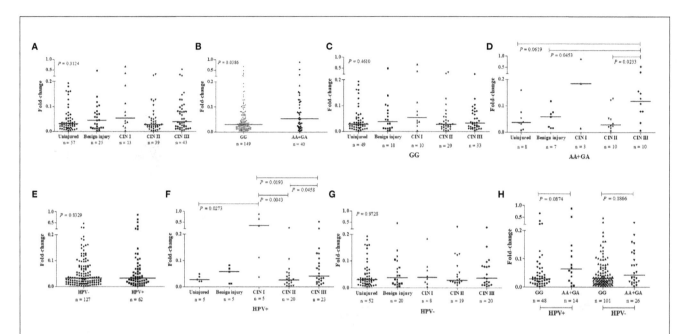

FIGURE 3 | *PDCD1* mRNA expression in exfoliative cervical cells of patients presenting normal (uninjured) and abnormal cytomorphological smear (injured) stratified according to the severity of the lesion, presence or absence of HPV infection, and the nucleotide variability at the promoter region *PDCD1*-606G>A polymorphic site (rs36084323). *PDCD1* expression was calculated by the qPCR comparative method using as reference the *GAPDH* gene and the SYRB green detection system, performed in duplicate. Fold-change differences were estimated by the Kruskal-Wallis or Mann-Whitney U tests. **(A)** *PDCD1* expression stratified according to the severity of the cervical lesion, **(B)** *PDCD1* expression stratified according to the presence of the -606GG and AA/GA genotypes, **(C)** *PDCD1* expression among carries of -606GG genotype, **(D)** and carries of -606 A allele in homo or heterozygosis stratified according to the severity of the cervical lesion, **(E)** *PDCD1* expression among women infected and non-infected by HPV, and stratified according to the severity of the cervical lesion in the presence **(F)** or absence **(G)** of HPV infection, and **(H)** *PDCD1* expression stratified according to the presence of the -606GG and AA/GA genotypes in the presence or absence of HPV infection.

primarily reflect the severity of inflammation associated with HPV infection (Yang et al., 2013), whereas the expression at the epithelium strongly indicates the role of PD-1 on the progression of the cervical lesions (Yang et al., 2017; Chang et al., 2018; Medeiros et al., 2018).

Considering that the magnitude of the *PDCD1* gene expression has been associated with the *PDCD1* -606 G>A polymorphic site (Ishizaki et al., 2010), we further investigated the relationship between alleles/genotypes with the magnitude of PD-1 cervical expression. First, we observed that the *PDCD1* -606AA genotype was rare in our population (1.1%), and according to the data reported at the 1000 Genomes Phase 3 database (The 1000 Genomes Project Consortium, 2015), the promoter region *PDCD1* -606G>A (rs36084323) polymorphic site presents diverse allele frequency distribution in worldwide populations (1000 Genomes Project Phase 3 Allele Frequencies rs36084323 Snp; Auton et al., 2015), being frequent in Asians (1000 Genomes Project Phase 3 Allele Frequencies rs36084323 Snp), particularly in Chinese (21.9%) and Japanese (25%) populations (Hua et al., 2011; Sasaki et al., 2014; Hou et al., 2017). The presence of the -606A allele was not associated with the risk for the development of HPV infection, probably because of the low frequency of the mutant allele in our population. According to the frequency of the -606A in our population, a cohort of 1,834 individuals would be necessary to discriminate susceptibility/protection alleles.

Women carrying the -606A allele in homozygosis or heterozygosis showed a significant increase in the *PDCD1* gene

expression and PD-1 protein level when compared to those who carry the -606G allele in homozygosis. In HPV-non-infected women, the *PDCD1* expression was irrespective of the severity of the lesion, but in the presence of HPV infection, the *PDCD1* expression was significantly increased in CIN I lesions, which may suggest a viral attempt to evade immune response against infection, favoring viral persistence (Yang et al., 2013). The PD-1 protein level in CIN I lesions was also high in HPV-infected women compared to non-infected women (*P*=0.0649). In contrast, HPV decreased the PD-1 protein levels in CIN III (*P*=0.0148), even though the protein levels remained significantly increased compared to the uninjured adjacent area, indicating that the HPV infection is associated with the cervical transformation (Martins et al., 2014). Noteworthy, the -606G>A variation site did not influence cervical PD-1 protein levels in adjacent uninjured tissue indicating that, besides the genetic background, local microenvironment factors such as local inflammation may have a role

The functional implications of the *PDCD1* -606G>A polymorphism on the magnitude of PD-1 production has been attributed to the target site of the ubiquitin-converting enzyme 2 (UCE-2) transcription regulator (GGCCG in position -610 to -606). The -606G allele was associated with higher relative expression of *PDCD1* mRNA in peripheral blood mononuclear cells of Japanese and Filipino patients exhibiting subacute sclerosing panencephalitis due to measles infection (Ishizaki et al., 2010), and with lower survival in patients with non-small cell lung cancer (Sasaki et al., 2014). Additionally, the -606GG genotype was associated with protection against the development

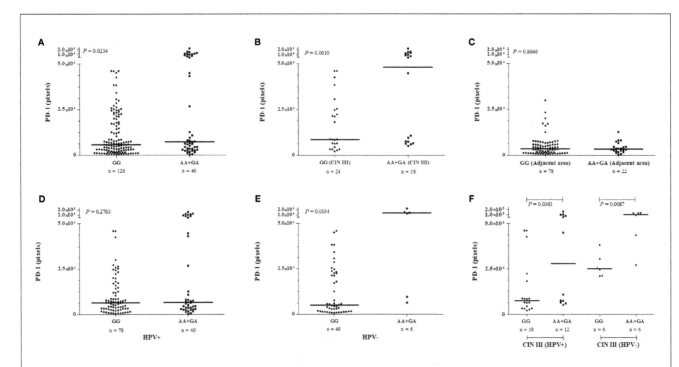

FIGURE 4 | PD-1 levels in cervical mucosa of samples obtained from patients exhibiting cervical lesions, stratified according to the severity of the lesion, presence or absence of HPV infection and according to the *PDCD1* -606G>A (rs36084323) polymorphism. The immunohistochemistry data were analyzed by two pathologists independently, and the intensity of labeling was quantified in three fields per slide. Data were presented as medians. The median differences were calculated using the Mann-Whitney test. **(A)** PD-1 protein levels were increased cervical mucosa of women encompassing the -606AA and -606GA genotypes when compared to the -606GG genotype, the difference is high among severe CIN III injury **(B)**, but not in the uninjured adjacent tissue **(C)**. In the presence of HPV infection **(D)**, the high PD-1 levels previously associated with the presence of the -606A allele **(E)** was not observed anymore; however, the influence of HPV infection on PD-1 levels continue to be observed for high-grade CIN III lesions even being in less magnitude **(F)**.

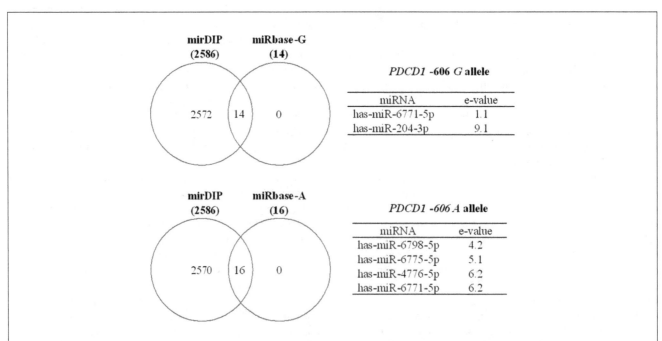

FIGURE 5 | Predicted miRNAs that target the *PDCD1* -606G>A (rs36084323) polymorphic site. Binding affinity was evaluated using miRbase and mirDIP software and expressed as e-values, in which high affinity is represented by low e-values and vice-versa.

and progression of breast cancer in women from Northeastern China; however, the A allele and the AA genotype were more frequent in patients exhibiting the p53 protein, a marker of biologically aggressive breast cancer (Hua et al., 2011). The *PDCD1* -606AA genotype was also associated with chronic hepatitis B virus (HBV) infection in the Chinese population, a viral infection that may progress to hepatocarcinoma (Hou et al., 2017). Altogether, these studies indicate a differential role of the *PDCD1* -606G>A polymorphic site according to the major subjacent cancer or viral disorder. In our study, we reported that the *PDCD1* expression and PD-1 protein levels were associated with the -606 A allele, and were modulated by HPV in severe tissue damage, suggesting that other mediators induced during the HPV infection progression may play an additional role.

Among the myriad of transcriptional and post-transcriptional elements that may differentially target gene polymorphic sites, the UCE-2 transcription regulator, which modulates the *PDCD1* -606 G>A polymorphic site (Ishizaki et al., 2010), has not been previously evaluated in the context of the progression of the HPV infection. On the other hand, several miRNAs have been associated with HPV lesion progression (Pardini et al., 2018; Pulati et al., 2019), and little is known regarding miRNA targeting the *PDCD1*-606 G>A region. Considering that virus infection may change the miRNA cell repertoire expression (Park et al., 2017; Chirayil et al., 2018; Del Mar Díaz-González et al., 2019), and that miRNA may also regulate gene expression at the transcriptional level (Lytle et al., 2007; Ørom et al., 2008; Place et al., 2008; Zhang et al., 2014), we conducted a bioinformatics analysis to predict miRNA interaction with the *PDCD1* -606G>A polymorphic site. Three miRNAs were predicted to bind to the mutant A allele: i) the hsa-MiR-6798-5p up-regulates decidual NK cells in recurrent spontaneous abortion (Sfera et al., 2015), ii) the hsa-MiR-6775 is reported to silence the transcription of the alpha 7-cholinergic nicotinic receptor gene (*CHRNA7*) expressed on lymphocyte surface and associated with lymphocyte anergy, T regulatory cell differentiation and immunologic tolerance, which consequently may predispose to cancer development (Li et al., 2018), and iii) the hsa-MiR-4776-5p specifically targets the nuclear factor Kappa B inhibitor beta (NFKBIB) mRNA in Influenza A virus-infected cells, leading to activation of NF-kB, and survival of infected cells (Othumpangat et al., 2017). The hsa-MiR-6771-5p binds to the -606 G alleles with high affinity (e-value = 1.1) and weakly to the mutant *A* allele (e-value = 6.2), and it is involved in ZIKA-associated microcephaly. This miRNA shares the same sequence of the ZIKV genome and human genes associated with microcephaly (McLean et al., 2017). Finally, the hsa-MiR-204-3p targets the wild *PDCD1* -606G allele, and several studies report that this miRNA is a protective factor against cancer development by

different cellular mechanisms depending upon the cell origin (Cui et al., 2014; Koga et al., 2018; Li et al., 2019; Xi et al., 2020). Besides targeting the *PDCD1* gene, these miRNAs may also be associated with cell transformation induced by viruses and may share sequences associated with virus infection complications. Therefore, a balance between transcriptional and post-transcription factors together with genetic variability may account for the final result that may halt or permit virus spread and cell transformation.

Concluding, this study showed that PD-1 protein levels are increased in HPV-induced cervical lesions, irrespective of the severity of the injury. In CIN I lesions, the highest PD-1 levels were observed in the inflammatory infiltrating cells of the stroma, whereas in high-grade CIN III lesions, the high PD-1 expression was observed in epithelial cells. In CIN I, the high levels of PD-1 were associated with increased *PDCD1* expression in HPV-infected samples, whereas in CIN III the presence of HPV induced a decrease in *PDCD1* expression and of PD-1 levels in carriers of the -606A allele, suggesting the possible gene regulation by miRNAs. Indeed, we identified some miRNAs specifically targeting the -606A allele region, which may be modulated by the presence of HPV, and may be involved in the progression of the cervical lesion. Future studies are needed to validate the role of these miRNAs in cervical cancer pathogenesis.

ETHICS STATEMENT

The studies involving human participants were reviewed and approved by Ethics Committee of the Aggeu Magalhães Institute (CAAE: 51111115.9.0000.5190). The patients/participants provided their written informed consent to participate in this study.

AUTHOR CONTRIBUTIONS

MS, FM, NL-S, and ED conceived, designed the study, did the formal analysis, and wrote the paper. MS, NS, FG, TG, CP, and MCS conducted the experimental work. LP, MR, MM, and SW followed-up patients and performed cytopathological and coloscopy evaluations. NL-S and ED applied for financial support and managed the project. All authors contributed to the article and approved the submitted version.

ACKNOWLEDGMENTS

We thank Viviane Carvalho for invaluable technical assistance and the Program for Technological Development in Tools for Health (PDTIS-FIOCRUZ).

REFERENCES

Ørom, U. A., Nielsen, F. C., and Lund, A. H. (2008). MicroRNA-10a Binds the 5'UTR of Ribosomal Protein mRNAs and Enhances Their Translation. *Mol. Cell* 30 (4), 460–471. doi: 10.1016/j.molcel.2008.05.001

Aggarwal, B. B., Shishodia, S., Sandur, S. K., Pandey, M. K., and Sethi, G. (2006). Inflammation and Cancer: How Hot is the Link? *Biochem. Pharmacol.* 72, 1605–1621. doi: 10.1016/j.bcp.2006.06.029

(2020) *1000 Genomes Project Phase 3 Allele Frequencies rs36084323 Snp*. Available at: http://www.ensembl.org/Homo_sapiens/Variation/Population?db=core;v=rs36084323;vdb=variation (Accessed in April 15, 2020).

Auton, A., Abecasis, G. R., Altshuler, D. M., Durbin, R. M., Bentley, D. R., Chakravarti, A., et al. (2015). A Global Reference for Human Genetic Variation. *Nature* 526, 68–74. doi: 10.1038/nature15393

Boussiotis, V. A. (2016). Molecular and Biochemical Aspects of the PD-1 Checkpoint Pathway. *N Engl. J. Med.* 375, 1767–1778. doi: 10.1056/NEJMra1514296

Chang, H., Hong, J. H., Lee, J. K., Cho, H. W., Ouh, Y. T., Min, K. J., et al. (2018). Programmed Death-1 (PD-1) Expression in Cervical Intraepithelial Neoplasia and its Relationship With Recurrence After Conization. *J. Gynecol. Oncol.* 29, 1–14. doi: 10.3802/jgo.2018.29.e27

Chirayil, R., Kincaid, R. P., Dahlke, C., Kuny, C. V., Dalken, N., Spohn, M., et al. (2018). Identification of Virus-Encoded microRNAs in Divergent Papillomaviruses. *PloS Pathog.* 14 (7), e1007156. doi: 10.1371/journal.ppat.1007156

Cui, Z. H., Shen, S. Q., Chen, Z. B., and Hu, C. (2014). Growth Inhibition of Hepatocellular Carcinoma Tumor Endothelial Cells by miR-204-3p and Underlying Mechanism. *World J. Gastroenterol.* 20 (18), 5493–5504. doi: 10.3748/wjg.v20.i18.5493

Del Mar Díaz-González, S., Rodríguez-Aguilar, E. D., Meneses-Acosta, A., Valadez-Graham, V., Deas, J., Gómez-Cerón, C., et al. (2019). Transregulation of microRNA miR-21 Promoter by AP-1 Transcription Factor in Cervical Cancer Cells. *Cancer Cell Int.* 19, 214. doi: 10.1186/s12935-019-0931-x

De Oliveira, C. M., Fregnani, J. H. T. G., and Villa, L. L. (2019). Hpv Vaccine: Updates and Highlights. *Acta Cytol.* 63, 159–168. doi: 10.1159/000497617

Grivennikov, S. I., Greten, F. R., and Karin, M. (2010). Immunity, Inflammation, and Cancer. *Cell* 140, 883–899. doi: 10.1016/j.cell.2010.01.025

Hemmat, N., and Bannazadeh Baghi, H. (2019). Association of Human Papillomavirus Infection and Inflammation in Cervical Cancer. *Pathog. Dis.* 77, ftz048. doi: 10.1093/femspd/ftz048

Hollander, P., Amini, R. M., Ginman, B., Molin, D., Enblad, G., and Glimelius, I. (2018). Expression of PD-1 and PD-L1 Increase in Consecutive Biopsies in Patients With Classical Hodgkin Lymphoma. *PloS One* 13, 1–16. doi: 10.1371/journal.pone.0204870

Hou, Z., Zhou, Q., Lu, M., Tan, D., and Xu, X. (2017). A Programmed Cell Death-1 Haplotype is Associated With Clearance of Hepatitis B Virus. *Ann. Clin. Lab. Sci.* 47, 334–343.

Hua, Z., Li, D., Xiang, G., Xu, F., Jie, G., Fu, Z., et al. (2011). PD-1 Polymorphisms are Associated With Sporadic Breast Cancer in Chinese Han Population of Northeast China. *Breast Cancer Res. Treat* 129, 195–201. doi: 10.1007/s10549-011-1440-3

Ishida, Y., Agata, Y., Shibahara, K., and Honjo, T. (1992). Induced Expression of PD-1, a Novel Member of the Immunoglobulin Gene Superfamily, Upon Programmed Cell Death. *EMBO J.* 11, 3887–3895. doi: 10.1002/j.1460-2075.1992.tb05481.x

Ishizaki, Y., Yukaya, N., Kusuhara, K., Kira, R., Torisu, H., Ihara, K., et al. (2010). PD1 as a Common Candidate Susceptibility Gene of Subacute Sclerosing Panencephalitis. *Hum. Genet.* 127, 411–419. doi: 10.1007/s00439-009-0781-z

Jiang, C., Cao, S. R., Li, N., Jiang, L., and Sun, T. (2019). PD-1 and PD-L1 Correlated Gene Expression Profiles and Their Association With Clinical Outcomes of Breast Cancer. *Cancer Cell Int.* 19, 1–9. doi: 10.1186/s12935-019-0955-2

Kawahara, T., Ishiguro, Y., Ohtake, S., Kato, I., Ito, Y., Ito, H., et al. (2018). PD-1 and PD-L1 are More Highly Expressed in High-Grade Bladder Cancer Than in Low-Grade Cases: PD-L1 Might Function as a Mediator of Stage Progression in Bladder Cancer 11 Medical and Health Sciences 1112 Oncology and Carcinogenesis. *BMC Urol.* 18, 1–6. doi: 10.1186/s12894-018-0414-8

Keir, M. E., Butte, M. J., Freeman, G. J., and Sharpe, A. H. (2008). PD-1 and Its Ligands in Tolerance and Immunity. *Annu. Rev. Immunol.* 26, 677–704. doi: 10.1146/annurev.immunol.26.021607.090331

Koga, T., Migita, K., Sato, T., Sato, S., Umeda, M., Nonaka, F., et al. (2018). MicroRNA-204-3p Inhibits Lipopolysaccharide-Induced Cytokines in Familial Mediterranean Fever Via the Phosphoinositide 3-Kinase γ Pathway. *Rheumatol. (Oxford).* 57 (4), 718–726. doi: 10.1093/rheumatology/kex451

Kozomara, A., Birgaoanu, M., and Griffiths-Jones, S. (2019). Mirbase: From microRNA Sequences to Function. *Nucleic Acids Res.* 47, D155–D162. doi: 10.1093/nar/gky1141

Lewinsky, H., Barak, A. F., Huber, V., Kramer, M. P., Radomir, L., Sever, L., et al. (2018). CD84 Regulates PD-1/PD-L1 Expression and Function in Chronic Lymphocytic Leukemia. *J. Clin. Invest.* 128, 5479–5488. doi: 10.1172/JCI96610

Li, D., Li, J., Jia, B., Wang, Y., Zhang, J., and Liu, G. (2018). Genome-Wide Identification of microRNAs in Decidual Natural Killer Cells From Patients With Unexplained Recurrent Spontaneous Abortion. *Am. J. Reprod. Immunol.* 80, e13052. doi: 10.1111/aji.13052

Li, X., Zhong, W., Xu, Y., Yu, B., and Liu, H. (2019). Silencing of Lncrna LINC00514 Inhibits the Malignant Behaviors of Papillary Thyroid Cancer Through miR-204-3p/CDC23 Axis. *Biochem. Biophys. Res. Commun.* 508 (4), 1145–1148. doi: 10.1016/j.bbrc.2018.12.051

Lytle, J. R., Yario, T. A., and Steitz, J. A. (2007). Target mRNAs are Repressed as Efficiently by microRNA-binding Sites in the 5' UTR as in the 3' Utr. *Proc. Natl. Acad. Sci. U. S. A.* 104 (23), 9667–9672. doi: 10.1073/pnas.0703820104

Manos, M., Ting, Y., Wright, D., Lewis, A., Broker, T., and Wolinsky, S. (1989). Use of Polymerase Chain Reaction Amplification for the Detection of Genital Human Papillomaviruses. *Cancer Cells: Mol. Diag. of Human Cancer* 7, 209–214.

Marinelli, O., Annibali, D., Aguzzi, C., Tuyaerts, S., Amant, F., Morelli, M. B., et al. (2019). The Controversial Role of PD-1 and Its Ligands in Gynecological Malignancies. *Front. Oncol.* 9:1073. doi: 10.3389/fonc.2019.01073

Martins, A. E. S., Lucena-Silva, N., Garcia, R. G., Welkovic, S., Barbosa, A., Menezes, M. L. B., et al. (2014). Prognostic Evaluation of DNA Index in HIV-HPV Co-Infected Women Cervical Samples Attending in Reference Centers for HIV-AIDS in Recife. *PloS One* 9, 1–8. doi: 10.1371/journal.pone.0104801

McLean, E., Bhattarai, R., Hughes, B. W., Mahalingam, K., and Bagasra, O. (2017). Computational Identification of Mutually Homologous Zika Virus miRNAs That Target Microcephaly Genes. *Libyan. J. Med.* 12:1. doi: 10.1080/19932820.2017.1304505

Medeiros, F. S., Martins, A. E. S., Gomes, R. G., De Oliveira, S. A. V., Welkovic, S., Maruza, M., et al. (2018). Variation Sites At the HLA-G 3' Untranslated Region Confer Differential Susceptibility to HIV/HPV Co-Infection and Aneuploidy in Cervical Cell. *PloS One* 13, 1–14. doi: 10.1371/journal.pone.0204679

Muenst, S., Läubli, H., Soysal, S. D., Zippelius, A., Tzankov, A., and Hoeller, S. (2016). The Immune System and Cancer Evasion Strategies: Therapeutic Concepts. *J. Intern. Med.* 279, 541–562. doi: 10.1111/joim.12470

Othumpangat, S., Bryan, N. B., Beezhold, D. H., and Noti, J. D. (2017). Upregulation of miRNA-4776 in Influenza Virus Infected Bronchial Epithelial Cells Is Associated With Downregulation of NFKBIB and Increased Viral Survival. *Viruses* 9:94. doi: 10.3390/v9050094

Pardini, B., De Maria, D., Francavilla, A., Di Gaetano, C., Ronco, G., and Naccarati, A. (2018). MicroRNAs as Markers of Progression in Cervical Cancer: A Systematic Review. *BMC Cancer.* 18 (1), 696. doi: 10.1186/s12885-018-4590-4

Park, S., Eom, K., Kim, J., Bang, H., Wang, H., Ahn, S., et al. (2017). MiR-9, miR-21, and miR-155 as Potential Biomarkers for HPV Positive and Negative Cervical Cancer. *BMC Cancer* 17 (1), 658. doi: 10.1186/s12885-017-3642-5

Place, R. F., Li, L. C., Pookot, D., Noonan, E. J., and Dahiya, R. (2008). MicroRNA-373 Induces Expression of Genes with Complementary Promoter Sequences. *Proc. Natl. Acad. Sci. U. S. A.* 105 (5), 1608–1613. doi: 10.1073/pnas.0707594105

Pulati, N., Zhang, Z., Gulimilamu, A., Qi, X., and Yang, J. (2019). Hpv16(+)-miRNAs in Cervical Cancer and the Anti-Tumor Role Played by Mir-5701. *J. Gene Med.* 21 (11), e3126. doi: 10.1002/jgm.3126

Salmaninejad, A., Khoramshahi, V., Azani, A., Soltaninejad, E., Aslani, S., Zamani, M. R., et al. (2018). PD-1 and Cancer: Molecular Mechanisms and Polymorphisms. *Immunogenetics* 70, 73–86. doi: 10.1007/s00251-017-1015-5

Sasaki, H., Tatemaysu, T., Okuda, K., Moriyama, S., Yano, M., and Fujii, Y. (2014). PD-1 Gene Promoter Polymorphisms Correlate With a Poor Prognosis in non-Small Cell Lung Cancer. *Mol. Clin. Oncol.* 2, 1035–1042. doi: 10.3892/mco.2014.358

Senba, M., and Mori, N. (2012). Mechanisms of Virus Immune Evasion Lead to Development From Chronic Inflammation to Cancer Formation Associated With Human Papillomavirus Infection. *Oncol. Rev.* 6, 135–144. doi: 10.4081/oncol.2012.e17

Sfera, A., Cummings, M., and Osorio, C. (2015). Non-Neuronal Acetylcholine: The Missing Link Between Sepsis, Cancer, and Delirium? *Front. Med.* 2:56. doi: 10.3389/fmed.2015.00056

Increased PD-1 Level in Severe Cervical Injury is Associated with the Rare Programmed Cell Death...

59

Shinohara, T., Tanowaki, M., Ishida, Y., Kawaichi, M., and Honjo, T. (1994). Structure and Chromosomal Localization of the Human Pd-1 Gene (Pdcd1). *Genomics* 23, 704–706. doi: 10.1006/geno.1994.1562

Tamura, K., Peterson, D., Peterson, N., Stecher, G., Nei, M., and Kumar, S. (2011). Mega5: Molecular Evolutionary Genetics Analysis Using Maximum Likelihood, Evolutionary Distance, and Maximum Parsimony Methods. *Mol. Biol. Evol.* 28, 2731–2739. doi: 10.1093/molbev/msr121

Tao, L. H., Zhou, X. R., Li, F. C., Chen, Q., Meng, F. Y., Mao, Y., et al. (2017). A Polymorphism in the Promoter Region of PD-L1 Serves as a Binding-Site for SP1 and is Associated With PD-L1 Overexpression and Increased Occurrence of Gastric Cancer. *Cancer Immunol. Immunother.* 66, 309–318. doi: 10.1007/s00262-016-1936-0

The 1000 Genomes Project Consortium. (2015). A global reference for human genetic variation. *Nature* 526, 68–74. doi: 10.1038/nature15393

Tokar, T., Pastrello, C., Rossos, A. E. M., Abovsky, M., Hauschild, A. C., Tsay, M., et al. (2018). MirDIP 4.1 - Integrative Database of Human microRNA Target Predictions. *Nucleic Acids Res.* 46, D360–D370. doi: 10.1093/nar/gkx1144

Wang, Y., Wang, H., Yao, H., Li, C., Fang, J. Y., and Xu, J. (2018). Regulation of PD-L1: Emerging Routes for Targeting Tumor Immune Evasion. *Front. Pharmacol.* 9:536. doi: 10.3389/fphar.2018.00536

Wieser, V., Gaugg, I., Fleischer, M., Shivalingaiah, G., Sprung, S., Lax, S. F., et al. (2018). BRCA1/2 and TP53 Mutation Status Associates With PD-1 and PD-L1 Expression in Ovarian Cancer. *OncoTargets* 9, 17501–17511. doi: 10.18632/oncotarget.24770

World Health Organization (2017). Human papillomavirus Vaccines: WHO Position Paper, May 2017-Recommendations. *Vaccine* 43, 5753–5755. doi: 10.1016/j.vaccine.2017.05.069

Xi, X., Teng, M., Zhang, L., Xia, L., Chen, J., and Cui, Z. (2020). MicroRNA-204-3p Represses Colon Cancer Cells Proliferation, Migration, and Invasion by Targeting HMGA2. *J. Cell Physiol.* 235 (2), 1330–1338. doi: 10.1002/jcp.29050

Yang, W., Lu, Y. P., Yang, Y. Z., Kang, J. R., Jin, Y. D., and Wang, H. W. (2017). Expressions of Programmed Death (PD)-1 and PD-1 Ligand (PD-L1) in Cervical Intraepithelial Neoplasia and Cervical Squamous Cell Carcinomas are of Prognostic Value and Associated With Human Papillomavirus Status. *J. Obstet. Gynaecol. Res.* 43, 1602–1612. doi: 10.1111/jog.13411

Yang, W., Song, Y., Lu, Y. L., Sun, J. Z., and Wang, H. W. (2013). Increased Expression of Programmed Death (PD)-1 and its Ligand PD-L1 Correlates With Impaired Cell-Mediated Immunity in High-Risk Human Papillomavirus-Related Cervical Intraepithelial Neoplasia. *Immunology* 139, 513–522. doi: 10.1111/imm.12101

Zhang, Y., Fan, M., Zhang, X., Huang, F., Wu, K., Zhang, J., et al. (2014). Cellular microRNAs Up-Regulate Transcription Via Interaction With Promoter TATA-box Motifs. *RNA* 20 (12), 1878–1889. doi: 10.1261/rna.045633.114

6

The *SAMHD1* rs6029941 (A/G) Polymorphism Seems to Influence the HTLV-1 Proviral Load and IFN-Alpha Levels

Maria Alice Freitas Queiroz[1], Ednelza da Silva Graça Amoras[1],
Tuane Carolina Ferreira Moura[1], Carlos Araújo da Costa[2], Maisa Silva de Sousa[2],
Sandra Souza Lima[1], Ricardo Ishak[1] and Antonio Carlos Rosário Vallinoto[1]*

[1] Laboratory of Virology, Institute of Biological Sciences, Federal University of Pará, Belém, Brazil, [2] Laboratory of Cellular and Molecular Biology, Tropical Medicine Center, Federal University of Pará, Belém, Brazil

*Correspondence:
Maria Alice Freitas Queiroz
alicefarma@hotmail.com

SAMHD1, a host dNTPase, acts as a retroviral restriction factor by degrading the pool of nucleotides available for the initial reverse transcription of retroviruses, including HTLV-1. Polymorphisms in the *SAMDH1* gene may alter the enzymatic expression and influence the course of infection by the virus. The present study investigated the effect of polymorphisms on HTLV-1 infection susceptibility and on progression to disease in 108 individuals infected by HTLV-1 (47 symptomatic and 61 asymptomatic) and 100 individuals in a control group. *SAMHD1* rs6029941 (G/A) genotyping and HTLV-1 proviral load measurements were performed using real-time PCR and plasma IFN-α was measured by ELISA. Polymorphism frequency was not associated with HTLV-1 infection susceptibility or with the presence of symptoms. The proviral load was significantly higher in symptomatic individuals with the G allele ($p = 0.0143$), which presented lower levels of IFN-α ($p = 0.0383$). *SAMHD1* polymorphism is associated with increased proviral load and reduced levels of IFN-α in symptomatic patients, and may be a factor that contributes to the appearance of disease symptoms.

Keywords: HTLV-1, SAMHD1, polymorphism, IFN-α, symptomatic

INTRODUCTION

HTLV-1 is responsible for the development of HTLV-1-associated myelopathy/tropical spastic paraparesis (HAM/TSP) and adult T-cell leukemia/lymphoma (ATLL) and is associated with other inflammatory syndromes, such as rheumatoid arthritis, dermatitis, and uveitis, in addition to autoimmune diseases (Quaresma et al., 2015). However, most infected individuals do not develop symptoms, and parameters for evaluating the clinical outcome of each carrier remain undefined (Bangham et al., 2015). Therefore, several studies have investigated factors, mainly genetic factors that can elucidate the course of HTLV-1 infection in the onset of infection-related symptoms (Talledo et al., 2010; Assone et al., 2018; Vallinoto et al., 2019).

SAMHD1 is a deoxynucleotide triphosphate triphosphohydrolase (dNTPase) that acts as an intrinsic factor of retroviral restriction, degrading the pool of nucleotides available for the initial reverse transcription, limiting the replication of retroviruses, including HTLV-1 (van Montfoort et al., 2014). Blocking this step prevents the synthesis of double-stranded DNA and disrupts the later stages of the viral replication cycle, including nuclear translocation and integration of DNA into the genome of the host cell (Sze et al., 2013b).

Genetic variations in the *SAMDH1* gene may alter the expression of the enzyme and influence the course of viral infection. A polymorphism in the *SAMHD1* 3′-UTR region, rs6029941 (A/G), seems to alter enzyme expression, where the A allele is associated with higher levels of *SAMHD1* expression and the G polymorphic allele is associated with lower levels (Zhu et al., 2018). In this regard, individuals infected by HTLV-1 with reduced SAMHD1 levels may have a greater proviral load, whereas increased enzyme expression may reduce viral replication and activate a potent type I IFN response, which would enable infection control (van Montfoort et al., 2014). The aim of the present study was to evaluate the effect of the *SAMHD1* polymorphism rs6029941 (A/G) on the proviral load and the development of symptoms of HTLV-1-associated diseases.

MATERIALS AND METHODS

Study Population and Sample Collection

The present study included blood samples from 108 individuals infected with HTLV-1 (22 clinically diagnosed with HAM/TSP, 18 with rheumatic manifestations, 3 with dermatitis, 1 with uveitis, 3 with more than one diagnosis and 61 asymptomatic) treated at the Tropical Medicine Center outpatient clinic of the Federal University of Pará. The patients were of both sexes, were older than 18 years of age and had not been treated with glucocorticoids. The control group included 100 individuals at risk of infection but not infected with the HTLV-1/2, HIV-1, hepatitis B or C, *Chlamydia trachomatis* or syphilis viruses, to compare polymorphism frequencies.

A 10 mL blood sample was collected by intravenous puncture using a vacutainer system containing ethylenediaminetetraacetic acid as an anticoagulant. The samples were centrifuged and separated into plasma and a leukocyte mass. The leukocyte samples were used to extract genomic DNA for analysis of the SAMHD1 rs6029941 (A/G) polymorphism and quantification of the proviral load.

DNA Extraction

DNA was extracted from peripheral blood leukocytes using the Puregene kit (Gentra Systems, Minneapolis, MN, USA) according to the manufacturer's protocol, which included cell lysis, protein precipitation, and DNA precipitation and rehydration. DNA was quantified using a Qubit® 2.0 fluorometer (Life Technologies, Carlsbad, CA, USA) and Qubit™ DNA assay kit reagents (Life Technologies, Carlsbad, CA, USA), following the protocol recommended by the manufacturer.

Quantification of HTLV-1 Proviral Load

Proviral load was quantified using a quantitative real-time PCR using three target sequences, synthesized through the TaqMan® system (Life Technologies, Foster City, CA, USA), according to a previously described protocol (Tamegão-Lopes et al., 2006). Samples containing 5 mL of whole blood were collected for leukocyte DNA extraction, followed by relative quantification using real-time PCR. The results were subsequently adjusted for the absolute proviral quantity, based on leukocyte counts per μL, and expressed as proviral DNA copies/μL.

Genotyping of *SAMHD*1 rs6029941 (A/G)

The polymorphism, located in the UTR3′ region of the gene, was genotyped by real-time PCR using a StepOnePLUS™ Real-Time PCR System. The reaction consisted of a commercial assay (C__29973868_10) containing primers and specific TaqMan® probes for amplification of the target sequence (Thermo Fisher, Carlsbad, California, USA). The reaction contained 1× MasterMix, H_2O, 20× C_11537906_20 assay buffer and 50 ng of DNA, which was subjected to the following cycling conditions: 10 min at 95°C and 40 cycles of 15 s at 95°C and 1 min at 60°C.

Quantification of Plasma IFN-α

Plasma IFN-α was measured by the enzyme-linked immunosorbent assay (ELISA) Invitrogen Human IFN alpha ELISA Kit (ThermoFisher, Carlsbad, CA, USA), which uses specific monoclonal antibodies to detect the cytokine and followed the manufacturer's instructions.

Statistical Analysis

The genotype frequencies were estimated by direct count. The allele frequency was calculated using the formula: F = 2 × number of homozygous individuals + number of heterozygous individuals/total number of individuals. The sum of the two alleles must equal 1. This is the standard form of scientific literature in the field of genetics to describe allele frequencies (the allele frequency described in the table not corresponding to "*n*" and %).

Differences between genotype frequencies observed in the investigated groups were calculated by the χ^2 (chi-square) test. The proviral load and plasma IFN-α were compared between groups using the non-parametric Kruskal-Wallis and Mann-Whitney test. All tests were performed using BioEstat 5.3 software. Associations with $p < 0.05$ were considered statistically significant.

RESULTS

The distributions of the allele and genotype frequencies of the rs6029941 (A>G) polymorphism were similar between individuals infected with HTLV-1 and the control group, with a higher frequency of the polymorphic allele (*SAMDH1**G) in individuals with the virus, but without statistical significance (**Table 1**). Among the infected individuals, no statistically significant difference was observed between the asymptomatic group and the patients with different symptom manifestations (including patients with HAM/TSP, rheumatic manifestations, dermatitis, and uveitis) (**Table 1**).

The proviral load test was performed only on 47 samples and the plasma measurement of IFN-α in 52 samples from individuals infected with HTLV-1, because not all samples were viable for these tests.

The median of proviral load was higher in individuals infected carrying the polymorphic allele (AA: 33.95, AG: 270.1 and GG: 424.2), and significant difference was observed between wild-type and polymorphic genotypes, AG and GG (**Figure 1A**; $p = 0.0100$ and $p = 0.0010$, respectively). In contrast, median IFN-α levels were lower in individuals with polymorphic genotypes

TABLE 1 | Genotype and allele frequencies of *SAMHD1* rs6029941 (A>G) polymorphism among HTLV-1 carriers and in the control group and among asymptomatic and symptomatic HTLV-1 carriers.

Genotypes and alleles	HTLV-1 n = 108 n (%)	Control n = 100 n (%)	p**	Asymptomatic n = 61 n (%)	Symptomatic n = 47 n (%)	p**
AA	48 (33.3)	52 (52.0)	0.3339	25 (41.0)	23 (48.9)	0.5236
AG	41 (50.0)	37 (40.0)		26 (42.6)	15 (31.9)	
GG	19 (16.7)	11 (11.0)		10 (16.4)	09 (19.2)	
*A	0.63	0.71	0.2925	0.62	0.64	0.8836
*G	0.37	0.29		0.38	0.36	

*n, number of individuals. **Chi-square test. *allele.*

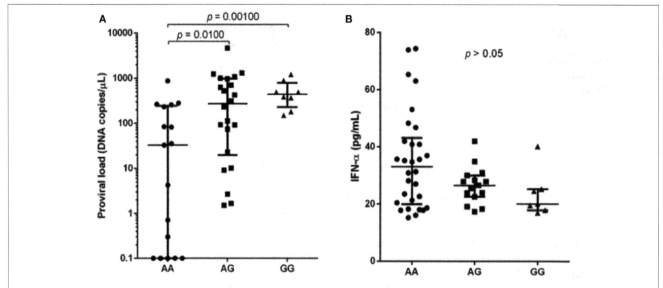

FIGURE 1 | Proviral load **(A)** and IFN-α levels **(B)** among HTLV-1 infected individuals with different genotypes for the SAMHD1 rs6029941 (A > G) polymorphism. Kruskal-Wallis test.

(AA: 33.04, AG: 26.52 and GG: 20.10) but without statistical significance (**Figure 1B**; $p = 0.1246$).

Analyzes of proviral load and IFN-alpha levels were performed among individuals with wild genotype (AA), related to greater expression of SAMHD1, compared to individuals with genotypes expressing the polymorphic allele (*G) in homo and heterozygosis (AG and GG), which are associated with reduced expression of the restriction factor. The viral load was significantly higher in symptomatic individuals with polymorphic genotypes, $p = 0.0143$ (**Figure 2A**), who had lower levels of IFN-α, $p = 0.0383$ (**Figure 2B**). Analysis of the asymptomatic group showed higher median levels of proviral load in individuals with polymorphic genotypes, although it is not statistically significant (**Figure 2C**). There was no difference in IFN-α levels (**Figure 2D**).

DISCUSSION

Restriction factors are important components of innate immunity that recognize specific patterns of retroviruses and inhibit viral replication. The main restriction factors associated with the inhibition of retroviruses include APOBEC3, TRIM5α, Tetherin, and SAMHD1 (Wilkins and Gale, 2010). The SAMHD1 enzyme restricts infection by degrading the pool of nucleotides available for viral reverse transcription. Furthermore, SAMHD1 undergoes specific conformational changes that promote signaling for the production of type I interferon and the expression of proinflammatory cytokines by the infected cell (van Montfoort et al., 2014).

In the present study, the frequency of the *SAMHD1* rs6029941 (A/G) polymorphism was not associated with infection susceptibility or with the presence of HTLV-1-related symptoms. These results may be related to the small sample size used in the study. Although the Amazon region is endemic for HTLV-2 infection, found mainly in the indigenous population (Ishak et al., 2003; Braço et al., 2019), the prevalence of HTLV-1 is low, approximately 0.9% among blood donors (Catalan-Soares et al., 2005). However, the sample size of the study corresponds to the number of patients who are attending the outpatient clinic at the Center for Tropical Medicine at the Federal University of

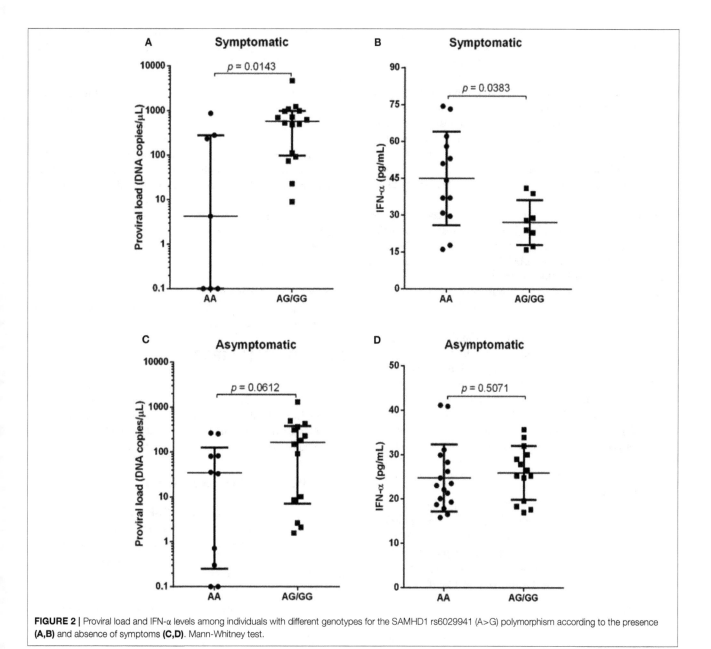

FIGURE 2 | Proviral load and IFN-α levels among individuals with different genotypes for the SAMHD1 rs6029941 (A>G) polymorphism according to the presence **(A,B)** and absence of symptoms **(C,D)**. Mann-Whitney test.

Pará, a place that monitors patients diagnosed with HTLV-1 in the city of Belém.

Another possibility of the lack of association of the frequency of *SAMHD1* rs6029941 (A/G) polymorphism with the symptoms of the diseases is that it may not be associated with the development of symptoms of all types of diseases associated with HTLV-1, because, although they are of inflammatory etiology, they activate different immunological mechanisms (Quaresma et al., 2015). Thus, these data show that frequency analysis alone is not sufficient to determine the influence of polymorphism on the development of HTLV-1 infection. To better assess this relationship, the levels of proviral load and IFN-α were analyzed, and the results showed that polymorphism could act as a possible factor that would contribute to the complex manifestations of the symptoms of the disease.

There was an association between the *SAMHD1* rs6029941 (A/G) polymorphism and variations in the HTLV-1 proviral load. The GG polymorphic genotype, related to lower enzyme levels (Zhu et al., 2018), was associated with a higher proviral load in individuals infected with HTLV-1, regardless of the presence or absence of infection-related symptoms. These results corroborate recent data indicating that this polymorphism reduces SAMHD1 gene expression (Zhu et al., 2018) because reduced SAMHD1 levels favor HTLV-1 replication, which results in an increased proviral load.

The AA genotype, which conferred greater expression of *SAMHD1*, was associated with lower levels of proviral load, which may be related to better control of HTLV-1 replication. Higher levels of SAMHD1 would restrict infection by degradation of the nucleotides pool for reverse transcription. Although it has been demonstrated that HTLV does not appear to be affected by SAMHD1, this finding could be related to a possible escape mechanism of the virus to the restriction factor (Gramberg et al., 2013). However, Sze et al. (2013a) observed that SAMHD1 inhibited reverse transcription in monocytes infected with HTLV-1, leading to the formation of reverse transcription intermediates, responsible for inducing apoptosis and limiting infection. Although the present study did not evaluate a specific type of cells, the results suggest that the polymorphism could favor escape mechanisms of the virus against the control of the innate immune system, influencing the evolution of the infection.

Mutations in the *SAMHD1* gene may alter enzyme synthesis and result in uncontrolled inflammatory responses, mainly mediated through the increased production of type I IFN (Rice et al., 2009). Mutations in the *SAMHD1* gene are associated with an autoimmune disorder through the irregular response of type I IFN, which characterizes Aicardi-Goutières syndrome, in which there is marked production of IL-12 and TNF-α (White et al., 2017).

An important aspect that needs to be considered is the genetic background of the population analyzed in this study, which results from interethnic crossbreeding of Europeans, Indians, and Africans (Santos et al., 2009). Therefore, these preliminary data seem to suggest that the *SAMHD1* rs6029941 (A/G) polymorphism may influence HTLV-1 infection in the evaluated tri-hybrid population. However, because this is the first study that investigated the association of polymorphism in HTLV-1 infection, it will also be necessary to analyze its relationship in other different infected ethnic groups to determine its relevance in other populations.

The choice of the SAMHD1 rs6029941 polymorphism (A/G) was based on its influence on changes in gene expression and because it has not yet been evaluated for HIV and HTLV infection. Although the frequency of polymorphism is not associated with the presence of disease symptoms, it was associated with a higher proviral burden in symptomatic patients,

and patients without symptoms, also had higher levels. Possibly, the polymorphism, related to the lower expression of SAMHD1, could promote less inhibition of reverse transcription, leading to the formation of few reverse transcription intermediates (RTIs) and low type I interferon production, resulting in a more productive infection, with a high proviral load (van Montfoort et al., 2014).

The findings found in the present study suggest that only *SAMHD1* rs6029941 (A/G) polymorphism is not able to induce the progression and worsening of the infection, but it would act as a factor that could increase the proviral load and contribute to the appearance of symptoms. Other studies, including the follow-up of asymptomatic patients with polymorphism, may better clarify its influence on the development of symptoms associated with HTLV-1.

In summary, the results suggest that the *SAMHD1* rs6029941 (A/G) polymorphism is associated with increased HTLV-1 proviral load and lower levels of IFN-α in symptomatic patients. Thus, the polymorphism could contribute to the development of the symptoms of the disease.

ETHICS STATEMENT

The studies involving human participants were reviewed and approved by the Research Ethics Committee of the Health Science Institute of the Federal University of Pará (protocol no. 2872434/2018). The patients/participants provided their written informed consent to participate in this study.

AUTHOR CONTRIBUTIONS

MQ and EA designed the study. TM, CC, and MS provided technical assistance and executed the experiments. MQ, EA, SL, and AV analyzed and interpreted the date. MQ, RI, and AV wrote the manuscript with input from all authors. All authors read and approved the final manuscript.

REFERENCES

Assone, T., Malta, F. M., Bakkour, S., Montalvo, L., Paiva, A. M., Smid, J., et al. (2018). Polymorphisms in HLA-C and KIR alleles are not associated with HAM/TSP risk in HTLV-1-infected subjects. *Virus Res.* 244, 71–74. doi: 10.1016/j.virusres.2017.11.010

Bangham, C. R., Araujo, A., Yamano, Y., and Taylor, G. P. (2015). HTLV-1-associated myelopathy/tropical spastic paraparesis. *Nat. Rev. Dis. Primers* 1:15012. doi: 10.1038/nrdp.2015.23

Braço, I. L. J., de Sá, K. S. G., Waqasi, M., Queiroz, M. A. F., da Silva, A. N. R., Cayres-Vallinoto, I. M. V., et al. (2019). High prevalence of human T-lymphotropic virus 2 (HTLV-2) infection in villages of the Xikrin tribe (Kayapo), Brazilian Amazon region. *BMC Infect. Dis.* 19:459. doi: 10.1186/s12879-019-4041-0

Catalan-Soares, B., Carneiro-Proietti, A. B. F., and Proietti, F. A. (2005). Interdisciplinary HTLV Research Group. Heterogeneous geographic distribution of human T-cell lymphotropic viruses I and II (HTLV-I / II): serological screening prevalence rates in blood donors from large urban areas in Brazil. *Cad. Saúde Pública* 21, 926–931. doi: 10.1590/S0102-311X2005000300027

Gramberg, T., Kahle, T., Bloch, N., Wittmann, S., Müllers, E., Daddacha, W., et al. (2013). Restriction of diverse retroviruses by SAMHD1. *Retrovirology* 10:26. doi: 10.1186/1742-4690-10-26

Ishak, V. A. C. R., Azevedo, V. N., and Guimarães Ishak, M. O. (2003). Epidemiological aspects of retrovirus (HTLV) infection among Indian populations in the Amazon Region of Brazil. *Cad. Saúde Pública* 19, 901–914. doi: 10.1590/S0102-311X2003000400013

Quaresma, J. A., Yoshikawa, G. T., Koyama, R. V., Dias, G. A., Fujihara, S., and Fuzii, H. T. (2015). HTLV-1, immune response and autoimmunity. *Viruses* 8:E5. doi: 10.3390/v8010005

Rice, G. I., Bond, J., Asipu, A., Brunette, R. L., Manfield, I. W., Carr, I. M., et al. (2009). Mutations involved in Aicardi-Goutières syndrome implicate SAMHD1 as regulator of the innate immune response. *Nat. Genet.* 41, 829–832. doi: 10.1038/ng.373

Santos, N. P., Ribeiro-Rodrigues, E. M., Ribeiro-Dos-Santos, A. K., Pereira, R., Gusmão, L., Amorim, A., et al. (2009). Assessing individual interethnic admixture and population substructure using a 48-insertion-deletion (INSEL) ancestry-informative marker (AIM) panel. *Hum. Mutat.* 31, 184–190. doi: 10.1002/humu.21159

Sze, A., Belgnaoui, S. M., Olagnier, D., Lin, R., Hiscott, J., and van Grevenynghe, J. (2013a). Host restriction factor SAMHD1 limits human T cell leukemia virus type 1 infection of monocytes via STING-mediated apoptosis. *Cell Host Microbe* 14, 422–434. doi: 10.1016/j.chom.2013.09.009

Sze, A., Olagnier, D., Lin, R., van Grevenynghe, J., and Hiscott, J. (2013b). SAMHD1 host restriction factor: a link with innate immune sensing of retrovirus infection. *J. Mol. Biol.* 425, 4981–4994. doi: 10.1016/j.jmb.2013.10.022

Talledo, M., López, G., Huyghe, J. R., Verdonck, K., Adaui, V., González, E., et al. (2010). Evaluation of host genetic and viral factors as surrogate markers for HTLV-1-associated myelopathy/tropical spastic paraparesis in Peruvian HTLV-1-infected patients. *J. Med. Virol.* 82, 460–466. doi: 10.1002/jmv.21675

Tamegão-Lopes, B. P., Rezende, P. R., Maradei-Pereira, L. M., and de Lemos, J. A. (2006). HTLV-1 and HTLV-2 proviral load: a simple method using quantitative real-time PCR. *Rev. Soc. Bras. Med. Trop.* 39, 548–552. doi: 10.1590/S0037-86822006000600007

Vallinoto, A. C. R., Cayres-Vallinoto, I., Freitas Queiroz, M. A., Ishak, M. O. G., and Ishak, R. (2019). Influence of immunogenetic biomarkers in the clinical outcome of HTLV-1 infected persons. *Viruses* 11:974. doi: 10.3390/v11110974

van Montfoort, N., Olagnier, D., and Hiscott, J. (2014). Unmasking immune sensing of retroviruses: interplay between innate sensors and host effectors. *Cytokine Growth Factor Rev.* 25, 657–668. doi: 10.1016/j.cytogfr.2014.08.006

White, T. E., Brandariz-Nuñez, A., Martinez-Lopez, A., Knowlton, C., Lenzi, G., Kim, B., et al. (2017). A SAMHD1 mutation associated with aicardi-goutières syndrome uncouples the ability of SAMHD1 to restrict HIV-1 from its ability to downmodulate type I interferon in humans. *Hum. Mutat.* 38, 658–668. doi: 10.1002/humu.23201

Wilkins, C., and Gale, M. Jr. (2010). Recognition of viruses by cytoplasmic sensors. *Curr. Opin. Immunol.* 22, 41–47. doi: 10.1016/j.coi.2009.12.003

Zhu, K. W., Chen, P., Zhang, D. Y., Yan, H., Liu, H., Cen, L. N., et al. (2018). Association of genetic polymorphisms in genes involved in Ara-C and dNTP metabolism pathway with chemosensitivity and prognosis of adult acute myeloid leukemia (AML). *J. Transl. Med.* 16:90. doi: 10.1186/s12967-018-1463-1

Clinical Experience of Personalized Phage Therapy Against Carbapenem-Resistant *Acinetobacter baumannii* Lung Infection in a Patient with Chronic Obstructive Pulmonary Disease

Xin Tan[1†], Huaisheng Chen[2†], Min Zhang[3,4], Ying Zhao[5], Yichun Jiang[2], Xueyan Liu[2], Wei Huang[3,4*] and Yingfei Ma[1*]

[1] Shenzhen Key Laboratory of Synthetic Genomics, Guangdong Provincial Key Laboratory of Synthetic Genomics, CAS Key Laboratory of Quantitative Engineering Biology, Shenzhen Institute of Synthetic Biology, Shenzhen Institute of Advanced Technology, Chinese Academy of Sciences, Shenzhen, China, [2] Department of Critical Care Medicine, Shenzhen People's Hospital (The Second Clinical Medical College of Jinan University, The First Affiliated Hospital of South University of Science and Technology), Shenzhen, China, [3] Shenzhen People's Hospital, Shenzhen Institute of Respiratory Diseases, Shenzhen, China, [4] Bacteriology and Antibacterial Resistance Surveillance Laboratory, Shenzhen People's Hospital (The Second Clinical Medical College, Jinan University, The First Affiliated Hospital, Southern University of Science and Technology), Shenzhen, China, [5] Department of Geriatrics, Shenzhen People's Hospital (The Second Clinical Medical College of Jinan University, The First Affiliated Hospital of South University of Science and Technology), Shenzhen, China

Correspondence:
Yingfei Ma
yingfei.ma@siat.ac.cn
Wei Huang
whuang_sz@163.com

[†] These authors have contributed equally to this work and share first authorship

Overuse of antibiotics in clinical medicine has contributed to the global spread of multidrug-resistant bacterial pathogens, including *Acinetobacter baumannii*. We present a case of an 88-year-old Chinese man who developed hospital-acquired pneumonia caused by carbapenem-resistant *A. baumannii* (CRAB). A personalized lytic pathogen-specific single-phage preparation was nebulized to the patient continuously for 16 days in combination with tigecycline and polymyxin E. The treatment was well tolerated and resulted in clearance of the pathogen and clinical improvement of the patient's lung function.

Keywords: carbapenem-resistant *Acinetobacter baumannii*, lung infection, personalized phage therapy, phage, endotoxin

INTRODUCTION

Infections caused by carbapenem-resistant *Acinetobacter baumannii* (CRAB) impose a major challenge in clinics (Perez et al., 2007; Maragakis and Perl, 2008; Wong et al., 2017). The most common CRAB infections, i.e., hospital-acquired pneumonia (HAP) and bloodstream infections, are often associated with extremely high mortality (Isler et al., 2019). The World Health Organization (WHO) designated CRAB as the critical-priority pathogen in the list of "priority pathogens", a group of bacteria that poses the greatest threat to human health. Novel strategies to treat CRAB infections are urgently needed (Tacconelli et al., 2018).

There have been increased initiatives to develop bacteriophage (phage) as an alternative or supplement to antibiotics in treating CRAB infections (Gordillo Altamirano and Barr, 2019; Kortright et al., 2019). Phage therapy has been applied in personalized therapy, and several examples of the successful treatment of infections caused by CRAB have been reported (Schooley et al., 2017; LaVergne et al., 2018). However, to the best of our knowledge, no case of lung infection with CRAB treated with phage therapy has been reported yet. Here, we present our clinical experience regarding phage therapy to treat CRAB lung infection in an 88-year-old Chinese man.

MATERIALS AND METHODS

Bacterial Strains

Clinical isolates were obtained from routine microbiological cultures of clinical samples: blood and bronchoalveolar lavage fluid (BALF). *A. baumannii* isolates were maintained in Luria-Bertani (LB) broth (Huankai Microbiol, Guangzhou, China) and stored in 15% glycerol at -80°C. Surveillance BALF cultures were screened for carbapenemase-producing (CP) *Enterobacteriales* by enrichment of non-selective LB medium and subsequent inoculation in selective chromogenic mSuperCARBA plate (CHROMagar, Paris, France). Creamy colonies were considered as the CP *A. baumannii* and re-identified by matrix-assisted laser desorption/ionization mass spectrometry (bioMérieux, Marcy-l'Étoile, France). The antimicrobial susceptibility testing was performed with the VITEK-2 compact system (bioMérieux, Marcy-l'Étoile, France). The results were interpreted based on the guidelines published by the Clinical and Laboratory Standards Institute (Institute CaLS, 2016).

Isolation of Phages

Phages used for this treatment were isolated and prepared at Shenzhen Institutes of Advanced Technology. Phages were isolated from various environmental samples by using routine isolation techniques, as previously described (Chen et al., 2018), except the cultures were incubated at 37°C. Briefly, *A. baumannii* clinical isolates obtained from the patient's BALF culture were used to isolate and propagate pathogen-specific phages. Following isolation, the phages were triple plaque-purified on their respective host bacterium. Finally, small-scale phage amplification on their corresponding host bacterium was performed to prepare the *A. baumannii*-specific phage library, which was subsequently stored at 4°C until required.

Phage DNA Extration, Genome Sequencing, and Assembly

Phage particles were precipitated with 10% polyethylene glycol 8,000 (PEG 8000) at 4°C overnight, centrifuged at 10,000x g for 15 min, and subsequently suspended in SM buffer (100 mM NaCl, 8 mM MgSO4, 50 mM Tris-HCl), then the concentrated phage particles were treated using DNase I and RNase A (New England BioLab, Massachusetts, USA) to remove bacterial nucleic acids, genomic phage DNA was extracted with Lambda Bacteriophage

Genomic DNA Rapid Extraction Kit (Aidlab, Beijing, China) following manufacturer's protocol (Chen et al., 2020). Whole-genome sequencing was performed at the Tianjing Sequencing Center (Novogene, Beijing, China) using the Illumina HiSeq system (Illumina Inc., San Diego, CA, USA). Reads were assembled with SOAPdenovo2 (Luo et al., 2012). The resulting contigs were uploaded into the RAST server using the RASTtk annotation workflow (Aziz et al., 2008). Putative functions of the ORFs were further identified with Blast-P based on amino acid sequences. A circular map of the phage was depicted using the CGView Server (Grant and Stothard, 2008).

Transmission Electron Microscopy

20 ul of phage suspension were placed onto a copper grid with carbon film, left for 3 to 5 min, and the excess liquid was removed using filter paper. Staining was performed with 2% phosphotungstic acid for 1 to 2 min, and the cuprum grids were observed under Transmission Electron Microscopy (HT7800, Hitachi, Tokyo, Japan).

Propagation and Purification of Therapeutic Phages

The phage preparations were processed in two different ways. The first batch phage preparation was purified with Amicon Ultra-15 centrifugal filter units (MWCO 100 K Da, Merck Milipore, Massachusetts, USA) (Bonilla et al., 2016). The second phage preparation was purified in a cesium chloride density gradient as previously described (Bachrach and Friedmann, 1971) and then dialyzed using a Spectra/Por RC membrane (MWCO 20 K Da, Spectrum, **New Jersey,** USA) in phosphate-buffered saline to remove cesium chloride. Dialysis reduced the cesium concentration to less than 210 parts per billion, as detected by inductively coupled plasma mass spectrometry (ICP-MS) (Dedrick et al., 2019). Phages were then sterilized through 0.22-µm filters. Then phages were titrated and evaluated for endotoxin with an End-point Chromogenic Endotoxin Test Kit (Bioendo, Xiamen, China). Phage preparations were subsequently stored at 4°C until required. The resulting titers and endotoxin levels were $5x10^8$ PFU/ml and 10^5 EU/ml, respectively, for the first batch, and $5x10^{10}$ PFU/ml and $1.3x10^4$ EU/ml for the second one.

Phage Therapy

The phage preparation was diluted with saline solution to 5 ml and administrated to the patient by a vibrating mesh nebulizer (Aerogen) every 12 h (about 30 min for each dose), except for the first 2 doses, which were given once daily. The first batch phage preparation was used initially for 13 days, then the second phage preparation was administrated for the rest time of phage therapy. See more details in the Results section.

Phage Quantification in Patient Samples

BALF samples were collected for measuring phage counts as follows: 0.5 ml sample was transferred to a 1.5 ml Eppendorf tube and 0.5 ml phage buffer was added. After vortexing, the sample was passed through a 0.22 µm filter, serially diluted, and 10 µl added to *A. baumannii* agar overlays.

RESULTS

Patient Clinical History

In June 2018, an 86-year-old Chinese man was admitted to our hospital for exacerbation of chronic obstructive pulmonary disease (COPD). The medical history of the patient was documented with a long history of type-2 diabetes. The patient suffered recurrent episodes of lung infections associated with repeated use of mechanical ventilation over the last 2 years during hospitalization. After resuscitation from cardiac arrest in April 2019, the patient had difficulty in weaning from mechanical ventilation.

In May 2020, the patient showed signs of lung infection. After almost one month of different episodes of antibiotic therapy (with ceftazidime and ciprofloxacin/amikacin) (**Figure 1A**), the

patient's condition was aggravated. Importantly, in June 2020, the CRAB-positive result of the bronchoalveolar lavage fluid (BALF) culture of this patient drew our attention (**Figure 1A**). The CRAB strains were resistant to all tested antibiotics, except tigecycline and polymyxin E (**Table S1**). Based on these facts, it seemed that the lung infection was most likely caused by this CRAB strain. However, the concentration of tigecycline in the lung is often relatively low (Ramirez et al., 2013). Besides, the patient showed reduced renal function (creatinine clearance at 32.38 ml/min, a normal level is 85–125 ml/min for a healthy male) and the rates of nephrotoxicity with polymyxin E are high (Zavascki and Nation, 2017). These facts indicated that these two antibiotics were not the best choice for the treatment any longer.

Phage therapy is a promising approach for infections caused by multidrug-resistant (MDR) pathogens, several examples of

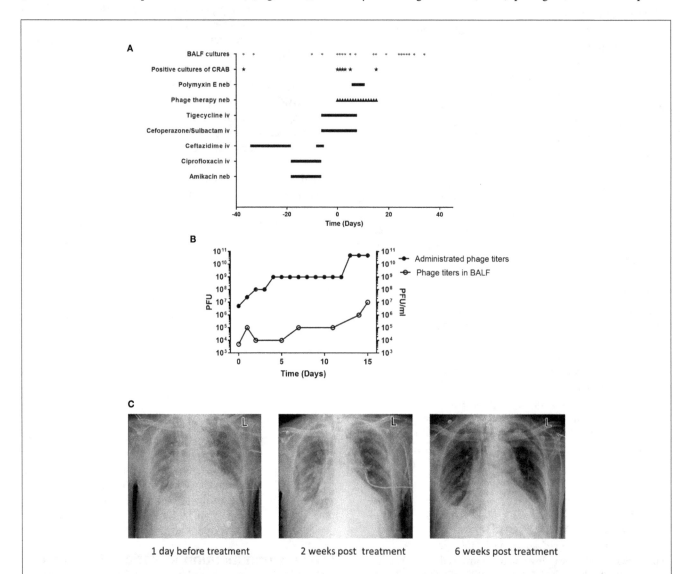

FIGURE 1 | Patient clinical data in phage therapy. **(A)** Timeline of bronchoalveolar lavage fluid (BALF) cultures, drug, and phage administration. BALF samples were collected as indicated (*), positive cultures of carbapenem-resistant *A. baumannii* (CRAB) have been marked (★). The timeline shows the administration of antibiotics and phage preparation, and the administration of drugs is indicated (day 0 indicates the time when phage therapy was initiated). Iv, intravenous; neb, nebulization. **(B)** Administrated phage titers and phage titers in BALF detected by plaque assays following the phage therapy. Left Y-axis represents the administrated phage titers and right Y-axis represents the phage titers in BALF. **(C)** Chest X-rays results on -1st day, 14th and 42nd day of phage treatment, respectively.

the successful treatment of infections caused by CRAB have been reported (Schooley et al., 2017; LaVergne et al., 2018). Hence, phage therapy was initiated upon the local hospital ethics committee's approval and the family's consent for this experimental treatment.

Phage Isolation and Characterization

In mid-June 2020, the *A. baumannii* isolates obtained from the BALF of the patient were sent to the lab of Shenzhen Institutes of Advanced Technology, Chinese Academy of Science for preparing a personalized, lytic phage preparation against the MDR *A. baumannii* strain. Ten *A. baumannii* phages *de novo* isolated from different sewage samples showed antibacterial activity. The phage candidate, Ab_SZ3, which showed the strongest antibacterial activity (according to the clearing of the lysis zone) as measured by spot assay was selected for inclusion in the therapeutic phage preparation (see **Figure S1**). Transmission Electron Microscopy studies were performed on the phage preparation and revealed a homogeneous population of phage particles belonging to the *Siphoviridae* morphological group. The virion revealed an icosahedral head structure of 62.2 nm and a contractile tail of 193.2 nm x 8.4 nm (**Figure 2A**).

Genome Sequence Analysis of Phage Ab_SZ3

The sequence of phage Ab_SZ3 has been deposited in the Genbank databases under accession number MW151244. The length of the phage's genome was 43,070-bp. Sequence-analysis indicated that it is affiliated to the *Caudovirales* order, *Siphoviridae* family, *Lokivirus* genus. This phage shared the highest identity (99% at the nucleotide level) with *Acinetobacter* phage vB_AbaS_D0 (GenBank: MK411820) and IME_AB3 (GenBank: KF811200).

The circular genetic map of Ab_SZ3 can be seen in **Figure 2B**. Analysis of the phage's whole genome shows that it possesses a series of genes encoding common phage-related features, including DNA polymerase, DNA helicase, tail, and head structure proteins. It also possesses two genes encoding the host lysis protein, endolysin, and holin. Importantly, the *in-silico* analysis did not reveal any putative virulence, antibiotic resistance, or integrase sequences in the genome of the phage.

Phage Therapy

Due to the sudden deterioration of the patient's condition, 50 mg tigecycline was given intravenously twice daily for 6 days before the phage therapy. From 16 July 2020, the personalized phage preparation was nebulized using a vibrating mesh nebulizer (Aerogen) to the patient every 12 h, except for the first 2 doses, which were given once daily. Administrated phage dose was gradually increased: day 0 at $5x10^6$ plaque-forming units (PFU), day 1 at $2.5x10^7$ PFU, day 2 at 10^8 PFU, day 4 at 10^9 PFU, and day 13 at $5x10^{10}$ PFU (**Figure 1B**). Intravenously tigecycline was given twice daily during the first 5 days of the phage therapy, then 50 million IU polymyxin E was administered by inhalation (separately from phage) twice daily for the subsequent 5 days. Antibiotic therapy was completely abolished in the following 6 days. The phage therapy lasted for 16 days in total (**Figure 1A**). Phage and bacterial titers in the lung were monitored by collecting BALF samples, and the inflammation factor profile was monitored by collecting blood samples. Phage particles were detected in BALF 1 h after the treatment started and reached with a titer of $5x10^3$ PFU/ml; phage titer gradually increased in BALF and had a relatively high phage titer (10^7 PFU/ml) in 15 days. This observation was consistent with the fact of increased administration dose of the phage (**Figure 1B**). Besides, it also suggested phage replication *in situ*.

Phage-resistant bacteria were isolated from BALF samples on day 2 and day 3 after phage therapy. However, it is plausible that phage-resistance could have been associated with fitness trade-offs.

Remarkably, on the 7th day of the phage therapy, for the first time, a culture of BALF did not yield any CRAB. From then on, and until the time of writing (January 2021), except for one culture of BALF on the 15th day of the phage therapy that was positive for CRAB (the isolate remains susceptible to phage Ab_SZ3, see Supplementary Material), all cultures from the patient's sputum/BALF were negative for CRAB (**Figure 1A**).

Importantly, the patient restored sinus rhythm on the 8th day after the phage therapy. Furthermore, the bilateral consolidations shown on pre-treatment chest X-rays (**Figure 1C**) gradually disappeared and the lung function improved. Additionally, the inflammation factor profile and the clinical signs of the patient showed no significant side-effect after phage therapy (**Figure 3**).

Patient Follow-up

In 1 month following phage therapy interruption, the patient was still hospitalized due to the difficulty in weaning from mechanical ventilation. The patient developed 1 episode of sepsis in August 2020, blood culture was positive for *Enterococcus faecium* and *Staphylococcus haemolyticus*, vancomycin was subsequently administered for 15 days. The patient also had 1 episode of a non-MDR *Pseudomonas aeruginosa* strain colonization during this period, although multiple BALF cultures were positive for *P. aeruginosa*, no clinical signs of respiratory infection were observed. Due to the patient's history of recurrent respiratory infections, amikacin was applied for the decolonization of the *P. aeruginosa* strain (see **Figure S2**). Despite the prolonged, antibiotic-driven selective pressure on the patient's lung microbiota and the protracted hospitalizations, we did not observe a reappearance of the CRAB. Till the time of writing (January 2021), the patient remains in stable condition.

DISCUSSION

To ensure the patient's safety, we started the phage therapy with relatively low phage concentrations compared to other studies (LaVergne et al., 2018; Dedrick et al., 2019). Due to the urgent need for efficacious products for the patient, we undertook a fast way to prepare the personalized phage preparation, in which the endotoxins level remained relatively high (10^5 EU/ml). However, we took the purified phage preparation (endotoxin levels at $1.3 x 10^4$ EU/ml) for treatment in the days that followed. Under the FDA-recommended endotoxin lipopolysaccharide limit of 5 EU/kg body

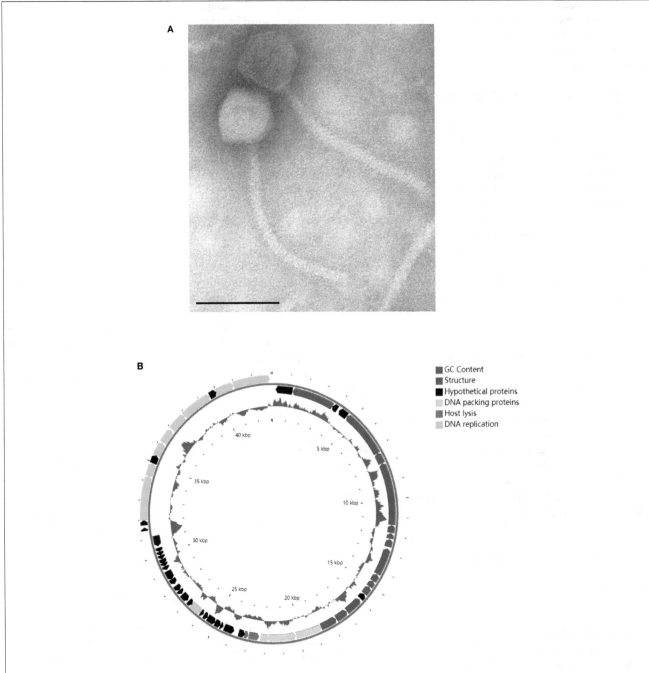

FIGURE 2 | Characterization of phage Ab_SZ3. **(A)** Transmission electron micrographs of the phage. Scale bar represents 100 nm. **(B)** Genome map of the phage. The color of the ORFs refers to five modules: phage structure, blue; host lysis, red; DNA packaging, light blue; DNA replication, green; and hypothetical proteins, black. GC content, purple.

weight per hour (LaVergne et al., 2018), we gave a relatively low dose of phages initially. Despite this, the endotoxin level in the phage preparation did not stricly follow the FDA recommendation. Our preparation was given by respiratory route instead of the intravenous route. Interestingly, the systemic inflammation factor profile and the clinical signs of the patient showed no significant side-effect after phage therapy. Our result indicates that a higher endotoxin level of the phage preparation for the respiratory route was tolerated in this COPD patient. However, these observations were not consistent with another study, where inhalation of nearly 5×10^4 EU of purified endotoxin were initially well tolerated by COPD patients, who then presented slightly increased systemic inflammation profiles at 24 h (Gupta et al., 2015). We presume that a non-significant change of systemic inflammation after exposure to the relatively high level of endotoxin could be due to this patient's special condition: age at 88-year-old and history of recurrent infection. Nonetheless, the standards of endotoxin level in phage preparation for clinical use require further investigation.

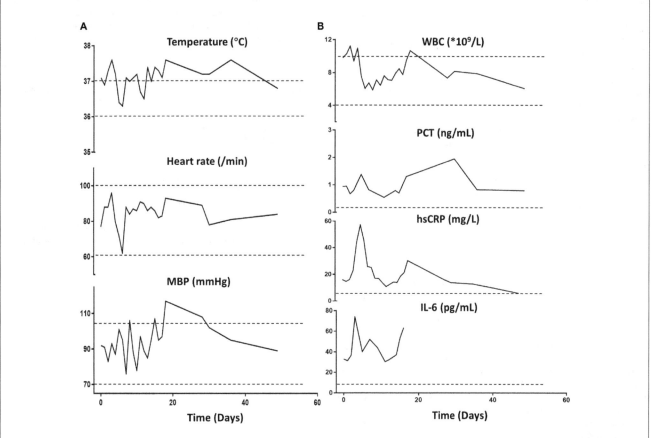

FIGURE 3 | Patient's clinical examination **(A)** and inflammatory factor profile **(B)**. No major alterations were observed (day 0 indicates the time when phage therapy was initiated). MBP, Mean blood pressure; WBC, white blood cells; PCT, procalcitonin; hs-CRP, high-sensitivity C-reactive protein. Normal ranges are presented between dotted lines in temperature, heart rate, MBP, and WBC; normal ranges are below the dotted line for PCT, hsCRP, and Il-6.

One of the major concerns regarding phage therapy is that phage-resistant bacteria might cause the failure of phage therapy (Oechslin, 2018). Herein, it is plausible that phage-resistance is associated with severe growth defect. Indeed, the trade-off between phage-resistance and fitness, such as antibiotic susceptibility or growth rate, has been reported elsewhere (Le et al., 2014; Gordillo Altamirano et al., 2021). In our opinion, the emergence of phage-resistance is an argument supporting the effective action of phages at the site of infection, since it implies that phages were able to provide a sufficiently-strong evolutionary pressure. This patient also received antibiotics that the strain was sensitive against during the phage therapy, we cannot exclude the role of antibiotics in the eradication of this pathogen. However, patients with similar clinical conditions typically have high morbidity and mortality under antibiotic monotherapy (Inchai et al., 2015). We also observed evidence suggesting phage replication *in situ*, as well as emergence of phage-resistant mutants. We therefore believe that phage therapy contributed to the clinical improvement of the patient.

In summary, this case demonstrates the clinical efficacy and safety of phage therapy in combination with antibiotics in the treatment of CRAB lung infection with COPD. However, more questions in molecular mechanisms (such as phage receptor, phage resistance, and immunogenicity of phage) involved in phage therapy remain unclear, and phage therapy deserves further evaluation in well-designed clinical trials in the era of increasing antimicrobial resistance.

ETHICS STATEMENT

The studies involving human participants were reviewed and approved by The Shenzhen People's Hospital Medical Ethics Committee. The patients/participants provided their written informed consent to participate in this study.

AUTHOR CONTRIBUTIONS

XT, HC, WH, and YM conceived and designed the study. XT, HC, and MZ performed the experiments and analysis. MZ and WH contributed with data and analysis. XT wrote the manuscript, with contributions and comments from all authors. All authors contributed to the article and approved the submitted version.

ACKNOWLEDGMENTS

We thank Prof. Hongping Wei and Dr. Junping Yu at the Wuhan Institute of Virology for their advice in this study. We thank Mr. Shunhui Lin for providing sewage water.

REFERENCES

Aziz, R. K., Bartels, D., Best, A. A., DeJongh, M., Disz, T., Edwards, R. A., et al. (2008). The RAST Server: rapid annotations using subsystems technology. *BMC Genomics* 9, 75.

Bachrach, U., and Friedmann, A. (1971). Practical procedures for the purification of bacterial viruses. *Appl. Microbiol.* 22 (4), 706–715.

Bonilla, N., Rojas, M. I., Netto Flores Cruz, G., Hung, S. H., Rohwer, F., and Barr, J. J. (2016). Phage on tap-a quick and efficient protocol for the preparation of bacteriophage laboratory stocks. *PeerJ.* 4, e2261.

Chen, L., Yuan, S., Liu, Q., Mai, G., Yang, J., Deng, D., et al. (2018). In Vitro Design and Evaluation of Phage Cocktails Against Aeromonas salmonicida. *Front. Microbiol.* 9, 1476.

Chen, L., Liu, Q., Fan, J., Yan, T., Zhang, H., Yang, J., et al. (2020). Characterization and Genomic Analysis of ValSw3-3, a New Siphoviridae Bacteriophage Infecting Vibrio alginolyticus. *J. Virol.* 94 (10), e00066–e00020.

Dedrick, R. M., Guerrero-Bustamante, C. A., Garlena, R. A., Russell, D. A., Ford, K., Harris, K., et al. (2019). Engineered bacteriophages for treatment of a patient with a disseminated drug-resistant Mycobacterium abscessus. *Nat. Med.* 25 (5), 730–733.

Gordillo Altamirano, F. L., and Barr, J. J. (2019). Phage Therapy in the Postantibiotic Era. *Clin. Microbiol. Rev.* 32 (2), e00066–e00018.

Gordillo Altamirano, F., Forsyth, J. H., Patwa, R., Kostoulias, X., Trim, M., Subedi, D., et al. (2021). Bacteriophage-resistant Acinetobacter baumannii are resensitized to antimicrobials. *Nat. Microbiol.* 6 (2), 157–161.

Grant, J. R., and Stothard, P. (2008). The CGView Server: a comparative genomics tool for circular genomes. *Nucleic Acids Res.* 36 (Web Server issue), W181–W184.

Gupta, V., Banyard, A., Mullan, A., Sriskantharajah, S., Southworth, T., and Singh, D. (2015). Characterization of the inflammatory response to inhaled lipopolysaccharide in mild to moderate chronic obstructive pulmonary disease. *Br. J. Clin. Pharmacol.* 79 (5), 767–776.

Inchai, J., Pothirat, C., Bumroongkit, C., Limsukon, A., Khositsakulchai, W., and Liwsrisakun, C. (2015). Prognostic factors associated with mortality of drug-resistant Acinetobacter baumannii ventilator-associated pneumonia. *J. Intensive Care* 3, 9.

Institute CaLS (2016). *Performance standards for antimicrobial susceptibility testing; twenty-sixth informational supplement. CLSI document M100-S26* (Wayne, PA: Clinical and Laboratory Standards Institute).

Isler, B., Doi, Y., Bonomo, R. A., and Paterson, D. L. (2019). New Treatment Options against Carbapenem-Resistant Acinetobacter baumannii Infections. *Antimicrob. Agents Chemother.* 63 (1), e01110–e01118.

Kortright, K. E., Chan, B. K., Koff, J. L., and Turner, P. E. (2019). Phage Therapy: A Renewed Approach to Combat Antibiotic-Resistant Bacteria. *Cell Host Microbe* 25 (2), 219–232.

LaVergne, S., Hamilton, T., Biswas, B., Kumaraswamy, M., Schooley, R. T., and Wooten, D. (2018). Phage Therapy for a Multidrug-Resistant Acinetobacter baumannii Craniectomy Site Infection. *Open Forum Infect. Dis.* 5 (4), ofy064.

Le, S., Yao, X., Lu, S., Tan, Y., Rao, X., Li, M., et al. (2014). Chromosomal DNA deletion confers phage resistance to Pseudomonas aeruginosa. *Sci. Rep.* 4, 4738.

Luo, R., Liu, B., Xie, Y., Li, Z., Huang, W., Yuan, J., et al. (2012). SOAPdenovo2: an empirically improved memory-efficient short-read de novo assembler. *Gigascience.* 1 (1), 18.

Maragakis, L. L., and Perl, T. M. (2008). Acinetobacter baumannii: epidemiology, antimicrobial resistance, and treatment options. *Clin. Infect. Dis.* 46 (8), 1254–1263.

Oechslin, F. (2018). Resistance Development to Bacteriophages Occurring during Bacteriophage Therapy. *Viruses.* 10 (7), 351.

Perez, F., Hujer, A. M., Hujer, K. M., Decker, B. K., Rather, P. N., and Bonomo, R. A. (2007). Global challenge of multidrug-resistant Acinetobacter baumannii. *Antimicrob. Agents Chemother.* 51 (10), 3471–3484.

Ramirez, J., Dartois, N., Gandjini, H., Yan, J. L., Korth-Bradley, J., and McGovern, P. C. (2013). Randomized phase 2 trial to evaluate the clinical efficacy of two high-dosage tigecycline regimens versus imipenem-cilastatin for treatment of hospital-acquired pneumonia. *Antimicrob. Agents Chemother.* 57 (4), 1756–1762.

Schooley, R. T., Biswas, B., Gill, J. J., Hernandez-Morales, A., Lancaster, J., Lessor, L., et al. (2017). Development and Use of Personalized Bacteriophage-Based Therapeutic Cocktails To Treat a Patient with a Disseminated Resistant Acinetobacter baumannii Infection. *Antimicrob. Agents Chemother.* 61 (10), e00954–e00917.

Tacconelli, E., Carrara, E., Savoldi, A., Harbarth, S., Mendelson, M., Monnet, D. L., et al. (2018). Discovery, research, and development of new antibiotics: the WHO priority list of antibiotic-resistant bacteria and tuberculosis. *Lancet Infect. Dis.* 18 (3), 318–327.

Wong, D., Nielsen, T. B., Bonomo, R. A., Pantapalangkoor, P., Luna, B., and Spellberg, B. (2017). Clinical and Pathophysiological Overview of Acinetobacter Infections: a Century of Challenges. *Clin. Microbiol. Rev.* 30 (1), 409–447.

Zavascki, A. P., and Nation, R. L. (2017). Nephrotoxicity of Polymyxins: Is There Any Difference between Colistimethate and Polymyxin B? *Antimicrob. Agents Chemother.* 61 (3), e02319–e02316.

8

Characterization of an *Enterococcus faecalis* Bacteriophage vB_EfaM_LG1 and its Synergistic Effect with Antibiotic

Min Song, Dongmei Wu, Yang Hu, Haiyan Luo and Gongbo Li *

Department of Neurology, The Second Affiliated Hospital of Chongqing Medical University, Chongqing, China

Correspondence:
Gongbo Li
ligongbo@hospital.cqmu.edu.cn

Enterococcus faecalis is a Gram-positive opportunistic pathogen that could cause pneumonia and bacteremia in stroke patients. The development of antibiotic resistance in hospital-associated *E. faecalis* is a formidable public health threat. Bacteriophage therapy is a renewed solution to treat antibiotic-resistant bacterial infections. However, bacteria can acquire phage resistance quite quickly, which is a significant barrier to phage therapy. Here, we characterized a lytic *E. faecalis* bacteriophage Vb_EfaM_LG1 with lytic activity. Its genome did not contain antibiotic resistance or virulence genes. Vb_EfaM_LG1 effectively inhibits *E. faecalis* growth for a short period, and phage resistance developed within hours. However, the combination of antibiotics and phage has a tremendous synergistic effect against *E. faecalis*, prevents the development of phage resistance, and disrupts the biofilm efficiently. Our results show that the phage-antibiotic combination has better killing efficiency against *E. faecalis*.

Keywords: bacteriophage, phage-antibiotic combination, *Enterococcus faecalis*, antibiotic resistance, phage therapy

INTRODUCTION

Enterococci are Gram-positive facultative anaerobes, examples of which include *E. faecalis* and *Enterococcus faecium*, which cause bacteremia, pneumonia, endocarditis, and urinary tract infections (Beganovic et al., 2018; Jabbari Shiadeh et al., 2019). In addition, *E. faecalis* is also one of the major pathogens for pneumonia and bacteremia in stroke patients, and the infection after stroke could lead to the death of the stroke patient (Hannawi et al., 2013; Dyal and Sehgal, 2015; Stanley et al., 2016). Moreover, the intrinsic and acquired antibiotic resistance of *Enterococci* is a formidable public health threat (Arias et al., 2011; Banla et al., 2018). *Enterococci* have evolved extensive drug resistance, including that to vancomycin, and could transmit antibiotic resistance among diverse bacteria (Palmer et al., 2010). Therefore, new therapeutic approaches are needed to treat *Enterococcal*-associated infections (Khalifa et al., 2015; Kortright et al., 2019; Bao et al., 2020).

Phages are viruses that infect and kill bacteria and are used to treat antibiotic-resistant bacteria (Barbu et al., 2016; Kortright et al., 2019; Dion et al., 2020). Phage therapy has several advantages over antibiotics. First, phages have a particular host range and only infect the targeted bacterium, so phage therapy would not affect other bacteria and did not interrupt the commensal microbes (Waters et al., 2017). Second, because of the different phage resistance and antibiotic resistance mechanisms in bacteria, phages could infect multidrug-resistant superbugs. Thus, phage therapy is being proceeded in many countries (Jault et al., 2018; Leitner et al., 2021).

Currently, numerous phages against pathogens had been characterized; however, there are only 63 sequenced *E. faecalis* bacteriophage deposited in NCBI (Chatterjee et al., 2021), which is relatively understudied compared with phages that infect other pathogens, such as *Pseudomonas aeruginosa* or *Staphylococcus aureus* phages (De Smet et al., 2017). More phages need to be characterized to provide more therapeutic options for treating the multidrug-resistant *E. faecalis*. Moreover, phage resistance is quite common for *E. faecalis*, which could be quickly selected because of the mutations of cell wall-associated polysaccharide or membrane protein (Duerkop et al., 2016; Banla et al., 2018; Chatterjee et al., 2019). Thus, a better strategy to hinder phage resistance should be investigated. In this study, we identified a phage infecting a broad range of *E. faecalis* strains and proved that phage-antibiotic synergism effectively inhibits phage resistance and disrupts biofilm.

RESULTS

The Biology of an *E. faecalis* Phage

A phage was isolated from the hospital sewage using *E. faecalis* strain ef118 as a host. It forms an obvious plaque on the host in the double layer agar plates (**Figure 1A**). The phage particle was extracted from the bacterial lysate and was observed by transmission electron microscopy. The head of the phage is a regular icosahedral structure with a diameter of approximately 80 nm, and it has a contractable tail with a length of approximately 110 nm (**Figure 1B**). Thus, the morphology of this phage conforms to the characteristics of the Myoviridae family, and it is named *Enterococcus faecalis* phage vB_EfaM_LG1 (refer as LG1 hereafter).

The phage titer reached the highest as 4×10^9 PFU/ml when the multiplicity of infection (MOI) was 0.001, the optimal MO of bacteriophage LG1 was 0.001 (**Figure 1C**). The one-step growth curve of LG1 was shown in **Figure 1D**. The latent phase was approximately 10 min, and then the titer of phages increased rapidly between 10 and 20 min, indicating a lysis period of approximately 20 min. The burst size was estimated as about 40 pfu per bacterium.

The adsorption rate of LG1 onto the host strain was determined by measuring the remaining phages in the supernatant. LG1 absorbed onto the host ef118 efficiently, and over 50% of the phage particles were adsorbed by the ef118 within 5 min, and approximately 80% of the phage could bind to the host within 20 min (**Figure 1E**).

Spot agar assays were performed to determine the phage infectivity against 10 *E. faecalis* clinically isolated strains. The formation of clear plaques indicates that the strain is sensitive to LG1, whereas the formation of blurred plaque or no spots is considered non-sensitive. LG1 infects 50% of the clinical isolated *E. faecalis* strains, representing a relatively broad host range, but LG1 cannot infect any *E. faecium* strain (**Table 1**).

Sequencing Analysis of an *E. faecalis* Phage LG1

Phage LG1 is a double-stranded (ds) DNA phage with a linear genome of 150,025 base pairs (bp). Its G + C content is 35.88%, and the genome is visualized by CPT Phage Galaxy (Ramsey et al., 2020).

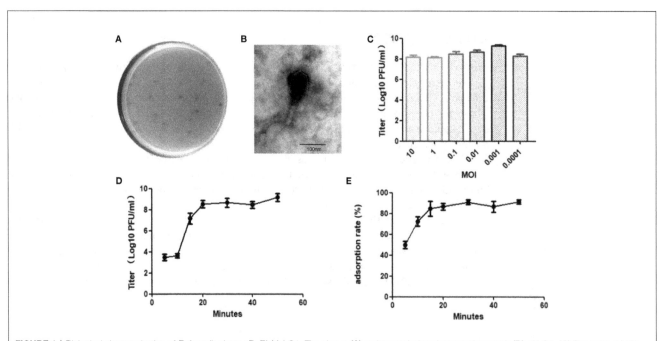

FIGURE 1 | Biological characterization of *E. faecalis* phage vB_EfaM_LG1. The plaque **(A)** and transmission electron micrograph **(B)** of LG1. **(C)** The optimal MOI test of phage. **(D)** The one-step growth curve of LG1. **(E)** The adsorption rate of LG1 against host strain ef118 within 60 min.

TABLE 1 | The host range of phage LG1.

Strain	Origin	LG1 sensitivity
Enterococcus faecalis ef118	Blood	+
Enterococcus faecalis ef122	Blood	−
Enterococcus faecalis ef153	Blood	−
Enterococcus faecalis ef177	Blood	+
Enterococcus faecalis ef134	Blood	+
Enterococcus faecalis ef189	Urine	−
Enterococcus faecalis ef101	Urine	+
Enterococcus faecalis ef116	Urine	−
Enterococcus faecalis ef126	Urine	+
Enterococcus faecalis ef148	Urine	−
Enterococcus faecium ef13	Blood	−
Enterococcus faecium ef14	Urine	−
Enterococcus faecium ef15	Blood	−
Enterococcus faecium ef16	Urine	−

+ indicates the strain is sensitive to phage LG1 and forms clear plaque; − indicates the strain is not sensitive to phage LG1.

There are 231 putative ORFs predicted by RAST (Overbeek et al., 2014), whereas most of the ORFs are functionally unknown. Also, LG1 encodes five tRNA genes. The annotated ORFs can be categorized into several functional modules, including phage replications, DNA metabolism/modifications, lysis, phage structural protein (**Figure 2**). LG1 encodes multiple ribonucleotide reductases, implying that LG1 could perform *de novo* DNA biosynthesis. Moreover, no antibiotic-resistant genes or virulence genes were predicted in the genome of LG1. BlastN searches of the non-redundant database at NCBI reveals that LG1 genome exhibits 90% to 98% nucleotide identity with a group of enterococcal phages, such as *Enterococcus* phage ECP3 and vB_EfaM_Ef2.1.

Stability of LG1

The optimal pH for storing LG1 was 7, and its viability was lost entirely when the pH was lower than 4 or higher than 11 (**Figure 3A**). The phage titers were further monitored when

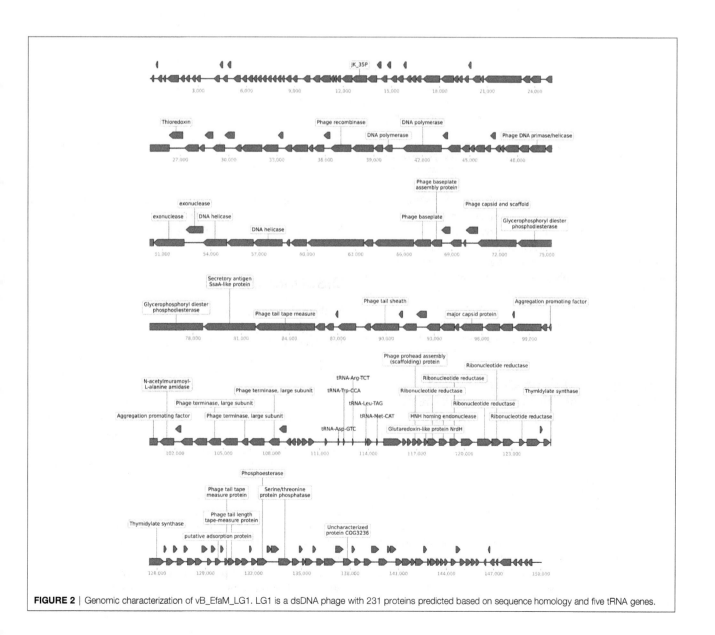

FIGURE 2 | Genomic characterization of vB_EfaM_LG1. LG1 is a dsDNA phage with 231 proteins predicted based on sequence homology and five tRNA genes.

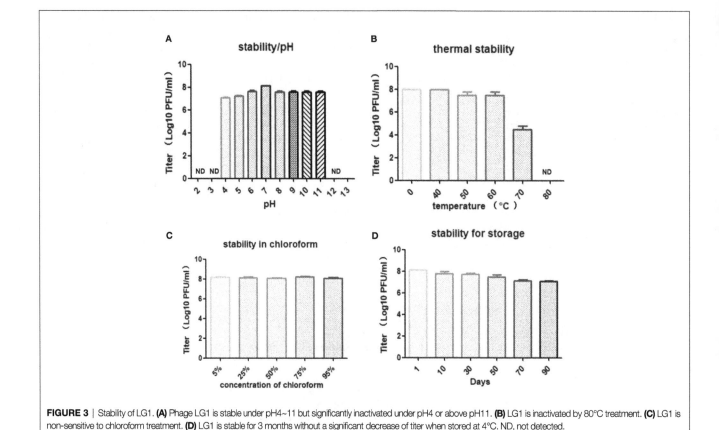

FIGURE 3 | Stability of LG1. **(A)** Phage LG1 is stable under pH4~11 but significantly inactivated under pH4 or above pH11. **(B)** LG1 is inactivated by 80°C treatment. **(C)** LG1 is non-sensitive to chloroform treatment. **(D)** LG1 is stable for 3 months without a significant decrease of titer when stored at 4°C. ND, not detected.

LG1 was incubated at different temperatures. It was found to be stable at different temperatures, maintained a titer of 10^5 after 60 min incubation at 70°C (**Figure 3B**), and was wholly inactivated over 80°C. Besides, chloroform treatment did not affect the phage titer, precluding the presence of lipid components on the phage surface (**Figure 3C**). Finally, the chloroform-treated phage was stored at 4°C, and its titer was monitored for 3 months (**Figure 3D**). And the titer of LG1 did not significantly decrease during this period, indicating LG1 was relatively stable at 4°C, and this feature is vital to produce phage agents.

The Phage-Antibiotic Combination Significantly Inhibits the Development of Phage Resistance and Disrupts the Biofilm

Phage resistance is quickly developed and is selected *in vitro* and *in vivo* (Labrie et al., 2010). And phage resistance in *E. faecalis* can be achieved through mutations of the receptors on the cell surface (Duerkop et al., 2016). As expected, in the liquid culture, phage LG1 was added to the log phase ef118 (OD600 = 0.5) to a final titer of 5×10^8 pfu/ml, and LG1 could only inhibit *E. faecalis* ef118 for several hours, and phage-resistant mutants regrow to a high density within 24 h (**Figure 4A**). The sensitive antibiotic cefotaxime (32 µg/ml) could inhibit the ef118, but the phage-antibiotic combination shows the best killing efficiency (**Figure 4A**). And in the *in vitro* biofilm model, cefotaxime (32 µg/ml) is less effective in disrupting the established biofilm

than phage ($5*10^8$ pfu/ml) alone, and the phage-antibiotic combination has a more significant effect in disrupting the biofilm than single treatment (**Figure 4B**).

DISCUSSION

With an ever-increasing amount of antibiotic-resistant strains of *E. faecalis* found in clinical and the difficulties in the treatment of those caused by the biofilm formation (Arias et al., 2011; Palmer et al., 2011). A better strategy to constrain *E. faecalis* infection is needed more than ever, and lytic bacteriophage is a promising alternative treatment to fight multidrug-resistant *E. faecalis* (Al-Zubidi et al., 2019). In this study, we isolated a dsDNA phage LG1, which effectively infects *E. faecalis* strains with a relatively broad host range. Transmission electron microscopy showed that the phage belongs to the Myoviridae family, and its genome sequence exhibited similarity to other *E. faecalis* phages in the Myoviridae family.

Phage stability is an essential parameter for manufacturing phage agents (Pires et al., 2020). In Phagoburn project, researchers found that the phage cocktail is significantly inactivated because of long-term storage, and the phage titer is as low as 10^2 pfu/ml per daily dose, which is one of the reasons for the failure of this phage therapy clinical trial (Jault et al., 2018). LG1 is stable under different conditions, including heat and pH, and it can be stored at 4°C without significant loss of the

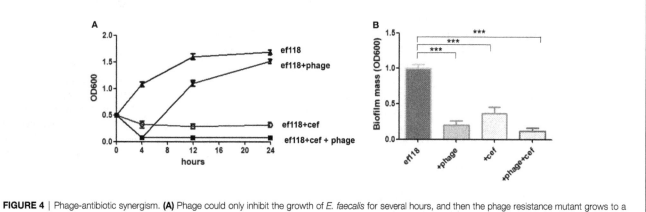

FIGURE 4 | Phage-antibiotic synergism. **(A)** Phage could only inhibit the growth of *E. faecalis* for several hours, and then the phage resistance mutant grows to a high density. **(B)** The phage-antibiotic combination has better efficacy in destroying the biofilm than phage or antibiotic alone (***$P < 0.05$).

titer for 3 months, which is an important parameter when LG1 is included in a phage cocktail agent.

Phage resistance is also an issue in phage therapy. Because bacteria are able to obtain phage resistance because of various mechanisms, including mutations of the receptor, restriction and modification systems, CRISPR-cas systems (Labrie et al., 2010; Goldfarb et al., 2015; Shen et al., 2018b; Azam and Tanji, 2019), and phage resistance have been reported in phage therapy cases (El Haddad et al., 2019; Bao et al., 2020), which is a severe issue in phage therapy. *E. faecalis* phage resistance has been investigated previously, mainly through the mutation of phage receptor, including membrane protein PIP for phage phiVPE25 (Duerkop et al., 2016) and enterococcal polysaccharide antigen for phage (Chatterjee et al., 2019). Various approaches had been suggested to inhibit the development of phage resistance. Phage-antibiotic is the well-acknowledged method in treating other pathogens, such as *P. aeruginosa* (Oechslin et al., 2017). This study also suggests that phage-antibiotic combination is a better strategy to treat *E. faecalis* infection.

Formation of biofilm is a severe issue in infections because the established biofilm is extremely difficult to disrupt, and the biofilm increases antibiotic resistance (Pires et al., 2017). Phage effectively disrupts biofilm because phage could penetrate the biofilm, and some phage encodes depolymerase to degrade the biofilm matrix to destroy further the biofilm. Depolymerases can be associated with the phage particle or be released during lysis of the host bacteria. Depolymerases are enzymes to degrade the extracellular polysaccharide. Therefore, it is particularly interesting in the removal of biofilms. (Wu et al., 2019; Ferriol-Gonzalez and Domingo-Calap, 2020).

Moreover, this experiment shows phage-antibiotic combination has better effects in treating biofilms, which would be a better approach to treat chronic *E. faecalis* when biofilm might have already formed. The phage-antibiotic synergism is mainly because of the different antibacterial targets. And under certain conditions, phages provide an adjuvating effect by lowering the minimum inhibitory concentration for drug-resistant strains to enhancing the effect of antibiotics (Liu et al., 2020). Overall, these data indicate phage-

antibiotic synergism has better treating efficiency than single phage therapy.

Experimental Procedures

Bacterial Strains, Phages, and Culture Conditions

The bacterial strains in this work were listed in **Table 1**. *Enterococcus* strains were collected from the Department of Clinical Laboratory Medicine and grown aerobically on Luria-Bertani (LB) broth at 37°C.

Bacteriophage LG1 was isolated from hospital sewage as previously described (Duerkop et al., 2016). Briefly, the sewage was pelleted, and the supernatant was filtered through a 0.45-μm pore-size filter to remove particles. Then, 50-μl sample was immediately mixed with 200 μl bacterial culture, and 4 ml of molten LB soft agar (0.7%) was added and poured onto LB agar plates, followed by overnight culture. Any formed plaque was picked using a pipette, deposited in 1 ml of LB, followed by 10-fold dilution, and double-layer agar assay to purify the phage. The phage was purified by three consecutive rounds. Then, one plaque from the third round was picked for this study.

Transmission Electron Microscopy

Phage particles were dropped on carbon-coated copper grids for 10 min. Then phosphotungstic acid (pH 7.0) was used to stain the sample for 15 s and examined under a Philips EM 300 electron microscope. The sizes of the phage were measured based on five randomly selected images using AxioVision LE.

Phage Titering and MOI Experiment

Phage titer was calculated by standard double-layer agar plate assay. Briefly, 10-fold dilutions of phage suspension were mixed with 200 μl host bacteria, then mixed with 5 ml molten 0.7% LB agar broth. Then poured on a 1.5% agar plate. After overnight incubation at 37°C, one plaque is calculated as a plaque-forming unit (pfu). MOI experiments were performed by mixing log-phase bacteria (OD600 = 0.5) with a different number of phages, and the coculture was incubated at 37°C with shaking for 5 h. Then the titer in the supernatant was calculated using a double-layer agar plate assay.

One-Step Growth

The one-step growth curve of LG1 was determined as described (Zhong et al., 2020). Briefly, 1 ml of log-phase bacteria and 1 ml of LG1 were mixed at an MOI of 1 and incubated at 37°C for 3 min. Then, the mixture was centrifuged at 4°C for 2min at a speed of 12,000g, and the pellet was resuspended in 10 ml LB medium. And samples were taken at the given time points, which are immediately pelleted, and phage titer in the supernatant was measured by directly using double-layer plate assay.

Adsorption Rate Experiments

Bacteriophage adsorption assay with various time points was performed as previously described (Al-Zubidi et al., 2019). Briefly, the log phase bacterial cultures were pelleted and resuspended in LB medium to a final concentration of 5×10^8 CFU/ml. Then, phage was added to a final titer of 5×10^5 pfu/ml. Then, the samples were cultured at 37°C for 60 min, and a 1-ml sample was collected at the set time point and centrifuged at 16,000g for 1 min. The phages in the supernatant were titered using the double-agar plating assays. At a given time point, the adsorption rate was calculated as (the original phage titer − the remaining phage titer)/the original phage titer.

Determination of Host Range

Ten *E. faecalis* and five *E. faecium* strains were selected as test strains. The host range of phage LG1 was determined using spot testing by dropping 1 μl of phage onto the double-layer soft agar premixed with the test strain and cultured at 37°C for 18 h. The formation of a clear plaque is considered as the sensitive host for phage LG1.

Isolation of Bacteriophage DNA

The phage DNA extraction is performed as previously described (Khan et al., 2021). Briefly, DNase I and RNase A were added to a final concentration of 5 and 1 μg/ml, respectively, and the purified phage particle was treated for 1 h at 37°C. Proteinase K (final concentration of 50 μg/ml), EDTA (pH 8.0), and 0.5% SDS were added and treated at 56°C for 1 h. Then, phage genome DNA was extracted with saturated phenol (pH 8.0). After centrifugation, the aqueous phase was extracted with chloroform and mixed with the same volume of isopropyl alcohol and stored at −20°C for 1 h. Then, phage DNA was precipitated by centrifugation and was washed with 70% ethanol and absolute ethanol, respectively. After drying, the precipitate was dissolved in TE solution, and the phage DNA was stored at −80°C.

Genome Sequencing and Annotation

Phage genomic DNA was sequenced using an Illumina Hiseq 2500 platform (~1 Gbp/sample). Fastp (Chen et al., 2018) was used for adapter trimming and quality filtering after demultiplexing the raw reads. The read data were assembled using the *de novo* assembly algorithm Newbler Version2.9 with default parameters, and the assembled genome was annotated by RAST. The DNA and protein sequences were checked for homologs with BLAST manually. The genome map was drawn by a phage genome visualization online software CPT Phage Galaxy (Ramsey et al., 2020). The sequence data are available in the NCBI under accession number MZ420150.

Stability Studies

To test the phage stability under various conditions, 10^8 pfu of LG1 was treated with different pH, temperature, or chloroform for 60 min, then the titer of the phage was calculated by double-layer agar assay. The LG1 was stored at 4°C, and its titer was determined at the given time points for 3 months.

Biofilm Assay

Biofilms were examined by the crystal violet staining method as previously described (Shen et al., 2018a). Briefly, 0.2 ml of log-phase bacterial culture were added to 96-well polystyrene microplates and incubated for 24 h at 37°C to establish biofilm. Then, the untreated control wells were washed with phosphate-buffered saline (PBS) and stained with crystal violet for 15 min, which was solubilized in 0.2 ml of 95% ethanol, and the biofilm biomass was estimated by measuring the OD 600, which was determined using a SpectraMax M3 multimode microplate reader. For the treatment groups, the wells were washed and PBS, then 0.2 ml of phage or antibiotic was added and incubated at 37°C for 4 h, the biofilm biomass was determined by crystal violet staining method.

Statistical Analysis

All the experiments were performed three times, and statistical analysis was performed using one-way ANOVA or t-test, and statistical significance was assumed if the P value was <0.05.

AUTHOR CONTRIBUTIONS

All the authors listed have made a substantial, direct and intellectual contribution to this work, and approved the submitted version for publication.

REFERENCES

Al-Zubidi, M., Widziolek, M., Court, E. K., Gains, A. F., Smith, R. E., Ansbro, K., et al. (2019). Identification of Novel Bacteriophages With Therapeutic Potential That Target Enterococcus Faecalis. *Infect. Immun.* 87 (11), e00512–19. doi: 10.1128/IAI.00512-19

Arias, C. A., Panesso, D., McGrath, D. M., Qin, X., Mojica, M. F., Miller, C., et al. (2011). Genetic Basis for *In Vivo* Daptomycin Resistance in Enterococci. *N Engl. J. Med.* 365, 892–900. doi: 10.1056/NEJMoa1011138

Azam, A. H., and Tanji, Y. (2019). Bacteriophage-Host Arm Race: An Update on the Mechanism of Phage Resistance in Bacteria and Revenge of the Phage With the Perspective for Phage Therapy. *Appl. Microbiol. Biotechnol.* 103, 2121–2131. doi: 10.1007/s00253-019-09629-x

Banla, I. L., Kommineni, S., Hayward, M., Rodrigues, M., Palmer, K. L., Salzman, N. H., et al. (2018). Modulators of Enterococcus Faecalis Cell Envelope Integrity and Antimicrobial Resistance Influence Stable Colonization of the Mammalian Gastrointestinal Tract. *Infect. Immun.* 86 (1), e00381-17. doi: 10.1128/IAI.00381-17

Bao, J., Wu, N., Zeng, Y., Chen, L., Li, L., Yang, L., et al. (2020). Non-Active Antibiotic and Bacteriophage Synergism to Successfully Treat Recurrent Urinary Tract Infection Caused by Extensively Drug-Resistant Klebsiella Pneumoniae. *Emerg. Microbes Infect.* 9, 771–774. doi: 10.1080/22221751.2020.1747950

Barbu, E. M., Cady, K. C., and Hubby, B. (2016). Phage Therapy in the Era of Synthetic Biology. *Cold Spring Harbor Perspect. Biol.* 8 (10), a023879. doi: 10.1101/cshperspect.a023879

Beganovic, M., Luther, M. K., Rice, L. B., Arias, C. A., Rybak, M. J., and LaPlante, K. L. (2018). A Review of Combination Antimicrobial Therapy for Enterococcus Faecalis Bloodstream Infections and Infective Endocarditis. *Clin. Infect. Dis: Off. Publ. Infect. Dis. Soc. America* 67, 303–309. doi: 10.1093/cid/ciy064

Chatterjee, A., Johnson, C. N., Luong, P., Hullahalli, K., McBride, S. W., Schubert, A. M., et al. (2019). Bacteriophage Resistance Alters Antibiotic-Mediated Intestinal Expansion of Enterococci. *Infect. Immun.* 87 (6), e00085-19. doi: 10.1128/IAI.00085-19

Chatterjee, A., Willett, J. L. E., Dunny, G. M., and Duerkop, B. A. (2021). Phage Infection and Sub-Lethal Antibiotic Exposure Mediate Enterococcus Faecalis Type VII Secretion System Dependent Inhibition of Bystander Bacteria. *PloS Genet.* 17, e1009204. doi: 10.1371/journal.pgen.1009204

Chen, S., Zhou, Y., Chen, Y., and Gu, J. (2021). Fastp: An Ultra-Fast All-In-One Fastq Preprocessor. *Bioinformatics* 34 (17), i884–i890. doi: 10.1093/bioinformatics/bty560

De Smet, J., Hendrix, H., Blasdel, B. G., Danis-Wlodarczyk, K., and Lavigne, R. (2017). Pseudomonas Predators: Understanding and Exploiting Phage-Host Interactions. *Nat. Rev. Microbiol.* 15, 517–530. doi: 10.1038/nrmicro.2017.61

Dion, M. B., Oechslin, F., and Moineau, S. (2020). Phage Diversity, Genomics and Phylogeny. *Nat. Rev. Microbiol.* 18, 125–138. doi: 10.1038/s41579-019-0311-5

Duerkop, B. A., Huo, W., Bhardwaj, P., Palmer, K. L., and Hooper, L. V. (2016). Molecular Basis for Lytic Bacteriophage Resistance in Enterococci. *mBio* 7 (4), e01304-16. doi: 10.1128/mBio.01304-16

Dyal, H. K., and Sehgal, R. (2015). The Catastrophic Journey of a Retained Temporary Epicardial Pacemaker Wire Leading to Enterococcus Faecalis Endocarditis and Subsequent Stroke. *BMJ Case Rep.* 2015, bcr2014206215. doi: 10.1136/bcr-2014-206215

El Haddad, L., Harb, C. P., Gebara, M. A., Stibich, M. A., and Chemaly, R. F. (2019). A Systematic and Critical Review of Bacteriophage Therapy Against Multidrug-Resistant ESKAPE Organisms in Humans. *Clin. Infect. Dis: Off. Publ. Infect. Dis. Soc. America* 69, 167–178. doi: 10.1093/cid/ciy947

Ferriol-Gonzalez, C., and Domingo-Calap, P. (2020). Phages for Biofilm Removal. *Antibiotics* 9 (5), 268. doi: 10.3390/antibiotics9050268

Goldfarb, T., Sberro, H., Weinstock, E., Cohen, O., Doron, S., Charpak-Amikam, Y., et al. (2015). BREX Is a Novel Phage Resistance System Widespread in Microbial Genomes. *EMBO J.* 34, 169–183. doi: 10.15252/embj.201489455

Hannawi, Y., Hannawi, B., Rao, C. P., Suarez, J. I., and Bershad, E. M. (2013). Stroke-Associated Pneumonia: Major Advances and Obstacles. *Cerebrovasc Dis.* 35, 430–443. doi: 10.1159/000350199

Jabbari Shiadeh, S. M., Pormohammad, A., Hashemi, A., and Lak, P. (2019). Global Prevalence of Antibiotic Resistance in Blood-Isolated Enterococcus Faecalis and Enterococcus Faecium: A Systematic Review and Meta-Analysis. *Infect. Drug Resist.* 12, 2713–2725. doi: 10.2147/IDR.S206084

Jault, P., Leclerc, T., Jennes, S., Pirnay, J. P., Que, Y. A., Resch, G., et al. (2018). Efficacy and Tolerability of a Cocktail of Bacteriophages to Treat Burn Wounds Infected by Pseudomonas Aeruginosa (PhagoBurn): A Randomised, Controlled, Double-Blind Phase 1/2 Trial. *Lancet Infect. Dis.* 19 (1), 35–45. doi: 10.1016/S1473-3099(18)30482-1

Khalifa, L., Brosh, Y., Gelman, D., Coppenhagen-Glazer, S., Beyth, S., Poradosu-Cohen, R., et al. (2015). Targeting Enterococcus Faecalis Biofilms With Phage Therapy. *Appl. Environ. Microbiol.* 81, 2696–2705. doi: 10.1128/AEM.00096-15

Khan, F. M., Gondil, V. S., Li, C., Jiang, M., Li, J., Yu, J., et al. (2021). A Novel Acinetobacter Baumannii Bacteriophage Endolysin LysAB54 With High Antibacterial Activity Against Multiple Gram-Negative Microbes. *Front. Cell Infect. Microbiol.* 11, 637313. doi: 10.3389/fcimb.2021.637313

Kortright, K. E., Chan, B. K., Koff, J. L., and Turner, P. E. (2019). Phage Therapy: A Renewed Approach to Combat Antibiotic-Resistant Bacteria. *Cell Host Microbe* 25, 219–232. doi: 10.1016/j.chom.2019.01.014

Labrie, S. J., Samson, J. E., and Moineau, S. (2010). Bacteriophage Resistance Mechanisms. *Nat. Rev. Microbiol.* 8, 317–327. doi: 10.1038/nrmicro2315

Leitner, L., Ujmajuridze, A., Chanishvili, N., Goderdzishvili, M., Chkonia, I., Rigvava, S., et al. (2021). Intravesical Bacteriophages for Treating Urinary Tract Infections in Patients Undergoing Transurethral Resection of the Prostate: A Randomised, Placebo-Controlled, Double-Blind Clinical Trial. *Lancet Infect. Dis.* 21, 427–436. doi: 10.1016/S1473-3099(20)30330-3

Liu, C., Green, S., Min, L., Clark, J., Salazar, K., Terwilliger, A., et al. (2020). Phage-Antibiotic Synergy Is Driven by a Unique Combination of Antibacterial Mechanism of Action and Stoichiometry. *mbio*, 01462–01420. doi: 10.1128/mBio.01462-20

Oechslin, F., Piccardi, P., Mancini, S., Gabard, J., Moreillon, P., Entenza, J. M., et al. (2017). Synergistic Interaction Between Phage Therapy and Antibiotics Clears Pseudomonas Aeruginosa Infection in Endocarditis and Reduces Virulence. *J. Infect. Dis.* 215, 703–712. doi: 10.1093/infdis/jiw632

Overbeek, R., Olson, R., Pusch, G. D., Olsen, G. J., Davis, J. J., Disz, T., et al. (2014). The SEED and the Rapid Annotation of Microbial Genomes Using Subsystems Technology (RAST). *Nucleic Acids Res.* 42, D206–D214. doi: 10.1093/nar/gkt1226

Palmer, K. L., Daniel, A., Hardy, C., Silverman, J., and Gilmore, M. S. (2011). Genetic Basis for Daptomycin Resistance in Enterococci. *Antimicrob. Agents Chemother.* 55, 3345–3356. doi: 10.1128/AAC.00207-11

Palmer, K. L., Kos, V. N., and Gilmore, M. S. (2010). Horizontal Gene Transfer and the Genomics of Enterococcal Antibiotic Resistance. *Curr. Opin. Microbiol.* 13, 632–639. doi: 10.1016/j.mib.2010.08.004

Pires, D. P., Costa, A. R., Pinto, G., Meneses, L., and Azeredo, J. (2020). Current Challenges and Future Opportunities of Phage Therapy. *FEMS Microbiol. Rev.* 44, 684–700. doi: 10.1093/femsre/fuaa017

Pires, D. P., Melo, L. D. R., Boas, D. V., Sillankorva, S., and Azeredo, J. (2017). Phage Therapy as an Alternative or Complementary Strategy to Prevent and Control Biofilm-Related Infections. *Curr. Opin. Microbiol.* 39, 48–56. doi: 10.1016/j.mib.2017.09.004

Ramsey, J., Rasche, H., Maughmer, C., Criscione, A., Mijalis, E., Liu, M., et al. (2020). Galaxy and Apollo as a Biologist-Friendly Interface for High-Quality Cooperative Phage Genome Annotation. *PloS Comput. Biol.* 16, e1008214. doi: 10.1371/journal.pcbi.1008214

Shen, M., Yang, Y., Shen, W., Cen, L., McLean, J. S., Shi, W., et al. (2018a). A Linear Plasmid-Like Prophage of Actinomyces Odontolyticus Promotes Biofilm Assembly. *Appl. Environ. Microbiol.* 84 (17), e01263-1. doi: 10.1128/AEM.01263-18

Shen, M., Zhang, H., Shen, W., Zou, Z., Lu, S., Li, G., et al. (2018b). Pseudomonas Aeruginosa MutL Promotes Large Chromosomal Deletions Through non-Homologous End Joining to Prevent Bacteriophage Predation. *Nucleic Acids Res.* 46, 4505–4514. doi: 10.1093/nar/gky160

Stanley, D., Mason, L. J., Mackin, K. E., Srikhanta, Y. N., Lyras, D., Prakash, M. D., et al. (2016). Translocation and Dissemination of Commensal Bacteria in Post-Stroke Infection. *Nat. Med.* 22, 1277–1284. doi: 10.1038/nm.4194

Waters, E. M., Neill, D. R., Kaman, B., Sahota, J. S., Clokie, M. R. J., Winstanley, C., et al. (2017). Phage Therapy is Highly Effective Against Chronic Lung Infections With Pseudomonas Aeruginosa. *Thorax* 72, 666–667. doi: 10.1136/thoraxjnl-2016-209265

Wu, Y., Wang, R., Xu, M., Liu, Y., Zhu, X., Qiu, J., et al. (2019). A Novel Polysaccharide Depolymerase Encoded by the Phage SH-KP152226 Confers Specific Activity Against Multidrug-Resistant Klebsiella Pneumoniae *via* Biofilm Degradation. *Front. Microbiol.* 10, 2768. doi: 10.3389/fmicb.2019.02768

Zhong, Q., Yang, L., Li, L., Shen, W., Li, Y., Xu, H., et al. (2020). Transcriptomic Analysis Reveals the Dependency of Pseudomonas Aeruginosa Genes for Double-Stranded RNA Bacteriophage phiYY Infection Cycle. *iScience* 23, 101437. doi: 10.1016/j.isci.2020.101437

9

CAR T Cells Beyond Cancer: Hope for Immunomodulatory Therapy of Infectious Diseases

Michelle Seif, Hermann Einsele and Jürgen Löffler*

Department of Internal Medicine II, University Hospital Wuerzburg, Würzburg, Germany

*Correspondence:
Jürgen Löffler
loeffler_j@ukw.de

Infectious diseases are still a significant cause of morbidity and mortality worldwide. Despite the progress in drug development, the occurrence of microbial resistance is still a significant concern. Alternative therapeutic strategies are required for non-responding or relapsing patients. Chimeric antigen receptor (CAR) T cells has revolutionized cancer immunotherapy, providing a potential therapeutic option for patients who are unresponsive to standard treatments. Recently two CAR T cell therapies, Yescarta® (Kite Pharma/Gilead) and Kymriah® (Novartis) were approved by the FDA for the treatments of certain types of non-Hodgkin lymphoma and B-cell precursor acute lymphoblastic leukemia, respectively. The success of adoptive CAR T cell therapy for cancer has inspired researchers to develop CARs for the treatment of infectious diseases. Here, we review the main achievements in CAR T cell therapy targeting viral infections, including Human Immunodeficiency Virus, Hepatitis C Virus, Hepatitis B Virus, Human Cytomegalovirus, and opportunistic fungal infections such as invasive aspergillosis.

Keywords: infectious diseases, mAb engineering, CAR T cells, HIV, HCV, CMV, invasive aspergillosis, HBV

INTRODUCTION

Viral and opportunistic fungal infections represent a major threat to chronically infected individuals and immunocompromised patients. Despite the availability of antifungal and antiviral drugs, the mortality rate is still significant in high-risk patients (1–3). Current anti-viral treatments fail to cure chronic viral infections (caused by, e.g., HIV, HBV, and HCV) due to the viral-reservoir composed of infected cells that can stay latent for several years and would restart producing infectious virus at any time (4, 5) and the occurrence of resistance (6, 7). Therapies providing long term control or able to eradicate the viral-reservoir are required.

Pathogen-specific effector T cells play a crucial role in the control of acute viral and fungal infections in immunocompetent individuals (8–12), making adoptive T cell therapy an attractive alternative to currently used anti-infectious therapies. Pathogen-specific T cells occur in low frequencies in the patient's blood, making them difficult to isolate and expand. Moreover, they have exhausted phenotypes and might be rendered inefficient by viral escape mutation mechanisms lowering the major histocompatibility complex (MHC) or mutating the targeted epitope (10, 13–15). Thus, Chimeric antigen receptors (CARs) T cells present an attractive alternative.

CAR T cells are considered as a major scientific breakthrough and an important turning point in cancer immunotherapy (16), especially in the treatment of B cell malignancies. Recently, the US Food and Drug Administration (FDA) then the European Commission have approved two CAR T-cell products, Kymriah® (Novartis) and Yescarta® (Kite Pharma/ Gilead) for the treatment of B-cell precursor acute lymphoblastic leukemia and aggressive B-cell lymphoma, respectively.

CAR T cells are described as having the targeting specificity of a monoclonal antibody combined with the effector functions of a cytotoxic T cell (17). They offer potential advantages over pathogen-specific T cells, the CAR allows antigen recognition independent of the MHC and can be designed to specifically target the conserved and essential epitopes of the antigen, which allows them to overcome pathogen escape mechanisms.

Few anti-infectious CARs were described in the literature so far, most of them targeting HIV. Here we review the progress and discuss the remaining challenges of making CAR T cell therapy a reality for individuals suffering from infectious diseases. The main anti-infectious CAR constructs are summarized in **Table 1**.

CAR T CELLS

CARs are synthetic receptors composed of a targeting element linked by a spacer to a transmembrane domain followed by an intracellular signaling domain. The targeting element is usually, but not exclusively composed by a single-chain variable fragment (scFv) (17). The spacer constitutes mainly of a full-length Fc receptor of an IgG (Hinge-CH_2-CH_3) or shorter parts like the Hinge region only or Hinge-CH_2 (37–40). Furthermore, parts of the extracellular domains of CD28 and CD8α were used as spacers (41, 42). Several transmembrane domains were used to anchor the receptor on the surface of a T cell, mainly derived from CD28, CD8α, or CD4 (42–44). The signaling domain consists of the intracellular part of CD3ζ from the TCR complex (45). Over the years, in order to improve the CAR functionality and persistence, several generations of CARs have been established differing in their intracellular signaling (17). First-generation CARs mediated T-cell activation only through the CD3ζ complex (45, 46). Second-generation CARs include an intracellular costimulatory domain, mainly CD28 or 4-1BB, leading to an enhanced expansion, and functionality (43, 47–52). These second-generation receptors are the origin of the recently approved CAR T-cell therapies (53). Third-generation CARs combine two costimulatory domains, mainly CD28, and 4-1BB (54). Finally, fourth-generation CARs, also called TRUCKs (T-cells redirected for universal cytokine-mediated killing), emerged, including an additional transgene for inducible cytokine secretion upon CAR activation [mainly IL-12 (55)]. Several other strategies for minimizing toxicity and enhancing versatility and control of CAR T cells were reviewed by others (17, 56).

CAR T CELLS SPECIFIC FOR HUMAN IMMUNODEFICIENCY VIRUS (HIV)

Studies on developing CAR T cell therapy to cure HIV infections are ongoing since the early 90th. The first findings were already reviewed by others (57–60). Here we shortly summarize the anti-HIV CAR T cell history and focus on the most recent achievements.

CD4 Based CARs

The concept of CAR T cells was initially described in the 90th when the cytotoxic T cells specificity was redirected toward HIV infected cells. The first CAR was specific for HIV envelope protein (Env) using the CD4 receptor as a targeting element fused to the CD3ζ chain for intracellular signaling (CD4ζCAR) (61, 62). Clinical trials with the CD4ζCAR showed that the concept is feasible and safe, but failed to reduce HIV viral burden permanently (63–66).

To improve the CAR T cell activity and persistence, CD4ζCAR was re-engineered into second-generation and third-generation CARs. While CAR T cells containing CD28 costimulatory domain promoted higher cytokine production and better control over HIV replication *in vitro*, the 4-1BB containing CARs were more potent in controlling HIV infection *in vivo*. When compared to first-generation CAR T cells, second-generation CAR T cells were more potent at suppressing HIV replication *in vitro*. Furthermore, in a humanized mouse model of HIV infection, they preserved the CD4$^+$ T cell count, reduced HIV burden, and expanded to a greater extent than first-generation CAR T cells (20).

However, it was shown that CD4-based CARs render the CAR T cells susceptible to HIV infection (18, 25). To overcome this limitation, CD4ζCAR was equipped with either a viral fusion inhibitor (C46 peptide) (18) or small hairpin RNAs to knock down HIV-1 co-receptor CC-chemokine receptor 5 (CCR5) and degrade viral RNA (19). Both methods successfully rendered CD4ζCAR T resistant to HIV infection and conferred them a long persistence and proper control of HIV infection *in vivo* (18, 19).

Moreover, several genome editing techniques were used to knock out CCR5 in T cells to confer them permanent resistance to HIV infection (67). These include the use of ZFNs (Zinc-finger nucleases) (68), which showed promising results in clinical trials (NCT00842634, NCT01044654, NCT01252641), TALEN (Transcription activator-like nucleases) (69, 70), and CRISPR-CAS 9 (71) in preclinical studies. These endonucleases were already used to produce universal CAR T cells by knocking down the TCR (72–77). It would be useful to test them to knock down CCR5 in HIV-CAR T cells.

scFvs Based CARs

To avoid using the CD4 as targeting element, novel CARs of several generations were designed using single-chain variable fragments (scFv) derived from broadly neutralizing antibodies (bNAbs) targeting Env.

Targets included the CD4-binding site, several antigens of glycoprotein 120 (gp120), the membrane-proximal region of gp41, the mannose-rich region, and variable glycan regions (20, 21, 24, 78).

Second-generation CARs for the different targets enabled the CAR T cells to kill HIV-1-infected cells. However, their antiviral activity was variable according to the virus strain (78). Second-generation anti-glycan CARs, in combination with CCR5 ablation, provided better control of viral replication than the CAR alone (24).

First-generation anti-gp120 CARs induced efficient activation and cytokine secretion by the gene-modified T cells and mediated

TABLE 1 | CAR design of the most promising anti-infectious CAR T-cells.

Pathogen	Targeted antigen	Targeting element	Spacer	Transmembrane domain	Costimulatory domain	Extra modification	References
HIV	CD4 binding site on gp-120	CD4	n.a.	CD4	n.a.	C46 peptide	(18)
	CD4 binding site on gp-120	CD4	n.a.	CD4	n.a.	CCR5 sh 1005; sh 516	(19)
	CD4 binding site on gp-120	CD4	n.a.	CD8α	CD28 or 4-1BB		(20)
	CD4 binding site on gp-120	VRC01-scFv	(GGGGS)$_3$	CD8α or CD28	CD28-4-1BB		(21)
	CD4 binding site on gp-120	105-scFv	CD8 hinge	CD3ζ	n.a.		(22)
	Env/gp120 glycans	CD4/ CRD	CD28	CD28	CD28		(23)
	V1/V2 glycan loop	PGT145-scFv	CD8α Hinge	CD8α	4-1BB	AAV6-CCR5	(24)
	CD4-induced epitope on gp120/CD4 binding site	17b-scFv/CD4	Tripeptide AAA	CD28	CD28		(25)
	CD4-induced epitope on gp120/CD4 binding site	mD1.22-G$_4$S-m36.4	CD8	CD8	4-1BB	C46 peptide	(26)
HBV	S HBV surface protein	C8-scFv	IgG1 Fc	CD28	CD28		(27–29)
	HBV surface antigen	19.79.6-scFv	IgG4 Fc mutated	CD28	CD28		(30)
HCV	HCV E2 glycoprotein	e137-scFv	IgG Fc	CD28	CD28		(31)
CMV	Glycoprotein B	27-287-scFv	Ig Hinge	CD28	CD28		(32–34)
	Virally encoded FcRs	IgG1 or IgG4 Fc mutated	n.a.	CD28	CD28		(35)
Aspergillus fumigatus	β-glucan	Dectin 1	IgG4 Fc mutated	CD28	CD28		(36)

lysis of envelope-expressing cells and HIV-1-infected CD4$^+$ T-lymphocytes in vitro (22). Third generation anti-gp120 CAR-T cells were more efficient than CD4 based CARs in lysing gp120 expressing cells in vitro. Furthermore, their interaction with cell-free HIV did not result in their infection. More importantly, they efficiently induced cytolysis of the reactivated HIV reservoir isolated from infected individuals. Thus, anti-gp120 third-generation CAR T cells might be a suitable candidate for therapeutic approaches aiming to eradicate the HIV reservoir (21).

However, one major drawback to developing scFvs-based CAR T cell therapy is the HIV viral escape mutation mechanism that can abrogate the antibody-binding site and render the CAR T cell therapy inefficient.

Bi- and Tri-specific CARs

In order to overcome the HIV mutation escape mechanism, bi-and tri-specific CAR-expressing T cells targeting up to three HIV antigens were designed to increase the specificity and affinity.

The CD4 segment was fused with an scFv specific for a CD4-induced epitope on gp120 (25) or the carbohydrate recognition domain (CRD) of a human C- type lectin binding to conserved glycans on Env (23). The CD4-anti gp120 scFv bispecific CAR had better suppressive activity against HIV than the CD4 alone. CD4-mannose binding lectin (MBL) CARs showed the best potency when compared to both CD4 alone and CD4-anti gp120 (23). However, since C- type lectins can bind glycans which are not specific for HIV infected cells and can be associated with healthy cells, off-targets cannot be excluded.

More recently, T cells were engineered with up to three functionally distinct HIV envelope-binding domains to form bispecific and tri-specific targeting anti-HIV CAR-T cells. These cells carry two distinct CARs expressed on one T cell or one CAR having tow targeting elements linked together. Targets included CD4-binding site on HIV gp120 and CD4-induced (CD4i) epitope on gp120 near the co-receptor binding site. Tri-specific CARs expressed the C46 peptide, which inhibits HIV viral fusion and thus can prevent the infection of CAR T cells. Bi-and tri-specific CAR T cells showed potent in vitro and in vivo anti-HIV effects, they efficiently killed HIV-infected cells in a humanized mouse model while protecting the CAR- T cells from infection (26).

Despite all the challenges faced, anti-HIV CAR T cell therapy made much progress toward enhancing the CAR T cell antiviral activity, protecting CAR T cells from HIV infection, and overcoming HIV escape mechanisms. Currently, at least two clinical trials are ongoing for latent reservoir eradication, one using a modified bNAb-based CAR-T cell therapy (NCT03240328) and one using CD4-based CAR-T cell therapy with CCR5 ablation (NCT03617198).

CAR T CELLS SPECIFIC FOR HEPATITIS B VIRUS (HBV)

Some preclinical studies are focusing on engineering second-generation CAR T cells to cure chronic hepatitis B and prevent the development of hepatocellular carcinoma (HCC). Cytotoxic T cells were redirected toward HBV surface and secreted antigens.

Second generation CAR T cells were designed to target HBV-surface proteins S and L, which are expressed continuously on the surface of HBV replicating cells. S and L specific CAR T cells were able to recognize soluble HBsAg and HBsAg-positive hepatocytes *in vitro* and subsequently secret IFNγ and IL-2. S-CAR T cells were activated faster and secreted higher cytokine levels than L-CAR T cells. This might be due to the higher expression of the S-protein on the surface of viral and subviral particles when compared with the L-protein (27).

Furthermore, both CAR T cells were able to lyse HBV transfected cells as well as selectively eliminated HBV-infected primary hepatocytes. However, even after the elimination of HBV-infected hepatocytes, HBV core protein and HBV rcDNA remained detectable. It is most probably because HBV rcDNA is localized in viral capsids and thus protected from caspase-activated DNAses (27). The S-CAR construct was tested *in vivo* in an immune-competent HBV transgenic mouse model. CD8$^+$ mouse T cells expressing the human S-CAR localized to the liver and effectively reduced HBV replication, causing only transient liver damage. Furthermore, contact of CAR T cells with circulating viral antigen did not lead to their functional exhaustion or excessive liver damage. However, the survival of the CAR T cells was limited due to the immune response triggered by the human CAR (28). In an immunocompetent mouse model tolerized with a signaling-deficient S-CAR, S-CAR T cells persisted and showed long-lasting antiviral effector function (29). However, the use of a transgene instead of cccDNA to transcribe HBV makes these mouse models unsuitable to judge whether S-CAR T cells can cure HBV infection (28, 29).

More recently, other novel second-generation CARs targeting HBsAg were designed with different spacer length. Only HBs-CAR T-cells equipped with a long spacer (HBs-G4m-CAR) recognized HBV-positive cell lines and HBsAg particles *in vitro* and subsequently produced significant amounts of IFN-γ, IL-2, and TNF-α. However, HBs-G4m-CAR T cells were not capable of killing HBV-positive cell lines *in vitro*. This might be due to HBsAg particles produced by HBV-positive cells that can bind to HBs-G4m-CAR T-cells and potentially inhibit CAR-T targeting or killing of infected cells. In a humanized HBV-infected mouse model, adoptive transfer of HBsAg-CAR T-cells led to the accumulation of the cells in the liver and an important reduction in plasma HBsAg and HBV-DNA levels. Furthermore, the absence of HBV core expression in a portion of human hepatocytes and the unchanged plasma human albumin levels indicated HBV clearance without destruction of the infected hepatocytes. However, no complete elimination of HBV was observed. Despite this limitation, HBs-G4m-CAR T cells had superior anti-HBV activity than HBV entry inhibitors (30).

These studies showed promising results; a direct comparison of S-CAR T cell and HBsAg-CAR T-cell would be interesting to test. Furthermore, a better mouse model more representative of the actual infection should be used to evaluate the CAR activity *in vivo*. Finally, combination therapy using CAR T-cells with reverse transcriptase inhibitors or hepatitis B immunoglobulin might be required to have better control of the HBV infection.

CAR T CELLS SPECIFIC FOR HEPATITIS C VIRUS (HCV)

Very recently, the first two CARs targeting HCV were designed based on a broadly cross-reactive and cross-neutralizing human monoclonal antibody specific for a conserved epitope of the HCV E2 glycoprotein (HCV/E2). Anti-HCV CAR T cells showed good anti-viral activity and lyzed HCV/E2-transfected as well as HCV-infected target cells (31).

This study showed that the concept of CAR T cells might also be suitable for the treatment of HCV. The described CAR should be evaluated *in vivo* in a suitable animal model. Furthermore, since HCV/E2 is the main target of the host immune response and is consequently very susceptible to mutations (32), targeting other conserved, and essential antigens might also be of interest.

CAR T CELLS SPECIFIC FOR HUMAN CYTOMEGALOVIRUS (CMV)

The first CAR targeting CMV was described in 2010 based on the anti-gB antibody. Second generation gB CAR T cells were activated when co-cultured with CMV-infected cells and secreted TNF α and IFN γ and subsequently inhibited CMV replication in infected cells (33–35). Moreover, they eliminated gB transfected cells (33) but were not always able to lyse infected cells, especially at later stages of the replication cycle. This might be due to HCMV-encoded anti-apoptotic proteins that are known to prevent the suicide of infected host cells (34, 35). This CAR T cell therapy was not tested *in vivo* due to the few sequence similarities between the murine CMV gB protein and the human one. An appropriate mouse model using a recombinant MCMV expressing HCMV-gB should be developed (33).

In a later study, it was shown that the long spacer (CH2–CH3 Fc domain from IgG1) usually used in CAR preparation could bind to virally encoded Fc binding receptors on the surface of infected cells and act as a receptor for CMV. The mutated form of the spacer is only recognized by viral FcRs and not the human ones. In this way, the long spacer can act as a receptor for CMV infected cells (35).

The gB-CAR with long and short spacer should be further tested *in vivo* in an appropriate animal model. More targeting elements should be tested. Finally, the combination of new targeting elements with a long spacer might confer a bispecific targeting of CMV infected cells.

CAR T CELLS SPECIFIC FOR EPSTEIN-BARR VIRUS (EBV)

To target Epstein-Barr virus (EBV) associated malignancies, a second-generation CAR specific for the EBV latent membrane protein 1 (LMP1) was described. EBV-CAR T cells were activated *in vitro* in co-culture with nasopharyngeal carcinoma cells overexpressing LMP1

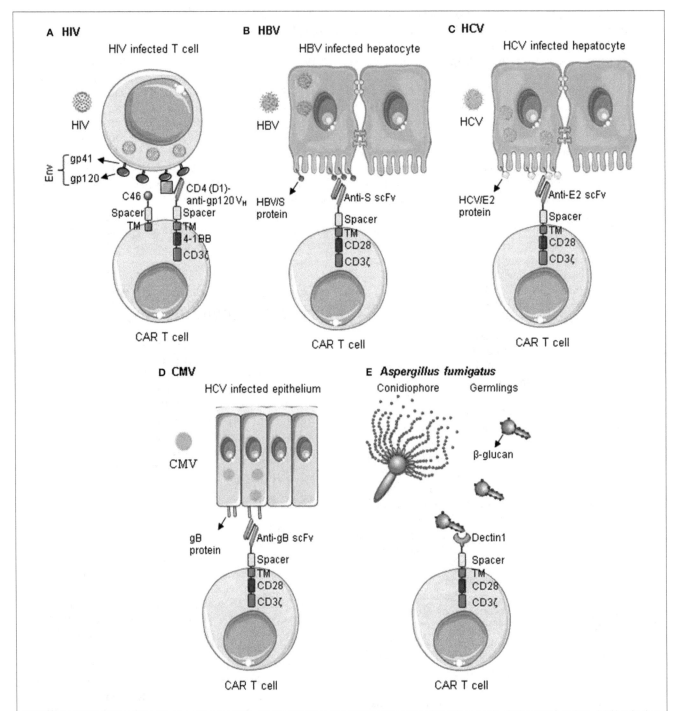

FIGURE 1 | CAR T cells targeting infectious diseases. **(A)** T cells are redirected against HIV by the expression of Env-specific CARs on their surface. Additionally, they are rendered resistant to HIV infection by expression of an anti-fusion peptide. Anti-HIV CAR T cells can successfully kill HIV infected cells and control HIV infection. **(B–D)** CAR T cells specific for HBV S protein, HCV/E2, or gB can recognize cells infected by HBV, HCV, and CMV, respectively. They can selectively kill the infected cells within the epithelium. **(E)** Dectin 1-CAR T cells can directly bind to *Aspergillus fumigatus* germlings and induce hyphal damage. Env, HIV envelope protein; Gp, Glycoprotein; TM, transmembrane; V_H, variable heavy chain; gB, Glycoprotein B.

and subsequently produced IFNɤ and IL-2. Intra-tumoral injection of EBV-CAR T cells in a xenograft mouse model having tumors overexpressing LMP1 reduced tumor growth (79).

CAR-T cell therapy for solid tumors is still facing many challenges, like the inability to reach the tumor and survive in the tumor microenvironment. These challenges and the developed strategies to overcome them were reviewed by others (80).

CAR T CELLS SPECIFIC FOR *Aspergillus fumigatus*

A second-generation CAR using the extracellular domain of Dectin-1 as targeting element called D-CAR was designed to target *Aspergillus fumigatus*. Dectin 1 is a C-type lectin receptor specific for ß-glucan, a motif expressed on the surface of many fungi (81). D-CAR T cells were activated by ß-glucan and subsequently secreted IFNγ and induced hyphal damage *in vitro*. In an immunocompromised invasive aspergillosis mouse model, D-CAR T cells reduced the fungal burden (36).

This study suggested that the application of CAR T cells might extend beyond cancer and chronic viral infections to acute fungal infections. Although promising results were shown for D-CAR T cells, Dectin 1 might not be the best targeting element to redirect the T cell specificity toward *Aspergillus fumigatus*. Since ß-glucans are not specific for *Aspergillus fumigatus* but rather a broad range of commensal and pathogenic microorganisms, off-target activity of the CAR T cells cannot be excluded (82). Using scFvs derived from fungal specific antibodies might provide better specificity and activity of the CAR. Moreover, strategies to significantly shorten the CAR T cell preparation time [currently time from leukapheresis to infusion of the CART product can take up to 3–4 weeks (83)] will be essential to allow their clinical use for acute infections.

REFERENCES

Heinz WJ, Vehreschild JJ, Buchheidt D. Diagnostic work up to assess early response indicators in invasive pulmonary aspergillosis in adult patients with haematologic malignancies. *Mycoses*. (2019) 62:486–93.doi:10.1111/myc.12860

Green ML. CMV viral load and mortality after hematopoietic cell transplantation: a cohort study in the era of preemptive therapy. *Lancet Haematol*. (2016) 3:e119–27.doi: 10.1016/S2352-3026(15)00289-6

Teira P, Battiwalla M, Ramanathan M, Barrett AJ, Ahn KW, Chen M, et al. Early cytomegalovirus reactivation remains associated with increased transplant-related mortality in the current era: a CIBMTR analysis. *Blood*. (2016) 127:2427–38.doi:10.1182/blood-2015-11-679639

Bongiovanni M, Adorni F, Casana M, Tordato F, Tincati C, Cicconi P, et al. Subclinical hypothyroidism in HIV-infected subjects. *J Antimicrob Chemother*. (2006) 58:1086–9.doi:10.1093/jac/dkl360

Wong JK, Hezareh M, Günthard HF, Havlir DV, Ignacio CC, Spina CA, et al. Recovery of replication-competent HIV despite prolonged suppression of plasma viremia. *Science*. (1997) 278:1291–5.doi:10.1126/science.278.5341.1291

Paydary K, Khaghani P, Emamzadeh-Fard S, Alinaghi SAS, Baesi K. The emergence of drug resistant HIV variants and novel anti-retroviral therapy. *Asian Pac J Trop Biomed*. (2013) 3:515–22.doi:10.1016/S2221-1691(13)60106-9

Margeridon-Thermet S, Shafer RW. Comparison of the mechanisms of drug resistance among HIV, hepatitis B, and hepatitis C. *Viruses*. (2010) 2:2696–739.doi:10.3390/v2122696

Neumann-Haefelin C, Thimme R. Adaptive immune responses in hepatitis C virus infection. *Curr Top Microbiol Immunol*. (2013) 369:243–62.doi:10.1007/978-3-642-27340-7_10

Klenerman P, Oxenius A. T cell responses to cytomegalovirus. *Nat Rev Immunol*. (2016) 16:367–77.doi:10.1038/nri.2016.38

Jones RB, Walker BD. Jones, Walker HIV-specific CD8 T cells and HIV eradication. *J Clin Invest*. (2016) 126:455–63.doi:10.1172/JCI80566

Maini MK, Boni C, Ogg GS, King AS, Reignat S, Chun Kyon Lee, et al. Direct *ex vivo* analysis of hepatitis B virus-specific CD8+ T cells associated with the control of infection. *Gastroenterology*. (1999) 117:1386–96.doi:10.1016/S0016-5085(99)70289-1

CONCLUSION AND PERSPECTIVES

CAR T-cell therapy has gained much interest since its clinical application was approved for cancer immunotherapy. Relying on the knowledge accumulated on CAR T cell engineering in cancer research, many efforts are being made toward developing similar therapies for patients affected by chronical viral and acute invasive fungal infections. While targets are more precise and unique to the pathogen, making it easier to avoid off-targets, pathogen escape mechanisms, and reservoirs are still major obstacles.

Several CARs targeting infectious diseases have been described; the most relevant ones are summarized in **Figure 1** and **Table 1**. Tremendous progress was made in anti-HIV CAR T cell therapy, which reached now clinical trials. CAR T cells targeting other viruses such as HBV, HCV, CMV, and opportunistic fungus are still in their early pre-clinical testing. So far, promising data were observed, providing a proof of concept of CAR T cell application. Nevertheless, considerable optimization work is still required regarding the safety and efficacy of the constructs. More targets should be evaluated *in vitro* and *in vivo* in relevant animal models.

AUTHOR CONTRIBUTIONS

MS wrote the manuscript. JL and HE reviewed and edited the manuscript. All authors approved the manuscript for publication.

Kumaresan PR, da Silva TA, Kontoyiannis DP. Methods of controlling invasive fungal infections using CD8 + T cells. *Front Immunol*. (2018) 8:1–14.doi: 10.3389/fimmu.2017.01939

Iijima S, Lee Y-J, Ode H, Arold ST, Kimura N, Yokoyama M, et al. A Non-canonical mu-1A-binding motif in the N terminus of HIV-1 nef determines its ability to downregulate major histocompatibility complex class I in T lymphocytes. *J Virol*. (2012) 86:3944–51.doi: 10.1128/JVI.06257-11

Boni C, Fisicaro P, Valdatta C, Amadei B, Di Vincenzo P, Giuberti T, et al. Characterization of hepatitis B virus (HBV)-specific T-cell dysfunction in chronic HBV infection. *J Virol*. (2007) 81:4215–25.doi: 10.1128/JVI.02844-06

Kurktschiev PD, Raziorrouh B, Schraut W, Backmund M, Wächtler M, Wendtner CM, et al. Dysfunctional CD8+ T cells in hepatitis B and C are characterized by a lack of antigen-specific T-bet induction. *J Exp Med*. (2014) 211:2047–59.doi: 10.1084/jem.20131333

Couzin-Frankel J. Cancer immunotherapy. *Crit Rev Clin Lab Sci*. (2016) 8363:167–89.doi: 10.1080/10408360902937809

Subklewe M, Von Bergwelt-Baildon M, Humpe A. Chimeric antigen receptor T cells: a race to revolutionize cancer therapy. *Transfus Med Hemotherapy*. (2019) 46:15–24.doi: 10.1159/000496870

Zhen A, Peterson CW, Carrillo MA, Reddy SS, Youn CS, Lam BB, et al. Long-term persistence and function of hematopoietic stem cell-derived chimeric antigen receptor T cells in a non-human primate model of HIV/AIDS. *PLoS Pathog*. (2017) 13:e1006753.doi: 10.1371/journal.ppat.1006753

Zhen A, Kamata M, Rezek V, Rick J, Levin B, Kasparian S, et al. HIV-specific immunity derived from chimeric antigen receptor-engineered stem cells. *Mol Ther*. (2015) 23:1358–67.doi: 10.1038/mt.2015.102

Leibman RS, Richardson MW, Ellebrecht CT, Maldini CR, Glover JA, Secreto AJ, et al. Supraphysiologic control over HIV-1 replication mediated by CD8 T cells expressing a re-engineered CD4-based chimeric antigen receptor. *PLoS Pathog*. (2017) 13:1–30.doi: 10.1371/journal.ppat.1006613

Liu B, Zou F, Lu L, Chen C, He D, Zhang X, et al. Chimeric antigen receptor T cells guided by the single-chain Fv of a broadly neutralizing antibody specifically and effectively eradicate virus reactivated from latency in CD4 T lymphocytes isolated from HIV-1- infected individuals receiving suppressive combined antiretroviral therapy. *J Virol*. (2016) 90:9712–24.doi: 10.1128/JVI.00852-16

Masiero S, Del Vecchio C, Gavioli R, Mattiuzzo G, Cusi MG, Micheli L, et al. T-cell engineering by a chimeric T-cell receptor with antibody-type specificity for the HIV-1 gp120. *Gene Ther.* (2005) 12:299–310.doi: 10.1038/sj.gt.3302413

Ghanem MH, Bolivar-Wagers S, Dey B, Hajduczki A, Vargas-Inchaustegui DA, Danielson DT, et al. Bispecific chimeric antigen receptors targeting the CD4 binding site and high-mannose Glycans of gp120 optimized for anti–human immunodeficiency virus potency and breadth with minimal immunogenicity. *Cytotherapy.* (2018) 20:407–19.doi: 10.1016/j.jcyt.2017. 11.001

Hale M, Mesojednik T, Ibarra GSR, Sahni J, Bernard A, Sommer K, et al. Engineering HIV-resistant, anti-HIV chimeric antigen receptor T cells. *Mol Ther.* (2017) 25:570–9.doi: 10.1016/j.ymthe.2016.12.023

Liu L, Patel B, Ghanem MH, Bundoc V, Zheng Z, Morgan RA, et al. Novel CD4-based bispecific chimeric antigen receptor designed for enhanced anti- HIV potency and absence of HIV entry receptor activity. *J Virol.* (2015) 89:6685–94.doi: 10.1128/JVI.00474-15

Anthony-Gonda K, Bardhi A, Ray A, Flerin N, Li M, Chen W, et al. Multispecific anti-HIV duoCAR-T cells display broad *in vitro* antiviral activity and potent *in vivo* elimination of HIV-infected cells in a humanized mouse model. *Sci Transl Med.* (2019) 11:eaav5685.doi: 10.1126/scitranslmed.aav5685

Bohne F, Chmielewski M, Ebert G, Wiegmann K, Kürschner T, Schulze A, et al. T cells redirected against hepatitis B virus surface proteins eliminate infected hepatocytes. *Gastroenterology.* (2008) 134:239–47.doi: 10.1053/j. gastro.2007.11.002

Krebs K, Böttinger N, Huang LR, Chmielewski M, Arzberger S, Gasteiger G, et al. T cells expressing a chimeric antigen receptor that binds hepatitis B virus envelope proteins control virus replication in mice. *Gastroenterology.* (2013) 145:456–65. doi: 10.1053/j.gastro.2013.04.047

Festag MM, Festag J, Fräßle SP, Asen T, Sacherl J, Schreiber S, et al. Evaluation of a fully human, hepatitis B virus-specific chimeric antigen receptor in an immunocompetent mouse model. *Mol Ther.* (2019) 27:947– 59.doi: 10.1016/j. ymthe.2019.02.001

Kruse RL, Shum T, Tashiro H, Barzi M, Yi Z, Whitten-Bauer C, et al. HBsAg-redirected T cells exhibit antiviral activity in HBV-infected human liver chimeric mice. *Cytotherapy.* (2018) 20:697–705.doi: 10.1016/j.jcyt.2018. 02.002

Sautto GA, Wisskirchen K, Clementi N, Castelli M, Diotti RA, Graf J, et al. Chimeric antigen receptor (CAR)-engineered t cells redirected against hepatitis C virus (HCV) E2 glycoprotein. *Gut.* (2016) 65:512– 23.doi:10.1136/ gutjnl-2014-308316

Sautto G, Tarr AW, Mancini N, Clementi M. Structural and antigenic definition of hepatitis C virus E2 glycoprotein epitopes targeted by monoclonal antibodies. *Clin Dev Immunol.* (2013) 2013:450963.doi: 10.1155/2013/450963

Full F, Lehner M, Thonn V, Goetz G, Scholz B, Kaufmann KB, et al. T cells engineered with a cytomegalovirus-specific chimeric immunoreceptor. *J Virol.* (2010) 84:4083–8.doi: 10.1128/JVI.02117-09

Proff J, Walterskirchen C, Brey C, Geyeregger R, Full F, Ensser A, et al. Cytomegalovirus-infected cells resist T cell mediated killing in an HLA-recognition independent manner. *Front Microbiol.* (2016) 7:1– 15.doi:10.3389/ fmicb.2016.00844

Proff J, Brey CU, Ensser A, Holter W, Lehner M. Turning the tables on cytomegalovirus : targeting viral Fc receptors by CARs containing mutated CH2 – CH3 IgG spacer domains. *J Transl Med.* (2018) 1– 12.doi: 10.1186/ s12967-018-1394-x

Kumaresan PR, Manuri PR, Albert ND, Maiti S, Singh H, Mi T, et al. Bioengineering T cells to target carbohydrate to treat opportunistic fungal infection. *Proc Natl Acad Sci USA.* (2014) 111:10660–5.doi: 10.1073/pnas.1312789111

Hudecek M, Lupo-Stanghellini MT, Kosasih PL, Sommermeyer D, Jensen MC, Rader C, et al. Receptor affinity and extracellular domain modifications affect tumor recognition by ROR1-specific chimeric antigen receptor T cells. *Clin Cancer Res.* (2013) 19:3153–64.doi: 10.1158/1078-0432.CCR- 13-0330

Hudecek M, Sommermeyer D, Kosasih PL, Silva-Benedict A, Liu L, Rader C, et al. The non-signaling extracellular spacer domain of chimeric antigen receptors is decisive for *in vivo* antitumor activity. *Cancer Immunol Res.* (2015) 3:125–35.doi: 10.1158/2326-6066.CIR-14-0127

James SE, Greenberg PD, Jensen MC, Lin Y, Wang J, Till BG, et al. Antigen sensitivity of CD22-specific chimeric TCR is modulated by target epitope distance from the cell membrane. *J Immunol.* (2008) 180:7028– 38.doi: 10.4049/ jimmunol.180.10.7028

Guest RD, Hawkins RE, Kirillova N, Cheadle EJ, Arnold J, O' Neill A, et al. The role of extracellular spacer regions in the optimal design of chimeric immune receptors. *J Immunother.* (2005) 28:203– 11.doi: 10.1097/01. cji.0000161397.96582.59

Milone MC, Fish JD, Carpenito C, Carroll RG, Binder GK, Teachey D, et al. Chimeric receptors containing CD137 signal transduction domains mediate enhanced survival of T cells and increased antileukemic efficacy *in vivo. Mol Ther.* (2009) 17:1453–64.doi: 10.1038/mt.2009.83

Kochenderfer JN, Feldman SA, Zhao Y, Xu H, Black MA, Morgan RA, et al. Construction and preclinical evaluation of an anti-CD19 chimeric antigen receptor. *J Immunother.* (2009) 32:689–702.doi: 10.1097/CJI.0b013e3181ac6138

Imai C, Mihara K, Andreansky M, Nicholson IC, Pui CH, Geiger TL, et al. Chimeric receptors with 4-1BB signaling capacity provoke potent cytotoxicity against acute lymphoblastic leukemia. *Leukemia.* (2004) 18:676– 84.doi: 10.1038/sj.leu.2403302

Jensen M, Tan G, Forman S, Wu AM, Raubitschek A. CD20 is a molecular target for scFvFc:ζ receptor redirected T cells: implications for cellular immunotherapy of CD10+ malignancy. *Biol Blood Marrow Transplant.* (1998) 4:75–83.doi: 10.1053/bbmt.1998.v4.pm9763110

Gong MC, Latouche JB, Krause A, Heston WDW, Bander NH, Sadelain M. Cancer patient T cells genetically targeted to prostate-specific membrane antigen specifically lyse prostate cancer cells and release cytokines in response to prostate-specific membrane antigen. *Neoplasia.* (1999) 1:123– 7.doi: 10.1038/ sj.neo.7900018

Brocker T, Karjalainen K. Signals through T cell receptor-ζ chain alone are insufficient to prime resting T lymphocytes. *J Exp Med.* (1995) 181:1653–9.doi: 10.1084/jem.181.5.1653

Maher J, Brentjens RJ, Gunset G, Rivière I, Sadelain M. Human T-lymphocyte cytotoxicity and proliferation directed by a single chimeric TCRζ/CD28 receptor. *Nat Biotechnol.* (2002) 20:70–5.doi: 10.1038/nbt0102-70

Krause A, Guo HF, Latouche JB, Tan C, Cheung NKV, Sadelain M. Antigen-dependent CD28 signaling selectively enhances survival and proliferation in genetically modified activated human primary T lymphocytes. *J Exp Med.* (1998) 188:619–26.doi: 10.1084/jem.188.4.619

Finney HM, Lawson AD, Bebbington CR, Weir AN. Chimeric receptors providing both primary and costimulatory signaling in T cells from a single gene product. *J Immunol.* (1998) 161:2791–7.

Finney HM, Akbar AN, Lawson ADG. Activation of resting human primary T cells with chimeric receptors: costimulation from CD28, inducible costimulator, CD134, and CD137 in series with signals from the TCRζ chain. *J Immunol.* (2004) 172:104–13.doi: 10.4049/jimmunol.172.1.104

Porter D, Levine BL, Kalos M, Bagg A, June CH. Chimeric antigen receptor-modified T cells in chronic lymphoid leukemia. *N Engl J Med.* (2011) 365:725–33.doi: 10.1056/NEJMoa1103849

van der stegen SJC, Hamieh M, Sadelain M. The pharmacology of second-generation chimeric antigen receptors. *Nat Rev Drug Discov.* (2015) 14:499–509.doi: 10.1038/nrd4597

Salmikangas P, Kinsella N, Chamberlain P. Chimeric antigen receptor T-cells (CAR T-cells) for cancer immunotherapy – moving target for industry? *Pharm Res.* (2018) 35:1–8.doi: 10.1007/s11095-018-2436-z

Wang J, Jensen M, Lin Y, Sui X, Chen E, Lindgren CG, et al. Optimizing adoptive polyclonal T cell immunotherapy of lymphomas, using a chimeric T cell receptor possessing CD28 and CD137 costimulatory domains. *Hum Gene Ther.* (2007) 18:712–25.doi: 10.1089/hum.2007.028

Chmielewski M, Abken H. CAR T cells transform to trucks: chimeric antigen receptor-redirected T cells engineered to deliver inducible IL-12 modulate the tumour stroma to combat cancer. *Cancer Immunol Immunother.* (2012) 61:1269–77.doi: 10.1007/s00262-012-1202-z

Fesnak AD, June CH, Levine BL. Engineered T cells: the promise and challenges of cancer immunotherapy. *Nat Rev Cancer.* (2016) 16:566– 81.doi: 10.1038/ nrc.2016.97

Maldini CR, Ellis GI, Riley JL. CAR T cells for infection, autoimmunity and allotransplantation. *Nat Rev Immunol.* (2018) 18:605–16.doi: 10.1038/s41577-018-0042-2

Wagner TA. Quarter century of Anti-HIV CAR T cells. (2015) 344:1173– 8.doi: 10.1007/s11904-018-0388-x

Liu B, Zhang W, Zhang H. Development of CAR-T cells for long-term eradication and surveillance of HIV-1 reservoir. *Curr Opin Virol.* (2019) 38:21–30.doi: 10.1016/j.coviro.2019.04.004

Kuhlmann AS, Peterson CW, Kiem HP. Chimeric antigen receptor T- cell approaches to HIV cure. *Curr Opin HIV AIDS.* (2018) 13:446– 53.doi: 10.1097/COH.0000000000000485

Romeo C, Seed B. Cellular immunity to HIV activated by CD4 fused to T cell or Fc receptor polypeptides. *Cell.* (1991) 64:1037–46.doi: 10.1016/0092-8674(91)90327-U

Roberts MR, Qin L, Zhang D, Smith DH, Tran AC, Dull TJ, et al. Targeting of human immunodeficiency virus-infected cells by CD8+ T lymphocytes armed with universal T-cell receptors. *Blood.* (1994) 84:2878– 89.doi: 10.1182/blood.V84.9.2878.bloodjournal8492878

Scholler J, Brady TL, Binder-Scholl G, Hwang WT, Plesa G, Hege K, et al. Decade-long safety and function of retroviral- modified chimeric antigen receptor T-cells. *Sci Transl Med.* (2012) 4:132ra53.doi: 10.1126/scitranslmed.3003761

Walker RE, Bechtel CM, Natarajan V, Baseler M, Hege KM, Metcalf JA, et al. Long-term *in vivo* survival of receptor-modified syngeneic T cells in patients with human immunodeficiency virus infection. *Blood.* (2000) 96:467–74. doi: 10.1182/blood.V96.2.467.014k34_467_474

Mitsuyasu RT, Anton PA, Deeks SG, Scadden DT, Connick E, Downs MT, et al. Prolonged survival and tissue trafficking following adoptive transfer of CD4ζ gene-modified autologous CD4+ and CD8+ T cells in human immunodeficiency virus-infected subjects. *Blood.* (2000) 96:785– 93.doi: 10.1182/blood.V96.3.785.015k10_785_793

Deeks SG, Wagner B, Anton PA, Mitsuyasu RT, Scadden DT, Huang C, et al. A phase II randomized study of HIV-specific T-cell gene therapy in subjects with undetectable plasma viremia on combination antiretroviral therapy. *Mol Ther.* (2002) 5:788–97.doi: 10.1006/mthe.2002.0611

Kwarteng A, Ahuno ST, Kwakye-Nuako G. The therapeutic landscape of HIV-1 via genome editing. *AIDS Res Ther.* (2017) 14:1–16.doi: 10.1186/s12981-017-0157-8

Perez EE, Wang J, Miller JC, Jouvenot Y, Kim KA, Liu O, et al. Establishment of HIV-1 resistance in CD4+ T cells by genome editing using zinc-finger nucleases. *Nat Biotechnol.* (2008) 26:808–16.doi: 10.1038/nbt1410

Mock U, MacHowicz R, Hauber I, Horn S, Abramowski P, Berdien B, et al. mRNA transfection of a novel TAL effector nuclease (TALEN) facilitates efficient knockout of HIV co-receptor CCR5. *Nucleic Acids Res.* (2015) 43:5560–71.doi: 10.1093/nar/gkv469

Shi B, Li J, Shi X, Jia W, Wen Y, Hu X, et al. TALEN-mediated knockout of CCR5 confers protection against infection of human immunodeficiency virus. *J Acquir Immune Defic Syndr.* (2017) 74:229–41.doi: 10.1097/QAI.0000000000001190

Wang W, Ye C, Liu J, Zhang D, Kimata JT, Zhou P. CCR5 gene disruption via lentiviral vectors expressing Cas9 and single guided RNA renders cells resistant to HIV-1 infection. *PLoS ONE.* (2014) 9:1– 26.doi: 10.1371/journal.pone.0115987

Torikai H, Reik A, Liu PQ, Zhou Y, Zhang L, Maiti S, et al. A foundation for universal T-cell based immunotherapy: T cells engineered to express a CD19-specific chimeric-antigen-receptor and eliminate expression of endogenous TCR. *Blood.* (2012) 119:5697–705.doi: 10.1182/blood-2012-01-405365

Qasim W, Zhan H, Samarasinghe S, Adams S, Amrolia P,Stafford S, et al. Molecular remission of infant B-ALL after infusion of universal TALEN gene-edited CAR T cells. *Sci Transl Med.* (2017) 9:1–9.doi: 10.1126/scitranslmed.aaj2013

Philip LPB, Schiffer-Mannioui C, Le Clerre D, Chion-Sotinel I, Derniame S, Potrel P, et al. Multiplex genome-edited T-cell manufacturing platform for "off-the-shelf" adoptive T-cell immunotherapies. *Cancer Res.* (2015) 75:3853–64. doi: 10.1158/0008-5472.CAN-1 4-3321

Berdien B, Mock U, Atanackovic D, Fehse B. TALEN-mediated editing of endogenous T-cell receptors facilitates efficient reprogramming of T lymphocytes by lentiviral gene transfer. *Gene Ther.* (2014) 21:539– 48.doi: 10.1038/gt.2014.26

Ren J, Liu X, Fang C, Jiang S, June CH, Zhao Y. Multiplex genome editing to generate universal CAR T cells resistant to PD1 inhibition. *Clin Cancer Res.* (2017) 23:2255–66.doi: 10.1158/1078-0432.CCR-16-1300

Ren J, Zhang X, Liu X, Fang C, Jiang S, June CH, et al. A versatile system for rapid multiplex genome-edited CAR T cell generation. *Oncotarget.* (2017) 8:17002–11.doi: 10.18632/oncotarget.15218

Ali A, Kitchen SG, Chen ISY, Ng HL, Zack JA, Yang OO. HIV-1- specific chimeric antigen receptors based on broadly neutralizing antibodies. *J Virol.* (2016) 90:6999–7006.doi: 10.1128/JVI.00 805-16

Tang X, Zhou Y, Li W, Tang Q, Chen R, Zhu J, et al. T cells expressing a LMP1-specific chimeric antigen receptor mediate antitumor effects against LMP1-positive nasopharyngeal carcinoma cells *in vitro* and *in vivo. J Biomed Res.* (2014) 28:468–75.doi: 10.7555/JBR.28.20140066

D'Aloia MM, Zizzari IG, Sacchetti B, Pierelli L, Alimandi M. CAR-T cells: the long and winding road to solid tumors review-article. *Cell Death Dis.* (2018) 9:282. doi: 10.1038/s41419-018-0278-6

Bowman SM, Free SJ. The structure and synthesis of the fungal cell wall. *BioEssays.* (2006) 28:799–808.doi: 10.1002/bies.20441

Iliev ID, Funari VA, Taylor KD, Nguyen Q, Reyes CN, Strom SP, et al. Interactions between commensal fungi and the C-type lectin receptor dectin-1 influence colitis. *Science.* (2012) 336:1314–7.doi: 10.1126/science.1221789

Buechner J, Kersten MJ, Fuchs M, Salmon F, Jäger U. Chimeric antigen receptor-T cell therapy: practical considerations for implementation in Europe. *HemaSphere.* (2018) 2:e18.doi: 10.1097/HS9.0000000000000018

Rapid Detection of *Enterocytozoon hepatopenaei* Infection in Shrimp with a Real-Time Isothermal Recombinase Polymerase Amplification Assay

Chao Ma[1†], Shihui Fan[1†], Yu Wang[1†], Haitao Yang[1], Yi Qiao[2], Ge Jiang[2], Mingsheng Lyu[1], Jingquan Dong[1*], Hui Shen[2*] and Song Gao[1*]

[1] Jiangsu Key Laboratory of Marine Biological Resources and Environment, Jiangsu Key Laboratory of Marine Pharmaceutical Compound Screening, Co-Innovation Center of Jiangsu Marine Bio-industry Technology, School of Pharmacy, Jiangsu Ocean University, Lianyungang, China, [2] Jiangsu Institute of Oceanology and Marine Fisheries, Nantong, China

*Correspondence:
Jingquan Dong
2018000029@jou.edu.cn
Hui Shen
darkhui@163.com
Song Gao
gaos@jou.edu.cn

[†]These authors have contributed equally to this work

Enterocytozoon hepatopenaei (EHP) infection has become a significant threat in shrimp farming industry in recent years, causing major economic losses in Asian countries. As there are a lack of effective therapeutics, prevention of the infection with rapid and reliable pathogen detection methods is fundamental. Molecular detection methods based on polymerase chain reaction (PCR) and loop-mediated isothermal amplification (LAMP) have been developed, but improvements on detection speed and convenience are still in demand. The isothermal recombinase polymerase amplification (RPA) assay derived from the recombination-dependent DNA replication (RDR) mechanism of bacteriophage T4 is promising, but the previously developed RPA assay for EHP detection read the signal by gel electrophoresis, which restricted this application to laboratory conditions and hampered the sensitivity. The present study combined fluorescence analysis with the RPA system and developed a real-time RPA assay for the detection of EHP. The detection procedure was completed in 3–7 min at 39°C and showed good specificity. The sensitivity of 13 gene copies per reaction was comparable to the current PCR- and LAMP-based methods, and was much improved than the RPA assay analyzed by gel electrophoresis. For real clinical samples, detection results of the real-time RPA assay were 100% consistent with the industrial standard nested PCR assay. Because of the rapid detection speed and the simple procedure, the real-time RPA assay developed in this study can be easily assembled as an efficient and reliable on-site detection tool to help control EHP infection in shrimp farms.

Keywords: *Enterocytozoon hepatopenaei*, recombinase polymerase amplification, recombination-dependent replication, spore wall protein gene, molecular detection

INTRODUCTION

Microsporidia are intracellular parasites which can infect a wide range of crustaceans and fish (Ning et al., 2019). Among Microsporidia, *Enterocytozoon hepatopenaei* (EHP) is an emerging pathogen and has been classified into the group of *Enterocytozoonidae*, suborder *Apansporoblastina*, phylum *Microsporidia*, and kingdom Fungi (Tourtip et al., 2009). In shrimp aquaculture industry, EHP can infect the hepatopancreas of different shrimp species including *Penaeus japonicas*, *Penaeus monodon*, and *Penaeus vannamei* (Tang et al., 2016; Thitamadee et al., 2016; Chaijarasphong et al., 2020). When infected, it causes stunted growth, soft shells, lethargy and white feces symptoms (Behera et al., 2019). In Asian countries including India, Thailand and China, EHP caused 10%–20% reduced production of shrimp annually leading to significant economic losses (Thamizhvanan et al., 2019). In the year 2015 in Jiangsu, China, EHP infections had caused 300 million CNY of loss for the shrimp farming industry. EHP has been considered a huge threat to farms in many shrimp-farming countries (Shen et al., 2019).

There are no specific clinical signs in EHP-infected shrimps, making it difficult to monitor EHP infection and to control the spreading. The feces of EHP-infected shrimp contain a large number of spores, which can infect healthy shrimp through horizontal transmission (Karthikeyan and Sudhakaran, 2019). In addition, there are no proven therapeutic methods for EHP infection (Chaijarasphong et al., 2020). Thus, it is very important to develop a rapid and simple detection method for EHP infection to prevent disease outbreaks and economic losses. To date, a number of diagnostic methods for the detection of EHP have been reported. These include loop-mediated isothermal amplification (LAMP), polymerase chain reaction (PCR), and quantitative PCR (qPCR) targeting the small subunit ribosomal RNA gene (SSU rRNA), nested PCR targeting the spore wall protein gene (*swp*) or *β-tubulin* gene, *in situ* hybridization assay, and histopathology (Jaroenlak et al., 2016; Han et al., 2018; Sathish et al., 2018; Piamsomboon et al., 2019). However, these methods have drawbacks like long detection time, need for trained personnel, and equipment dependence. Although the LAMP method takes only 45 min for the reaction, it still requires an accurate temperature-controlled machine (Sathish et al., 2018). These methods are not suitable for use in remote areas.

The isothermal recombinase polymerase amplification (RPA) assay derived from the recombination-dependent DNA replication (RDR) mechanism of bacteriophage T4 is a potentially suitable method (Li et al., 2018; Lobato and O'Sullivan, 2018; Dong et al., 2020; Hu et al., 2020; Wang et al., 2020). The RPA system uses several enzymes from bacteriophage T4, including the strand-exchange protein UvsX, the mediator protein UvsY, and the single-strand binding protein gp32, to mimic the bacteriophage T4 RDR system *in vitro*. UvsX and UvsY anchor on a DNA single strand and search for homologous sequences on another double-stranded DNA. Once a homologous sequence is found, a recombination event occurs and one strand of the double-stranded DNA is displaced

by the single strand. The displaced strand is stabilized by gp32. The 3'-end of the displacing strand is extended by the *Bsu* DNA polymerase (Piepenburg et al., 2006). By mimicking the T4 RDR mechanism, the RPA system solves the low-temperature strand opening problem and amplifies the target DNA fragment isothermally at 37–42°C. Researchers have tried to apply the RPA technology to the detection of EHP infection in shrimp and, indeed, simplified the procedure because a thermocycler was no longer required. However, the analysis of amplification products by gel electrophoresis did not free the assay from the laboratory for field use, and the sensitivity was also limited by gel imaging tools (Zhou et al., 2020).

The amplification products of RPA can be analyzed with better convenience by lateral flow chromatography or fluorescence (Li et al., 2018). Among these two options, fluorescence analysis makes real-time reading of the signal possible and this "real-time RPA" assay has a good combination of speed, portability, and accessibility. Briefly, the real time RPA reaction contains an "exo probe" that anneals to one of the amplified strands and recruits an exonuclease to cleave off the tetrahydrofuran (THF) substitution on the probe to separate the fluorophore and the quenching group at the two adjacent sites of THF on the probe, emitting the fluorescence signal (**Figure 1**) (Piepenburg et al., 2006).

In this study, a real-time RPA assay for rapid detection of EHP has been established. This method finished the detection in 10 min with good specificity. The limit of detection was 13 gene copies per reaction. Detection results were 100% consistent with the established nested PCR assay for real clinical samples. The real-time RPA assay is simple and reliable, and can be widely deployed for the detection of EHP infection in remote areas.

MATERIALS AND METHODS

Infected Shrimp Samples, Bacterial Strains, and Clinical Samples

A collection of shrimps infected by *Enterocytozoon hepatopenaei* (EHP), white spot syndrome virus (WSSV), shrimp hemocyte iridescent virus (SHIV), and a *Vibrio parahaemolyticus* strain causing acute hepatopancreatic necrosis disease (AHPND) (referred to as VP_{AHPND} in this study), and reference strains of *Vibrio vulnificus* and *Vibrio parahaemolyticus* (not AHPND-causative, referred to as non-VP_{AHPND} in this study) were obtained from Jiangsu Institute of Oceanology and Marine Fisheries (Nantong, China). Clinical shrimp samples at different growing stages were collected from shrimp farms of different areas in China, including Qingdao, Rudong, Yancheng, Qidong, Lianyungang, and Rizhao. DNA of infected shrimp samples or clinical samples was extracted by the Magnetic Universal Genomic DNA Kit using the handheld 3rd Gen. TGrinder (Tiangen Biotech Co., Ltd., Beijing, China) and quantified with a Qubit 4 fluorometer (Thermo Fisher Scientific Inc, Wilmington, DE, USA). DNA from the infected shrimp samples were confirmed for the presence of infection agents by qPCR as described previously (Zhu and Quan, 2012;

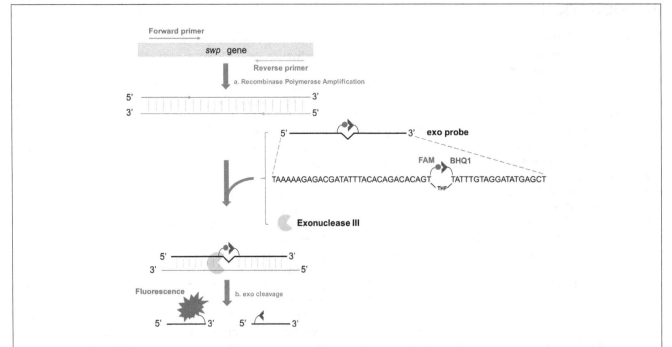

FIGURE 1 | Schematic representation of the real-time RPA assay. Fragment of the target gene (*swp* gene in case of EHP detection) is isothermally amplified by recombinase polymerase amplification (event a). To one of the amplified strands, the exo probe anneals, and the Exonuclease III (exo) cleaves at the THF site once the bases flanking it have paired (event b). On the exo probe, the two T bases adjacent the THF site have been substituted by FAM-dT (fluorescent group) and BHQ1-dT (quenching group), respectively. The exo cleavage separates the two groups to allow fluorescence emission. There is a SpC3 group (not shown in this diagram) at the 3'-end of the exo probe to block the undesired extension of the probe.

Liu et al., 2018; Qiu et al., 2018; Zheng et al., 2018). The reference bacterial strains were confirmed by 16S rRNA sequencing (Hiergeist et al., 2016).

Design of Primers and Probes

An NCBI Primer-BLAST (https://www.ncbi.nlm.nih.gov/tools/primer-blast) search was conducted using the FASTA sequence of the *swp* gene of EHP (GenBank accession no. KX258197.1). For parameter settings, the product size was set as minimum at 100 bp and maximum at 200 bp. The organism was set as *Enterocytozoon hepatopenaei* (taxid: 646526). The primer size was set at a minimum of 30 bases and a maximum of 35 bases. The primer GC content was set at a minimum of 20% and a maximum of 70%. The maximal self-complementarity was set as any at 4 and 3' at 1. The maximal pair complementarity was set as any at 4 and 3' at 1. Other parameters were set as default. For the probe design, the sequence defined by the primer pair was input into the Primer Premier 5 software. The size of the probe was set at a minimum of 46 bases and a maximum of 51 bases. The melting temperature (*Tm*) was set at a minimum of 57°C and a maximum of 63°C. The GC content was set at a minimum of 20% and a maximum of 80%. The maximum hairpin score was set as 1. The maximum primer-dimer score was set as 1. The maximum poly-X was set as 3. Other parameters were set as default. The probe had a C3 spacer (SpC3) at the 3'-end that could block strand extension and a tetrahydrofuran (THF) group at the middle to facilitate exonuclease III (exo) cutting. The two T bases adjacent the THF site were substituted by FAM (6-corboxy-fluorescein)-dT and BHQ1 (Black Hole Quencher 1)-

dT (**Figure 1**). Primers and probes were synthesized by General Biosystems Co., Ltd., Anhui, China. The sequences are shown in **Table 1**.

Construction of the Plasmid Standard

DNA extracted from the EHP-infected shrimp was used as the template and a pair of primers (SWP_1F and SWP_1R) was used for PCR amplification to obtain the target fragment of the *swp* gene (**Table 1**) (Jaroenlak et al., 2016). The PCR product was cloned into a pMD18-T vector (Takara Biomedical Technology Co., Ltd., Beijing, China) and verified by sequencing. The recombinant plasmid was extracted from the correct clone and quantified with a Qubit 4 fluorometer (Thermo Fisher Scientific Inc, Wilmington, DE, USA). The plasmid copy number was calculated based on its size (3,206 bp). The standard plasmid was tenfold serially diluted and used as templates for qPCR with the specific primers SWP_1F and SWP_2R targeting the *swp* gene fragment. The correlation of the *Ct* value with the copy number of the *swp* gene fragment was calculated from the qPCR results.

Real-Time RPA Procedure

Real-time RPA reactions were performed according to the manufacturer instructions of the TwistAmp DNA Amplification exo Kit (TwistDx Inc., Maidenhead, United Kingdom). The reaction mixture contained 29.5 µl of rehydration buffer, 2.1 µl of each primer (10 µM), 0.6 µl of probe (10 µM), 12.2 µl of distilled water, 1 µl of the template, and a dried enzyme pellet. The reaction was initiated by adding 2.5 µl of magnesium acetate (280 mM) to the mixture. The reaction was conducted on a Roche

LightCycler 480 II qPCR machine at 39°C in the FAM channel with signal reads at 15-s intervals for 20 min.

Nested PCR

The nested PCR detection of EHP was performed as previously reported (Jaroenlak et al., 2016). Primers SWP_1F and SWP_1R were used for the 1st PCR step with an expected amplicon size of 514 bp. From the reaction mixture of the 1st PCR step, 1 µl was directly used for the 2nd PCR step with primers SWP_2F and SWP_2R (**Table 1**). The expected amplicon size of the 2nd PCR step was 147 bp. The amplicons were analyzed on a 1.5% agarose gel.

RESULTS

Determination of Copy Number of the *swp* Gene Fragment in Extracted DNA

To determine the copy number of the *swp* gene fragment in the extracted DNA of EHP-infected shrimp, a standard plasmid containing the gene fragment was constructed (**Supplementary Figure S1**), purified, and quantified spectrophotometrically. Tenfold serial dilutions of the standard plasmid from 10^9 to 10^3 copies/µl were used as the template for qPCR, and the Ct value for each concentration was determined. A standard curve was built showing a good correlation between the DNA copy number and the Ct value (R^2 = 0.9982) (**Figure 2**). This correlation was used to determine the copy number of the *swp* gene fragment in the extracted DNA of EHP-infected shrimp.

Limit of Detection of the Real-Time RPA Assay

DNA was extracted from the EHP-infected shrimp and quantified by qPCR using the standard curve. The quantified DNA was diluted to final concentrations of 10^4 to 10^0 copies/µl of the gene fragment and used to evaluate the limit of detection of the real-time RPA assay. The results showed that the signal of 10^1 copies per reaction could be observed (**Figure 3A**). Reactions were conducted for eight independent repeats; 10^2 copies and above per reaction were detected in all the eight repeats and 10^1 copies per reaction were detected in seven of the eight repeats. A probit regression analysis was conducted and the limit of detection was calculated to be 13 copies/reaction in 95% of cases (**Figure 3B**). Semi-log regression analysis of the data of the eight repeats showed that the reaction time lengths of the

real-time RPA assay to observe the signal were 3 to 7 min for 10^4 to 10^1 copies (**Figure 3C**).

Detection Specificity of the Real-Time RPA Assay

To evaluate the specificity of the real-time RPA assay, shrimp samples infected with different viruses and microbes were tested (EHP, WSSV, SHIV, and VP_{AHPND}). Also tested were reference strains of *V. vulnificus* and *V. parahaemolyticus* (non-VP_{AHPND}). DNA extracted from the healthy shrimp (*P. vannamei*) was used as the control. The DNA concentrations were normalized to 10 ng/µl and used as the templates. For the two reference bacterial strains, incubation cultures of 10^6 colony-forming unit (CFU)/ml were boiled at 100°C for 10 min and immediately used as the templates. Only the DNA from EHP-infected shrimp was positive, indicating good specificity of the real-time RPA assay toward EHP (**Table 2**).

Application of the Real-Time RPA Assay for EHP Detection

A total of 32 clinical shrimp samples at different growth stages from several shrimp farms were tested for EHP with the real-time RPA assay and the nested PCR assay. A total of 22 EHP-positive samples were detected and the results of real-time RPA assay were 100% consistent with the nested PCR assay (**Tables 3, 4**, and **Supplementary Figure S2**). These results indicated that the real-time RPA assay was effective for real clinical samples.

DISCUSSION

Enterocytozoon hepatopenaei (EHP) has emerged as a serious threat to shrimp aquaculture worldwide (Thitamadee et al., 2016). EHP infection in farmed shrimps does not cause mass mortality, but inflicts significant economic loss due to stunted growth and reduced feed consumption (Aranguren Caro et al., 2020) . Noting the lack of pharmacological interventions for EHP, a rapid and accurate detection assay of EHP infection in shrimp is significant for the shrimp farming industry as prevention is the only currently available control method. The currently available detection methods, including the nested PCR, qPCR, and LAMP, cannot fulfill the demand for rapidness and accessibility, especially in remote areas. Nested PCR and qPCR take several hours and require a precise temperature-controlled

TABLE 1 | Primers and probe used in this study.

Method	Description	Sequence (5'-3')	Length (bp)	Amplicon Size (bp)	Amplification target on Gene	GenBank No. of Gene
Real-time RPA	RPA-F	ACAATTTCAAACACTGTAAACCTTAAAGCA	30	176	79..254	KX258197.1
	RPA-P	TAAAAAGAGACGATATTTACACAGACACAG[FAM-dT][THF][BHQ1-dT]ATTTGTAGGATATGAGCT	46			*(swp)*
	RPA-R	TCATTCATTTTCCTTTTATCTTCTGATATG	30			
Nested PCR	SWP_1F	TTGCAGAGTGTTGTTAAGGGTTT	23	514	1..514	
(Jaroenlak et al., 2016)	SWP_1R	CACGATGTGTCTTTGCAATTTTC	23			
	SWP_2F	TTGGCGGCACAATTCTCAAACA	22	147	38..184	
	SWP_2R	GCTGTTTGTCTCCAACTGTATTTGA	25			

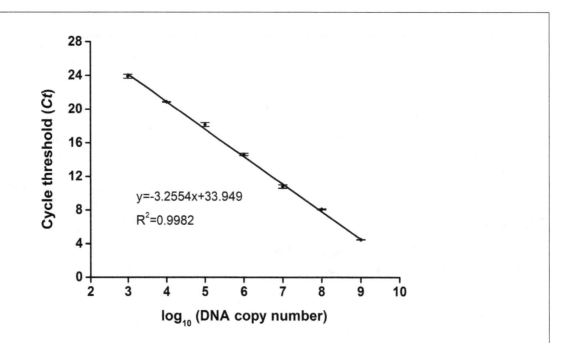

FIGURE 2 | Standard curve of *swp* gene fragment by qPCR. For each reaction, 1 μl of the standard plasmid between 10^3 and 10^9 copies/μl was used as the template. The standard curve representing the correlation between the DNA copy number and the qPCR cycle threshold (*Ct*) value was built using GraphPad Prism 8.0 (GraphPad Software Inc, San Diego, CA). The function of the standard curve and the R^2 value are indicated. The error bars represent the mean and standard error of three qPCR repeats.

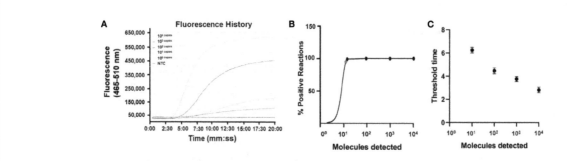

FIGURE 3 | Limit of detection of the real-time RPA assay. **(A)** The fluorescence history diagram of the results of real-time RPA with different amounts (in copies) of the *swp* gene fragment. The amounts tested are indicated with different colors. The NTC is the no-template control. The diagram was one typical outcome of eight independent experiments. **(B)** Probit regression analysis of the data collected from the eight real-time RPA repeats using SPSS software (IBM, Armonk, NY, USA). The limit of detection at 95% probability (13 copies/reaction) is depicted by a red rhomboid. **(C)** Semi-logarithmic regression analysis of the data collected from the eight real-time RPA repeats using GraphPad Prism 8.0 (GraphPad Software Inc). The run time (threshold time) of the real-time RPA was 3–7 min for the templates at 10^4–10^0 copies/reaction.

thermocycler. LAMP can finish the detection within an hour, but an accurately controlled thermal source is still needed.

The RDR mechanism of bacteriophage T4 provided a good strategy to open the double strands of DNA without the need for temperature elevation (Alberts and Frey, 1970; Kodadek et al., 1988). By assembly of the RDR system *in vitro* with UvsX, UvsY, and gp32 of bacteriophage T4 and a strand-displacing DNA polymerase from *Bacillus subtilis* (*Bsu*), the DNA amplification cycle, including strand opening, primer pairing, and chain extension, can be conducted under one constant temperature between 37 and 42°C. Exponential amplification of DNA is achieved very rapidly, usually within 30 min (Li et al., 2018).

This RPA system derived from bacteriophage T4 has been commercialized and widely applied to molecular diagnosis for many infectious diseases (Dong et al., 2020; Hu et al., 2020; Wang et al., 2020). An effort has been made to apply the RPA technology for the detection of EHP infection that targeted the SSU rRNA gene, but the analysis of the amplification signal was performed by gel electrophoresis, which not only hampered the sensitivity (8×10^2 gene copies per reaction) but also restrained the detection assay to the laboratory (Zhou et al., 2020).

Using fluorescence signal reading, this study described the development and evaluation of a real-time RPA assay for the detection of EHP infection in shrimp. The assay targeted the *swp*

TABLE 2 | Information of shrimp samples and bacteria strains used in this study.

Infection agent	Sample type	Source/designation	Real-time RPA
Enterocytozoon hepatopenaei (EHP)	Infected shrimp (*Penaeus vannamei*)	Nantong, China	+
White spot syndrome virus (WSSV)	Infected shrimp (*Penaeus vannamei*)	Nantong, China	–
Shrimp hemocyte iridescent virus (SHIV)	Infected shrimp (*Penaeus vannamei*)	Nantong, China	–
Vibrio parahaemolyticus (VP_{AHPND})	Infected shrimp (*Penaeus vannamei*)	Nantong, China	–
Vibrio vulnificus	Reference strain	ATCC 27562	–
Vibrio parahaemolyticus (non-VP_{AHPND})	Reference strain	ATCC 17802	–
None	Healthy shrimp (*Penaeus vannamei*)	Nantong, China	–

(+, positive result; –, negative result).

TABLE 3 | Detection of *Enterocytozoon hepatopenaei* (EHP) infection in clinical samples.

No.	Sample type	Sample species	Length of shrimp (cm)	Source	Detection results	
					Nested PCR	Real-time RPA
1	Shrimp	*Penaeus vannamei*	0.5–3	Qingdao, China	+	+
2	Shrimp	*Penaeus vannamei*	0.5–3	Qingdao, China	+	+
3	Shrimp	*Penaeus vannamei*	0.5–3	Rudong, China	+	+
4	Shrimp	*Penaeus vannamei*	0.5–3	Rudong, China	+	+
5	Shrimp	*Penaeus vannamei*	4–5	Yancheng, China	+	+
6	Shrimp	*Penaeus vannamei*	8–9	Rudong, China	+	+
7	Shrimp	*Penaeus vannamei*	8–9	Rudong, China	+	+
8	Shrimp	*Penaeus vannamei*	0.5–3	Rudong, China	+	+
9	Shrimp	*Penaeus vannamei*	0.5–3	Rudong, China	–	–
10	Shrimp	*Penaeus vannamei*	5–6	Qidong, China	+	+
11	Shrimp	*Penaeus vannamei*	5–6	Yancheng, China	+	+
12	Shrimp	*Penaeus vannamei*	0.5–3	Lianyungang, China	+	+
13	Shrimp	*Penaeus vannamei*	0.5–3	Lianyungang, China	+	+
14	Shrimp	*Penaeus vannamei*	7–8	Yancheng, China	–	–
15	Shrimp	*Penaeus vannamei*	7–8	Yancheng, China	+	+
16	Shrimp	*Penaeus vannamei*	0.5–3	Rudong, China	+	+
17	Shrimp	*Penaeus vannamei*	0.5–3	Rudong, China	–	–
18	Shrimp	*Penaeus vannamei*	0.5–3	Rizhao, China	+	+
19	Shrimp	*Penaeus vannamei*	5–6	Rizhao, China	–	–
20	Shrimp	*Penaeus vannamei*	5–6	Lianyungang, China	+	+
21	Shrimp	*Penaeus vannamei*	0.5–3	Lianyungang, China	+	+
22	Shrimp	*Penaeus vannamei*	5–6	Rizhao, China	+	+
23	Shrimp	*Penaeus vannamei*	0.5–3	Rizhao, China	+	+
24	Shrimp	*Penaeus vannamei*	4–5	Qidong, China	–	–
25	Shrimp	*Penaeus vannamei*	7–8	Qidong, China	–	–
26	Shrimp	*Penaeus vannamei*	0.5–3	Rudong, China	+	+
27	Shrimp	*Penaeus vannamei*	0.5–3	Qidong, China	–	–
28	Shrimp	*Penaeus vannamei*	0.5–3	Rudong, China	+	+
29	Shrimp	*Penaeus vannamei*	0.5–3	Yancheng, China	–	–
30	Shrimp	*Penaeus vannamei*	4–5	Lianyungang, China	–	–
31	Shrimp	*Penaeus vannamei*	7–8	Rizhao, China	–	–
32	Shrimp	*Penaeus vannamei*	4–5	Rizhao, China	+	+

(+, positive result; –, negative result).

gene encoding the spore wall protein of EHP. This gene is considered a better molecular diagnosis biomarker than the SSU rRNA gene and has been used as the target in the previously established nested PCR method, which has been recognized as an industrial standard of shrimp farming (Jaroenlak et al., 2016). The results in this study confirmed the good specificity of this gene toward EHP detection.

The real-time RPA assay showed good detection sensitivity that was comparable to the nested PCR method and much better than the RPA assay using the gel electrophoresis analysis. The limit of detection was 13 copies/reaction in 95% of the cases. As referenced in other reports, the limit of detection of EHP was 10^1 copies/reaction with the nested PCR method as well as with the qPCR- and LAMP-

based methods (Liu et al., 2018; Ma et al., 2019). Comparing with the RPA assay using the gel electrophoresis analysis, the sensitivity of real-time RPA has improved for ~60 folds. Moreover, the real-time RPA results of real clinical samples are 100% consistent with the nested PCR method, indicating good reliability.

Besides the good sensitivity, the rapid and simple procedure is the advantage of the real-time RPA method. The detection procedure could be finished in 3–7 min at a conveniently low temperature of 39°C. For the pretreatment of the samples, DNA was extracted with a magnetic bead-based commercialized kit that only needs a magnet to perform the extraction. For the signal reading, although we used a qPCR machine to read the fluorescence signal in

TABLE 4 | Detection of *Enterocytozoon hepatopenaei* (EHP) infection in clinical samples (summarized).

Sample information	Number of samples	Number of positive samples detected	
		Nested PCR	Real-time RPA
Shrimp (0.5-3 cm)	17	13	13
Shrimp (4-5 cm)	4	2	2
Shrimp (5-6 cm)	5	4	4
Shrimp (7-8 cm)	4	1	1
Shrimp (8-9 cm)	2	2	2
Total	32	22	22

this study, portable tube scanners had been developed for field applications, such as the Genie III scanner from Beijing Suntrap Science & Technology Co., Ltd, China, the ESE Quant tube scanner from ESE Gmbh, Stockach, Germany, and the TwistDx tube-scanner from TwistDx Inc (Yi et al., 2014; Mondal et al., 2016; Geng et al., 2019). These small-sized, battery-powered fluorescence tube scanners are good replacements of qPCR machines for on-site real-time RPA detections. Because of the low dependence on equipment and power source, the real-time RPA assay can be easily assembled into a mobile suitcase laboratory for transport and use in the field (Mondal et al., 2016).

In conclusion, a real-time RPA assay was developed for rapid detection of EHP infection in shrimp. It can be applied as an efficient and reliable on-site detection tool to help control EHP infection in shrimp farms.

AUTHOR CONTRIBUTIONS

JD, HS, and SG designed the research. CM, SF, YW, and HY conducted the research. CM, YQ, GJ, and ML analyzed the data. CM and SG wrote the manuscript. All authors contributed to the article and approved the submitted version.

ACKNOWLEDGMENTS

We thank LetPub (www.letpub.com) for its linguistic assistance during the preparation of this manuscript.

REFERENCES

Alberts, B. M., and Frey, L. (1970). T4 Bacteriophage Gene 32: A Structural Protein in the Replication and Recombination of DNA. *Nature* 227, 1313–1318. doi: 10.1038/2271313a0

Aranguren Caro, L. F., Mai, H., Pichardo, O., Cruz-Flores, R., Hanggono, B., and Dhar, A. K. (2020). Evidences supporting *Enterocytozoon hepatopenaei* association with white feces syndrome in farmed Penaeus vannamei in Venezuela and Indonesia. *Dis. Aquat. Organ.* 141, 71–78. doi: 10.3354/dao03522

Behera, B. K., Das, A., Paria, P., Sahoo, A. K., Parida, P. K., Abdulla, T., et al. (2019). Prevalence of microsporidian parasite, *Enterocytozoon hepatopenaei* in cultured Pacific White shrimp, *Litopenaeus vannamei* (Boone 1931) in West Bengal, East Coast of India. *Aquacult. Int.* 27, 609–620. doi: 10.1007/s10499-019-00350-0

Chaijarasphong, T., Munkongwongsiri, N., Stentiford, G. D., Aldama, D. J., Thansa, K., Flegel, T. W., et al. (2020). The shrimp microsporidian *Enterocytozoon hepatopenaei* (EHP): Biology, pathology, diagnostics and control. *J. Invertebr. Pathol.* 1, 107458. doi: 10.1016/j.jip.2020.107458

Dong, Y., Zhao, P., Chen, L., Wu, H., Si, X., Shen, X., et al. (2020). Fast, simple and highly specific molecular detection of *Vibrio alginolyticus* pathogenic strains using a visualized isothermal amplification method. *BMC Vet. Res.* 16, 76–76. doi: 10.1186/s12917-020-02297-4

Geng, Y., Tan, K., Liu, L., Sun, X. X., Zhao, B., and Wang, J. (2019). Development and evaluation of a rapid and sensitive RPA assay for specific detection of *Vibrio parahaemolyticus* in seafood. *BMC Microbiol.* 19, 186. doi: 10.1186/s12866-019-1562-z

Han, J. E., Tang, K. F. J., and Kim, J. H. (2018). The use of beta-tubulin gene for phylogenetic analysis of the microsporidian parasite *Enterocytozoon hepatopenaei* (EHP) and in the development of a nested PCR as its diagnostic tool. *Aquaculture* 495, 899–902. doi: 10.1016/j.aquaculture.2018.06.059

Hiergeist, A., Reischl, U., and Gessner, A. (2016). Multicenter quality assessment of 16S ribosomal DNA-sequencing for microbiome analyses reveals high inter-center variability. *Int. J. Med. Microbiol.* 306, 334–342. doi: 10.1016/j.ijmm.2016.03.005

Hu, J., Wang, Y., Ding, H., Jiang, C., Geng, Y., Sun, X., et al. (2020). Recombinase polymerase amplification with polymer flocculation sedimentation for rapid detection of *Staphylococcus aureus* in food samples. *Int. J. Food Microbiol.* 331, 108691. doi: 10.1016/j.ijfoodmicro.2020.108691

Jaroenlak, P., Sanguanrut, P., Williams, B. A., Stentiford, G. D., Flegel, T. W., Sritunyalucksana, K., et al. (2016). A Nested PCR Assay to Avoid False Positive Detection of the Microsporidian *Enterocytozoon hepatopenaei* (EHP) in Environmental Samples in Shrimp Farms. *PLoS One* 11, e0166320. doi: 10.1371/journal.pone.0166320

Karthikeyan, K., and Sudhakaran, R. (2019). Experimental horizontal transmission of *Enterocytozoon hepatopenaei* in post-larvae of whiteleg shrimp, Litopenaeus vannamei. *J. Fish Dis.* 3, 397–404. doi: 10.1111/jfd.12945

Kodadek, T., Wong, M., and Alberts, B. (1988). The mechanism of homologous DNA strand exchange catalyzed by the bacteriophage T4 uvsX and gene 32 proteins. *J. Biol. Chem.* 263, 9427–9436. doi: 10.1016/S0021-9258(19)76558-2

Li, J., Macdonald, J., and Stetten, F. (2018). Review: a comprehensive summary of a decade development of the recombinase polymerase amplification. *Analyst* 144, 31–67. doi: 10.1039/c8an01621f

Liu, Y., Qiu, L., Sheng, A., Wan, X., Cheng, D., and Huang, J. (2018). Quantitative detection method of *Enterocytozoon hepatopenaei* using TaqMan probe real-time PCR. *J. Invertebr. Pathol.* 151, 191–196. doi: 10.1016/j.jip.2017.12.006

Lobato, I. M., and O'Sullivan, C. K. (2018). Recombinase polymerase amplification: Basics, applications and recent advances. *Trends Analyt. Chem.* 98, 19–35. doi: 10.1016/j.trac.2017.10.015

Ma, B., Yu, H., Fang, J., Sun, C., and Zhang, M. (2019). Employing DNA binding dye to improve detection of *Enterocytozoon hepatopenaei* in real-time LAMP. *Sci. Rep.* 9, 15860. doi: 10.1038/s41598-019-52459-0

Mondal, D., Ghosh, P., Khan, M. A. A., Hossain, F., Böhlken-Fascher, S., Matlashewski, G., et al. (2016). Mobile suitcase laboratory for rapid detection of Leishmania donovani using recombinase polymerase amplification assay. *Parasit. Vectors* 9, 281. doi: 10.1186/s13071-016-1572-8

Ning, M., Wei, P., Shen, H., Wan, X., Jin, M., Li, X., et al. (2019). Proteomic and metabolomic responses in hepatopancreas of whiteleg shrimp Litopenaeus vannamei infected by microsporidian *Enterocytozoon hepatopenaei*. *Fish Shellfish Immunol.* 87, 534–545. doi: 10.1016/j.fsi.2019.01.051

Piamsomboon, P., Choi, S. K., Hanggono, B., Nuraini, Y. L., Wati, F., Tang, K. F. J., et al. (2019). Quantification of *Enterocytozoon hepatopenaei* (EHP) in Penaeid Shrimps from Southeast Asia and Latin America Using TaqMan Probe-Based Quantitative PCR. *Pathog. (Basel Switzerland)* 8:233. doi: 10.3390/pathogens8040233

Piepenburg, O., Williams, C. H., Stemple, D. L., and Armes, N. A. (2006). DNA detection using recombination proteins. *PloS Biol.* 4, e204. doi: 10.1371/journal.pbio.0040204

Qiu, L., Chen, M., Wan, X., Zhang, Q., Li, C., Dong, X., et al. (2018). Detection and quantification of shrimp hemocyte iridescent virus by TaqMan probe based real-time PCR. *J. Invertebr. Pathol.* 154, 95–101. doi: 10.1016/j.jip.2018.04.005

Sathish, K. T., Navaneeth, K. A., Joseph, S. R. J., Makesh, M., Jithendran, K. P., Alavandi, S. V., et al. (2018). Visual loop-mediated isothermal amplification (LAMP) for the rapid diagnosis of Enterocytozoon hepatopenaei (EHP) infection. *Parasitol. Res.* 117, 1485–1493. doi: 10.1007/s00436-018-5828-4

Shen, H., Qiao, Y., Wan, X., Jiang, G., Fan, X., Li, H., et al. (2019). Prevalence of shrimp microsporidian parasite *Enterocytozoon hepatopenaei* in Jiangsu Province, China. *Aquacult. Int.* 27, 675–683. doi: 10.1007/s10499-019-00358-6

Tang, K. F. J., Han, J. E., Aranguren, L. F., White-Noble, B., Schmidt, M. M., Piamsomboon, P., et al. (2016). Dense populations of the microsporidian *Enterocytozoon hepatopenaei* (EHP) in feces of *Penaeus vannamei* exhibiting white feces syndrome and pathways of their transmission to healthy shrimp. *J. Invertebr. Pathol.* 140, 1–7. doi: 10.1016/j.jip.2016.08.004

Thamizhvanan, S., Sivakumar, S., Santhosh Kumar, S., Vinoth Kumar, D., Suryakodi, S., Balaji, K., et al. (2019). Multiple infections caused by white spot syndrome virus and *Enterocytozoon hepatopenaei in* pond-reared *Penaeus vannamei* in India and multiplex PCR for their simultaneous detection. *J. Fish Dis.* 42, 447–454. doi: 10.1111/jfd.12956

Thitamadee, S., Prachumwat, A., Srisala, J., Jaroenlak, P., Salachan, P. V., Sritunyalucksana, K., et al. (2016). Review of current disease threats for cultivated penaeid shrimp in Asia. *Aquaculture* 452, 69–87. doi: 10.1016/j.aquaculture.2015.10.02

Tourtip, S., Wongtripop, S., Stentiford, G. D., Bateman, K. S., Sriurairatana, S., Chavadej, J., et al. (2009). *Enterocytozoon hepatopenaei* sp. nov. (Microsporida: Enterocytozoonidae), a parasite of the black tiger shrimp *Penaeus monodon* (Decapoda: Penaeidae): Fine structure and phylogenetic relationships. *J. Invertebr. Pathol.* 102, 21–29. doi: 10.1016/j.jip.2009.06.004

Wang, L., Zhao, P., Si, X., Li, J., Dai, X., Zhang, K., et al. (2020). Rapid and Specific Detection of *Listeria monocytogenes* With an Isothermal Amplification and Lateral Flow Strip Combined Method That Eliminates False-Positive Signals From Primer–Dimers. *Front. Microbiol.* 10, 2959. doi: 10.3389/fmicb.2019.02959

Yi, M., Ling, L., Neogi, S. B., Fan, Y., Tang, D., Yamasaki, S., et al. (2014). Real time loop-mediated isothermal amplification using a portable fluorescence scanner for rapid and simple detection of Vibrio parahaemolyticus. *Food Control.* 41, 91–95. doi: 10.1016/j.foodcont.2014.01.005

Zheng, Z., Aweya, J., Wang, F., Yao, D., Lun, J., Li, S., et al. (2018). Acute Hepatopancreatic Necrosis Disease (AHPND) related microRNAs in Litopenaeus vannamei infected with AHPND-causing strain of Vibrio parahemolyticus. *BMC Genomics* 19, 335. doi: 10.1186/s12864-018-4728-4

Zhou, S., Wang, M., Liu, M., Jiang, K., Wang, B., and Wang, L. (2020). Rapid detection of *Enterocytozoon hepatopenaei in* shrimp through an isothermal recombinase polymerase amplification assay. *Aquaculture* 521:734987. doi: 10.1016/j.aquaculture.2020.734987

Zhu, F., and Quan, H. (2012). A new method for quantifying white spot syndrome virus: Experimental challenge dose using TaqMan real-time PCR assay. *J. Virol. Methods* 184, 121–124. doi: 10.1016/j.jviromet.2012.05.026

11

Characterisation of Bacteriophage-Encoded Depolymerases Selective for Key *Klebsiella pneumoniae* Capsular Exopolysaccharides

George Blundell-Hunter[1], Mark C. Enright[2], David Negus[3], Matthew J. Dorman[4], Gemma E. Beecham[1], Derek J. Pickard[5], Phitchayapak Wintachai[6], Supayang P. Voravuthikunchai[6], Nicholas R. Thomson[4,7] and Peter W. Taylor[1]*

[1] School of Pharmacy, University College London, London, United Kingdom, [2] Department of Life Sciences, Manchester Metropolitan University, Manchester, United Kingdom, [3] School of Science & Technology, Nottingham Trent University, Nottingham, United Kingdom, [4] Parasites and Microbes Programme, Wellcome Sanger Institute, Hinxton, United Kingdom, [5] Department of Medicine, University of Cambridge, Addenbrooke's Hospital, Cambridge, United Kingdom, [6] Faculty of Science, Prince of Songkla University, Songkhla, Thailand, [7] Department of Infectious and Tropical Diseases, London School of Hygiene & Tropical Medicine, London, United Kingdom

*Correspondence:
Peter W. Taylor
peter.taylor@ucl.ac.uk

Capsular polysaccharides enable clinically important clones of *Klebsiella pneumoniae* to cause severe systemic infections in susceptible hosts. Phage-encoded capsule depolymerases have the potential to provide an alternative treatment paradigm in patients when multiple drug resistance has eroded the efficacy of conventional antibiotic chemotherapy. An investigation of 164 K. pneumoniae from intensive care patients in Thailand revealed a large number of distinct K types in low abundance but four (K2, K51, K1, K10) with a frequency of at least 5%. To identify depolymerases with the capacity to degrade capsules associated with these common K-types, 62 lytic phage were isolated from Thai hospital sewage water using K1, K2 and K51 isolates as hosts; phage plaques, without exception, displayed halos indicative of the presence of capsule-degrading enzymes. Phage genomes ranged in size from 41–348 kb with between 50 and 535 predicted coding sequences (CDSs). Using a custom phage protein database we were successful in applying annotation to 30 - 70% (mean = 58%) of these CDSs. The largest genomes, of so-called jumbo phage, carried multiple tRNAs as well as CRISPR repeat and spacer sequences. One of the smaller phage genomes was found to contain a putative Cas type 1E gene, indicating a history of host DNA acquisition in these obligate lytic phage. Whole-genome sequencing (WGS) indicated that some phage displayed an extended host range due to the presence of multiple depolymerase genes; in total, 42 candidate depolymerase genes were identified with up to eight in a single genome. Seven distinct virions were selected for further investigation on the basis of host range, phage morphology and WGS. Candidate genes for K1, K2 and K51 depolymerases were expressed and purified as his6-tagged soluble protein and enzymatic activity demonstrated against K. pneumoniae capsular polysaccharides by gel electrophoresis and Anton-Paar rolling ball viscometry. Depolymerases completely removed the capsule in K-type-specific fashion from *K. pneumoniae* cells. We conclude that broad-host range phage carry multiple enzymes, each with the capacity to degrade a single K-type, and any future use of these enzymes as therapeutic agents will require enzyme cocktails for utility against a range of *K. pneumoniae* infections.

Keywords: *Klebsiella pneumoniae*, bacteriophage, capsule depolymerase, whole-genome sequencing (WGS), jumbo phage, capsular polysaccharide, alternative antibacterial therapy

INTRODUCTION

Extracellular polysaccharide and polypeptide capsules are major virulence determinants of Gram-positive and Gram-negative pathogens, aiding colonisation of mucosal surfaces and protecting invasive bacteria from immune recognition and killing by cellular and humoral immune mechanisms during infection of susceptible hosts. They are key contributors to the enormous diversity of bacterial surfaces and provide the interface >with their immediate external environment (Roberts, 1996; Mostowy and Holt, 2018). The rising incidence of antibiotic resistance in both nosocomial and community-acquired pathogenic bacteria poses a serious threat to global health, compounded by the paucity of new antibiotics in the drug development pipeline, and has sparked renewed interest in alternative, non-antibiotic modes of treatment for bacterial infections, including the therapeutic use of bacteriophage (Lin D. M. et al., 2017), stimulation of immune cellular functions (Haney and Hancock, 2013) and the development of agents that advantageously modify the antibiotic resistance and virulence of bacterial pathogens (Mellbye and Schuster, 2011; Taylor, 2017).

There is growing evidence that rapid removal of the protective capsule during infection facilitates elimination of the invading pathogen from the host. This approach, which circumvents the consequences of acquisition of genes conferring antibiotic resistance, was initially investigated in the pre-antibiotic era by Dubos and Avery using an enzyme preparation from cultures of a peat soil bacterium to selectively remove the polysaccharide capsule from the surface of type III pneumococci (Avery and Dubos, 1930; Avery and Dubos, 1931; Dubos and Avery, 1931; Goodner et al., 1932; Francis et al., 1934). The enzyme selectively degraded the capsule; administration to mice prior to challenge with type III pneumococci gave rise to type III-specific protection; the enzyme terminated normally fatal type III pneumococcal dermal infection in rabbits and abrogated spread of the pneumonic lesion in infected cynomolgus monkeys. More recently, a depolymerase from an environmental bacterium was shown to prevent lethal infection in mice infected with a highly virulent strain of *Bacillus anthracis* (Negus et al., 2015).

Bacteriophage, predominantly of the *Podovirdae*, *Siphoviridae* and *Myoviridae* families, are a primary source of depolymerase. These enzymes usually manifest as structural proteins such as tail fibres and baseplates but may also be present as soluble proteins during the lytic cycle; they facilitate initial binding to the host bacterium and effect degradation of the capsule to initiate phage infection (Pires et al., 2016; Knecht et al., 2020). These enzymes show promise as putative therapeutic agents. Endosialidase E derived from an *Escherichia coli* K1-specific phage rapidly and selectively degraded the polysialic acid K1 capsule that enables these bacteria to cause potentially lethal sepsis and meningitis in the neonate (Tomlinson and Taylor, 1985); intraperitoneal administration of the enzyme interrupted the transit of *E. coli* K1 from gut to brain *via* the blood circulation in colonised neonatal rat pups, abrogated meningeal inflammation and prevented death from systemic infection (Mushtaq et al., 2004; Zelmer et al., 2010; Birchenough et al., 2017). Other investigations have also shown that phage-derived depolymerases have wide utility. For example, phage-encoded capsule depolymerase sensitised extensively drug-resistant *Acinetobacter baumannii* to complement and rescued normal and immunocompromised mice from lethal peritoneal sepsis (Liu et al., 2019). Depolymerase increased survival of mice infected with a lethal bolus of *Pasteurella multocida* (Chen et al., 2018) and alginate-selective enzymes can disrupt a number of bacterial biofilms (Sutherland et al., 2004).

Extended-spectrum β-lactamase-producing clones of *K. pneumoniae* have emerged as a global threat to the health of hospitalised patients and, increasingly, to otherwise healthy individuals in the community (Paczosa and Mecsas, 2016; Wyres et al., 2020). The therapeutic challenge has been compounded by the recent emergence of hypervirulent *K. pneumoniae* clones associated with pyogenic liver abscesses, pneumonia, and meningitis in young, healthy patients (Paczosa and Mecsas, 2016). In consequence, a number of reports describe the characterisation of *K. pneumoniae*-selective capsule depolymerases (recently reviewed by Knecht et al., 2020) and they demonstrate efficacy in *Galleria* (Majkowska-Skrobek et al., 2016) and murine models of infection (Lin et al., 2014, Lin H. et al., 2017; Wang et al., 2019). We have characterised 164 recent clinical isolates of *K. pneumoniae* from three hospitals in Thailand by whole-genome sequencing and phenotypic assays for virulence markers and defined the frequency of capsular (K) chemotypes (Loraine et al., 2018) with a view to developing a palette of depolymerases that would address the most abundant pathogens in intensive care settings in Thailand. A large number of distinct K types were found in low abundance although four (K2, K51, K1 and K10) were found with a frequency of >5%. Here, we report on the isolation and molecular characterisation of phage specific for K1, K2 and K51 *K. pneumoniae* and describe the properties of their depolymerases that selectively disrupt capsules associated with these serotypes.

MATERIALS AND METHODS

Reagents

All reagents were supplied by Sigma-Aldrich, Gillingham, UK unless otherwise specified.

Bacteria

K. pneumoniae clinical isolates used in this study are detailed in **Table 1**. The majority of isolates were from Thammasat University Hospital (Pathum Thani Province), Siriraj Hospital (Bangkok) and Songklanagarind Hospital (Hat Yai, Songkhla Province); these are major tertiary care hospitals in Thailand. All Thai isolates were obtained in 2016 (Loraine et al., 2018). *K. pneumoniae* isolate NTUH-K2044 has been described by Fang et al. (2004) and ATCC-43816 by Broberg et al. (2014). Bacteria were cultured in tryptic soy broth (TSB) and stored at -80°C.

Phage Isolation, Amplification and Host Range

Sewage water samples were collected from the Thai hospitals: 10 ml aliquots of sewage water sample were mixed with 0.3 g TSB powder, inoculated with 100 μl overnight bacteria culture and incubated overnight at 37°C in an orbital incubator (200 rpm). After centrifugation (4,000 rpm; 20 min) supernatants were filtered (0.45 μm Merck Millipore filter) and maintained at 4°C prior to use. Individual plaques were obtained using tenfold dilutions (10^{-1} to 10^{-8}) of supernatants with the double-layer agar method (Kropinski et al., 2009): 100 μl overnight culture was mixed with top agar and poured over a tryptic soy agar (TSA) plate, 10 μl supernatant was dropped onto the surface and the plates incubated overnight at 37°C. Plaques were picked with a sterile tip and transferred to 300 μl sterile SM buffer (Cold Spring Harbour, 2006) and maintained at 4°C overnight. Serial dilutions were prepared in SM buffer and used to inoculate TSB containing 200 μl logarithmic phase culture, which was then mixed with top agar, poured onto TSA plate and the plate incubated overnight at 37°C. Single plaque isolation was repeated three times: plaques from the third cycle were picked from the plates, transferred to 300 μl sterile SM buffer, maintained at 4°C overnight, serially diluted in SM buffer prior to inoculation into TSB containing 200 μl logarithmic phase bacteria, dilutions mixed with top agar and mixtures poured onto TSA for overnight incubation at 37°C. For collection of phage, 10 μl of phage stock was added to 10 ml logarithmic phase bacteria in TSB and the mixture incubated overnight at 37°C in an orbital incubator at 200 rpm. The culture was centrifuged (4,000 rpm; 4°C; 30 min) and supernatants filtered (0.45 μm). Suspensions were stored at 4°C. Phage host range was determined by spot test; 100 μl logarithmic phase bacterial culture was mixed with 10 ml 0.75% TSA, the mixture poured onto 10 ml 1.5% TSA plates and 10 μl phage lysate (~10^{9} pfu/ml) spotted onto the plate prior to overnight incubation at 37°C. All host range assays were performed in triplicate.

Visualisation of Phage

For transmission electron microscopy (TEM), formvar/carbon grids (Agar Scientific Ltd., Stansted, UK) were prepared by glow discharge (10 mA, 10 s) using a Q150R ES sputter coater (Quorum Technologies Ltd., Lewes, UK). Bacteriophage suspensions (15 μl) were pipetted onto the surface of the grids for 30 s before removal with Whatman filter paper. Samples were then stained by pipetting 15 μl 2% phosphotungstic acid onto the grids. Excess stain was removed with Whatman filter paper and grids air dried. Samples were visualised using a JOEL JEM-2100Plus transmission electron microscope at an accelerating voltage of 160 Kv.

Genomic DNA Extraction and Sequencing

Phage DNA was extracted using protocol 3.3.3 described by Pickard (2009). Briefly, 1.8 ml phage lysate was incubated with

TABLE 1 | *K. pneumoniae* isolates used in this study.

Isolate	Location/source	Sequence type	O type	K type
SR7	Siriraj Hospital	ST23	O1v2	K1
SR65	Siriraj Hospital	ST23	O1v2	K1
TU37	Tammasat University Hospital	ST23	O1v2	K1
NTUH-K2044	National Taiwan University Hospital	ST23	O1v?	K1
SR3	Siriraj Hospital	ST14	O1v1	K2
TU18	Tammasat University Hospital	ST14	O1v1	K2
TU30	Tammasat University Hospital	ST14	O1v1	K2
SG44	Songklanagarind Hospital	ST14	O1v1	K2
SG46	Songklanagarind Hospital	ST65	O1v2	K2
SR10	Siriraj Hospital	ST65	O1v2	K2
SR51	Siriraj Hospital	ST86	O1v1	K2
ATCC-43816	American Type Culture Collection	ST493	?	K2
SR57	Siriraj Hospital	ST16	O3s	K51
TU16	Tammasat University Hospital	ST16	O3s	K51
SG43	Songklanagarind Hospital	ST16	O3s	K51
SG45	Songklanagarind Hospital	ST16	O3s	K51
SG79	Songklanagarind Hospital	ST16	O3s	K51
SR54	Siriraj Hospital	ST231	O1v2	K51
TU9	Tammasat University Hospital	ST231	O1v2	K51
TU29	Tammasat University Hospital	ST45	O3s	K10
SR4	Siriraj Hospital	ST147	O3l	K10
SG95	Songklanagarind Hospital	ST629	O3l*	K10
TU1	Tammasat University Hospital	ST36	O2v2	K102
SG41	Songklanagarind Hospital	ST307	O2v2	K102
SG56	Songklanagarind Hospital	ST307	O2v2	K102

10 μg/ml DNase I and 50 μg/ml RNase A for 30 min, then incubated for a further 30 min with 10 μg/ml Proteinase K and 0.5% SDS, both at 37°C. Mixtures were transferred to phase-lock Eppendorf tubes, mixed with 500 μl phenol:chloroform:isoamyl alcohol (25:24:1), centrifuged (1,500 g; 5 min), the aqueous phase moved to fresh phase-lock tubes and the extraction repeated. Aqueous phases were then moved to fresh phase-lock tubes and mixed with 500μl chloroform:isoamyl alcohol (24:1), centrifuged (6,000 g; 5 min), the aqueous phase removed, mixed with 45 μl 3M sodium acetate (pH 5.2) and 500 μL isopropanol, maintained at room temperature for 20 min, centrifuged (14,000 rpm; 20 min), the pellet washed twice with 70% ethanol, left to dry and suspended in TE buffer. DNA quality was assessed by restriction digestion with HindIII-HF (New England Biolabs UK) followed by electrophoresis on 0.8% agarose gels. In all cases, clear bands indicated absence of contamination with bacterial DNA; no ethanol contamination was detected when DNA was subjected to nanodrop analysis. Phage genomic DNA (~0.5 μg) was sequenced using Illumina HiSeq X10 paired-end sequencing. Annotated assemblies were produced according to Page et al. (2016). Sequence reads were assembled *de novo* with Velvet v1.2 (Zerbino and Birney, 2008) and VelvetOptimiser v2.2.5 (Gladman and Seemann, 2008). Assemblies were also made using SPades v1.3.1. (Nurk et al., 2017) with the -meta option to identify prophage. Reads were annotated using PROKKA v1.14.6 (Seemann, 2014) using a custom Caudovirales gene database provided by Dr Andrew Millard, University of Leicester. The stand-alone scaffolder SSPACE (Boetzer et al., 2011) was used to refine contig assembly; sequence gaps were filled using GapFiller (Boetzer and Pirovano, 2012). Phylogenetic trees were prepared using Archaeopteryx (https://sites.google.com/site/cmzmasek/home/software/archaeopteryx).

Protein Expression and Purification

Putative depolymerase gene coding sequences were cloned directly from phage genomes using PCR (conditions in **Supplementary Table 1**) by ligation into the pET26b+ expression vector (Merck KGaA, Darmstadt, Germany) between NdeI-XhoI or HindIII-XhoI depending on the presence or absence of the pelB leader sequence to aid protein solubility. All expressed proteins carried a C-terminal-his$_6$ tag. Plasmid sequences are shown in **Supplementary Data Sheet 1**. Proteins were expressed in T7 express cells (ER2766, NEB) by IPTG induction at OD$_{600}$ ~0.4. Cells were collected by centrifugation (5,000 g; 4°C; 15 min), the pellet suspended in 40 ml binding buffer (50 mM NaH$_2$PO$_4$; 300 mM NaCl; 10 mM imidazole; pH 7.4) and one protease inhibitor cocktail tablet (Roche Applied Science) together with 100 μg/ml lysozyme. After maintenance on ice for 30 min, the lysate was centrifuged (10,000 g; 4°C; 30 min) and the supernatant loaded onto a 5 ml Histrap column housed in an AKTAprime FPLC system (Cytiva, Amersham, UK). Proteins were eluted with a 30 ml gradient of loading buffer into elution buffer (binding buffer with 500 mM imidazole), dialysed against storage buffer (binding buffer, no imidazole; 5 ml eluate against 5 l buffer), filtered (0.22 μM) and stored at -80°C. Protein concentration was determined by Bradford assay.

Enzyme Characterisation

Klebsiella pneumoniae capsules were prepared essentially as described by Domenico et al. (1989): 200 ml bacterial culture was mixed with 40 ml 1% Zwittergent 3-14 detergent in 100 mM citric acid (pH 2.0) for 30 min at 50°C. Bacteria were removed by centrifugation (16,000 g; 2 min), supernatants mixed with ice cold ethanol to a final ethanol concentration of 80%, and maintained at 4°C for 30 min. After centrifugation (16,000 g; 5 min) pellets were air dried, suspended in 40 ml H$_2$O and treated with DNase and RNase (both 30 μg/ml) for 30 min at 37°C. Preparations were lyophilised after heat inactivation (65°C; 10 min).

To determine the impact of depolymerase on capsule viscosity, enzyme aliquots (final protein concentrations: GBH001_056, 25 ng/μl; GBH038_054, 22.2 ng/μl; GBH019_279, 1.6 ng/μl) were mixed with 400 μg polymer in 1 ml protein storage buffer and incubated for 1 h at 37°C; reactions were terminated by maintenance at 98°C for 5 min and, if required, samples stored at −20°C before viscometric analysis. Polymer viscosity was determined using an Anton Paar rolling ball microviscometer (Anton Paar, Graz, Austria); samples were transferred to a glass viscometry 1.6 mm diameter capillary containing a solid steel ball. Viscosity was determined as the time taken for the ball to fall 25 cm through the sample at an angle of 20° to the horizontal; each automated, timed determination was performed six times. Degradation of polysaccharide substrate was also determined by gel electrophoresis. Enzyme aliquots were mixed with 7.5 μg of substrate in 22.5 μl reaction volume, the reactions terminated as described above and after electrophoresis using 10% SDS-PAGE, gels were washed (10% acetic acid; 25% ethanol) after 5, 10 and 15 min at 50°C, stained with 0.1% Alcian blue in 10% acetic acid and 25% ethanol for 30 min at 50°C and de-stained with wash buffer at room temperature overnight. Enzyme activity was also monitored by spotting 10 μl depolymerase onto agar plates seeded with appropriate *K. pneumoniae* strains (spot tests). The capacity of recombinant depolymerases to remove capsule from the surface of *K. pneumoniae* was examined by preparation of turbid bacterial suspensions (OD$_{600}$ ~ 1) in 100 μl PBS, enzyme added to give a final concentration of 1 μg/ml and incubation for 90 min at 37°C. Negative controls were incubated with PBS. Bacterial suspensions were combined with nigrosin and examined by phase contrast microscopy. Area occupied by the capsule was determined using the microbeJ application of ImageJ (https://imagej.net/Welcome).

RESULTS

Phage Isolation

K. pneumoniae isolates TU37 (capsule K1), TU18 (K2), TU30 (K2), SG44 (K2), SG46 (K2), TU9 (K51), SG43 (K51), SG45 (K51) and SG79 (K51) (**Table 1**) were used to isolate phage selective for these capsule types from three filtered sewage water samples. Sixty-two phage were isolated, encompassing a variety of distinct host range patterns (**Supplementary Table 2**); 28 of these were chosen for further study, based on divergent morphology, host range, genome size and sequence similarity, and were ordered into seven groups based on a high degree (>95%) of nucleotide sequence identity (**Table 2**). In general, phage producing plaques on a host carrying the target K-type lysed other clinical isolates of the same K type, although there were exceptions as detailed in **Supplementary Table 2** and **Table 2**. The majority did not have absolute specificity for K-type: for example, GBH013 and GBH017, isolated on and with specificity for isolates carrying the K2 capsule type, were able to lyse all four K1 indicator strains, and the six phage isolated on and active against K51 strains also lysed two of three K102 indicator strains, producing incomplete lysis of the third. Incomplete lysis was independent of virion concentration and is therefore not due to "lysis from without". All lytic plaques on fully-susceptible host strains were surrounded by halos after overnight incubation at 37°C followed by 3-4 days storage at 4°C, indicating diffusion of soluble (non-virion) capsule depolymerase into the surrounding bacterial lawn (Adams and Park, 1956). Representative phage from each of the seven groups shown in **Table 2** were also examined against *K. pneumoniae* expressing capsular K-types K5, K20, K15-1, K21, K24, K25, K28, K54, K103 and K122. GBH029 and GBH054 lysed the K21 isolate SR95 and GBH001, GBH014, GBH029 and GBH033 lysed the K28 isolate SR33; in all other cases no lytic activity was noted.

The genetic relatedness of the 28 phage genomes sequenced in this study (**Figure 1A**) in comparison to the 314 from published studies of *Klebsiella* phage is shown in **Figure 1B**. **Figure 1A** uses formal designations for the phage (e.g., vB_KpnA_GBH001) but here and elsewhere in this study the abbreviated form has been used (e.g., GBH001) for clarity (Adriaenssens and Brister, 2017). The *Klebsiella* phage genome diversity found in our study paralleled that in studies of previously sequenced phage (Santiago and Donlan, 2020; Townsend et al., 2021). A combination of genome sequence comparison and TEM was employed to classify the phage in accord with the most recent International Committee on Taxonomy of Viruses (ICTV) guidelines (Adriaenssens et al., 2020); five (GBH054, GBH055, GBH056, GBH060, GBH061) were assigned to the family *Siphoviridae* (order *Caudovirales*), five (GBH019, GBH020, GBH023, GBH033, GBH035) to the *Myoviridae* (order *Caudovirales*), fifteen (GBH001, GBH002, GBH003, GBH005, GBH007, GBH013, GBH014, GBH017, GBH018, GBH038, GBH039, GBH045, GBH046, GBH049, GBH050) to the *Autographiviridae* (order *Tubulavirales*) and three (GBH026, GBH027, GBH029), to the *Drexlerviridae* (order *Tubulavirales*). There was complete concordance between assignments based on genome sequence and morphology as determined by TEM; representative images from each phage family together with corresponding plaque morphology are shown in **Figure 2**.

From the genome sequence data the 28 phage showed a wide range of genome sizes (**Table 2**). Four phage selective for either capsular K1 or K2 strains possessed genomes of <50 kb, seven genomes of 50-100 kb and seven genomes of 100-200 kb. Three K51-selective phage displayed non-identical genomes of 348 kb and consequently fell into the category of jumbo (Yuan and Gao, 2017) also known as huge (Al-Shayeb et al., 2020) phage characterised by genomes of >200 kb. As isolation-based methods select against large phage (Yuan and Gao, 2017), only 94 jumbo phage have been described following isolation and only three of these, with a high degree of sequence similarity, are *Klebsiella* spp virions (Šimoliūnas et al., 2013; Pan et al., 2017; Mora et al., 2021): these have genomes of 345.8 kb, making phage

GBH019, GBH020 and GBH023 (**Table 2**) amongst the largest *Klebsiella* phage described and sequenced to date.

Phage Genome Analysis

The 28 phage selected for sequencing were found to belong to seven groups with members sharing MASH (Ondov et al., 2016) DNA sequence similarity of >95%. These groups are exemplified by phage GBH001 (45 kb), GBH014 (41 kb), GBH019 (348 kb), GBH029 (50 kb), GBH033 (166 kb), GBH038 (44 kb) and GBH054 (59 kb). Phage GBH038 and GBH50 share 96.5% MASH sequence identity but have divergent gene orders. As others have noted (Townsend et al., 2021), analysis of genome assemblies using metaSPAdes showed the presence of prophage in sequenced lysate preparations of lytic phage GBH001 (prophage genome size 48.6 kb) and GBH029 (43.4 kb) and closely related phage. However, these were low coverage assemblies compared to those of the lytic phage with coverage depths of <7% compared to the main phage assembly. Presumably these prophage were released from the host genome during phage lysate preparation. Prophage from *K. pneumoniae* on which GBH001 formed plaques were 48.6 kb in length and contained genes associated with integration and excision from host genomes such as integrases and transposases, and a *cro* repressor protein. GBH029 and similar phage contain a prophage of 43.4 kb whose genomes contain integrase, transposase and putative excisionase genes.

Jumbo Phage GBH019

The genome of phage GBH019, at 347,546 bp, is the largest of any *K. pneumoniae* phage sequenced to date. It contains 534 CDSs and six tRNA genes with a coding gene density of 90.2% and GC% of 32.0. Annotations were attributed to 141 CDSs (shown in colour in **Figure 3**) leaving a total of 393 (73.6%) CDSs of unknown function. GBH019 shows high similarity to previously described jumbo phage Muenster (Mora et al., 2021), K64-1 (Pan et al., 2017) and vB_KleM-RaK2 (Šimoliūnas et al., 2013) with DNA similarity values calculated using MASH of 98.2–98.4% but with highly dissimilar gene organisation (**Supplementary Figure 1**). Examination of the pangenome of these four phage using Roary 3.13 (Page et al., 2015) showed that 384 genes were common to all genomes (BLASTP > 90%). The genome of GBH019 has three putative tail fibre protein genes (**Figure 3**) as well as tail spike and other tail-associated protein genes. These genes encode structures involved in host receptor recognition and binding, and the presence of several such structures in the genomes of these large phage is associated with extended host ranges (Pan et al., 2017). One of these putative tail fibre genes, corresponding to GBH019 gene 00383 is common to all four phage and is highly conserved (>98% DNA sequence identity, determined by Clustal Φ).

GBH019 contains six tRNA genes in common with those of phage Muenster, with K64-1 having seven and KleM-RaK2 eight. GBH019 also has many genes involved in nucleotide metabolism, DNA transcription, replication and repair including a DNA polymerase and DNA and RNA ligases and at least two endonucleases (**Figure 3**). These genes are presumably

TABLE 2 | *K. pneumoniae* phage isolates sequenced in this study, showing patterns of lytic activity against various *K. pneumoniae* K-types.

Phage	Host[a]	kb[b]	SR7	SR65	TU37	NTUH-K2044	SR3	TU18	SG44	SR10	SR51	ATCC-43816	SR57	TU16	SG45	SR45	TU9	TU29	SR4	SG95	TU1	SG41	SG56
					K1					K2					K51				K10			K102	
GBH001	**TU37**	**45.96**	++[c]	+	++	++	−	−	−	−	−	−	−	+	−	−	−	−	−	−	−	−	−
GBH002	TU37	45.97	++	+	++	++	−	−	−	+	−	−	−	+	−	−	−	−	−	−	−	−	−
GBH003	TU37	45.96	++	+	++	+	−	−	−	−	−	−	−	+	−	−	+	−	−	−	−	−	−
GBH005	TU37	45.96	++	+	++	++	−	−	−	−	−	−	−	+	−	−	−	−	−	−	−	−	−
GBH007	TU37	45.96	++	+	++	++	−	−	+	++	−	++	−	+	−	−	−	−	−	−	−	−	−
GBH014	**SG44**	**41.70**	+	−	−	−	++	++	++	++	++	++	−	−	+	+	−	−	−	−	−	−	−
GBH013	SG44	41.70	++	++	++	++	++	++	++	++	++	++	−	+	++	++	++	−	−	−	+	++	++
GBH017	SG44	41.09	++	++	++	++	++	++	++	++	++	++	−	++	++	++	++	−	−	−	+	++	++
GBH018	SG44	40.87	−	−	−	−	++	++	+	++	−	++	−	++	−	−	−	−	−	−	−	+	−
GBH019	**TU9**	**347.55**	−	−	−	−	−	−	−	−	−	−	++	++	++	++	++	−	−	−	+	++	++
GBH020	TU9	347.54	−	−	−	−	−	−	−	−	−	−	++	++	++	++	++	−	−	−	+	++	++
GBH023	TU9	347.55	−	−	−	−	−	−	−	−	−	−	++	++	++	++	++	−	−	−	+	++	++
GBH029	**SG43**	**49.92**	−	−	−	−	−	−	++	+	−	+	−	++	+	+	+	−	+	−	−	+	−
GBH026	SG43	50.49	−	−	−	−	−	++	++	+	−	++	−	++	+	+	+	−	+	−	+	+	−
GBH027	SG43	50.49	−	−	−	−	−	++	++	+	−	+	−	++	+	+	+	−	+	−	+	+	−
GBH033	**SG45**	**165.75**	−	−	−	−	−	++	+	−	++	+	−	++	+	+	−	−	−	−	−	−	−
GBH035	SG45	165.75	−	−	−	−	−	++	++	++	++	+	−	++	+	+	−	−	−	−	−	−	−
GBH038	**SG46**	**43.73**	−	−	−	−	++	++	++	++	++	++	−	++	+	+	++	−	−	−	−	−	++
GBH039	SG46	43.73	−	−	−	−	++	++	++	++	++	++	−	++	++	++	++	−	−	−	−	−	−
GBH045	TU18	44.03	−	−	−	−	++	++	++	++	++	++	−	++	++	++	++	−	−	−	−	−	−
GBH046	TU18	44.65	−	−	−	−	++	++	++	++	++	++	−	++	++	++	−	−	−	−	−	−	−
GBH049	TU30	44.22	−	−	−	−	++	++	++	++	++	++	−	−	++	−	−	−	−	−	−	−	−
GBH050	TU30	44.20	−	−	−	−	++	++	++	++	+	++	−	−	++	++	−	−	−	−	−	−	−
GBH054	**SG79**	**58.59**	−	−	−	−	−	++	++	++	−	−	+	++	++	+	++	−	−	−	−	−	−
GBH055	SG79	58.52	−	−	−	−	−	++	++	++	−	−	+	++	++	+	++	−	−	−	−	−	−
GBH056	SG79	58.52	−	−	−	−	−	++	++	+	−	−	+	++	+	−	++	−	+	−	−	−	−
GBH060	SG79	58.52	−	−	−	−	−	−	++	++	−	−	−	++	++	+	++	−	−	−	−	−	−
GBH061	SG79	58.52	−	−	−	−	−	+	+	++	−	−	++	++	++	+	++	−	−	−	−	−	−

[a] clinical isolates detailed in **Table 1**.

[b] genome length determined from whole-genome data.

[c] clear plaque, ++; +, incomplete lysis; −, no lysis. Determined by spot assay, phage concentration ~10_{10} virions/ml.

The 28 phages selected fell into seven groups based on sequence similarity of >95%. Exemplars for each group in bold.

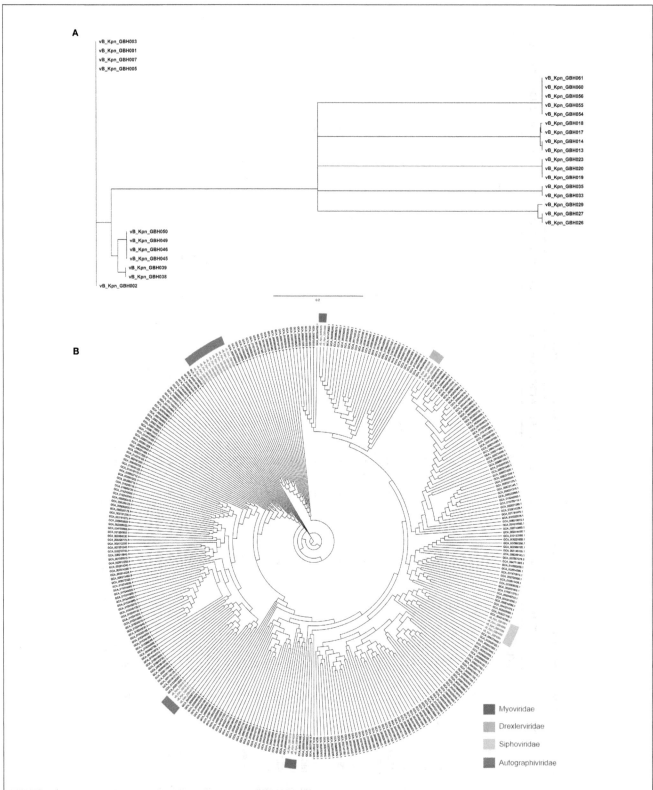

FIGURE 1 | Phylogeny of Thai *K pneumoniae*- selective phage. **(A)** MASH tree with degree of genetic similarity amongst the 28 phage genomes sequenced in this study. **(B)** Phylogenetic tree prepared using Archaeopteryx showing the relationship of the 28 phage genomes (in red) to 314 published *Klebsiella* phage genomes.

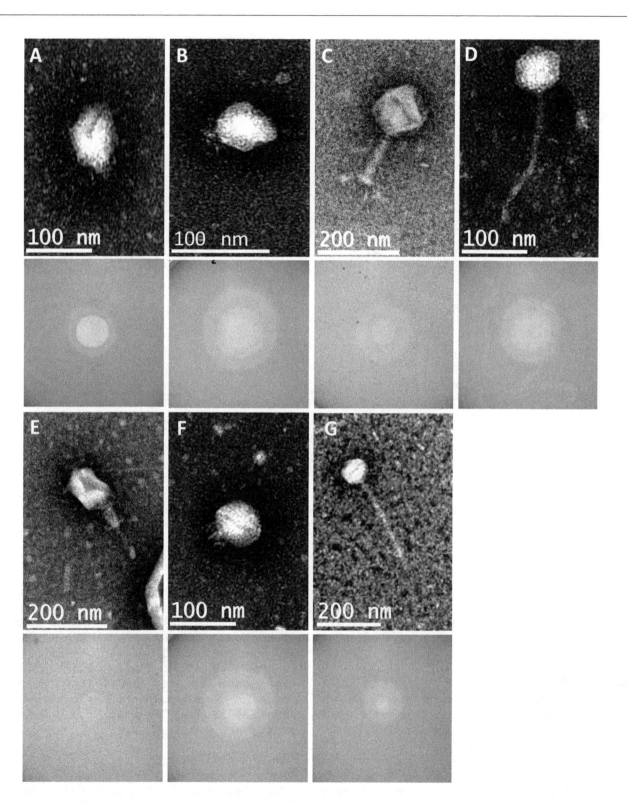

FIGURE 2 | Representative transmission electron micrographs and plaque morphology of the seven exemplars for each of the genetically distinct phage groups defined in this study and shown in **Table 2**. **(A)** GBH001 (mean capsid diameter 63.4 nm; mean tail length N/A; *n* = 10) **(B)** GBH014 (64.0 nm; N/A; *n* = 7) **(C)** GBH019 (132.7 nm; 163.4 nm; *n* = 9) **(D)** GBH029 (73.8 nm; 188.8 nm; *n* = 7) **(E)** GBH033 (86.7 nm; 105.2 nm; *n* = 8) **(F)** GBH038 (72.0 nm; N/A; *n* = 6) **(G)** GBH054 (81.2 nm; 256.4 nm; *n* = 11).

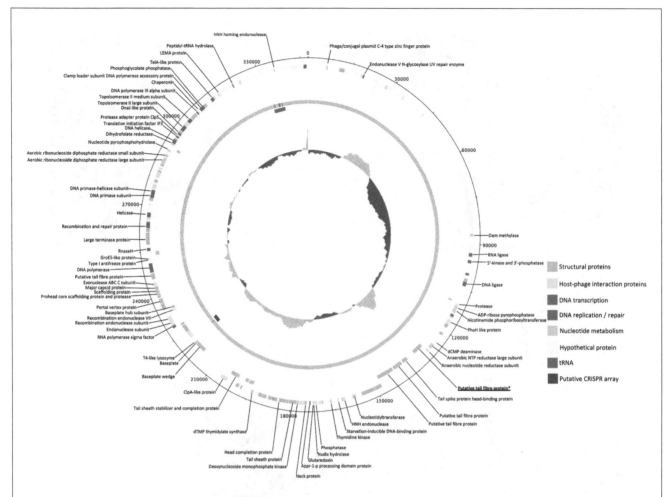

FIGURE 3 | Circular genomic map of Jumbo phage GBH019. Genes involved in virion structure (orange), host interaction (green), nucleotide metabolism (pink), DNA replication and repair (blue), and DNA transcription (magenta) are shown as the positions of six tRNAs (red) and a putative CRISPR array (purple). %GC is shown in the centre of the figure. Hypothetical proteins are shown in cream. Figure generated using DNA Plotter release 18.1.0.

involved in sophisticated re-purposing of the host DNA and protein synthesis machinery to phage particle biosynthesis. GBH019, in common with the three other similar phage has a putative CRISPR array of the sequence CCCAGTATTCATGC GGGTTGTAGGAATTAGGGACAC although no Cas genes are present in these genomes.

Phage GBH033

With the second largest phage genome in this study (165,752bp), GBH033 is similar to several *Myoviridae* genomes (>95% BLASTN nucleotide similarity) including *Klebsiella* virus JD18 (Genbank accession number KT239446). It has an AT-rich genome with %GC of 39.5 and contains 290 CDSs which we annotated with functions or putative functions. The genome of GBH033 contains 16 tRNA genes, the same number as found in the genome of phage JD18.

Phage GBH001 and GBH038

Phage GBH001 and GBH038 have genome sizes of 44,964 and 43,726 bp respectively. They share 93.4% DNA similarity,

determined using MASH, and have 56 and 54 CDSs respectively. We ascribed functions or putative functions to 31 of 56 GBH001 and 29 of 54 GBH038 genes. Their genomes are more GC-rich than that of GBH019 with GC% of 54.2 and 54.3, compared to 32.2. The most closely related genomes of both phage determined by BLASTN homology are phage of the family *Autographiviridae* (subfamily *Slopekvirinae*, genus *Drulisvirus*) whose genomes share <92% BLASTN DNA similarity and therefore both phage may represent a new species within this subfamily as <95% BLASTN similarity equates to new species (Adriaenssens et al., 2020).

Phage GBH014

The genome length of phage GBH014 is 40,697 bp, with GC% of 53.2, and the phage shares 96.2% BLASTN similarity (over 85% of its genome) with the *Klebsiella Autographidae* phage 066028 (Genbank accession MW042796.1) that is currently designated as an unclassified *Przondovirus*. However, GBH014 may represent a new species of *Klebsiella* phage as it shares <5% DNA similarity over its whole genome with any phage genome described thus far.

We were able to annotate functions or putative functions to 25 of the 51 predicted CDSs in the GBH014 genome.

Phage GBH029

GBH029 has a genome of 49,924 bp, a GC% of 51.2% and is most similar to *Klebsiella* phage Sweeney (Genbank accession NC_049839.1) which is an unclassified *Webervirus* in the family *Drexlerviridae*. Functions or putative functions were annotated to 35 of the 77 CDSs in this genome.

Phage GBH054

The genome of phage GBH054 is 58,588 bp long and has a GC% of 56.2. Functions or putative functions could only be annotated to 28 of 79 CDSs in this genome. This genome is most similar to that of the *Siphoviridae* phage Soft (Genbank accession MN106244.1). BLASTN comparison of both genomes revealed 93.84% sequence identity over 84% of the GBH054 genome, indicating that this phage may be a new species of *Siphovirus*.

Identification and Expression of Phage Depolymerase Genes

To identify genes encoding depolymerases with the capacity to degrade capsular polysaccharides produced by *K. pneumoniae* K1, K2 and K51 isolates, BLASTX (States and Gish, 1994) was used to search a customised library (**Supplementary Table 3**) of 25 published phage-encoded *K. pneumoniae* capsule depolymerases.

Phage GBH001 displayed lytic activity against the four clinical isolates of K1 capsule type (**Table 2**). The search identified two potential GBH001-encoded depolymerase genes, GBH001_048 (541 residues) and GBH001_056 (651 residues). The former was matched to multiple tail fibre and tail spike proteins, and to other putative depolymerase proteins using JACKHMMER (Finn et al., 2015); we also identified an N-terminal match with a tail fibre protein using the EMBL protein family database InterProScan (Quevillon et al., 2005). It was cloned and expressed as described in *Materials and Methods* but displayed no capsule depolymerase activity against K1 capsule. The latter showed >96% identity with known K1-selective depolymerases, was matched to tail fibre proteins using JACKHMMER (Finn et al., 2015) with the reference proteomes database and contained a pectin-lyase fold (residues 265-568) as determined with the EMBL protein family database InterProScan. GBH001_056 was inserted between pET26b+ NdeI and XhoI sites and grown for 16 h at 26°C following induction with 0.01 mM IPTG at OD_{600} ~0.4. Spot tests indicated that the his_6-tagged, affinity-purified protein possessed depolymerase activity against the K1 capsule but not against K2, K51, K10 and K102 capsules (**Table 3**). Depolymerase GBH001_056 possessed no activity against Thai clinical isolates expressing the K20, K24, K15-1, K21, K25, K103, K122, K28, K5, K54, K62 and K74 capsules; these K-types were found with relatively high frequency (incidence >1.5%) in clinical isolates from our Thai *K. pneumoniae* collection (Loraine et al., 2018).

Phage GBH014 and GBH038 were both able to lyse the six *K. pneumoniae* K2 isolates examined (**Table 2**). BLASTX revealed three potential K2 depolymerase candidate genes, GBH014_001 (215 residues) and GBH014_051 (433 residues) from phage GBH014 and GBH038_054 (577 residues) from phage

TABLE 3 | Spot tests showing the capacity of individual depolymerases to degrade the most common *K. pneumoniae* K-types encountered in Thai hospitals (Loraine et al., 2018).

Depolymerase																					
								Strain/isolate; capsule (K) type													
			K1				K2						K51				K10			K102	
	SR7	SR65	TU37	NTUH-K2044	SR3	TU18	SG44	SR10	SR51	ATCC-43816	SR57	TU16	SG45	SR54	TU9	TU29	SR4	SG95	TU1	SG41	SG56
GBH001_056	+	+	+	+	–	–	–	–	–	–	–	–	–	–	–	–	–	–	–	–	–
GBH038_054	–	–	–	–	+	+	+	+	+	+	–	–	–	–	–	–	–	–	–	–	–
GBH019_279	–	–	–	–	–	–	–	–	–	–	+	+	+	+	+	–	–	–	–	–	–

TSA plates were seeded with bacteria and 10 μl phage lysate (~10^9 pfu/ml) spotted onto the plate prior to overnight 37°C.

GBH038. With GBH014_001, JACKHMMER showed matches to phage tailspikes and tail fibres, and to tailspike 63D sialidase from phage 1611E-K2-1, shown to be an active K2 depolymerase (Wang et al., 2020). In addition, a galactose binding domain (residues 65-214) was identified by InterProScan; galactose is a constituent of the K2 capsular polysaccharide (Clements et al., 2008). GBH014_051 showed matches to tail fibres using JACKHMMER and to serralysin metalloprotease using InterProScan. We were unable to purify and test this protein. GBH014_001 was cloned into pET26b+ both with and without a *pelB* tag on the N-terminus to migrate the protein to the periplasm and aid folding. GBH014_001 expressed better without the addition of the *pelB* tag, but could not be purified without denaturation of the protein. Refolded protein possessed no depolymerase activity when tested against K1, K2 and K51 capsules. GBH038_054 (577 residues) showed >98% amino acid homology with vP_KpnP_KpV74_564, the sole K2 depolymerase published to date (Solovieva et al., 2018) and was inserted between the HindIII and XhoI sites of pET26b+ with and without N-terminal *pelB* and grown for 16 h at 16°C following induction with 0.01 mM IPTG at OD_{600} ~0.4. The gene was expressed only in the presence of *pelB*. In spot tests, affinity-purified protein degraded the K2 capsule, but not K1, K51, K10 or K102 capsules (**Table 3**), or any of the capsules described in the preceding paragraph.

Only jumbo phage GBH019 and closely related phage were able to lyse the five *K. pneumoniae* K51 isolates examined (**Table 2**). Putative depolymerase genes were restricted to a 30,000 bp section of the GBH019 genome (125,000-155,000 bp) where eight CDSs (278-285) were located in series; such clustering of depolymerase genes is consistent with a recent study of jumbo *K. pneumoniae* phage phiK64-1 (Pan et al., 2017). There are currently no published K51 depolymerase sequences and none of the eight putative depolymerases showed sufficient homology with currently available sequences to guide the identification of a K51 depolymerase gene. Attempts were therefore made to clone and express these eight genes. Although all showed some degree of alignment with sequences in the protein database (**Supplementary Table 3**), the majority could not be expressed as enzymatically active protein. GBH019_279 (809 residues) showed limited alignment with tail fibre and tail spike proteins within the first 200 residues. This was supported by InterProScan analysis which predicted a pectin-lyase fold between residues 139 and 532, and Phyre2 modelling (Kelley et al., 2015) which predicted a hydrolase with 98.7% confidence, suggesting potential depolymerase activity but with no link to the specific K51 capsule target. BH019_279 was cloned into pET26b+ with *pelB*, the gene inserted between HindIII and XhoI sites, grown for 16 h at 16°C following induction with 0.01 mM IPTG at OD_{600} ~0.4 and the protein affinity-purified in soluble form. Spot tests indicated that this gene product degraded the K51 capsule but had no effect on any other capsule types in our K-type panel described above.

GBH001_056 (K1 depolymerase), GBH038_054 (K2 depolymerase) and GBH019_279 (K51 depolymerase) were assigned molecular weights of 71 kDa, 66 kDa and 93 kDa respectively using SDS-PAGE and were in line with values predicted from the size of the coding region of each gene.

Characterisation of K1, K2 and K51 Depolymerases

The capacity of each depolymerase to degrade their respective primary substrates was determined by observing reductions in polysaccharide molecular mass and polysaccharide viscosity. Capsular substrates were purified from two K1 (SR7 & SR65), two K2 (SR3 & SR10) and two K51 (TU16 & SR54) clinical isolates. Essentially identical results were obtained for each K-type-specific pair so only data for the SR65, SR3 and TU16 polymers is presented in **Figure 4**. The three enzymes rapidly reduced the molecular mass with evidence of degradation after less than 1 min incubation time. After 60 min incubation each polymer appeared substantially degraded although depolymerisation of K2 and K51 polymers appeared greater than for K1. Reduction in molecular mass was accompanied in all cases by a large decrease in polymer viscosity using an Anton-Paar rolling ball viscometer. *K. pneumoniae* SR65 (K1), SR3 (K2) and TU16 (K51) were also employed to examine the capacity of the three depolymerases to remove the primary target capsule. The area occupied by the capsule was determined before addition of enzyme (final concentration 25 ng/μl for K1 depolymerase, 25 ng/μl for K2 depolymerase and 1.6 ng/μl for K51 depolymerase) and after 90 min incubation at 37°C following addition of the respective depolymerase. As noted in an earlier study (Loraine et al., 2018), there were significant differences in capsule size between each of the clinical isolates. K1, K2 and K51 depolymerases removed completely the capsules surrounding, respectively, isolates SR65, SR3 and TU16 (**Figure 5**). No significant differences were seen between bacteria prior to incubation and following 90 min incubation with PBS. Phase contrast images for *K. pneumoniae* SR65 are also shown in **Figure 5**.

DISCUSSION

The ideal candidate for capsule depolymerase therapy would be a difficult-to-treat infection caused by a single bacterial infectious agent producing a protective capsule that does not vary in its chemical composition between isolates and is essential for pathogenesis. Inhalation anthrax, due to *B. anthracis* strains that universally produce a poly-γ-D-glutamic acid capsule that is absolutely required for systemic, often lethal infection (Mock and Fouet, 2001), is probably the only infectious condition in which these tenets hold, so capsule depolymerisation as a principle for the therapy of other bacterial infections will be conditioned by a degree of structural variability, sometimes very large, at the cell surface. Our study confirms previous work showing that the host range of *K. pneumoniae* phage is to a large extent governed by carriage of distinct capsule depolymerases, each with a narrow substrate specificity (reviewed by Knecht et al., 2020). In a particularly illustrative example of this principal, the capacity of phage ΦK64-1 to infect *K. pneumoniae* belonging to eight capsule chemotypes was facilitated by carriage by the phage of eight capsule depolymerases, each capable of degrading only one structurally distinct capsule (Pan et al., 2017). Strains of *K. pneumoniae* elaborate a wide array of different capsule types (Wyres et al.,

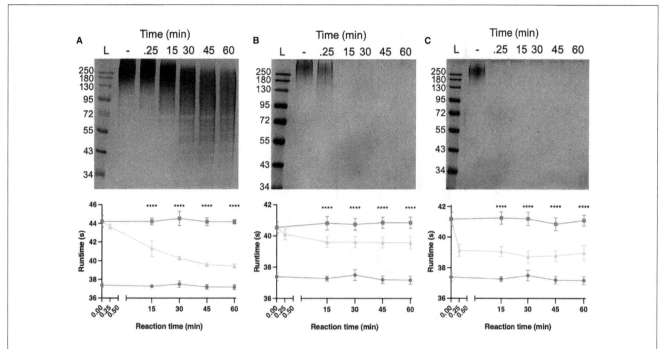

FIGURE 4 | Degradation of high-molecular-weight capsular polysaccharide from *K. pneumoniae* SR65 **(A)**, SR3 **(B)** and TU16 **(C)** following incubation at 37°C with the corresponding K1, K2 and K51 depolymerases. 10% SDS-PAGE gels; 5 μl Color Prestained Protein Standard, Broad Range (10-250 kDa) (New England Biolabs UK) as ladder; 22.5 μl loaded into each lane. Enzyme-mediated reductions in polymer viscosity as determined by Anton-Paar rolling ball viscometry are also shown alongside the corresponding gels. No polymer degradation was observed in the absence of enzyme. ****P = < 0.0001 (unpaired t-test with Welch's correction between treated and untreated groups).

2020) and this population diversity was reflected in the large number of distinct K-types we found in our analysis of Thai nosocomial isolates (Loraine et al., 2018); only one K-type (K2) was found in more than 10% of total isolates and only six were found with an incidence of 4.5% or more. Successful application of depolymerase therapy will therefore require a cocktail of enzymes in much the same way as proposed from phage therapy of *Klebsiella* infections (Townsend et al., 2021), unless personalised therapy can be augmented in tandem with rapid and accurate strain identification and K-typing.

Although bacteria have been exploited as occasional sources of capsule depolymerase (Avery and Dubos, 1930; Scorpio et al., 2007; Stabler et al., 2013), phage remain the primary source of O-glycosyl hydrolases and lyases with the capacity to selectively degrade a wide range of capsules (Knecht et al., 2020), including those from *K. pneumoniae*, and for the dispersal of biofilms (Rumbaugh and Sauer, 2020). The capsular diversity of *K. pneumoniae* correlates to a correspondingly high degree of variation of phage genotypes that have evolved a lifestyle enabling lytic cycles within specific K-type hosts, with the consequence that we were able to isolate a diverse selection of phage, belonging to four families and displaying a wide range of genome sizes (41-348 kb), from hospital sewage using three different K-types as host. The majority of these phage were distinct from, but genomically related to, phage described in previous studies (**Figure 1B**). Plaques from all phage developed halos when plated on their primary and on the majority of secondary hosts, indicating the presence of a soluble form of

capsule depolymerase that diffuses into the surrounding agar from the plaque during incubation. Genomic analyses were complicated by the presence of prophage sequences in a small number of DNA preparations that were presumably released from the host genome during phage lysate preparation as a consequence of host DNA damage, or prophage may have been induced by the lytic phage (Raya and Hebert, 2009; Townsend et al., 2021). It is however unlikely that this low level of contamination would have compromised the host range determined in this study (**Table 2** and **Supplementary Table 2**).

Phage-encoded capsule depolymerases are predominantly located in receptor binding proteins (RBPs) structured as tail fibres or tailspikes. *In situ*, these structures form trimers and each unit generally consists of a conserved N-terminal anchor domain that aids phage self-assembly, a K-type-variable central β-helical domain for host recognition and catalysis, and a C-terminal domain responsible for trimerisation and receptor recognition (Latka et al., 2017; Latka et al., 2019). Although direct evidence is lacking, it is generally accepted that both the soluble and integrated forms of RBP can freely diffuse through an agar matrix and that soluble and integrated monomers are structurally identical (Latka et al., 2017). However, due to their aggregative properties and multi-domain structure, RBPs are likely to form aqueous microparticulate dispersions rather than true solutions (Chi et al., 2003) and this may compromise high yield RBP expression. In the current study, as well as in our previous work (Leggate et al., 2002; Negus and Taylor, 2014), issues of solubility and low yield were encountered which in the

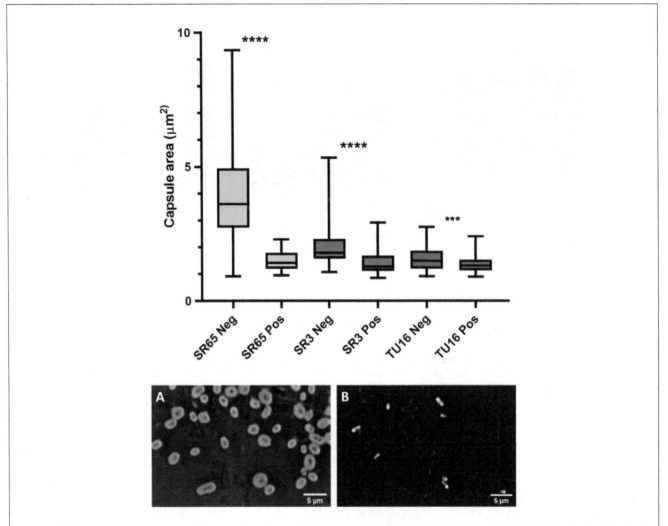

FIGURE 5 | Box and whiskers plot of the impact on capsules of the target *K. pneumoniae* isolates SR65 (K1), SR3 (K2) and TU16 (K51) following 90 min incubation at 37°C with the corresponding K1, K2 and K51 depolymerases. SR65 Neg, negative control (PBS incubation), n = 319, mean capsule area µm^2 3.41 ± 1.00 (Mean ± 1SD); SR65 Pos, K1 depolymerase-exposed, n = 74, 1.49 ± 0.34; SR3 Neg, n = 119, 1.96 ± 0.58; SR3 Pos, n = 66, 1.41 ± 0.42; TU16 Neg, n = 84, 1.54 ± 0.42; TU16 Pos, n = 170, 1.36 ± 0.31. ****P = < 0.0001, ***P = < 0.002 (unpaired t-test with Welch's correction between treated and untreated groups). Also shown: phase contrast microscopy images of nigrosin staining for isolate SR65 (K1) after 90 min incubation in PBS **(A)** and with K1 depolymerase **(B)**. Capsule can be seen in **(A)** as a bright halo around the cell.

current study were in part overcome by introduction of the *pelB* leader sequence into the plasmid vector, which directs the protein to the bacterial periplasm. Even so, a number of putative depolymerase genes identified in our screen could not be expressed as active protein in spite of repeated efforts: one possible way towards simplification of expression of a range of highly catalytic depolymerases could involve excision of the central catalytic domain of the RBP, where expression is more likely to lead to a fully soluble, enzymatically active polypeptide (Squeglia et al., 2020).

All seven exemplary phage that we studied in detail were closely related to other, previously described *Klebsiella* virions (**Figure 1B**), even though they were isolated from widely dispersed geographical regions. Of interest was the isolation of the jumbo phage GBH019, the source of the K51 depolymerase described herein, that counts amongst the largest *Klebsiella*

phage isolated to date. In common with other jumbo phage, the GBH019 genome contained multiple putative depolymerase genes and this phage may be a source of enzymes for the degradation of the less abundant K-types that we encountered in our study of nosocomial Thai isolates (Loraine et al., 2018). Although relatively few jumbo phage have been isolated and characterised to date, direct sequencing of phage DNA from diverse ecosystems has revealed that they are highly abundant (Al-Shayeb et al., 2020) and as they are excluded from typical phage preparations processed using membrane filters (Yuan and Gao, 2017) they are unlikely to be recovered unless special precautions are employed during their isolation. In common with other jumbo phage, the GBH019 genome carries a large number of genes for *de novo* synthesis of purines and pyrimidines, DNA and RNA polymerases and interconversion of nucleotide phosphorylation states (**Figure 3**). As has been previously noted (Al-Shayeb et al., 2020) these gene sets are similar to those of small bacteria and archaea with restricted symbiotic lifestyles (Castelle et al., 2018), may reduce the dependence of jumbo phage on their bacterial hosts and broaden their host range by acquisition of new genetic information, as reflected by the presence of multiple depolymerase genes. The presence of CRISPR-Cas systems is also a feature of jumbo phage and may be involved in the redirection of bacterial host biosynthesis toward phage-encoded functions as well as contribute to host-directed elimination of incoming phage. Indeed, the first description of phage-encoded CRISPR-Cas showed the system was able to counteract a phage inhibitory chromosomal island of the bacterial host (Seed et al., 2013).

The increasing number of *Klebsiella* phage genomes in the public domain show certain trends in their genome sequences. Whereas most of the phage genomes in this study and in public databases have genomes with %GC of 50-55, similar to that of their bacterial host (56-57), jumbo phage genomes had markedly more AT–rich genomes with ~32% GC. A group of phage genomes, including that of phage GBH033 from this study, are also relatively AT-rich with GC% of ~40%. These two groups of phages are notable for their content of multiple tRNA genes that may serve to lessen the possible impact of divergent codon usages in their genomes when subverting their hosts' metabolism. Comparative genomic analyses of our phage genomes with those in the databases revealed a number of phages that may represent novel phage species (with >5% sequence divergence and other differences) according to recent guidance from the ICTV (Adriaenssens et al., 2020). The increasing number of *Klebsiella* phage genomes deposited in databases increases our basic knowledge of gene composition and key phage phenotypic characteristics such as host range if appropriate metadata is available. However, difficulties in assigning functions to the majority of *Klebsiella* phage genes is an issue that is especially marked in jumbo phage genomes, where approximately three quarters of genes have no annotated function.

The trend toward untreatable, invasive *K. pneumoniae* infections shows no signs of abating and is being driven by the emergence and rapid spread of multi-drug-resistant forms. The problem is particularly acute in Asia, where hypervirulent *K. pneumoniae* clones associated with pyogenic liver abscesses, pneumonia, and meningitis in younger, otherwise healthy patients were first recognised, and as a consequence we have focused our efforts on finding alternative approaches to *Klebsiella* infections using recent clinical isolates from intensive care patients in Thailand (Loraine et al., 2018). There are clear advantages as well as obvious disadvantages in targeting capsule removal as an alternative therapeutic paradigm. Although there is substantial data from animal models showing that administration of capsule depolymerase under tightly controlled conditions during the early phase of infection with a known pathogen can rapidly resolve infection and prevent symptoms and death, there is no evidence that the approach would reduce morbidity and mortality in immunocompromised patients with established infections who are sick enough to be cared for in intensive care units. The complex array of surface-structure-related phenotypes of *K. pneumoniae* encountered in nosocomial infections will also complicate therapy. However, the capsule is the major determinant of virulence in *Klebsiella*, conferring a high degree of resistance to complement (Merino et al., 1992; Short et al., 2020) and to phagocytosis (Williams et al., 1983) and is rapidly and efficiently destroyed, *in vitro* and *in situ*, by each enzyme that we evaluated.

AUTHOR CONTRIBUTIONS

PT conceived the study. GB-H, ME, NR, DN and PT designed experimental procedures. GB-H, ME, DN, DP, GB, MD and PW performed the experiments, analysed and curated the data. SV, PW and GB-H assembled the phage collection. PT and ME wrote the manuscript. All authors contributed to the article and approved the submitted version.

ACKNOWLEDGMENTS

The National Institute for Health Research University College London Hospitals Biomedical Research Centre provided infrastructural support. We acknowledge expert informatics support from the Pathogen Informatics team at the Wellcome Sanger Institute.

SUPPLEMENTARY MATERIAL

Supplementary Figure 1 | Genomic comparison of four *K. pneumoniae* jumbo phage: Muenster (top), GBH019, K64-1, and vB_KleM-RaK2 (bottom) highlighting regions of gene similarity and synteny. Red bars indicate >99% BLASTN similarity between pairs of phage strains. Generated using Artemis Comparison Tool (Carver et al., 2005) with pairwise BLASTN comparisons using default parameters for highly similar sequences.

Supplementary Table 1 | Primers and conditions for cloning of depolymerase genes.

Supplementary Table 2 | Host range of 62 K. *pneumoniae* phage isolated from Thai sewage.

Supplementary Table 3 | Published protein sequences of phage-encoded *K. pneumoniae* depolymerases employed for BLASTX search of Thai *K. pneumoniae* phage genomes.

Supplementary Table 4 | Accession numbers for sequenced phage. Formal numbering of phage is affirmed in this table.

Supplementary Data Sheet 1 | Sequences of plasmids used in this study.

REFERENCES

Adams, M. H., and Park, B. H. (1956). An Enzyme Produced by a Phage Host-Cell System. II. The Properties of the Polysaccharide Depolymerase. *Virology* 2, 719–736. doi: 10.1016/0042-6822(56)90054-x

Adriaenssens, E., and Brister, J. R. (2017). How to Name and Classify Your Phage: An Informal Guide. *Viruses* 9, 70. doi: 10.3390/v9040070

Adriaenssens, E. M., Sullivan, M. B., Knezevic, P., van Zyl, L. J., Sarkar, B. L., Dutilh, B. E., et al. (2020). Taxonomy of Prokaryotic Viruses: 2018-2019 Update From the ICTV Bacterial and Archaeal Viruses Subcommittee. *Arch. Virol.* 165, 1253–1260. doi: 10.1007/s00705-020-04577-8

Al-Shayeb, B., Sachdeva, R., Chen, L. X., Ward, F., Munk, P., Devoto, A., et al. (2020). Clades of Huge Phages From Across Earth's Ecosystems. *Nature* 578, 425–431. doi: 10.1038/s41586-020-2007-4

Avery, O. T., and Dubos, R. (1930). The Specific Action of a Bacterial Enzyme on Pneumococci of Type III. *Science* 72, 151–152. doi: 10.1126/science.72.1858.151

Avery, O. T., and Dubos, R. (1931). The Protective Action of a Specific Enzyme Against Type III Pneumococcus Infection in Mice. *J. Exp. Med.* 54, 73–89. doi: 10.1084/jem.54.1.73

Birchenough, G. M. H., Dalgakiran, F., Witcomb, L. A., Johansson, M. E., McCarthy, A. J., Hansson, G. C., et al. (2017). Postnatal Development of the Small Intestinal Mucosa Drives Age-Dependent, Regio-Selective Susceptibility to *Escherichia Coli* K1 Infection. *Sci. Rep.* 7, 83. doi: 10.1038/s41598-017-00123-w

Boetzer, M., Henkel, C. V., Jansen, H. J., Butler, D., and Pirovano, W. (2011). Scaffolding Pre-Assembled Contigs Using SSPACE. *Bioinformatics* 27, 578–579. doi: 10.1093/bioinformatics/btq683

Boetzer, M., and Pirovano, W. (2012). Toward Almost Closed Genomes With Gapfiller. *Genome Biol.* 13, R56. doi: 10.1186/gb-2012-13-6-r56

Broberg, C. A., Wu, W., Cavalcoli, J. D., Miller, V. L., and Bachman, M. A. (2014). Complete Genome Sequence of *Klebsiella Pneumoniae* Strain ATCC 43816 KPPR1, a Rifampin-Resistant Mutant Commonly Used in Animal, Genetic, and Molecular Biology Studies. *Genome Announc* 2, e00924–e00914. doi: 10.1128/genomeA.00924-14

Carver, T. J., Rutherford, K. M., Berriman, M., Rajandream, M. A., Barrell, B. G., and Parkhill, J. (2005). ACT: The Artemis Comparison Tool. *Bioinformatics* 21, 3422–3423. doi: 10.1093/bioinformatics/bti553

Castelle, C. J., Brown, C. T., Anantharaman, K., Probst, A. J., Huang, R. H., and Banfield, J. F. (2018). Biosynthetic Capacity, Metabolic Variety and Unusual Biology in the CPR and DPANN Radiations. *Nat. Rev. Microbiol.* 16, 629–645. doi: 10.1038/s41579-018-0076-2

Chen, Y., Sun, E., Yang, L., Song, J., and Wu, B. (2018). Therapeutic Application of Bacteriophage PHB02 and Its Putative Depolymerase Against *Pasteurella Multocida* Capsular Type A in Mice. *Front. Microbiol.* 9, 1678. doi: 10.3389/fmicb.2018.01678

Chi, E. Y., Krishnan, S., Randolph, T. W., and Carpenter, J. F. (2003). Physical Stability of Proteins in Aqueous Solution: Mechanism and Driving Forces in non-Native Protein Aggregation. *Pharm. Res.* 20, 1325–1336. doi: 10.1023/A:1025771421906

Clements, A., Gaboriaud, F., Duval, J. F., Farn, J. L., Jenney, A. W., Lithgow, T., et al. (2008). The Major Surface-Associated Saccharides of *Klebsiella Pneumoniae* Contribute to Host Cell Association. *PloS One* 3, e3817. doi: 10.1371/journal.pone.0003817

Cold Spring Harbor Protocol (2006). doi: 10.1101/pdb.rec8111

Domenico, P., Schwartz, S., and Cunha, B. A. (1989). Reduction of Capsular Polysaccharide Production in *Klebsiella Pneumoniae* by Sodium Salicylate. *Infect. Immun.* 57, 3778–3782. doi: 10.1128/IAI.57.12.3778-3782.1989

Dubos, R., and Avery, O. T. (1931). Decomposition of the Capsular Polysaccharide of Pneumococci Type III by a Bacterial Enzyme. *J. Exp. Med.* 54, 51–71. doi: 10.1084/jem.54.1.51

Fang, C. T., Chuang, Y. P., Shun, C. T., Chang, S. C., and Wang, J. T. (2004). A Novel Virulence Gene in *Klebsiella Pneumoniae* Strains Causing Primary Liver Abscess and Septic Metastatic Complications. *J. Exp. Med.* 199, 697–705. doi: 10.1084/jem.20030857

Finn, R. D., Clements, J., Arndt, W., Miller, B. L., Wheeler, T. J., Schreiber, F., et al. (2015). HMMER Web Server: 2015 Update. *Nucleic Acids Res.* 43, W30–W38. doi: 10.1093/nar/gkv397

Francis, T., Terrell, E. E., Dubos, R., and Avery, O. T. (1934). Experimental Type III Pneumococcus Infection in Monkeys: II. Treatment With an Enzyme Which Decomposes the Specific Capsular Polysaccharide of Pneumococcus Type III. *J. Exp. Med.* 59, 641–667. doi: 10.1084/jem.59.5.641

Gladman, S., and Seemann, T. (2008). *Velvet Optimiser*. Available at: https://github.com/tseemann/VelvetOptimiser (Accessed April/May, 2020).

Goodner, K., Dubos, R., and Avery, O. T. (1932). The Action of a Specific Enzyme Upon the Dermal Infection of Rabbits With Type III Pneumococcus. *J. Exp. Med.* 55, 393–404. doi: 10.1084/jem.55.3.393

Haney, E. F., and Hancock, R. E. W. (2013). Peptide Design for Antimicrobial and Immunomodulatory Applications. *Biopolymers* 100, 572–583. doi: 10.1002/bip.22250

Kelley, L. A., Mezulis, S., Yates, C. M., Wass, M. N., and Sternberg, M. J. (2015). The Phyre2 Web Portal for Protein Modeling, Prediction and Analysis. *Nat. Protoc.* 10, 845–858. doi: 10.1038/nprot.2015.053

Knecht, L. E., Veljkovic, M., and Fieseler, L. (2020). Diversity and Function of Phage Encoded Depolymerases. *Front. Microbiol.* 10, 2949. doi: 10.3389/fmicb.2019.02949

Kropinski, A. M., Mazzocco, A., Waddell, T. E., Lingohr, E., and Johnson, R. P. (2009). Enumeration of Bacteriophages by Double Agar Overlay Plaque Assay. *Methods Mol. Biol.* 501, 69–76. doi: 10.1007/978-1-60327-164-6_7

Latka, A., Leiman, P. G., Drulis-Kawa, Z., and Briers, Y. (2019). Modeling the Architecture of Depolymerase-Containing Receptor Binding Proteins in *Klebsiella* Phages. *Front. Microbiol.* 10, 2649. doi: 10.3389/fmicb.2019.02649

Latka, A., Maciejewska, B., Majkowska-Skrobek, G., Briers, Y., and Drulis-Kawa, Z. (2017). Bacteriophage-encoded Virion-Associated Enzymes to Overcome the Carbohydrate Barriers During the Infection Process. *Appl. Microbiol. Biotechnol.* 101, 3103–3119. doi: 10.1007/s00253-017-8224-6

Leggate, D. R., Bryant, J. M., Redpath, M. B., Head, D., Taylor, P. W., and Luzio, J. P. (2002). Expression, Mutagenesis and Kinetic Analysis of Recombinant K1E Endosialidase to Define the Site of Proteolytic Processing and Requirements for Catalysis. *Mol. Microbiol.* 44, 749–760. doi: 10.1046/j.1365-2958.2002.02908.x

Lin, T. L., Hsieh, P. F., Huang, Y. T., Lee, W. C., Tsai, Y. T., Su, P. A., et al. (2014). Isolation of a Bacteriophage and Its Depolymerase Specific for K1 Capsule of *Klebsiella Pneumoniae*: Implication in Typing and Treatment. *J. Infect. Dis.* 210, 1734–1744. doi: 10.1093/infdis/jiu332

Lin, D. M., Koskella, B., and Lin, H. C. (2017). Phage Therapy: An Alternative to Antibiotics in the Age of Multi-Drug Resistance. *World J. Gastrointest Pharmacol. Ther.* 8, 162–173. doi: 10.4292/wjgpt.v8.i3.162

Lin, H., Paff, M. L., Molineux, I. J., and Bull, J. J. (2017). Therapeutic Application of Phage Capsule Depolymerases Against K1, K5, and K30 Capsulated E. Coli in Mice. *Front. Microbiol.* 8, 2257. doi: 10.3389/fmicb.2017.02257

Liu, Y., Leung, S. S. Y., Guo, Y., Zhao, L., Jiang, N., Mi, L., et al. (2019). The Capsule Depolymerase Dpo48 Rescues *Galleria Mellonella* and Mice From *Acinetobacter Baumannii* Systemic Infections. *Front. Microbiol.* 10, 545. doi: 10.3389/fmicb.2019.00545

Loraine, J., Heinz, E., De Sousa Almeida, J., Milevskyy, O., Voravuthikunchai, S. P., Srimanote, P., et al. (2018). Complement Susceptibility in Relation to Genome Sequence of Recent *Klebsiella Pneumoniae* Isolates From Thai Hospitals. *mSphere* 3, e00537–e00518. doi: 10.1128/mSphere.00537-18

Majkowska-Skrobek, G., Łątka, A., Berisio, R., Maciejewska, B., Squeglia, F., Romano, M., et al. (2016). Capsule-Targeting Depolymerase, Derived From *Klebsiella* KP36 Phage, as a Tool for the Development of Anti-Virulent Strategy. *Viruses* 8, 324. doi: 10.3390/v8120324

Mellbye, B., and Schuster, M. (2011). The Sociomicrobiology of Antivirulence Drug Resistance: A Proof of Concept. *mBio* 2, e00131–e00111. doi: 10.1128/mBio.00131-11

Merino, S., Camprubí, S., Albertí, S., Benedí, V. J., and Tomás, J. M. (1992). Mechanisms of *Klebsiella Pneumoniae* Resistance to Complement-Mediated Killing. *Infect. Immun.* 60, 2529–2535. doi: 10.1128/IAI.60.6.2529-2535.1992

Mock, M., and Fouet, A. (2001). Anthrax. *Annu. Rev. Microbiol.* 55, 647–671. doi: 10.1146/annurev.micro.55.1.647

Mora, D., Lessor, L., Le, T., Clark, J., Gill, J. J., and Liu, M. (2021). Complete Genome Sequence of *Klebsiella Pneumoniae* Jumbo Phage Miami. *Microbiol. Resour. Announc* 10, e01404–e01420. doi: 10.1128/MRA.01404-20

Mostowy, R. J., and Holt, K. E. (2018). Diversity-generating Machines: Genetics of Bacterial Sugar-Coating. *Trends Microbiol.* 26, 1008–1021. doi: 10.1016/j.tim.2018.06.006

Mushtaq, N., Redpath, M. B., Luzio, J. P., and Taylor, P. W. (2004). Prevention and Cure of Systemic *Escherichia Coli* K1 Infection by Modification of the Bacterial Phenotype. *Antimicrob. Agents Chemother.* 48, 1503–1508. doi: 10.1128/aac.48.5.1503-1508.2004

Negus, D., and Taylor, P. W. (2014). A Poly-γ-(D)-Glutamic Acid Depolymerase that Degrades the Protective Capsule of *Bacillus anthracis*. *Mol. Microbiol.* 91, 1136–1147. doi: 10.1111/mmi.12523

Nurk, S., Meleshko, D., Korobeynikov, A., and Pevzner, P. A. (2017). metaSPAdes: A New Versatile Metagenomic Assembler. *Genome Res.* 27, 824–834. doi: 10.1101/gr.213959.116

Ondov, B. D., Treangen, T. J., Melsted, P., Mallonee, A. B., Bergman, N. H., Koren, S., et al. (2016). Mash: Fast Genome and Metagenome Distance Estimation Using Minhash. *Genome Biol.* 17, 132. doi: 10.1186/s13059-016-0997-x

Paczosa, M. K., and Mecsas, J. (2016). *Klebsiella Pneumoniae*: Going on the Offense With a Strong Defense. *Microbiol. Mol. Biol. Rev.* 80, 629–661. doi: 10.1128/MMBR.00078-15

Page, A. J., Cummins, C. A., Hunt, M., Wong, V. K., Reuter, S., Holden, M. T., et al. (2015). Roary: Rapid Large-Scale Prokaryote Pan Genome Analysis. *Bioinformatics* 31, 3691–3693. doi: 10.1093/bioinformatics/btv421

Page, A. J., De Silva, N., Hunt, M., Quail, M. A., Parkhill, J., Harris, S. R., et al. (2016). Robust High-Throughput Prokaryote *De Novo* Assembly and

Improvement Pipeline for Illumina Data. *Microb. Genom.* 2, e000083. doi: 10.1099/mgen.0.000083

Pan, Y. J., Lin, T. L., Chen, C. C., Tsai, Y. T., Cheng, Y. H., Chen, Y. Y., et al. (2017). *Klebsiella* Phage ΦK64-1 Encodes Multiple Depolymerases for Multiple Host Capsular Types. *J. Virol.* 91, e02457–e02416. doi: 10.1128/JVI.02457-16

Pickard, D. J. (2009). Preparation of Bacteriophage Lysates and Pure DNA. *Methods Mol. Biol.* 502, 3–9. doi: 10.1007/978-1-60327-565-1_1

Pires, D. P., Oliveira, H., Melo, L. D. R., Sillankorva, S., and Azeredo, J. (2016). Bacteriophage-encoded Depolymerases: Their Diversity and Biotechnological Applications. *Appl. Microbiol. Biotechnol.* 100, 2141–2151. doi: 10.1007/s00253-015-7247-0

Quevillon, E., Silventoinen, V., Pillai, S., Harte, N., Mulder, N., Apweiler, R., et al. (2005). InterProScan: Protein Domains Identifier. *Nucleic Acids Res.* 33, W116–W120. doi: 10.1093/nar/gki442

Raya, R. R., and Hebert, E. M. (2009). Isolation of Phage Via Induction of Lysogens. *Methods Mol. Biol.* 501, 23–32. doi: 10.1007/978-1-60327-164-6_3

Roberts, I. S. (1996). The Biochemistry and Genetics of Capsular Polysaccharide Production in Bacteria. *Annu. Rev. Microbiol.* 50, 285–315. doi: 10.1146/annurev.micro.50.1.285

Rumbaugh, K. P., and Sauer, K. (2020). Biofilm Dispersion. *Nat. Rev. Microbiol.* 18, 571–586. doi: 10.1038/s41579-020-0385-0

Santiago, A., and Donlan, R. (2020). Bacteriophage infections of biofilms of health care-associated pathogens: *Klebsiella pneumoniae*. *EcoSal Plus*. doi: 10.1128/ecosalplus.ESP-0029-2019

Scorpio, A., Chabot, D. J., Day, W. A., O'Brien, D. K., Vietri, N. J., Itoh, Y., et al. (2007). Poly-γ-Glutamate Capsule-Degrading Enzyme Treatment Enhances Phagocytosis and Killing of Encapsulated *Bacillus Anthracis*. Antimicrob. *Agents Chemother.* 51, 215–222. doi: 10.1128/AAC.00706-06

Seed, K. D., Lazinski, D. W., Calderwood, S. B., and Camilli, A. (2013). A Bacteriophage Encodes its Own CRISPR/Cas Adaptive Response to Evade Host Innate Immunity. *Nature* 494, 489–491. doi: 10.1038/nature11927

Seemann, T. (2014). Prokka: Rapid Prokaryotic Genome Annotation. *Bioinformatics* 30, 2068–2069. doi: 10.1093/bioinformatics/btu153

Short, F. L., Di Sario, G., Reichmann, N. T., Kleanthous, C., Parkhill, J., and Taylor, P. W. (2020). Genomic Profiling Reveals Distinct Routes to Complement Resistance in *Klebsiella Pneumoniae*. *Infect. Immun.* 88, e00043–e00020. doi: 10.1128/IAI.00043-20

Šimoliūnas, E., Kaliniene, L., Truncaitė, L., Zajančkauskaitė, A., Staniulis, J., Kaupinis, A., et al. (2013). *Klebsiella* Phage vB_KleM-RaK2 - A Giant Singleton Virus of the Family *Myoviridae*. *PloS One* 8, e60717. doi: 10.1371/journal.pone.0060717

Solovieva, E. V., Myakinina, V. P., Kislichkina, A. A., Krasilnikova, V. M., Verevkin, V. V., Mochalov, V. V., et al. (2018). Comparative Genome Analysis of Novel Podoviruses Lytic for Hypermucoviscous *Klebsiella Pneumoniae* of K1, K2, and K57 Capsular Types. *Virus Res.* 243, 10–18. doi: 10.1016/j.virusres.2017.09.026

Squeglia, F., Maciejewska, B., Łątka, A., Ruggiero, A., Briers, Y., Drulis-Kawa, Z., et al. (2020). Structural and Functional Studies of a Klebsiella Phage Capsule Depolymerase Tailspike: Mechanistic Insights Into Capsular Degradation. *Structure* 28, 613–624.e4. doi: 10.1016/j.str.2020.04.015

Stabler, R. A., Negus, D., Pain, A., and Taylor, P. W. (2013). Draft Genome Sequences of *Pseudomonas Fluorescens* BS2 and *Pusillimonas Noertemanii* BS8, Soil Bacteria That Cooperate to Degrade the Poly-γ-D-glutamic Acid Anthrax Capsule. *Genome Announc* 1, e00057–e00012. doi: 10.1128/genomeA.00057-12

States, D. J., and Gish, W. (1994). Combined Use of Sequence Similarity and Codon Bias for Coding Region Identification. *J. Comp. Biol.* 1, 39–50. doi: 10.1089/cmb.1994.1.39

Sutherland, I. W., Hughes, K. A., Skillman, L. C., and Tait, K. (2004). The Interaction of Phage and Biofilms. *FEMS Microbiol. Lett.* 232, 1–6. doi: 10.1016/S0378-1097(04)00041-2

Taylor, P. W. (2017). Novel Therapeutics for Bacterial Infections. *Emerg. Top. Life Sci.* 1, 85–92. doi: 10.1042/ETLS20160017

Tomlinson, S., and Taylor, P. W. (1985). Neuraminidase Associated With Coliphage E That Specifically Depolymerizes the *Escherichia Coli* K1 Capsular Polysaccharide. *J. Virol.* 55, 374–378. doi: 10.1128/JVI.55.2.374-378.1985

Townsend, E., Kelly, L., Gannon, L., Muscatt, G., Dunstan, R., Michniewski, S., et al. (2021). Isolation and Characterisation of *Klebsiella* Phages for Phage Therapy. *Phage* 2, 26–42. doi: 10.1089/phage.2020.0046

Wang, C., Li, P., Niu, W., Yuan, X., Liu, H., Huang, Y., et al. (2019). Protective and Therapeutic Application of the Depolymerase Derived From a Novel KN1 Genotype of *Klebsiella pneumoniae* Bacteriophage in Mice. *Res. Microbiol.* 170, 156–164. doi: 10.1016/j.resmic.2019.01.003

Wang, J. T., Wu, S. H., and Wu, C. (2020). *Klebsiella Pneumoniae* Capsule Polysaccharide Vaccines. U.S. Patent Application No 20200038497 (Washington DC: U.S. Patent and Trademark Office).

Williams, P., Lambert, P. A., Brown, M. R. W., and Jones, R. J. (1983). The Role of the O and K Antigens in Determining the Resistance of *Klebsiella Aerogenes* to Serum Killing and Phagocytosis. *J. Gen. Microbiol.* 129, 2181–2191. doi: 10.1099/00221287-129-7-2181

Wyres, K. L., Lam, M. M. C., and Holt, K. E. (2020). Population Genomics of *Klebsiella pneumoniae*. *Nat. Rev. Microbiol.* 18, 344–359. doi: 10.1038/s41579-019-0315-1

Yuan, Y., and Gao, M. (2017). Jumbo Bacteriophages: An Overview. *Front. Microbiol.* 8, 403. doi: 10.3389/fmicb.2017.00403

Zelmer, A., Martin, M. J., Gundogdu, O., Birchenough, G., Lever, R., Wren, B. W., et al. (2010). Administration of Capsule-Selective Endosialidase E Minimizes Upregulation of Organ Gene Expression Induced by Experimental Systemic Infection With *Escherichia Coli* K1. *Microbiology* 156, 2205–2215. doi: 10.1099/mic.0.036145-0

Zerbino, D. R., and Birney, E. (2008). Velvet: Algorithms for *De Novo* Short Read Assembly Using De Bruijn Graphs. *Genome Res.* 18, 821–829. doi: 10.1101/gr.074492.107

12

Using Omics Technologies and Systems Biology to Identify Epitope Targets for the Development of Monoclonal Antibodies Against Antibiotic-Resistant Bacteria

Antonio J. Martín-Galiano and Michael J. McConnell*

Intrahospital Infections Laboratory, National Centre for Microbiology, Instituto de Salud Carlos III, Majadahonda, Spain

*Correspondence:
Michael J. McConnell
michael.mcconnell@isciii.es

Over the past few decades, antimicrobial resistance has emerged as an important threat to public health due to the global dissemination of multidrug-resistant strains from several bacterial species. This worrisome trend, in addition to the paucity of new antibiotics with novel mechanisms of action in the development pipeline, warrants the development of non-antimicrobial approaches to combating infection caused by these isolates. Monoclonal antibodies (mAbs) have emerged as highly effective molecules for the treatment of multiple diseases. However, in spite of the fact that antibodies play an important role in protective immunity against bacteria, only three mAb therapies have been approved for clinical use in the treatment of bacterial infections. In the present review, we briefly outline the therapeutic potential of mAbs in the treatment of bacterial diseases and discuss how their development can be facilitated when assisted by "omics" technologies and interpreted under a systems biology paradigm. Specifically, methods employing large genomic, transcriptomic, structural, and proteomic datasets allow for the rational identification of epitopes. Ideally, these include those that are present in the majority of circulating isolates, highly conserved at the amino acid level, surface-exposed, located on antigens essential for virulence, and expressed during critical stages of infection. Therefore, these knowledge-based approaches can contribute to the identification of high-value epitopes for the development of effective mAbs against challenging bacterial clones.

Keywords: monoclonal antibodies, antibiotic resistance, multidrug resistance, systems biology, big data, immunoinformatics, bound rationality

DO WE NEED MONOCLONAL ANTIBODIES AGAINST ANTIBIOTIC-RESISTANT BACTERIA?

In recent years, there has been an explosive increase in the emergence and dissemination of antimicrobial resistance. Multiple factors have likely contributed to this phenomenon, including the overuse of existing antibiotics in the clinical setting, non-human use of antibiotics, and increased international travel. A report commissioned by the United Kingdom in 2014 estimated that deaths directly attributable to antimicrobial resistance will increase to 10 million annually by 2050, as compared to the 700,000 deaths currently produced by these infections per year (1).

The predicted economic expense caused by antimicrobial resistance is also significant, as the same study projected that the cumulative worldwide loss of Gross Domestic Product (GDP) between 2014 and 2050 would be higher than the current yearly GDP of all countries combined. Although these extreme scenarios represent projections based on current trends, there is little doubt that antimicrobial resistance will be a major public health threat in the near future. Importantly, the clinical management of multidrug-resistant (MDR) infections is complicated by the lack of currently approved antimicrobials that retain sufficient activity against MDR strains, particularly the so-called ESKAPE microorganisms, which include *Enterococcus faecium*, *Staphylococcus aureus*, *Klebsiella pneumoniae*, *Acinetobacter baumannii*, *Pseudomonas aeruginosa*, and *Enterobacter* spp. (2). Recent sporadic reports from different geographic regions describing pan-drug resistant isolates, with resistance to all clinically-available antibiotics, are cause for particular concern (3–5). In this context, the need to develop new antibiotics, ideally with novel mechanisms of action not affected by cross-resistance to existing mechanisms, is apparent. Unfortunately, while there have been recent approvals of new antibiotics for clinical use, very few antimicrobials with completely novel mechanisms of action have been developed over the last 40 years.

While new antibiotics will be key players in combating resistance, it is likely that treatment and prevention approaches fighting on alternative fronts will need to be explored. In this regard, a recent report summarizing the portfolio of alternatives to antibiotics that are currently under development identified antibody-based therapies, probiotics, phage therapy, immune stimulation, and vaccines as "Tier 1," based on their stage of development and probability of success (6). Among these approaches, therapies based on monoclonal antibodies (mAbs) have a number of characteristics that may make them ideally suited for the treatment and prevention of infections caused by MDR bacteria, including (a) absence of susceptibility to existing resistance mechanisms and lack of selection for resistance to existing antibiotics, (b) facilitating immune-mediated clearance of bacterial pathogens, (c) high specificity and therefore minimal effects on non-target bacteria present in the human microbiota, (d) safety and efficiency in humans, and (e) passive immunization, which, in contrast to active immunization with vaccines, has potential to provide immediate protective immunity against infection, which may be particularly important in critically-ill patients with decreased immune function. In this review, we assess the potential of omics technologies and systems biology approaches to enhance the rational identification of epitopes for the development of mAbs against MDR bacteria.

CHALLENGES TO DEVELOPING MABS FOR RESISTANT BACTERIA

MAbs are highly directed therapeutics that embody the magic bullet ideal of specifically targeting a particular pathogen. However, despite the fact that a large number of therapeutic mAbs have been successfully developed for multiple different human pathologies, most notably for rheumatologic and oncologic diseases, only three mAb therapies have been approved for bacterial infections. Raxibacumab and obiltoxaximab have been developed for inhalational anthrax (7, 8), while bezlotoxumab was recently approved for the prevention of *Clostridium difficile* infection (9). The relative paucity of mAbs for bacterial infections is especially noteworthy given the key role played by antibodies in bacterial clearance during natural infection and vaccine-induced immunity. However, the difference in the rate of increase in approved antibodies for different disease types may be partially due to the fact that the features of the underlying biology being targeted by mAbs for non-infectious diseases are very different from those in pathogenic bacteria. In the former cases, highly conserved human proteins, either cancer antigens or immune effector molecules (e.g., cytokines), are targeted. In stark contrast, antibacterial mAbs target rapidly dividing microorganisms with high genetic plasticity. Bacteria have the ability to downregulate or even completely abolish the expression of molecules containing targeted epitopes, in a process generally known as epitope masking (10). Moreover, these microorganisms can exert epitope switching since they are able to modify and tolerate severe amino acid changes in epitopes that reduce antibody affinity through recombination with externally-acquired DNA or via mutations that do not produce significant changes in virulence and fitness (11, 12). This is a consequence of confronting double Darwinian pressure in search of an equilibrium between keeping important functions for (patho)biology and the evasion of host immunity. By doing so, bacterial pathogens have evolved to avoid detection and neutralization by antibodies.

In the three aforementioned antibacterial mAbs, disease is prevented due to the neutralization of toxins via binding to highly conserved epitopes on toxin subunits. This approach is effective for anthrax and *C. difficile* infection due to the fact that these pathologies are mediated by the action of potent toxins. However, this is not the case for most bacterial pathogens, particularly for MDR-associated species. MAbs for these infections will most likely need to target epitopes present on the bacterial cell and facilitate clearance by the immune system to be effective. In this regard, bacterial epitopes that would be ideal targets for mAbs may need to meet most, if not all, of the following criteria: (a) high conservation between circulating strains, (b) expression during bacterial infection and/or colonization, (c) surface exposure in order to permit antibody binding, and (d) antigenically distinct compared to epitopes on human proteins and the normal human microbiota to prevent cross-reactivity.

The biological function of the molecule containing the targeted epitope may be of particular importance. MAbs that target epitopes on molecules that participate in essential bacterial processes for viability or virulence may be less susceptible to the generation of escape mutants, given that reduced expression or sequence variation in these molecules may be detrimental to bacterial survival. It is worth noting that MDR organisms consist of a series of interacting molecular elements, a functional network, with emergent properties only approachable as a whole by systems biology and high-throughput "omics" techniques (13). One of the emergent properties of scale-free networks is the tolerance to failures that, in this case, means that many essential bacterial processes are subject to total or partial functional redundancy (14). Bacteria can increase fitness mainly by gathering genes that exert functions efficiently but that can be, at least partially, covered by other means. For example, 30 alternative sugar transporters (15) and seven plasminogen-binding proteins have been identified in *Streptococcus pneumoniae* (16) that ensure that these important tasks required for infection are performed under many conditions. Likewise, antigenic proteins rarely act in isolation but rather as part of functional sub-networks that exert simultaneous or sequential activities leading to colonization and/or disease (13). In this respect, epitope switching by mutation or down-regulation of a single participant targeted by mAbs in one of these pathways may not greatly affect the ability of the bacteria to replicate and produce infection if this change can be adequately compensated for elsewhere in the interactome. Thus, non-overlapping irreplaceable elements of the pathofunctional sub-networks, i.e., virulence hubs, should be prioritized. This may present particular challenges in identifying a single epitope for mAb development that is less susceptible to the generation of escape mutants.

USING OMICS TECHNOLOGY AND SYSTEMS BIOLOGY FOR MAB DEVELOPMENT

Omics Data and Systems Biology Basics

Although there are significant challenges to developing broadly effective mAb-based therapies for bacterial infections, it is conceivable that the availability of multiple large data sets involving genomic sequences and global profiling experiments (e.g., transcriptomics, proteomics, and interactomics; the latter defined as the global pool of physical and/or functional connections between molecules in a cell) may serve as raw material for elucidating high-value epitopes. **Table 1** lists the different omics approaches that are discussed in the sections below and how they can be employed for mAb development. Omics technologies can be considered as those that characterize molecules and their states at a holistic level through the collective characterization of molecular profiles, e.g., transcriptomics, the whole set of transcripts under defined conditions. Omics cover virtually all kinds of biological molecules, and their accumulated outcome volumes approximate to the range of big data, i.e., so massive that they are unable to be stored and managed by ordinary computer users. For instance, central repositories such as the European Bioinformatics Institute store over 160 petabytes of data (17).

While processing large biological data sets could be considered mere brute force, it is important to underscore that the data needed for translational medicine are those that contribute to achieving precise clinical goals, so-called "smart data" (18). Systems biology approaches move in that direction by permitting a more comprehensive and contextual interpretation of the information, given that they can identify not only epitopes meeting certain criteria but also the interplay between different

TABLE 1 | Use of omics technologies and systems biology in antibacterial mAb development.

Technology	Use in identifying epitopes/antigens
Comparative genomics	- Identification of epitopes with highly conserved sequences - Identification of epitopes present in the majority of strains within a species - Clonal distribution of epitopes - Avoidance of cross-reaction with microbiota and human proteins
Transcriptomics	- Identification of antigens preferentially expressed during infection
Proteomics	- Identification of antigens highly expressed during infection - Identification of epitopes on the bacterial cell surface
Molecular modeling and dynamics	- Identification of surface-exposed epitopes - Assessment of the stability of surface exposure of the epitope and its binding to the antigen
Interactomics/systems biology	- Identification of optimal synergistic mixtures of epitopes (for use in developing mAb cocktails) - Identification of epitopes/antigens that participate in essential bacterial processes that involve molecular connections

essential criteria (19). The integration of multivariate data for rational vaccine purposes is far from trivial (20); clearly the challenge here is converting large quantities of data into information with biological value that can be used for the development of mAb therapeutics. As data volumes become larger and more varied due to the availability of multi-omics experiments, it is here that systems biology can be of great value in responding to biological problems of great complexity. Systems biology then becomes a natural analysis option that captures emergent properties of bacteria as a whole that cannot be studied by isolated reductionist protocols. The complexity of the immune response to vaccines has been monitored and analyzed through an analogous approach called systems vaccinology, a branch of systems immunology concentrated on the intrinsic responses of the host to vaccines (21). Parallels can be drawn to reverse vaccinology (RV), which employs both genomics and structural biology to reveal the fraction of the molecular space of a pathogen appropriate for vaccine development (22). It is noteworthy that RV has already yielded successes, most notably in the development of a vaccine for *Neisseria meningitidis* (23). In contrast to RV for vaccines, which can operate at the antigen level, omics and computational approaches for mAb development must be performed at the epitope level, potentially adding increased stringency and complexity to the identification process. Thus, RV is confronted with a significant challenge in the design of mAbs, and the question arises of whether such obstacles hamper knowledge-based solutions. This situation evokes the "bounded rationality" idea (24, 25), in which rational approaches are inefficient due to limited understanding of the inherent complexity of the task.

In the following sections, we assess how the availability of huge and variable data sets can be harnessed, together with systems biology, to enhance RV when oriented to epitope selection for mAb development.

Comparative Genomics: Whole Species and Clone-Specific Epitope Conservation

A common challenge in developing immunoprotective approaches for bacterial infections is that these microorganisms exhibit a high rate of escape from vaccine formulations at the whole species level. Thus, the ideal of identifying immutable antigenic proteins as part of the core proteome of target species and absent from other species is difficult to achieve and may be confined to the aforementioned exotoxins that have already been exploited for mAb development (7–9). Nevertheless, the availability of up to thousands of draft genome sequences for the most important MDR pathogens may enable the assessment of

epitope conservation at intra-clonal resolution with sufficient depth (**Figure 1A**). A plausible strategy may be to focus on the development of mAbs tailored to circulating hypervirulent and/or hyperresistant clones for which the recognized epitope is conserved. This is, for instance, the case for mAbs directed against *K. pneumoniae* O-antigen from the ST258 clone, since it is a recurrent infective lineage and a strong producer of this endotoxin (26). In addition, such clonal specificity preserves the microbiota, highlighting one of the advantages of immunological interventions with respect to antibiotics (27).

Identifying Epitopes Highly Expressed During Infection and/or Colonization

Epitopes of interest for mAb development must be expressed during the course of colonization or infection. Rather than

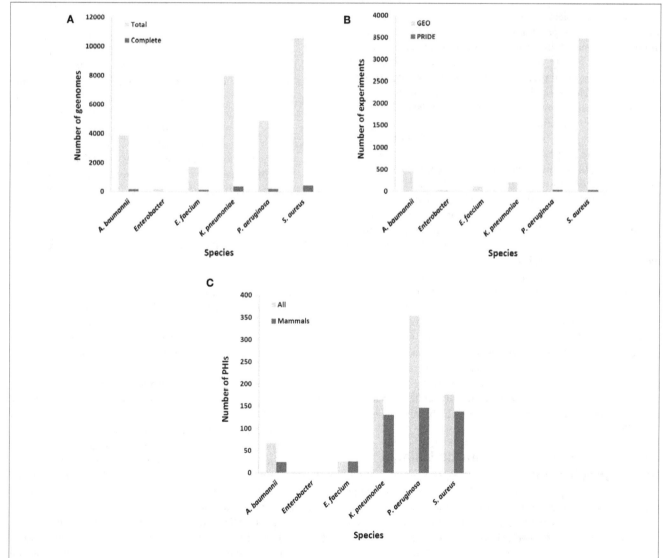

FIGURE 1 | Coverage of ESKAPE organisms by omics databases utilized in rational mAb development. **(A)** Number of available complete and draft/scaffold genomes; **(B)** number of expression experiments, either transcriptomic (GEO database) or proteomic (PRIDE database); **(C)** number of identified molecular interactions between pathogen and host (total and those involving only mammal hosts).

constitutive, the expression of many immunogenic proteins is tightly repressed in order to reduce metabolic expense and overexposure to the host immune system, unless the bacterium senses the right environmental signals for its production (28). To include this important issue in the mAb production pipeline, results from a number of transcriptomic and proteomic experiments stored in databases such as GEO and PRIDE (29), respectively, should be taken into account. MDR microorganisms are well-covered in this respect (**Figure 1B**), including the upregulation of potentially antigenic proteins for mAbs *in vivo* or under *in vitro* conditions that mimic infection, such as bacteremia (30), biofilm (sessile)-to-planktonic transition (31), and iron limitation (32).

Exposure of the Epitope

MAbs must not only fulfill the basic RV principle of being directed against surface or secreted proteins but must also be directed toward epitopes that are exposed on these proteins. This poses a problem on two levels. First, accessible—either secreted or surface—proteins can be detected by the presence of motifs and domains linked to secretion and surface anchoring, in most cases readily detectable by sensitive hidden-Markov models thanks to optimized heuristics adapted to huge protein datasets (33). However, these computational strategies cannot cope with accessible proteins lacking identifiable labels, and must therefore be complemented with experimental high-throughput protein detection on fractionated samples, including cell-free medium for the exoproteome (34) or the outer membrane (35) and cell wall (36) for the surface proteome. On the other hand, the prediction of non-linear epitopes and their location on the solvent-oriented zone of the protein is facilitated by structural information (37). Resolving a structure is labor-intensive, but the combined effort of small scientific groups and large structural genomics consortia (38) has promoted the inclusion of structural biology to the biological pool of large data volumes. The central structural repository, the Protein Data Bank (PDB), currently contains 142,433 proteins (44,971 non-redundant, last accessed: 05/Jul/2019). Likewise, the SwissModel archive reached 1.6 million pre-built structural models (39) covering 62% of *S. aureus* and 72% of *P. aeruginosa* proteins. Once reliable structural information is available for the candidate antigen, epitopes that are highly solvent-accessible can be identified. Dynamic simulations by simulator packages such as GROMACS additionally permit assessment of the dynamic stability of epitope exposure and even of mAb-protein binding when co-crystalized (40).

Design of Anti-virulence mAbs Using Functional Information

As a rational approach, functional information regarding the essentiality of a protein carrying the candidate mAb epitope or its involvement in virulence is invaluable. If these essential/virulence-associated epitopes are not targeted, there is high risk of epitope masking or switching, leading to rapid circumvention of the monoclonal therapy. Specialized resources such as PATRIC, VFDB, and Victors (41–43) compile virulence factors at the species level from dedicated research reports.

Laboratory and animal-model screenings, such as signature-tagged mutagenesis (44), permit the explicit detection of potential genes essential for pathogenesis in a high-throughput manner. Such relevant information would be a promising starting point for antigen selection and prioritization to block virulence traits with mAbs in a precise knowledge-based way. Considering that most virulence factors are not essential for fundamental viability, neutralization by mAbs is akin to blocking virulence rather than the viability of the pathogen and follows the anti-virulence drug paradigm, in contrast to lethal antibiotics (45). Currently licensed mAbs that block the activity of exotoxins can be considered virulence-blocking therapies.

Interactomics

According to systems biology principles, the pathogen and host exhibit a dense network of inter-species molecular interactions throughout their relationship (46). The identification of these interactions has permitted the design of protective strategies in viruses (47). This information may be used to design mAbs that impede connections between pathogen and host molecules that are central to infection progression. A proficient resource for this information is the PHI-base database (48), but of the 12,466 interactions included (Last accessed, 5 Sep 2019), only 467 pertain to connections between the six ESKAPE bacteria and mammals, suggesting that the volume of useful information could still be increased to facilitate the prediction of network tolerance in a global manner (**Figure 1C**). A possible exception is those pathogens whose virulence is almost fully dependent upon the activity of potent exotoxins, which indicates that successful mAb strategies at present are those that circumvent the pitfall of pathogenic network tolerance.

OMICS-SYSTEMS BIOLOGY VS. OTHER STRATEGIES

A fundamental controversy may arise when systemic computational approaches in the RV framework are compared to empirical screenings (49) or the low-throughput selection of antigen/epitope targets (50) by microbiology experts. Each of these strategies has advantages and pitfalls based on their underlying assumptions (**Table 2**), but it is worth noting that the only mAb products that have been approved or are in the clinical phases of testing were developed using the latter two approaches. This may call into question the use of rational approaches based on RV strategies for identifying epitopes for mAb development. More empirical approaches may have achieved their previous successes because experimental screenings are better equipped to accommodate the degenerate and flexible nature of the immune system. Nevertheless, massive data and systemic approaches have likely not yet been successful, not because of their lack of potential, but because of the interpretation of results (51, 52). In addition, there is room for improvement for rational approaches through the collection of new data, algorithms, and paradigms, and this is a continuous process, whereas screening and expert selection are probably closer to their respective plateaus. Moreover, different methods of omics data integration

TABLE 2 | Pros and cons of systems biology/big data/reverse vaccinology approaches vs. empirical screening vs. expert selection for mAb development.

Aspects related to mAb development	Omics/systems biology	Empirical screening	Expert selection
Use for mAb cocktail development	++	−	−
Reduced cost	+	−	++
Time required	+	−	++
Focus on clinical clones	++	+	+
Requires bioinformatics expertise	−	++	++
Requires computational infrastructure	−	++	++
Requires experimental infrastructure	++	−	+
Intrinsic experimental validation	−	++	++
Rational selection	++	−	++
Resistance to "bound rationality"	−	++	+
Room for improvement	++	+	+
Scalability to many targets	++	+	−
Species completeness	++	+	+
Systemic view	++	−	−
Transferability to other species	++	−	−

++ Highly efficient.
+ Moderately efficient.
− Low efficiency.

can be developed in order to identify targets for biomedical applications (13). Conceivably, hybrid approaches that combine the strengths of all of these methods may achieve the highest performances. For instance, a list of the candidate mAb epitopes that have a complex list of features could be revealed from large data sets, verified by experts, and then refined by screenings methods.

An option that may also ease the "bound rationality" of RV is the design of mAb cocktails. The advantages of increasing valence by using mAb combinations are multiple: (1) a net increment in the success rate of neutralization of a process

by reducing the network tolerance of the pathogen; (2) lower chances of future immune evasion since several concerted epitope switches are exponentially more difficult to achieve than individual ones; (3) the possibility of designing complex blocking strategies concentrated on the same (pathogen siege) or sequential (pathogen exhaustion) stages of infection, thus applying a more comprehensive molecular view of the virulent process. Knowing this, the bottleneck in mAb development against bacteria may not lie in the experimental efficiency of mAb identification but in scaling processes required for the production of a mature pharmaceutical product.

CONCLUSIONS AND FUTURE DIRECTIONS

In contrast to cancer, rheumatologic diseases, and viral infections, the limited use of mAbs for MDR bacterial pathogens may be due to several technical and biological constraints. In this context, rational approaches based on large-scale data/systems biology methodologies may facilitate the identification of high-value epitopes for mAb development, perhaps in concert with traditionally used empirical strategies. The extreme challenge associated with finding ideal, immutable epitopes may support the development of mAb cocktails. This could require improvement in the efficiency (development and scaling) of mAb production, i.e., within a reasonable timeframe and at a reasonable cost, at the service of holistic paradigms that consider the molecular pathobiology of the targeted species. We envisage that the large data/systems biology combination will find its utility in RV approaches applied to mAb development as more information is collected.

AUTHOR CONTRIBUTIONS

MM and AM-G planned the manuscript content, wrote the manuscript, and approved the final version.

REFERENCES

Review on Antimicrobial Resistance. *Antimicrobial Resistance: Tackling A Crisis for the Health and Wealth of Nations.* (2014). Available online at: https://amr-review.org/sites/default/files/AMR%20Review%20Paper%20-%20Tackling%20a%20crisis%20for%20the%20health%20and%20wealth%20of%20nations_1.pdf
Boucher HW, Talbot GH, Bradley JS, Edwards JE, Gilbert D, Rice LB, et al. Bad bugs, no drugs: no ESKAPE! An update from the Infectious Diseases Society of America. *Clin Infect Dis.* (2009) 48:1–12. doi: 10.1086/595011
Avgoulea K, Di Pilato V, Zarkotou O, Sennati S, Politi L, Cannatelli A, et al. Characterization of extensively drug-resistant or pandrug-resistant sequence Type 147 and 101 OXA-48-producing *Klebsiella pneumoniae* causing bloodstream infections in patients in an intensive care unit. *Antimicrob Agents Chemother.* (2018) 62:e02457-17. doi: 10.1128/AAC.02457-17
Brennan-Krohn T, Kirby JE. Synergistic combinations and repurposed antibiotics active against the pandrug-resistant *Klebsiella pneumoniae* nevada strain. *Antimicrob Agents Chemother.* (2019) 63:e01374-19. doi:10.1128/AAC.01374-19
Nowak J, Zander E, Stefanik D, Higgins PG, Roca I, Vila J, et al. High incidence of pandrug-resistant *Acinetobacter baumannii* isolates collected from patients with ventilator-associated pneumonia in Greece, Italy and Spain as part of the MagicBullet clinical trial. *J Antimicrob Chemother.* (2017) 72:3277–82. doi: 10.1093/jac/dkx322

Czaplewski L, Bax R, Clokie M, Dawson M, Fairhead H, Fischetti VA, et al. Alternatives to antibiotics-a pipeline portfolio review. *Lancet Infect Dis.* (2016) 16:239–51. doi: 10.1016/S1473-3099(15)00466-1
Hou AW, Morrill AM. Obiltoxaximab: adding to the treatment arsenal for bacillus anthracis infection. *Ann Pharmacother.* (2017) 51:908–13. doi: 10.1177/1060028017713029
Tsai CW, Morris S. Approval of raxibacumab for the treatment of inhalation anthrax under the US Food and Drug Administration "animal rule." *Front Microbiol.* (2015) 6:1320. doi: 10.3389/fmicb.2015.01320
Kufel WD, Devanathan AS, Marx AH, Weber DJ, Daniels LM. Bezlotoxumab: a novel agent for the prevention of recurrent clostridium difficile infection. *Pharmacotherapy.* (2017) 37:1298–308. doi: 10.1002/phar.1990
Zhang Q, Wise KS. Coupled phase-variable expression and epitope masking of selective surface lipoproteins increase surface phenotypic diversity in *Mycoplasma hominis. Infect Immun.* (2001) 69:5177–81. doi: 10.1128/IAI.69.8.5177-5181.2001
Georgieva M, Kagedan L, Lu YJ, Thompson CM, Lipsitch M. Antigenic variation in *Streptococcus pneumoniae* PspC promotes immune escape in the presence of variant-specific immunity. *mBio.* (2018) 9:e00264-18. doi:10.1128/mBio.00264-18
Palmer GH, Bankhead T, Seifert HS. Antigenic variation in bacterial pathogens.

Microbiol Spectr. (2016) 4. doi: 10.1128/microbiolspec.VMBF-0005-2015

Kim CY, Lee M, Lee K, Yoon SS, Lee I. Network-based genetic investigation of virulence-associated phenotypes in methicillin-resistant *Staphylococcus aureus*. *Sci Rep.* (2018) 8:10796. doi: 10.1038/s41598-018-29120-3

Albert R, Jeong H, Barabasi AL. Error and attack tolerance of complex networks. *Nature.* (2000) 406:378–82. doi: 10.1038/35019019

Bidossi A, Mulas L, Decorosi F, Colomba L, Ricci S, Pozzi G, et al. A functional genomics approach to establish the complement of carbohydrate transporters in *Streptococcus pneumoniae*. *PLoS ONE.* (2012) 7:e33320. doi:10.1371/journal.pone.0033320

Meinel C, Sparta G, Dahse HM, Horhold F, Konig R, Westermann M, et al. *Streptococcus pneumoniae* from patients with hemolytic uremic syndrome binds human plasminogen via the surface protein PspC and uses plasmin to damage human endothelial cells. *J Infect Dis.* (2018) 217:358–70. doi: 10.1093/infdis/jix305

Cook CE, Lopez R, Stroe O, Cochrane G, Brooksbank C, Birney E, et al. The European Bioinformatics Institute in 2018: tools, infrastructure and training. *Nucleic Acids Res.* (2019) 47:D15–22. doi: 10.1093/nar/gky1124

Geerts H, Dacks PA, Devanarayan V, Haas M, Khachaturian ZS, Gordon MF, et al. Big data to smart data in Alzheimer's disease: the brain health modeling initiative to foster actionable knowledge. *Alzheimer's Dement.* (2016) 12:1014–21. doi: 10.1016/j.jalz.2016.04.008

Kitano, H. Systems biology: a brief overview. *Science.* (2002) 295:1662–4. doi: 10.1126/science.1069492

Weiner J 3rd, Kaufmann SH, Maertzdorf J. High-throughput data analysis and data integration for vaccine trials. *Vaccine.* (2015) 33:5249–55. doi: 10.1016/j.vaccine.2015.04.096

Pulendran B. Learning immunology from the yellow fever vaccine: innate immunity to systems vaccinology. *Nat Rev Immunol.* (2009) 9:741–7. doi: 10.1038/nri2629

Rappuoli R, Bottomley MJ, D'Oro U, Finco O, De Gregorio E. Reverse vaccinology 2.0: human immunology instructs vaccine antigen design. *J Exp Med.* (2016) 213:469–81. doi: 10.1084/jem.20151960

Parikh SR, Andrews NJ, Beebeejaun K, Campbell H, Ribeiro S, Ward C, et al. Effectiveness and impact of a reduced infant schedule of 4CMenB vaccine against group B meningococcal disease in England: a national observational cohort study. *Lancet.* (2016) 388:2775–82. doi:10.1016/S0140-6736(16)31921-3

Van Regenmortel MH. Basic research in HIV vaccinology is hampered by reductionist thinking. *Front Immunol.* (2012) 3:194. doi: 10.3389/fimmu.2012.00194

Van Regenmortel MH. Requirements for empirical immunogenicity trials, rather than structure-based design, for developing an effective HIV vaccine. *Arch Virol.* (2012) 157:1–20. doi: 10.1007/s00705-011-1145-2

Szijarto V, Guachalla LM, Hartl K, Varga C, Badarau A, Mirkina I, et al. Endotoxin neutralization by an O-antigen specific monoclonal antibody: a potential novel therapeutic approach against *Klebsiella pneumoniae* ST258. *Virulence.* (2017) 8:1203–15. doi: 10.1080/21505594.2017. 1279778

Bloom DE, Black S, Salisbury D, Rappuoli R. Antimicrobial resistance and the role of vaccines. *Proc Natl Acad Sci USA.* (2018) 115:12868–71. doi:10.1073/pnas.1717157115

Delaune A, Dubrac S, Blanchet C, Poupel O, Mader U, Hiron A, et al. The WalKR system controls major staphylococcal virulence genes and is involved in triggering the host inflammatory response. *Infect Immun.* (2012) 80:3438–53. doi: 10.1128/IAI.00195-12

Vizcaino JA, Csordas A, del-Toro N, Dianes JA, Griss J, Lavidas I, et al. 2016 update of the PRIDE database and its related tools. *Nucleic Acids Res.* (2016) 44:D447–56. doi: 10.1093/nar/gkv1145

Murray GL, Tsyganov K, Kostoulias XP, Bulach DM, Powell D, Creek DJ, et al. Global gene expression profile of *Acinetobacter baumannii* during bacteremia. *J Infect Dis.* (2017) 215(Suppl_1):S52–7. doi: 10.1093/infdis/jiw529

Guilhen C, Charbonnel N, Parisot N, Gueguen N, Iltis A, Forestier C, et al. Transcriptional profiling of *Klebsiella pneumoniae* defines signatures for planktonic, sessile and biofilm-dispersed cells. *BMC Genom.* (2016) 17:237. doi:10.1186/s12864-016-2557-x

Holden VI, Wright MS, Houle S, Collingwood A, Dozois CM, Adams MD, et al. Iron acquisition and siderophore release by carbapenem-resistant sequence type 258 *Klebsiella pneumoniae*. *mSphere.* (2018) 3:e00125-18. doi: 10.1128/mSphere.00125-18

Eddy SR. Accelerated profile HMM searches. *PLoS Comput Biol.* (2011) 7:e1002195. doi:10.1371/journal.pcbi.1002195

Sengupta N, Alam SI, Kumar B, Kumar RB, Gautam V, Kumar S, et al. Comparative proteomic analysis of extracellular proteins of *Clostridium perfringens* type A and type C strains. *Infect Immun.* (2010) 78:3957–68. doi:10.1128/IAI.00374-10

Li H, Zhang DF, Lin XM, Peng XX. Outer membrane proteomics of kanamycin-resistant *Escherichia coli* identified MipA as a novel antibiotic resistance-related protein. *FEMS Microbiol Lett.* (2015) 362:fnv074. doi:10.1093/femsle/fnv074

Wang W, Jeffery CJ. An analysis of surface proteomics results reveals novel candidates for intracellular/surface moonlighting proteins in bacteria. *Mol Biosyst.* (2016) 12:1420–31. doi: 10.1039/C5MB00550G

Haste Andersen P, Nielsen M, Lund O. Prediction of residues in discontinuous B-cell epitopes using protein 3D structures. *Protein Sci.* (2006) 15:2558–67. doi: 10.1110/ps.062405906

Grabowski M, Niedzialkowska E, Zimmerman MD, Minor W. The impact of structural genomics: the first quindecennial. *J Struct Funct Genom.* (2016) 17:1–16. doi: 10.1007/s10969-016-9201-5

Bienert S, Waterhouse A, de Beer TA, Tauriello G, Studer G, Bordoli L, et al. The SWISS-MODEL Repository-new features and functionality. *Nucleic Acids Res.* (2017) 45:D313–9. doi: 10.1093/nar/gkw1132

Ebrahimi Z, Asgari S, Ahangari Cohan R, Hosseinzadeh R, Hosseinzadeh G, et al. Rational affinity enhancement of fragmented antibody by ligand- based affinity improvement approach. *Biochem Biophys Res Commun.* (2018) 506:653–9. doi: 10.1016/j.bbrc.2018.10.127

Liu B, Zheng D, Jin Q, Chen L, Yang J. VFDB 2019: a comparative pathogenomic platform with an interactive web interface. *Nucleic Acids Res.* (2019) 47:D687–92. doi: 10.1093/nar/gky1080

Mao C, Abraham D, Wattam AR, Wilson MJ, Shukla M, Yoo HS, et al. Curation, integration and visualization of bacterial virulence factors in PATRIC. *Bioinformatics.* (2015) 31:252–8. doi: 10.1093/bioinformatics/btu631

Sayers S, Li L, Ong E, Deng S, Fu G, Lin Y, et al. Victors: a web-based knowledge base of virulence factors in human and animal pathogens. *Nucleic Acids Res.* (2019) 47:D693–700. doi: 10.1093/nar/gky999

Hensel M, Shea JE, Gleeson C, Jones MD, Dalton E, Holden DW. Simultaneous identification of bacterial virulence genes by negative selection. *Science.* (1995) 269:400–3. doi: 10.1126/science.7618105

Rasko DA, Sperandio V. Anti-virulence strategies to combat bacteria- mediated disease. *Nat Rev Drug Discov.* (2010) 9:117–28. doi: 10.1038/nrd3013

Sen R, Nayak L, De RK. A review on host-pathogen interactions: classification and prediction. *Eur J Clin Microbiol Infect Dis.* (2016) 35:1581–99. doi: 10.1007/s10096-016-2716-7

Rahim MN, Klewes L, Zahedi-Amiri A, Mai S, Coombs KM. Global interactomics connect nuclear mitotic apparatus protein NUMA1 to influenza virus maturation. *Viruses.* (2018) 10:731. doi: 10.3390/v10120731

Urban M, Cuzick A, Rutherford K, Irvine A, Pedro H, Pant R, et al. PHI-base: a new interface and further additions for the multi-species pathogen-host interactions database. *Nucleic Acids Res.* (2017) 45:D604–10. doi: 10.1093/nar/gkw1089

Rossmann FS, Laverde D, Kropec A, Romero-Saavedra F, Meyer-Buehn M, Huebner J. Isolation of highly active monoclonal antibodies against multiresistant gram-positive bacteria. *PLoS ONE.* (2015) 10:e0118405. doi: 10.1371/journal.pone.0118405

DiGiandomenico A, Keller AE, Gao C, Rainey GJ, Warrener P, Camara MM, et al. A multifunctional bispecific antibody protects against *Pseudomonas aeruginosa*. *Sci Transl Med.* (2014) 6:262ra155. doi:10.1126/scitranslmed.3009655

13

A Lytic *Yersina pestis* Bacteriophage Obtained from the Bone Marrow of *Marmota himalayana* in a Plague-Focus Area in China

Junrong Liang[1†], Shuai Qin[1†], Ran Duan[1†], Haoran Zhang[1], Weiwei Wu[1,2], Xu Li[3], Deming Tang[1], Guoming Fu[4], Xinmin Lu[5], Dongyue Lv[1], Zhaokai He[1], Hui Mu[1], Meng Xiao[1], Jinchuan Yang[1], Huaiqi Jing[1] and Xin Wang[1*]

[1] State Key Laboratory of Infectious Disease Prevention and Control, National Institute for Communicable Disease Control and Prevention, Chinese Center for Disease Control and Prevention, Beijing, China, [2] Sanitary Inspection Center, Xuzhou Municipal Centre for Disease Control and Prevention, Xuzhou, China, [3] School of Light Industry, Beijing Technology and Business University, Beijing, China, [4] Sanitary Inspection Center, Subei Mongolian Autonomous County Center for Disease Control and Prevention, Jiuquan, China, [5] Sanitary Inspection Center, Akesai Kazakh Autonomous County Center for Disease Control and Prevention, Jiuquan, China

*Correspondence:
Xin Wang
wangxin@icdc.cn

[†] These authors have contributed equally to this work

A lytic *Yersinia pestis* phage vB_YpP-YepMm (also named YepMm for briefly) was first isolated from the bone marrow of a *Marmota himalayana* who died of natural causes on the Qinghai-Tibet plateau in China. Based on its morphologic (isometric hexagonal head and short non-contractile conical tail) and genomic features, we classified it as belonging to the *Podoviridae* family. At the MOI of 10, YepMm reached maximum titers; and the one-step growth curve showed that the incubation period of the phage was about 10 min, the rise phase was about 80 min, and the lysis amount of the phage during the lysis period of 80 min was about 187 PFU/cell. The genome of the bacteriophage YepMm had nucleotide-sequence similarity of 99.99% to that of the *Y. pestis* bacteriophage Yep-phi characterized previously. Analyses of the biological characters showed that YepMm has a short latent period, strong lysis, and a broader lysis spectrum. It could infect *Y. pestis*, highly pathogenic bioserotype 1B/O:8 *Y. enterocolitica*, as well as serotype O:1b *Y. pseudotuberculosis*—the ancestor of *Y. pestis*. It could be further developed as an important biocontrol agent in pathogenic *Yersinia* spp. infection.

Keywords: bacteriophage, Yersinia pestis, Marmota himalayana, natural plague focus, Qinghai-Tibet plateau

INTRODUCTION

Bacteriophages are the most abundant organisms on earth that can interactions with myriad bacterial hosts (Bergh et al., 1989). Lytic bacteriophages have been used as agents for identification and therapeutic of infections in animals and humans (Mukerjee et al., 1963; Gorski et al., 2009; Muniesa et al., 2012; Chhibber et al., 2013; Moojen, 2013; Doub, 2020). Integrity of the bacteriophage tail is essential for the viability of tailed phages, which belong to the *Caudovirales* (Hardy et al., 2020). The tail protein of *Caudovirales* has an important role in the interaction between bacteriophages and host bacteria, which can serve as an adsorption device, a host cell wall-perforating machine, and a genome delivery pathway (Flayhan et al., 2014; Zhang et al., 2018).

In the bacteria of the genus *Yersinia*, bacteriophages have also been used for typing and diagnostics. Bacteriophages ΦYeO3-12 and phiYe-F10 are specific for the *Yersina enterocolitica* serotype O:3 (Kiljunen et al., 2003; Liang et al., 2016); PhiA1122 and Yep-phi are used as a diagnostic agent to confirm the identification of *Yersina pestis*; YpsP-G and YpP-R have been reported to diagnose *Yersina pseudotuberculosis* infection. Many genomes of *Y. pestis* bacteriophages have been fully sequenced, including the *Podoviridae* bacteriophages phiA1122, Yep-phi, Berlin, Yepe2, YpP-R, YpP-G, YpsP-G, Yps-Y, and the *Myoviridae* bacteriophages L-413C, PY100, YpsP-PST, and phiD1 (Garcia et al., 2003; Kiljunen et al., 2011; Rashid et al., 2012; Zhao and Skurnik, 2016).

Qinghai-Tibet plateau is one of the most active natural plague focus in China with *M. himalayana* as the primary host in this area (**Figure 1A**) (**Figure 1E** shows a healthy *Marmota himalayana* in a plague-focus area of the Qinghai-Tibet plateau). The high altitude and harsh climate in the Qinghai-Tibet plateau show that there are few human inhabitants, and the local ecology is relatively stable. Local *M. himalayana* carries a significantly high seropositivity rate of *Y. pestis* F1 antibody, which can be witnessed by continuous outbreaks of plague in animals (*M. himalayana*) and occasionally spreading to humans

(Wang et al., 2011; Ge et al., 2015; Wang et al., 2017). With one human case in 2004, two cases in 2007, one case in 2010, and three cases in 2014 (Ge et al., 2015) among the natural-focus area of Qilian Mountain (**Figure 1B**). There is no report about the *Y. pestis* bacteriophage that naturally existed in the host animals of natural plague foci. So we try to isolate *Y. pestis* bacteriophage from different sources in Qinghai-Tibet plateau and investigate the characterization and subsequent employment of the phages.

In the present study, the bacteriophage vB_YpP-YepMm obtained from the bone marrow of self-died *Marmota himalayana*. The bacteriophage YepMm could lyse three human pathogenic *Yersinia* species and can be used as a biocontrol agent.

MATERIALS AND METHODS

Bacteriophage Isolation

In the routine prevalence surveillance for *Y. pestis* in China, a *Marmota himalayana* that had died of natural causes (**Figure 1C**) was collected from a plague-focus area in the Qinghai-Tibet plateau in China at an altitude of 3076.85 m (39°52′ N, 95°03′ E). *Yersinia* species-selective Cefsulodin–Irgasan–Novobiocin (CIN) agar (Oxoid, Basingstoke, UK) was used to detect the host strain

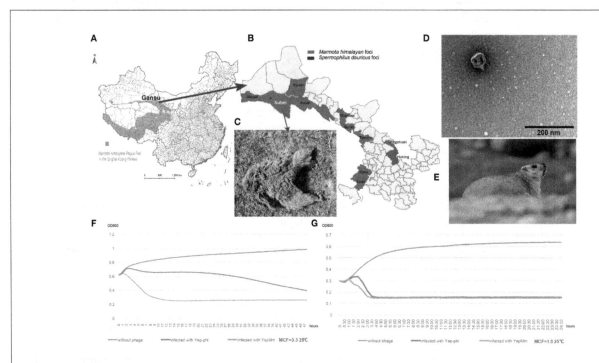

FIGURE 1 | Characteristics of the *Y. pestis* bacteriophage YepMm. **(A)** *Marmota himalayana* in a plague-area focus in Qinghai-Tibet plateau in China. **(B)** *Marmota himalayana* in a plague-area focus in Gansu Province, China. **(C)** The *Marmota himalayana* (who died of natural causes) from which we isolated a lytic *Y. pestis* bacteriophage: YepMm. **(D)** Electron microscopy of YepMm. **(E)** A healthy *Marmota himalayana* in a plague-focus area of the Qinghai-Tibet plateau. **(F)** Growth curves of *Y. pestis* EV76 at 25°C, with MCF = 3.3 in the initial culture. Approximately 3.0 ± 0.2 × 10⁷ PFU of the bacteriophages YepMm and Yep-phi in 30 μl were mixed with 300 μl of the bacterial culture (MCF = 3.3), respectively, and allowed to incubate for 24 h at 25°C. Each group had three duplicates. The OD₆₀₀ value of each group was measured every 30 min. The blue line shows the growth curve of strains without bacteriophage infection. The orange line shows the growth curve of strains infected with the bacteriophage Yep-phi. The gray line shows the growth curve of strains infected with the bacteriophage YepMm. **(G)** Growth curves of *Y. pestis* EV76 at 25°C, with MCF = 1.0 in the initial culture. Approximately 3.0 ± 0.2 × 10⁷ PFU of the bacteriophages YepMm and Yep-phi in 30 μl were mixed with 300 μl of the bacterial culture (MCF = 1.0), and incubated for 24 h at 25°C. Each group had three duplicates. The OD₆₀₀ of each group was measured every 30 min. The blue line shows the growth curve of strains without bacteriophage infection. The orange line shows the growth curve of strains infected with the bacteriophage Yep-phi. The gray line show the growths curve of strains infected with the bacteriophage YepMm.

Y. pestis. The *Y. pestis*–specific phage can lyse the host strains to form transparent plaques on it. The phage YepMm and its original host strain (*Y. pestis* dcw-bs-007) were isolated together from the same bone-marrow samples of *M. himalayana*. The lytic bacteriophage (vB_YpP-YepMm) was propagated and spotted on CIN agar plates after incubating for 24 h at 25°C. Subsequently, a single-lysis zone of bacteriophage was picked with a sterile truncated tip and amplified in the presence of *Y. pestis* EV76 in *Brucella* medium for 24 h at 37°C. The solution was filtered through a sterile 0.22-μm syringe filter. Afterward, the filtered fluid and EV76 were poured on top of the agar plate to obtain purified bacteriophage.

Electron Microscopy

Crude bacteriophage lysates (~5×10^{10} PFU/mL) were filter-sterilized using a 0.22-μm membrane (Millipore, Waltham, MA, USA) and then pelleted at 25,000g for 1 h at 4°C using a high-speed centrifuge (Beckman Coulter, Palo Alto, CA, USA). The bacteriophage pellet was resuspended in 150 μl of SM-buffer supplemented with CaCl$_2$ (5 mM) after washing twice in a neutral solution of ammonium acetate (0.1 M). Bacteriophage particles were deposited onto a carbon-coated Formvar film on copper grids and stained with 20 μl of 2% potassium phosphotungstate (pH 7.2). After dye removal with filter paper, bacteriophage particles were examined under a transmission electron microscope (TECNAI 12; FEI, Hillsboro, OR, USA) at 120 kEv. Images were collected and analyzed using Digital Micrograph™ (Gatan, Pleasanton, CA, USA). Taxonomic assignments were made according to the classification scheme for bacteriophages developed by Ackermann and Berthiaume (Berthiaume and Ackermann, 1977) and the International Committee on the Taxonomy of Viruses.

Genome Sequencing of Bacteriophage DNA, Assembly, and Bioinformatics Analysis

Bacteriophage DNA was obtained from purified 2.4 × 10^9 PFU/ml bacteriophage particles as described previously (Shubeita et al., 1987). We tested the quality of the whole genome of bacteriophages with Qubit3.0 (Life Technologies, Carlsbad, CA, USA). A random "shotgun" library was constructed using the NEBNext DNA ultra II protocol. Whole-genome sequencing was carried out using the HiSeq2500 Genome Analyzer (Illumina, San Diego, CA, USA). Generated reads were assembled using the SPAdes algorithm. The average nucleotide identity (ANI) was determined among all pairwise combinations of phage genomes. The assembly sequence was evaluated and corrected with PhageTerm (Hu et al., 2020), putative open reading frame (ORF) was predicted by Prokka 1.1.3. The annotated genome sequence of the bacteriophage YepMm has been deposited into the National Center for Biotechnology Information GenBank database under the accession numbers MW767996 and BankIt 2439990.

Determination of Host Ranges

The host range of the bacteriophage YepMm was estimated using the classical plaque assay. The infectivity of the membrane-filtered phage lysate (2.4×10^9 PFU/ml) was tested on the bacterial strains listed in **Table 1**. All experiments with viable *Y. pestis* except EV76 were undertaken in a Biosafety Level-3

laboratory. The formation of lysis zone was determined using a double-layer plaque at 25°C or 37°C after 24 h of incubation.

Optimal Multiplicity of Infection Determination and One-Step Growth Assays

To estimate MOI, different amounts of phages were serially diluted and incubated with host bacteria EV76 (2 × 10^8 CFU/ml) (at different MOI of 100, 10, 1, 0.1, 0.01, 0.001) at 37°C for 3 h. After incubation, the phage titer of each MOI phage-host assay group was examined. The highest phage titer group was the optimal MOI. Three parallel experiments were performed for this MOI assay.

The one-step growth assay was carried out as follows: equivalent ratios of overnight cultures of EV76 were mixed with YepMm suspension at an MOI=10. After incubation at 37°C for 15 min, the mixture was centrifuged at 11,000g for 30 s. The pellet was then resuspended in 10-ml fresh media. The phage titer was tested with 5-min intervals at the first 30 min and 10-min intervals at the last 90 min by a double-layer agar method.

Comparison of the Lytic Ability of the Bacteriophages YepMm and Yep-phi

The growth conditions and lytic ability of the bacteriophages YepMm and Yep-phi were tested on host strain *Y. pestis* EV76. EV76 was grown in *Brucella* medium at 27°C to reach McFarland turbidity (MCF) of 3.3 and 1.0, respectively. Each MCF culture solution was divided into three groups (with 300 μl of bacterial culture in each group). Group A was mixed with 30 μl of the bacteriophage YepMm (~3.0 × 10^7 PFU), group B was mixed with 30 μl of the bacteriophage Yep-phi (~3.2×10^7 PFU), group C was mixed with 30 μl of phosphate-buffered saline in EV76 culture solution. Each group with three duplicates was allowed to incubate for 48 h, and OD$_{600}$ for each group was measured every 30 min. Experiments were carried out at 25°C and 37°C, respectively. Data are the mean ± SD of three independent experiments.

RESULTS

Electron Microscopy and Biological Characteristic

Purified phages YepMm was examined using transmission electron microscopy after negative staining (**Figure 1D**). The virions showed hexagonal outlines with isometric, hexagonal heads and short, noncontractile, conical tails and were classified as members of the *Podoviridae* family.

The optimal multiplicity of infection for phage vB_YpP-YepMm was 10 (**Table S1**), and the one-step growth curve showed that the incubation period of the phage was about 10 min, the rise phase was about 80 min, and the lysis amount of the phage during the lysis period of 80 min was about 187 PFU/Cell (**Figure S1**).

Sensitivity Test

Three *Y. pseudotuberculosis* strains were sensitive to the bacteriophage YepMm: O:1b and O:14 were sensitive at 25°C and 37°C; O:1a was sensitive at 37°C but not at 25°C. The bacteriophage YepMm could lyse *Y. pestis* and strains of the

TABLE 1 | Lytic activity of the bacteriophages Yep-phi and YepMm at 37°C and 25°C.

Species	Serotype (Bioserotype for *Y.e*)	Strain	YepMm		Yep-phi	
			37°C	25°C	37°C	25°C
Y. pestis	/	Azi30	+	+	+	+
	/	Azi32	+	+	+	+
	/	Azi34	+	+	+	+
	/	Azi36	+	+	+	+
	/	Azi39	+	+	+	+
	/	Azi42	+	+	+	+
	/	EV76	+	+	+	+
Y. enterocolitica	1B/O:8	YE92010	+	−	−	−
	1B/O:8	Pa12986	+	+	−	−
	1B/O:8	WA	+	+	−	−
	1B/O:8	52211	+	+	−	−
	1A/O:8	JS2012-xz034	−	−	−	−
	1A/O:8	JS1986-Y40	−	−	−	−
	2/O:9	2 strains	−	−	−	−
	3/O:3	3 strains	−	−	−	−
	1A/O:5,27	3 strains	−	−	−	−
Y. pseudotuberculosis	O:14	YP014	+	+	+	+
	O:1a	53512	+	−	−	−
	O:1b	PTB3	+	+	−	−
	O:2a	53517	−	−	−	−
	O:3	YP3	−	−	−	−
	O:3b	YP2B	−	−	−	−
	O:4b	YP4B	−	−	−	−
	O:6	YP6	−	−	−	−
	O:8	YP09	−	−	−	−
	O:10	YO010	−	−	−	−
	O:15	YP15	−	−	−	−
Escherichia coli	EPEC	2 strains	−	−	−	−
	EIEC	2 strains	−	−	−	−
	ETEC	2 strains	−	−	−	−
	EAEC	2 strains	−	−	−	−
	EHEC	2 strains	−	−	−	−
Shigella species	*Shigella flexneria*	5 strains	−	−	−	−
	Shigella sonnei	5 strain	−	−	−	−
Salmonella species		10 strains	−	−	−	−

no serotype for Y. pestis.

highly pathogenic *Y. enterocolitica* bioserotype 1B/O:8 at both temperatures (**Table 1**). However, the bacteriophage Yep-phi can only lyse *Y. pestis* and O:14 *Y. pseudotuberculosis*. YepMm can form larger plaques at 25°C than at 37°C (data not shown), indicating (as expected) a temperature-dependent response.

Genome Sequencing and Bioinformatics Analyses

The complete nucleotide sequence of YepMm is 38,512 bp, with G+C content of 47.1 mol%. It was assembled as a circular molecule and contains no RNA genes. The lysis genes encoding the holin (33,704 to 33,910 bp), endolysin (9,108 to 9,563 bp), and so on existed; no genes associated with lysogenic cycle were founded, such as integrase, lysis repressor. In total, 43 gene products were predicted in the YepMm genome; functions were assigned to 42 of them based on the similarities of the predicted products to known proteins. Genomic comparisons indicated that the genome of some lytic *Y. pestis* phages was highly similar. Bacteriophage YepMm shares 99.99% nucleotide sequence identity with Yep-phi, 97.91% with Berlin, 96.46% with Yepe2, 96.35% with YpP-G, but only 67.48% nucleotide sequence identity with phiA1122 (**Figure 2**). The

genome sequences of YepMm and Yep-phi had exactly similar genetic organization, which all contain 222-bp direct repeats at the termini of the mature DNAs and both had head and tail genes in the same relative positions. There are 43 new open reading frame (ORFs) in genome sequence of YepMm and 41 ORFs are 100% identical to Yep-phi, except for the new ORF -29 (phage capsid and scaffold, 21,255 to 21,419 bp) and ORF-43 (**Figure 3A** and **Table S2**). All together, the mutations were primarily for 104 bp deletions in the intergenic and six short nucleotide polymorphisms (SNPs) in the coding regions. Among the six SNPs of YepMm, one at 21,330 bp located in the new ORF-29, which encoded phage capsid and scaffold; one at 37,921 bp of ORF-43 encoded hypothetical protein; and the rest four SNPs located at the direct repeats (DR) terminal regions (216, 217, 38,610, and 38,611 bp). The SNP at 21,330 bp located in the upstream activating sequence of tail tubular protein A (TTPA) in genome of phage Yep-phi; however, a new ORF-encoded phage capsid and scaffold generated by this SNP in the genome of YepMm (**Figure 3B**). The missense mutation of 21,330 bp caused the termination codon to change to Glu amino acid; 37,921 bp caused the Ile to change to Leu amino acid (**Figure 3C**).

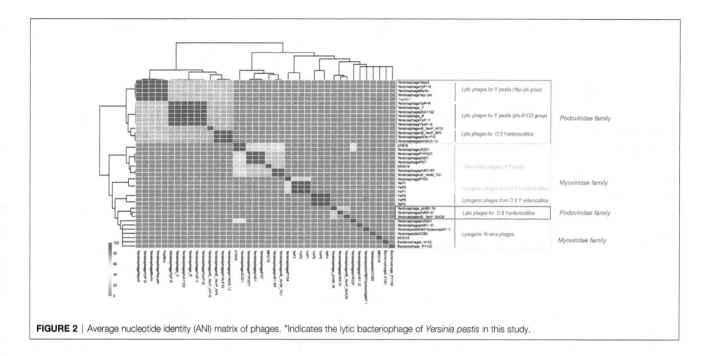

FIGURE 2 | Average nucleotide identity (ANI) matrix of phages. *Indicates the lytic bacteriophage of *Yersinia pestis* in this study.

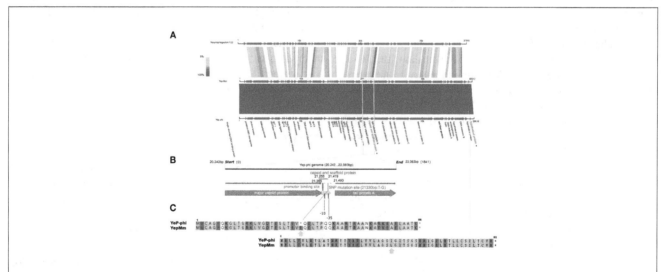

FIGURE 3 | The biological sequence analysis of the bacteriophages YepMm, Yep-phi, and phiA1122. **(A)** Pairwise comparison of the nucleotide sequences of bacteriophages YepMm, Yep-phi, and phiA1122 (the two different ORFs were indicated in asterisks). **(B)** The main difference between the two *Y. pestis* phages of YepMm, Yep-phi. The intergenic region and new ORFs with SNP mutation of YepMm was indicated in yellow rectangle. **(C)** The amino acid similarity alignment of the new ORF-29 of bacteriophages YepMm and Yep-phi.

Compared with the lytic phages for *Y. pestis* characterized previously, the nine available genome sequences could be divided into two subgroups (**Figure 2**). The genome of YepMm clustered with the bacteriophages Yep-phi, Berlin (GenBank accession number, AM183667.1), YpP-G (JQ965702.1), and Yepe2 (EU734170.1), and these bacteriophages comprised subgroup A. The other subgroup comprised *Yersinia* phage YpP-R (GenBank accession number, JQ965701.1), *Yersinia* phage_Y (JQ957925.1), *Yersinia* phage phiA1122 (AY247822.1), *Yersinia* phage_R (JX000007.1), *Yersinia* phage YpP-Y (Q965700.1), and *Yersinia* phage YpsP-G (JQ965703.1).

Lytic Abilities and Efficiency of the Bacteriophages YepMm and Yep-phi on the Host Strain EV76

Every half hour, the optical density at 600 nm (OD_{600}) value was plotted to generate a growth curve for each group. The OD_{600} of EV76 increased initially and then decreased rapidly upon bacteriophage addition. The growth curve decreased more rapidly after infection with the bacteriophage YepMm compared with that in infection with the bacteriophage Yep-phi. With the initial concentration of MCF = 3.3, the OD_{600} of culture solution infected with bacteriophage YepMm began to descend at 2 h later compared with 4.3 h after being infected with bacteriophage Yep-phi. When with the initial concentration of MCF=1.0, the OD_{600} of culture solution infected with bacteriophage YepMm began to descend at 1.3 h later compared with 2.3 h after being infected with bacteriophage Yep-phi. Hence, the lytic ability of the bacteriophage YepMm was more efficient than that of the bacteriophage Yep-phi. Statistical analysis showed the difference is significant at the 0.05 level (**Table S3** and **Figures 1F, G**). The culture solution infected with bacteriophage YepMm lyse absolutely within three and half hours with the initial concentration of MCF=1.0, shorter than initial concentration of MCF=3.3 (almost within 10 h) (**Figures 1F, G**).

DISCUSSION

Y. pestis is the causative agent of plague. It emerged from the enteropathogen O:1b *Y. pseudotuberculosis* 3,000 years ago by losing many genes and the horizontal acquisition of several genetic elements (Wren, 2003). Lytic bacteriophages have been used as therapeutic and prophylactic agents for controlling bacterial infections. Over the past 100 years, lytic bacteriophages have been used for the diagnosis of *Y. pestis* infections and to identify plagues caused by *Y. pestis* (D'Herelle and Malone, 1927; Duckworth, 1976).

We isolated, for the first time, the lytic bacteriophages of *Y. pestis* from an epidemic-focus area of *Y. pestis* in China. Our study on the bacteriophage YepMm showed a very broad range of hosts for bacteria of the genus *Yersinia*. This range included all of the three human pathogenic *Yersinia* species: *Y. pestis*, *Y. pseudotuberculosis* (O:1a, O:1b, and O:14), and the highly pathogenic *Y. enterocolitica* bioserotype 1B/O:8. Even though the genomes of YepMm and Yep-phi are almost identical, they varied in their ability to lyse bacteria of the genus *Yersinia*. Analyses of the host range showed that YepMm could infect not only *Y. pestis* strains but also the strains of the highly pathogenic *Y. enterocolitica* bioserotype 1B/O:8 and several strains of *Y. pseudotuberculosis*. However, Yep-phi is a *Y. pestis*-specific lytic bacteriophage (Zhao et al., 2011). The different phage receptors for adsorption are one of the important reasons to different bacteriolytic efficacy (Liang et al., 2016; Zhao and Skurnik, 2016). Our findings suggest that a sense mutation of an upstream activating sequence of TTPA generate a new ORF, which may modify phage tail protein and cause differences in host sensitivity. TTPA has been described as a structural protein of a bacteriophage tail. It forms an attachment for tail spikes to mediate infection through sensing the deflection of side fibers upon cell-wall binding. During infection by bacteria, TPPA can bind with bacterial receptors to mediate bacteriophage adsorption and subsequent bacterial lysis (Hu et al., 2020; Pyra et al., 2020a; Pyra et al., 2020b). If differences occur specifically in

the genes encoding the tail fibers, then recognition of the cell target will change (Vacheron et al., 2021). How a mutation in the upstream activating sequence of TTPA modifies its expression merits investigation.

We discovered that YepMm could form plaques on two more strains (*Y. enterocolitica* YE92010 and *Y. pseudotuberculosis* 53512) at 37°C than at 25°C (**Table 1**). This finding was likely because of the receptors being recognized specifically at a higher temperature, with a reduced ability of the bacteriophage (and parental bacteriophage) to infect and grow on host strains at a lower temperature. Despite the almost identical genome sequences of the bacteriophages YepMm and Yep-phi, they varied in their ability to lyse host bacteria among *Yersinia* species, which suggests that they might use different receptors for adsorption. The bacteriophages Yep-phi and φA1122 have been used as a diagnostic agent *Y. pestis* infection (Hu et al., 2020). Unlike the bacteriophage YepMm, the bacteriophage Yep-phi infects *Y. pestis* exclusively and is inactive toward other *Yersinia* species, irrespective of the growth temperature (Zhao et al., 2011; Zhao and Skurnik, 2016); the phage A1122 only grows on *Y. pseudotuberculosis* at 37°C and not at 25°C. Obviously, the phage YepMm has the broadest host range. Interestingly, strains of the highly pathogenic *Y. enterocolitica* bioserotype 1B/O:8 differed markedly in their susceptibility to the bacteriophage YepMm and had a temperature-dependent response.

Bacteriophage control is the most environmentally friendly method used to eradicate pathogens from food products. The lytic properties and activity of the bacteriophage YepMm in controlling infection from *Yersinia* species will be studied in the future.

ETHICS STATEMENT

The animal study was reviewed and approved by Ethics Committee of National Institute for Communicable Disease Control and Prevention, Chinese Center for Disease Control and Prevention.

AUTHOR CONTRIBUTIONS

JL, XW, SQ, RD preparing manuscript, writing, and correction this manuscript, JL, ZH, and XuL did designed figures. HJ, HZ, WW, DT, GF, XML, DL generated experimental data and wrote the manuscript. HM, MX, JY, JL, SQ, RD, HJ, XW conceived the work and critically review the manuscript. All authors contributed to the article and approved the submitted version.

ACKNOWLEDGMENTS

We thank Charlesworth author services (Paper#:79684) for their critical editing and helpful comments regarding our manuscript.

REFERENCES

Bergh, O., Borsheim, K. Y., Bratbak, G., and Heldal, M. (1989). High Abundance of Viruses Found in Aquatic Environments. *Nature* 340, 467–468. doi: 10.1038/340467a0

Berthiaume, L., and Ackermann, H. W. (1977). Classification of Actinophages. *Pathol. Biol. (Paris)* 25, 195–201.

Chhibber, S., Kaur, T., and Sandeep, K. (2013). Co-Therapy Using Lytic Bacteriophage and Linezolid: Effective Treatment in Eliminating Methicillin

Resistant Staphylococcus Aureus (MRSA) From Diabetic Foot Infections. *PloS One* 8, e56022. doi: 10.1371/journal.pone.0056022

D'Herelle, F., and Malone, R. H. (1927). A Preliminary Report of Work Carried Out by the Cholera Bacteriophage Enquiry. *Ind. Med. Gaz* 62, 614–616.

Doub, J. B. (2020). Bacteriophage Therapy for Clinical Biofilm Infections: Parameters That Influence Treatment Protocols and Current Treatment Approaches. *Antibiotics (Basel)* 9, 799. doi: 10.3390/antibiotics9110799

Duckworth, D. H. (1976). "Who Discovered Bacteriophage?". *Bacteriol Rev.* 40, 793–802. doi: 10.1128/br.40.4.793-802.1976

Flayhan, A., Vellieux, F. M., Lurz, R., Maury, O., Contreras-Martel, C., Girard, E., et al. (2014). Crystal Structure of Pb9, the Distal Tail Protein of Bacteriophage T5: A Conserved Structural Motif Among All Siphophages. *J. Virol.* 88, 820–828. doi: 10.1128/JVI.02135-13

Garcia, E., Elliott, J. M., Ramanculov, E., Chain, P. S., Chu, M. C., and Molineux, I. J. (2003). The Genome Sequence of Yersinia Pestis Bacteriophage Phia1122 Reveals an Intimate History With the Coliphage T3 and T7 Genomes. *J. Bacteriol* 185, 5248–5262. doi: 10.1128/JB.185.17.5248-5262.2003

Ge, P., Xi, J., Ding, J., Jin, F., Zhang, H., Guo, L., et al. (2015). Primary Case of Human Pneumonic Plague Occurring in a Himalayan Marmot Natural Focus Area Gansu Province, China. *Int. J. Infect. Dis.* 33, 67–70. doi: 10.1016/j.ijid.2014.12.044

Gorski, A., Miedzybrodzki, R., Borysowski, J., Weber-Dabrowska, B., Lobocka, M., Fortuna, W., et al. (2009). Bacteriophage Therapy for the Treatment of Infections. *Curr. Opin. Investig. Drugs* 10, 766–774. doi: 10.1117/12.895292

Hardy, J. M., Dunstan, R. A., Grinter, R., Belousoff, M. J., Wang, J., Pickard, D., et al. (2020). The Architecture and Stabilisation of Flagellotropic Tailed Bacteriophages. *Nat. Commun.* 11, 3748. doi: 10.1038/s41467-020-17505-w

Hu, M., Zhang, H., Gu, D., Ma, Y., and Zhou, X. (2020). Identification of a Novel Bacterial Receptor That Binds Tail Tubular Proteins and Mediates Phage Infection of Vibrio Parahaemolyticus. *Emerg. Microbes Infect.* 9, 855–867. doi: 10.1080/22221751.2020.1754134

Kiljunen, S., Datta, N., Dentovskaya, S. V., Anisimov, A. P., Knirel, Y. A., Bengoechea, J. A., et al. (2011). Identification of the Lipopolysaccharide Core of Yersinia Pestis and Yersinia Pseudotuberculosis as the Receptor for Bacteriophage Phia1122. *J. Bacteriol* 193, 4963–4972. doi: 10.1128/JB.00339-11

Kiljunen, S., Vilen, H., Savilahti, H., and Skurnik, M. (2003). Transposon Mutagenesis of the Phage Phi YeO3-12. *Adv. Exp. Med. Biol.* 529, 245–248. doi: 10.1007/0-306-48416-1_47

Liang, J., Li, X., Zha, T., Chen, Y., Hao, H., Liu, C., et al. (2016). DTDP-Rhamnosyl Transferase RfbF, Is a Newfound Receptor-Related Regulatory Protein for Phage phiYe-F10 Specific for Yersinia Enterocolitica Serotype O:3. *Sci. Rep.* 6, 22905. doi: 10.1038/srep22905

Moojen, D. J. F. (2013). Exploring New Strategies for Infection Treatment. *J. Bone Joint Surg. Am.* 95 (2), e11. doi: 10.2106/JBJS.L.01419

Mukerjee, S., Roy, U. K., and Rudra, B. C. (1963). Studies on Typing of Cholera Vibrios by Bacteriophage. V. Geographical Distribution of Phage-Types of Vibrio Cholerae. *Ann. Biochem. Exp. Med.* 23, 523–530.

Muniesa, M., Lucena, F., Blanch, A. R., Payan, A., and Jofre, J. (2012). Use of Abundance Ratios of Somatic Coliphages and Bacteriophages of Bacteroides Thetaiotaomicron GA17 for Microbial Source Identification. *Water Res.* 46, 6410–6418. doi: 10.1016/j.watres.2012.09.015

Pyra, A., Filik, K., Szermer-Olearnik, B., Czarny, A., and Brzozowska, E. (2020a). New Insights on the Feature and Function of Tail Tubular Protein B and Tail Fiber Protein of the Lytic Bacteriophage Phiyeo3-12 Specific for Yersinia Enterocolitica Serotype O:3. *Molecules* 25, 4392. doi: 10.3390/molecules 25194392

Pyra, A., Urbanska, N., Filik, K., Tyrlik, K., and Brzozowska, E. (2020b). Biochemical Features of the Novel Tail Tubular Protein A of Yersinia Phage Phiyeo3-12. *Sci. Rep.* 10, 4196. doi: 10.1038/s41598-020-61145-5

Rashid, M. H., Revazishvili, T., Dean, T., Butani, A., Verratti, K., Bishop-Lilly, K. A., et al. (2012). A Yersinia pestis-specific, Lytic Phage Preparation Significantly Reduces Viable Y. pestis on various hard surfaces experimentally contaminated with the bacterium. *Bacteriophage* 2, 168–177. doi: 10.4161/bact.22240

Shubeita, H. E., Sambrook, J. F., and McCormick, A. M. (1987). Molecular Cloning and Analysis of Functional cDNA and Genomic Clones Encoding Bovine Cellular Retinoic Acid-Binding Protein. *Proc. Natl. Acad. Sci. U.S.A.* 84, 5645–5649. doi: 10.1073/pnas.84.16.5645

Vacheron, J., Heiman, C. M., and Keel, C. (2021). Live Cell Dynamics of Production, Explosive Release and Killing Activity of Phage Tail-Like Weapons for Pseudomonas Kin Exclusion. *Commun. Biol.* 4, 87. doi: 10.1038/s42003-020-01581-1

Wang, H., Cui, Y., Wang, Z., Wang, X., Guo, Z., Yan, Y., et al. (2011). A Dog-Associated Primary Pneumonic Plague in Qinghai Province, China. *Clin. Infect. Dis.* 52, 185–190. doi: 10.1093/cid/ciq107

Wang, X., Wei, X., Song, Z., Wang, M., Xi, J., Liang, J., et al. (2017). Mechanism Study on a Plague Outbreak Driven by the Construction of a Large Reservoir in Southwest China (Surveillance From 2000-2015). *PloS Negl. Trop. Dis.* 11, e0005425. doi: 10.1371/journal.pntd.0005425

Wren, B. W. (2003). The Yersiniae–a Model Genus to Study the Rapid Evolution of Bacterial Pathogens. *Nat. Rev. Microbiol.* 1, 55–64. doi: 10.1038/nrmicro730

Zhang, Z., Tian, C., Zhao, J., Chen, X., Wei, X., Li, H., et al. (2018). Characterization of Tail Sheath Protein of N4-Like Phage Phiaxp-3. *Front. Microbiol.* 9, 450. doi: 10.3389/fmicb.2018.00450

Zhao, X., and Skurnik, M. (2016). Bacteriophages of Yersinia Pestis. *Adv. Exp. Med. Biol.* 918, 361–375. doi: 10.1007/978-94-024-0890-4_13

Zhao, X., Wu, W., Qi, Z., Cui, Y., Yan, Y., Guo, Z., et al. (2011). The Complete Genome Sequence and Proteomics of Yersinia Pestis Phage Yep-Phi. *J. Gen. Virol.* 92, 216–221. doi: 10.1099/vir.0.026328-0

14

A Novel *Acinetobacter baumannii* Bacteriophage Endolysin LysAB54 with High Antibacterial Activity Against Multiple Gram-Negative Microbes

Fazal Mehmood Khan [1,2], Vijay Singh Gondil [1], Changchang Li [1,2], Mengwei Jiang [1], Junhua Li [1], Junping Yu [1,2], Hongping Wei [1,2]* and Hang Yang [1,2]*

[1] CAS Key Laboratory of Special Pathogens and Biosafety, Center for Biosafety Mega-Science, Wuhan Institute of Virology, Chinese Academy of Sciences, Wuhan, China, [2] International College, University of Chinese Academy of Sciences, Beijing, China

*Correspondence:
Hongping Wei
hpwei@wh.iov.cn
Hang Yang
yangh@wh.iov.cn

The rapid spread and emergence of multidrug-resistant *Acinetobacter baumannii* and other pathogenic Gram-negative bacteria spurred scientists and clinicians to look for alternative therapeutic agents to conventional antibiotics. In the present study, an *A. baumannii* bacteriophage p54 was isolated and characterized. Morphological and genome analysis revealed that bacteriophage p54 belongs to Myoviridae family with a genome size of 165,813 bps. A novel endolysin, namely LysAB54, showing low similarity with other well-known related endolysins, was cloned, expressed, and characterized from the bacteriophage p54. LysAB54 showed significant bactericidal activity against multidrug-resistant *A. baumannii* and other Gram-negative bacteria, including *Pseudomonas aeruginosa*, *Klebsiella pneumoniae*, and *Escherichia coli*, in the absence of outer membrane permeabilizers. Based on all those observations, LysAB54 could represent a potential agent for the treatment of multidrug-resistant Gram-negative superbugs.

Keywords: bacteriophage, endolysin, *Acinetobacter baumannii*, Gram-negative "superbugs", antimicrobial resistance

INTRODUCTION

Bacterial infections deleteriously impact human health and are a leading cause of mortality worldwide. The emergence of antibiotic-resistant bacterial strains further exaggerates the present situation and alarming for humankind in various aspects of daily life. The occurrence of multi-drug resistant (MDR) Gram-negative bacterial pathogens, which mainly includes antibiotic-resistant strains of *Acinetobacter baumannii*, *Pseudomonas aeruginosa*, *Klebsiella pneumoniae*, and *Escherichia coli*, may lead to serious complications and nosocomial infections (Bonomo and Szabo, 2006; Spellberg et al., 2013; Heron, 2017; Collaborators, 2018). *A. baumannii* is an opportunistic Gram-negative pathogen that can initiate several serious nosocomial infections, which majorly includes wound infections, urinary tract infections, ventilator related pneumonia, and secondary meningitis. The high resistance of *A. baumannii* toward conventional antibiotics makes their management very cumbersome (Valencia et al., 2009; Pendleton et al., 2013; Potron et al., 2015). The high degree of antibiotic resistance conferred by *A. baumannii* and other pathogenic bacteria spurred scientists and clinicians to look for alternative therapeutic agents to antibiotics (Magiorakos et al., 2012).

Among various available alternative agents, bacteriophage encoded peptidoglycan hydrolases, popularly known as endolysins or lysins, represent a promising alternative for the treatment of drug-resistant bacteria. Endolysins are enzymatic proteins that are produced inside the bacterial host at the later stage of bacteriophage replication and can lyse bacterial hosts when applied externally (Fischetti, 2008; Nelson et al., 2012; Schmelcher et al., 2012; Yang et al., 2014; Gondil et al., 2020). Endolysin renders numerous advantages over other alternative antibacterial agents, including high activity against drug-resistant pathogens, low chances of resistance, and high specificity towards target bacterium (Loessner et al., 2002; Schuch et al., 2002; Fischetti, 2008; Briers et al., 2009). Several endolysin have been reported to harbor broad-spectrum activity against Gram-positive bacteria *in vitro* and *in vivo*, such as PlyC (Nelson et al., 2006), ClyR (Yang et al., 2015a), Cpl-1 (Loeffler et al., 2003), ClyJ (Yang et al., 2020), and ClyV (Huang et al., 2020).

On the Contrary, due to the presence of protective bacterial outer membrane, most endolysins fail to exhibit prominent activity against Gram-negative bacteria (Fischetti, 2005; Rodríguez-Rubio et al., 2016). However, treatment bacteria with outer membrane permeabilizers (OMPs), such as citric acid, trichloroethane (CHCl₃), Triton X-100, and EDTA, can improve the antibacterial activity of endolysins and conquer the hindrance presented by the outer membrane of Gram-negative bacteria (Helander and Mattila-Sandholm, 2000; Briers et al., 2007; Briers et al., 2011; Briers et al., 2014; Yang et al., 2015b; Guo et al., 2017). In this context, several endolysins have showed improved or synergistic bactericidal activity against MDR *A. baumannii* and *P. aeruginosa* in the presence of OMPs, including LysSS (Kim et al., 2020b), Abtn-4 (Yuan et al., 2020), LysPA26 (Guo et al., 2017), PlyA (Yang et al., 2015b), ABgp46 (Oliveira et al., 2016), and OBPgp279 (Walmagh et al., 2012). However, lysins with OMP-independent antibacterial activity against Gram-negative microbes still un-adequately addressed since few of them are demonstrated effective in animal infection models.

In the present study, we report the comprehensive characterization of a novel *A. baumannii* bacteriophage p54 and its endolysin, namely, LysAB54. Our results demonstrated that LysAB54 has a high and rapid antibacterial activity against a range of antibiotic-resistant Gram-negative bacterial strains in the absence of OMPs.

MATERIALS AND METHODS

Collection of Water Sample for Bacteriophage Isolation
The water sample was collected in sterile 50 ml screw tubes from the Tongji Hospital, Wuhan, Hubei Province, China. The water samples were kept in an ice bucket box to preserve the specimen. After removing the impurities by sterile syringe filter, samples were kept in 4°C for further use.

Isolation of Bacteriophage p54
The stored water sample was mixed 1:1 with phage buffer (50 mM Tris-HCl, 150 mM NaCl, 10 mM MgCl₂, 2 mM CaCl₂, pH 7.5). The *A. baumannii* strain WHG3083 was cultured in lysogeny broth (LB) at 37°C to logarithmic phase and then transferred to the conical flask. Conical flask solution containing water sample, phage buffer, and bacteria were incubated aerobically in shaking incubator on 160 rpm at 37°C for 2–3 days. After incubation, solution was centrifuged (1,000 rpm for 10 min, 4°C) and filtered through a sterile 0.22 μm syringe filter (Guangzhou Jet bio-filtration Co., Ltd). Then, 500 μl of the filtrate was mixed with 500 μl of *A. baumannii* in a sterile 1.5 ml microcentrifuge tube and incubated aerobically in a shaking incubator on 160 rpm at 37°C for 15–20 min. The mixture was mixed with 4 ml of 0.7% soft agar (approximately 50°C) in a sterile 15 ml tube (Guangzhou Jet bio-filtration Co., Ltd) and poured onto the LB agar plates and incubated overnight at 37°C.

Purification of the Bacteriophage p54
A single plaque was picked and resuspended in the phage buffer in a sterile 1.5 microcentrifuge tube. The microcentrifuge tube containing plaque was vortexed for approximately 2–3 min. The vortexed solution was further filtered through a sterile 0.22 μm syringe filter. 10 μl of the filtered solution (10-fold serially diluted) was mixed with the 1 ml of *A. baumannii* cell suspension and incubated on 160 rpm at 37°C for 15–30 min. Afterwards, bacterium-phage mixture was mixed with 4 ml of soft agar and poured onto LB agar plates and incubated overnight at 37°C. This cycle was repeated for five times to obtain purified bacteriophage p54.

Bacteriophage p54 Genome Extraction and Sequencing Analysis
The bacteriophage p54 genome was extracted and sequenced following the protocol and procedures as previously described (Kering et al., 2020). The sequenced genome was compared with the available whole genome sequences of *A. baumannii* bacteriophages by the Neighbor-Joining method (Saitou and Nei, 1987). The bootstrap consensus tree inferred from 1,000 replicates is taken to represent the evolutionary history of the taxa analyzed (Felsenstein, 1985). Branches corresponding to partitions reproduced in less than 50% bootstrap replicates are collapsed. The percentage of replicate trees in which the associated taxa clustered together in the bootstrap test (1,000

replicates) are shown next to the branches (Felsenstein, 1985). The evolutionary distances were computed using the p-distance method and are in the units of the number of base differences per site. This analysis involved 10 nucleotide sequences and the codon positions included were 1st+2nd+3rd+Noncoding. All ambiguous positions were removed for each sequence pair. There was a total of 16,5813 positions in the final dataset. Evolutionary analyses were conducted in MEGA X software (Kumar et al., 2018).

Transmission Electron Microscopy (TEM) of the Bacteriophage p54

The bacteriophage p54 was purified and concentrated using cesium chloride density gradient ultracentrifugation on 35,000 rpm for 2 h at 4°C. The concentrated bacteriophage was stained with freshly prepared phosphotungstic acid solution (2%) for 3 min and spot dried on the copper grid for 2 h. The samples were examined on H-7000FA transmission electron microscope (Hitachi, Japan).

Bacterial Culture Conditions

All bacterial strains were cultured in LB broth aerobically at 37°C. The stocks of bacterial strains containing 20% glycerol was store in -80°C refrigerator for long time storage. E. coli BL21(DE3) (Takara) cells were used for cloning and protein expression.

Cloning of LysAB54 in the Expression Vector

The open-reading frame (ORF) encoding the putative endolysin LysAB54 was amplified by Polymerase Chain Reaction (PCR) with the primers (5′ to 3′): 54-Forward: TATACCATG GACGTTAAACCATTTTTTG (NcoI) and 54-Reverse: TATACTCGAGTTGTTCAAAATACGCTTTCTC (XhoI). The purified (Omega Bio-tek®) PCR product was digested with restriction endonuclease enzymes NcoI and XhoI (Thermo Scientific). Purified PCR product was ligated into pET28a (+) and transformed to the competent E. coli BL21(DE3) cells. The inserted gene was further confirmed by Sanger sequencing (Sangon Biotech, Shanghai).

Protein Expression and Purification

E. coli BL21 (DE3) containing the pET28a-LysAB54 was grown in 500 ml LB with 100 mg/ml of kanamycin for approximately 2–3 h until the OD_{600} reached to 0.5–0.6. Protein expression was induced with 1 mM Isopropyl-beta-D-thiogalactopyranoside (IPTG; Thermo Scientific) at 16°C for 16 h. The bacterial culture was harvested by centrifugation at 10,000 rpm at 4°C for 10 min. Bacterial cells were washed once by PBS (pH7.4) and centrifuged at 10,000 rpm at 4°C for 10 min. Cells were disrupted through sonication in ice cold environment. The insoluble cell fragments were removed through centrifugation at 10,000 rpm at 4°C for 10 min and the supernatant was collected by filter through 0.22 μm syringe filter. His-tagged LysAB54 was purified using nickel nitrilotriacic acid affinity column

chromatography (GE Healthcare, US) with gradient of imidazole solutions. After purification, proteins were dialyzed overnight at 4°C against Tris buffer (pH 7.4). The purity of protein was assessed using SDS-PAGE.

Antibacterial Activity Assay of Endolysin LysAB54

Antibacterial activity of endolysin LysAB54 was determined as defined previously (Yang et al., 2015b) with minor modifications. To determine the antibacterial activity of LysAB54, the bacteria were cultured in LB broth at 37°C for both the logarithmic phase (OD_{600} = 0.6–0.8) and stationary phase (OD_{600} = 1.4–1.6). Bacterial culture was centrifuged at 8,000 rpm at 4°C for 5 min and bacterial cells were washed and re-suspended in Tris buffer (pH 7.4). LysAB54 was added into bacterial suspension and incubated aerobically at 37°C for 60 min. Groups treated with the same amount of Tris buffer instead of LysAB54 were used as negative controls. The mixture was then serially diluted than plated on the LB agar petri dishes, incubated overnight aerobically at 37°C.

Killing Range of LysAB54

To evaluate the bactericidal activity of endolysin LysAB54 against clinical Gram-negative isolates, logarithmic phase bacteria were treated with 100 μg/ml of LysAB54 at 37°C for 1 h. The reduction in bacterial count in term of LogCFU/mL was defined as the antibacterial activity of LysAB54 against tested isolate.

The Activity of LysAB54 in Complex Medium

To test the antibacterial activity of endolysin LysAB54 against A. baumannii in complex medium, logarithmic phase bacteria were re-suspended in LB broth and human-serum (Sigma Aldrich, Shanghai, China), and treated with 100 μg/ml of LysAB54 at 37° C for 1 h. The mixture was serially diluted and plated on LB agar Petri dishes for viable cell count.

Statistical Analysis

The data were analyzed using GraphPad prism Version 5 software on Microsoft Windows 2019 operating system. All the experiments were performed in triplicates on different time points. The data was expressed in term of Mean ± Standard Deviation (SD) for statistical considerations.

RESULTS

Characterization of Bacteriophage p54

Bacteriophage p54 was isolated and purified from the hospital water sample. Double-layer agar assay showed clear plaques on A. baumannii lawn postulating the lytic potential of isolated

A

B

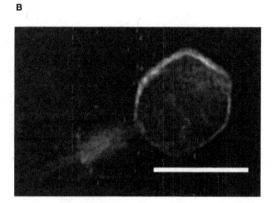

FIGURE 1 | Characteristics of bacteriophage p54. **(A)** Double layer agar assay of the isolated bacteriophage p54 with host bacterium. **(B)** Morphological analysis of the bacteriophage p54 by transmission electron microscopy (TEM). Scale bar: 25 µm.

bacteriophage p54 (**Figure 1A**). Morphological analysis showed that the bacteriophage p54 contains an icosahedral head and a short tail, with a particle size of 24.4×55.8 nm (**Figure 1B**). Based on these observations, bacteriophage p54 can be classified to the family of Myoviridae according to the latest classification by the International Committee on the Taxonomy of Viruses (ICTV).

Genome Sequencing and ORF Annotation of Bacteriophage p54

Full genome sequencing analysis showed that bacteriophage p54 consists 165,813 bps with a GC content of 36.3%. A Blast-P analysis further revealed that bacteriophage p54 contains 248 predicted ORFs, with putative functions categorized into multiple functional modules, including phage structure, host lysis, phage DNA metabolism and modifications (**Figure 2**). Whole-genome based phylogenetic analysis showed that bacteriophage p54 possesses maximum similarity with *A. baumannii* phage AP22 (NCBI No: HE806280) among various phages analyzed (**Figure S1**), indicating the novelty of bacteriophage p54.

Bioinformatics Analysis of the Endolysin LysAB54

The putative endolysin LysAB54 of bacteriophage p54, i.e., ORF159 (120,967–121,530 bp), comprised 187 amino acids with a putative lysozyme activity. As shown in **Figure 3A**, a phylogenetic analysis of LysAB54 and other Gram-negative endolysins showed that LysAB54 has similarity with the other reported endolysin containing lysozyme domain, such as LysPA26 of *A. baumannii* phage (Guo et al., 2017). The similarity of LysAB54 with other closely related endolysins was further performed by the MultAlign server and revealed a lower level of similarity with known related endolysins, postulating the novelty of LysAB54 (**Figure 3B**). Phyre2 server-based structural prediction showed that LysAB54 contains multiple alpha-helix domains with the absence of predictable beta plated sheets (**Figure 3C**).

LysAB54 Shows High Bactericidal Activity Against *A. baumannii*

SDS-PAGE analysis showed a single band of LysAB54 after purification (**Figure 4A**), which was consistent with its predicted molecular mass of 24 kDa. The time-killing assay showed that the LysAB54 (100 µg/ml) could kill logarithmic *A. baumannii* with 0.6 logs of reduction in the first 1 min of incubation, while up to 4 logs of decrement in bacterial count was achieved after incubation for 10 min. These results showed that the LysAB54 exhibits robust as well as rapid bactericidal activity (**Figure 4B**).

Antibacterial Activity of LysAB54 Against Logarithmic Phase Gram-Negative Bacteria

The antibacterial activity of LysAB54 in Tris buffer against each ten different clinical isolates of *A. baumannii*, *P. aeruginosa*, *E. coli*, and *K. pneumoniae* was investigated. As shown in **Figure 5**, LysAB54 showed high bactericidal activity against all isolates of *A. baumannii*, *E. coli*, and *K. pneumoniae* tested. Moreover, 8 out of 10 *P. aeruginosa* strains were found to be highly susceptible to LysAB54 (**Figure 5B**). The difference in antibacterial activity of log reduction against these clinical strains may be due to the difference in the molecular architecture of the bacterial outer membrane. Notably, reduction of 4 logs (from 4.2 to 0), 2.17 logs (from 5.77 to 3.60), 2 logs (from 4.22 to 2.16), and 2.33 log (from 3.86 to 1.53) were observed in *A. baumannii* WHG 40090, *P. aeruginosa* WHG50023, *E. coli* WHG11023, and *K. pneumoniae* WHG11004, respectively. These results suggested that LysAB54 has a wide range of antibacterial activity against multi-drug resistant Gram-negative microbes.

Antibacterial Activity of LysAB54 Under Various Conditions

Previous reports showed that multiple Gram-negative endolysins have good activity against the logarithmic phase bacteria but less

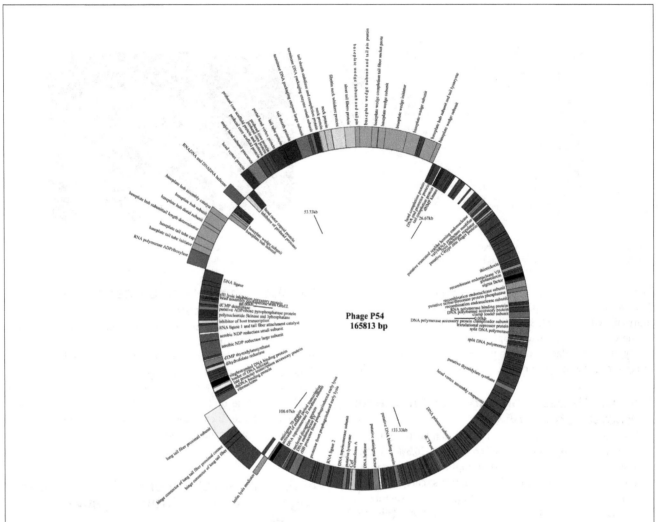

FIGURE 2 | Genome map of the bacteriophage p54. Genes on the positive chain of the genome (Outer ring); Gene on the negative chain of the genome (Inner ring). The genome direction from 5' to 3' in the figure is drawn counterclockwise. Functions of putative open-reading frames (ORFs) are marked.

or rare active against the stationary bacteria (Yang et al., 2015b; Guo et al., 2017). Therefore, we first evaluated the bactericidal activity of LysAB54 with bacteria under different growth phases. Results showed that LysAB54 showed similar antibacterial activity against both logarithmic as well as stationary phase of *A. baumannii* (**Figure 6**). These results indicates that the bacterial phase have minor effect on the antibacterial activity of LysAB54.

Another challenge for application of Gram-negative endolysin is the reduced or abolished killing activity in a complex medium like serum. Most of the reported endolysins lose their activity in serum. In this context, we checked out the antibacterial activity of LysAB54 against the logarithmic phase of *A. baumannii* in complex medium, including LB broth and human serum. As reported previously, insignificant bactericidal activity of LysAB54 was observed in the complex mediums (**Figure S2**). The possible reason for loss of bactericidal activity is the ion exchange in these complex media which can potentially

neutralize the interaction between endolysin and the negatively charged outer membrane.

DISCUSSION

The increasing infections caused by drug-resistant Gram-negative bacteria is a public health concern worldwide (Chopra et al., 2008; Scallan et al., 2011; Gondil et al., 2019). The Gram-negative bacterium *A. baumannii* which is responsible for multiple infections is an alarming threat to human health. Due to its intrinsic resistance and the overuse of antibiotics, some isolates of *A. baumannii* are now resistant to almost all known antibiotics (Manchanda et al., 2010). The increasing trend of antibiotic resistance in pathogenic bacteria necessitate the search for alternative antimicrobial agents to treat and cure such resistant pathogens mediated infections (Magiorakos et al., 2012). Currently, a very limited solutions are available in the

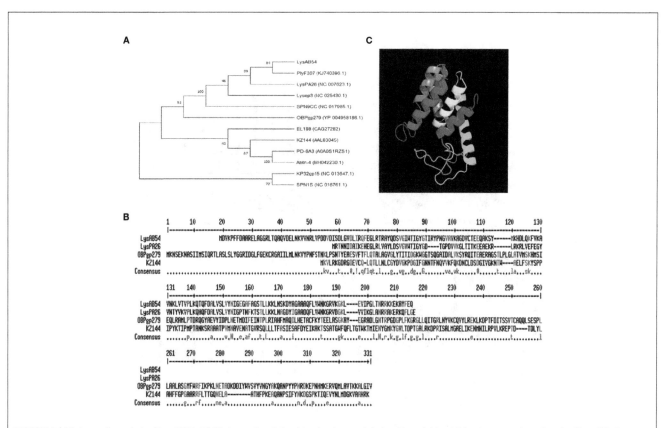

FIGURE 3 | Phylogenetic analysis of LysAB54. **(A)** Phylogenetic relationship of various endolysins. The neighbor-joining trees were based on the ClustalW alignment of DNA sequences by MEGAX software. **(B)** Multi-alignment analysis of LysAB54 with other closely related Gram-negative endolysins. **(C)** Predicted three-dimensional structure of LysAB54. Three-dimensional structure model by Phyre2 web server. NORMAL mode. Confidence in the model: 100.0%. 148 residues (79% of sequence) have been modeled with 100.0% confidence by the single highest scoring template. Model dimensions (Å): X: 35.277, Y: 41.465, Z: 46.142.

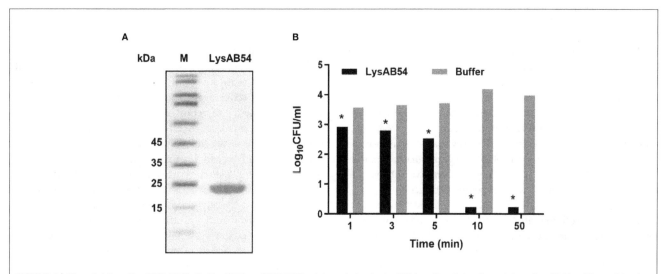

FIGURE 4 | Characteristics of LysAB54. **(A)** Purified LysAB54 on SDS-PAGE gel. Lane 1 showing LysAB54 and lane 2 showing protein marker. **(B)** Time-killing activity of LysAB54 against logarithmic phase of A. baumannii WHG 40090 in Tris buffer. Data are shown as means ± standard deviations. *p < 0.05.

treatment of MDR *A. baumannii* in clinical settings (Fischetti, 2010). Endolysin is a class of novel antimicrobial agents to treat and cure antibiotic-resistant bacteria due to its rapid bactericidal activity and low chances of antibiotic resistance (Nelson et al.,

2012). Currently, several endolysins are being evaluated in clinical trials to explore their potential in treating Gram-positive bacterial infections (Kim et al., 2018). On the contrary, endolysins for Gram-negative bacterial infections are still under

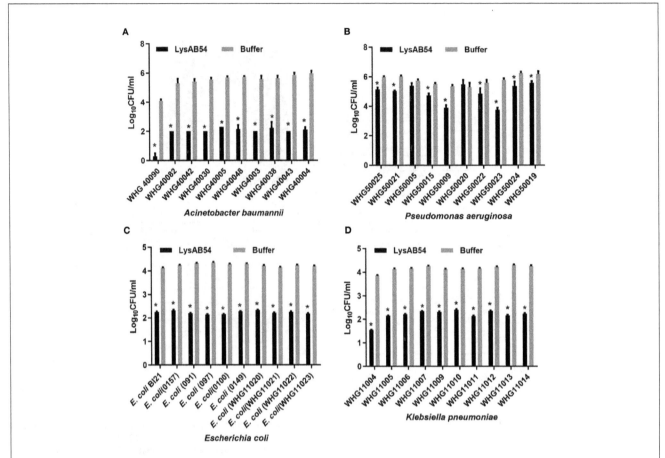

FIGURE 5 | Antibacterial activities of LysAB54 against logarithmic phase of Gram-negative microbes in Tris buffer. Logarithmic phase strains of *A baumannii* **(A)**, *P. aeruginosa* **(B)**, *E. coli* **(C)**, and *K pneumoniae* **(D)** were treated with 100 µg/ml of LysAB54 for 1 h at 37°C. The viable cell number was calculated on the LB agar plates. Data are shown as means ± standard deviations. *$p < 0.05$.

development. Although few studies have reported positive results in treating infections caused by Gram-negative bacteria *in vitro* and *in vivo*, including *A. baumannii* and *P. aeruginosa* (Ghose and Euler, 2020).

In this study, we characterized a novel bacteriophage endolysin LysAB54 encoded by a novel *A. baumannii* bacteriophage p54, which showed a broad range of antibacterial activity against Gram-negative bacteria irrespective of their growth phases, suggesting that the naturally occurring endolysin could be a promising alternative antimicrobial agent against number of MDR Gram-positive pathogens.

One excellent merit of the LysAB54 is its robust bactericidal activity against both logarithmic and stationary phase of Gram-negative bacteria in the absence of OMPs. Encouragingly, a reduction of over 4 logs in viable bacterial number was observed after treatment of *A. baumannii* cells with 100 µg/ml LysAB54 for 10 min.

To our knowledge, it is unconventional for an endolysin to render such rapid antibacterial activity against various antibiotic-resistant Gram-negative bacteria. Several natural known endolysins also exhibited antibacterial activity against Gram-negative bacteria in the absence of OMPs, such as

OBPgp279 against *P. aeruginosa*, PlyF307 and LysAB21 against *A. baumannii* (Lai et al., 2011; Walmagh et al., 2012; Lood et al., 2015). It is demonstrated with increasing evidence that several endolysins are active against multiple Gram-negative bacteria, and few of them are reported active against Gram-positive pathogens *in vitro*, such as Abtn-4 (Yuan et al., 2020), LysSAP26 (Kim et al., 2020a), and LysSS (Kim et al., 2020b). Such lysins with broad host-range are commonly contain a lysozyme or glycoside hydrolase catalytic activity, which cleaves the β-1,4-glycosidic linkage between N-acetylmuramic acid (NAM) and N-acetylglucosamine (NAG) in peptidoglycans that is generally shared by various bacteria (Ghose and Euler, 2020). In this context, LysAB54 was predicted to contain a lysozyme activity, which is possibly the reason for its broad antibacterial activity against several other antibiotic-resistant Gram-negative bacteria, which includes *P. aeruginosa*, *K. pneumoniae*, and *E. coli*.

It is well known that environmental factors such as salts and proteins have a significant effect on the activity of Gram-negative endolysins. Our results showed that LysAB54 completely loses its antibacterial activity in the complex medium like LB broth and

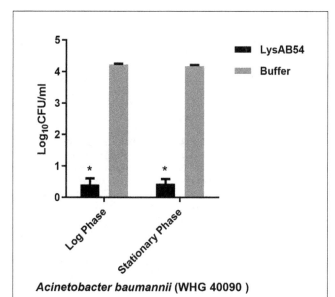

FIGURE 6 | Antibacterial activities of LysAB54 against the logarithmic and stationary phase of *A. baumannii*. *A. baumannii* WHG 40090 cells under different growth phases were treated with 100 µg/ml of LysAB54 for 1 h at 37°C. The viable cell number was calculated on the LB agar plates. Data are shown as means ± standard deviations. *$p < 0.05$.

serum, which narrows down its application to topical infections, such as burn wound, or suture infections. One possible reason for the loss of LysAB54 activity in these media may be due to ions

exchanging of endolysin in these environments, which could possibly neutralize the antibacterial activity of endolysins (Yang et al., 2015b).

In conclusion, our study demonstrates the morphological and genomic characteristics of a newly isolated *A. baumannii* bacteriophage p54 and the bactericidal activity of its endolysin, LysAB54, against multiple drug-resistant Gram-negative bacteria under various growth phases and conditions. The OMP-independent activity of LysAB54 makes it a potential candidate for the treatment of infections caused by multiple drug resistant Gram-negative pathogens. However, molecular dissection and validation of LysAB54 in biofilms and animal models still need to be established to reveal the enigmatic aspects of the present endolysin.

AUTHOR CONTRIBUTIONS

HY and HW designed the study. FK, VG, CL, MJ, and JL performed the experiments. FK, VG, JY, and HY performed data analysis. HY and HW contributed with reagents and/or funds for research. FK and VG wrote the draft manuscript. HY revised the manuscript. All authors contributed to the article and approved the submitted version.

ACKNOWLEDGMENTS

We thank Mrs. Pei Zhang from the Core Facility and Technical Support, Wuhan Institute of Virology for her assistance in microscopy analysis.

REFERENCES

Bonomo, R. A., and Szabo, D. (2006). Mechanisms of multidrug resistance in Acinetobacter species and. *Pseudomonas Aeruginosa Clin. Infect. Dis.* 43 Suppl 2, S49–S56. doi: 10.1086/504477

Briers, Y., Volckaert, G., Cornelissen, A., Lagaert, S., Michiels, C. W., Hertveldt, K., et al. (2007). Muralytic activity and modular structure of the endolysins of *Pseudomonas aeruginosa* bacteriophages phiKZ and EL. *Mol. Microbiol.* 65, 1334–1344. doi: 10.1111/j.1365-2958.2007.05870.x

Briers, Y., Schmelcher, M., Loessner, M. J., Hendrix, J., Engelborghs, Y., Volckaert, G., et al. (2009). The high-affinity peptidoglycan binding domain of Pseudomonas phage endolysin KZ144. *Biochem. Biophys. Res. Commun.* 383, 187–191. doi: 10.1016/j.bbrc.2009.03.161

Briers, Y., Walmagh, M., and Lavigne, R. (2011). Use of bacteriophage endolysin EL188 and outer membrane permeabilizers against *Pseudomonas aeruginosa*. *J. Appl. Microbiol.* 110, 778–785. doi: 10.1111/j.1365-2672.2010.04931.x

Briers, Y., Walmagh, M., Van Puyenbroeck, V., Cornelissen, A., Cenens, W., Aertsen, A., et al. (2014). Engineered endolysin-based "Artilysins". *Combat Multidrug-Resist. Gram-negative Pathog. mBio* 5, e01379–e01314. doi: 10.1128/mBio.01379-14

Chopra, I., Schofield, C., Everett, M., O'neill, A., Miller, K., Wilcox, M., et al. (2008). Treatment of health-care-associated infections caused by Gram-negative bacteria: a consensus statement. *Lancet Infect. Dis.* 8, 133–139. doi: 10.1016/S1473-3099(08)70018-5

Collaborators, G.B.D.L.R.I. (2018). Estimates of the global, regional, and national morbidity, mortality, and aetiologies of lower respiratory infections in 195 countrie-2016: a systematic analysis for the Global Burden of Disease Study 2016. *Lancet Infect. Dis.* 18, 1191–1210. doi: 10.1016/S1473-3099(18)30310-4

Felsenstein, J. (1985). Confidence limits on phylogenies: an approach using the bootstrap. *Evolution* 39, 783–791. doi: 10.1111/j.1558-5646.1985.tb00420.x

Fischetti, V. A. (2005). Bacteriophage lytic enzymes: novel anti-infectives. *Trends Microbiol.* 13, 491–496. doi: 10.1016/j.tim.2005.08.007

Fischetti, V. A. (2008). Bacteriophage lysins as effective antibacterials. *Curr. Opin. Microbiol.* 11, 393–400. doi: 10.1016/j.mib.2008.09.012

Fischetti, V. A. (2010). Bacteriophage endolysins: a novel anti-infective to control Gram-positive pathogens. *Int. J. Med. Microbiol.* 300, 357–362. doi: 10.1016/j.ijmm.2010.04.002

Ghose, C., and Euler, C. W. (2020). Gram-Negative Bacterial Lysins. *Antibiotics (Basel)* 9(2), 74. doi: 10.3390/antibiotics9020074

Gondil, V. S., Kalaiyarasan, T., Bharti, V. K., and Chhibber, S. (2019). Antibiofilm potential of Seabuckthorn silver nanoparticles (SBT@AgNPs) against *Pseudomonas aeruginosa*. *3 Biotech.* 9, 402. doi: 10.1007/s13205-019-1947-6

Gondil, V. S., Harjai, K., and Chhibber, S. (2020). Endolysins as emerging alternative therapeutic agents to counter drug-resistant infections. *Int. J. Antimicrob. Agents* 55, 105844. doi: 10.1016/j.ijantimicag.2019.11.001

Guo, M., Feng, C., Ren, J., Zhuang, X., Zhang, Y., Zhu, Y., et al. (2017). A novel antimicrobial endolysin, LysPA26, against *Pseudomonas aeruginosa*. *Front. Microbiol.* 8, 293. doi: 10.3389/fmicb.2017.00293

Helander, I. M., and Mattila-Sandholm, T. (2000). Fluorometric assessment of gram-negative bacterial permeabilization. *J. Appl. Microbiol.* 88, 213–219. doi: 10.1046/j.1365-2672.2000.00971.x

Heron, M. (2017). Deaths: Leading Causes for 2015. *Natl. Vital. Stat. Rep.* 66, 1–76.

Huang, L., Luo, D., Gondil, V. S., Gong, Y., Jia, M., Yan, D., et al. (2020). Construction and characterization of a chimeric lysin ClyV with improved bactericidal activity against *Streptococcus agalactiae* in vitro and in vivo. *Appl. Microbiol. Biotechnol.* 104, 1609–1619. doi: 10.1007/s00253-019-10325-z

Kering, K. K., Zhang, X., Nyaruaba, R., Yu, J., and Wei, H. (2020). Application of adaptive evolution to improve the stability of bacteriophages during storage. *Viruses* 12(4), 423. doi: 10.3390/v12040423

Kim, N. H., Park, W. B., Cho, J. E., Choi, Y. J., Choi, S. J., Jun, S. Y., et al. (2018). Effects of phage endolysin SAL200 combined with antibiotics on *Staphylococcus aureus* infection. *Antimicrob. Agents Chemother.* 62(10), e00731–18. doi: 10.1128/AAC.00731-18

Kim, S., Jin, J. S., Choi, Y. J., and Kim, J. (2020a). LysSAP26, a new recombinant phage endolysin with a broad spectrum antibacterial activity. *Viruses* 12(11), 1340. doi: 10.3390/v12111340

Kim, S., Lee, D. W., Jin, J. S., and Kim, J. (2020b). Antimicrobial activity of LysSS, a novel phage endolysin, against *Acinetobacter baumannii* and *Pseudomonas aeruginosa*. *J. Glob. Antimicrob. Resist.* 22, 32–39. doi: 10.1016/j.jgar.2020.01.005

Kumar, S., Stecher, G., Li, M., Knyaz, C., and Tamura, K. (2018). MEGA X: Molecular Evolutionary Genetics Analysis across Computing Platforms. *Mol. Biol. Evol.* 35, 1547–1549. doi: 10.1093/molbev/msy096

Lai, M. J., Lin, N. T., Hu, A., Soo, P. C., Chen, L. K., Chen, L. H., et al. (2011). Antibacterial activity of *Acinetobacter baumannii* phage φAB2 endolysin (LysAB2) against both gram-positive and gram-negative bacteria. *Appl. Microbiol. Biotechnol.* 90, 529–539. doi: 10.1007/s00253-011-3104-y

Loeffler, J. M., Djurkovic, S., and Fischetti, V. A. (2003). Phage lytic enzyme Cpl-1 as a novel antimicrobial for pneumococcal bacteremia. *Infect. Immun.* 71, 6199–6204. doi: 10.1128/IAI.71.11.6199-6204.2003

Loessner, M. J., Kramer, K., Ebel, F., and Scherer, S. (2002). C-terminal domains of *Listeria monocytogenes* bacteriophage murein hydrolases determine specific recognition and high-affinity binding to bacterial cell wall carbohydrates. *Mol. Microbiol.* 44, 335–349. doi: 10.1046/j.1365-2958.2002.02889.x

Lood, R., Winer, B. Y., Pelzek, A. J., Diez-Martinez, R., Thandar, M., Euler, C. W., et al. (2015). Novel phage lysin capable of killing the multidrug-resistant gram-negative bacterium *Acinetobacter baumannii* in a mouse bacteremia model. *Antimicrob. Agents Chemother.* 59, 1983–1991. doi: 10.1128/AAC.04641-14

Magiorakos, A. P., Srinivasan, A., Carey, R. B., Carmeli, Y., Falagas, M. E., Giske, C. G., et al. (2012). Multidrug-resistant, extensively drug-resistant and pandrug-resistant bacteria: an international expert proposal for interim standard definitions for acquired resistance. *Clin. Microbiol. Infect.* 18, 268–281. doi: 10.1111/j.1469-0691.2011.03570.x

Manchanda, V., Sanchaita, S., and Singh, N. (2010). Multidrug resistant acinetobacter. *J. Glob. Infect. Dis.* 2, 291–304. doi: 10.4103/0974-777X.68538

Nelson, D., Schuch, R., Chahales, P., Zhu, S., and Fischetti, V. A. (2006). PlyC: a multimeric bacteriophage lysin. *Proc. Natl. Acad. Sci. U. S. A.* 103, 10765–10770. doi: 10.1073/pnas.0604521103

Nelson, D. C., Schmelcher, M., Rodriguez-Rubio, L., Klumpp, J., Pritchard, D. G., Dong, S., et al. (2012). Endolysins as antimicrobials. *Adv. Virus Res.* 83, 299–365. doi: 10.1016/B978-0-12-394438-2.00007-4

Oliveira, H., Vilas Boas, D., Mesnage, S., Kluskens, L. D., Lavigne, R., Sillankorva, S., et al. (2016). Structural and enzymatic characterization of ABgp46, a novel phage endolysin with broad anti-gram-negative bacterial activity. *Front. Microbiol.* 7, 208. doi: 10.3389/fmicb.2016.00208

Pendleton, J. N., Gorman, S. P., and Gilmore, B. F. (2013). Clinical relevance of the ESKAPE pathogens. *Expert Rev. Anti Infect. Ther.* 11, 297–308. doi: 10.1586/eri.13.12

Potron, A., Poirel, L., and Nordmann, P. (2015). Emerging broad-spectrum resistance in *Pseudomonas aeruginosa* and *Acinetobacter baumannii*: Mechanisms and epidemiology. *Int. J. Antimicrob. Agents* 45, 568–585. doi: 10.1016/j.ijantimicag.2015.03.001

Rodríguez-Rubio, L., Chang, W. L., Gutiérrez, D., Lavigne, R., Martínez, B., Rodríguez, A., et al. (2016). 'Artilysation' of endolysin λSa2lys strongly improves its enzymatic and antibacterial activity against streptococci. *Sci. Rep.* 6, 35382. doi: 10.1038/srep35382

Saitou, N., and Nei, M. (1987). The neighbor-joining method: a new method for reconstructing phylogenetic trees. *Mol. Biol. Evol.* 4, 406–425. doi: 10.1093/oxfordjournals.molbev.a040454

Scallan, E., Griffin, P. M., Angulo, F. J., Tauxe, R. V., and Hoekstra, R. M. (2011). Foodborne illness acquired in the United States–unspecified agents. *Emerg. Infect. Dis.* 17, 16–22. doi: 10.3201/eid1701.P21101

Schmelcher, M., Donovan, D. M., and Loessner, M. J. (2012). Bacteriophage endolysins as novel antimicrobials. *Future Microbiol.* 7, 1147–1171. doi: 10.2217/fmb.12.97

Schuch, R., Nelson, D., and Fischetti, V. A. (2002). A bacteriolytic agent that detects and kills *Bacillus anthracis*. *Nature* 418, 884–889. doi: 10.1038/nature01026

Spellberg, B., Bartlett, J. G., and Gilbert, D. N. (2013). The future of antibiotics and resistance. *N. Engl. J. Med.* 368, 299–302. doi: 10.1056/NEJMp1215093

Valencia, R., Arroyo, L. A., Conde, M., Aldana, J. M., Torres, M. J., Fernández-Cuenca, F., et al. (2009). Nosocomial outbreak of infection with pan-drug-resistant *Acinetobacter baumannii* in a tertiary care university hospital. *Infect. Control. Hosp. Epidemiol.* 30, 257 263. doi: 10.1086/595977

Walmagh, M., Briers, Y., Dos Santos, S. B., Azeredo, J., and Lavigne, R. (2012). Characterization of modular bacteriophage endolysins from Myoviridae phages OBP, 201φ2-1 and PVP-SE1. *PLoS One* 7, e36991. doi: 10.1371/journal.pone.0036991

Yang, H., Yu, J., and Wei, H. (2014). Engineered bacteriophage lysins as novel anti-infectives. *Front. Microbiol.* 5, 542. doi: 10.3389/fmicb.2014.00542

Yang, H., Linden, S. B., Wang, J., Yu, J., Nelson, D. C., and Wei, H. (2015a). A chimeolysin with extended-spectrum streptococcal host range found by an induced lysis-based rapid screening method. *Sci. Rep.* 5, 17257. doi: 10.1038/srep17257

Yang, H., Wang, M., Yu, J., and Wei, H. (2015b). Antibacterial activity of a novel peptide-modified lysin against *Acinetobacter baumannii* and *Pseudomonas aeruginosa*. *Front. Microbiol.* 6, 1471. doi: 10.3389/fmicb.2015.01471

Yang, H., Luo, D., Etobayeva, I., Li, X., Gong, Y., Wang, S., et al. (2020). Linker editing of pneumococcal lysin ClyJ conveys improved bactericidal activity. *Antimicrob. Agents Chemother.* 64(2), e01610–19. doi: 10.1128/AAC.01610-19

Yuan, Y., Li, X., Wang, L., Li, G., Cong, C., Li, R., et al. (2020). The endolysin of the Acinetobacter baumannii phage vB_AbaP_D2 shows broad antibacterial activity. *Microb. Biotechnol.* doi: 10.1111/1751-7915.13594

15

Pharmacokinetics and Pharmacodynamics of a Novel Virulent Klebsiella Phage Kp_Pokalde_002 in a Mouse Model

Gunaraj Dhungana[1]*, Roshan Nepal[1,2†], Madhav Regmi[1] and Rajani Malla[1]

[1] Central Department of Biotechnology, Tribhuvan University, Kirtipur, Nepal, [2] Adelaide Medical School, Faculty of Health and Medical Sciences, The University of Adelaide, Adelaide, SA, Australia

*Correspondence:
Gunaraj Dhungana
grdhungana79@gmail.com

†Present address:
Roshan Nepal,
Adelaide Medical School,
Faculty of Health and Medical
Sciences, The University of Adelaide,
Adelaide, SA, Australia

Phage therapy is one of the most promising alternatives to antibiotics as we face global antibiotic resistance crisis. However, the pharmacokinetics (PK) and pharmacodynamics (PD) of phage therapy are largely unknown. In the present study, we aimed to evaluate the PK/PD of a locally isolated virulent novel øKp_Pokalde_002 (*Podoviridae*, C1 morphotype) that infects carbapenem-resistant *Klebsiella pneumoniae* (Kp56) using oral and intraperitoneal (IP) route in a mouse model. The result showed that the øKp_Pokalde_002 rapidly distributed into the systemic circulation within an hour *via* both oral and IP routes. A higher concentration of phage in plasma was found after 4 h (2.3 x 10^5 PFU/ml) and 8 h (7.3 x 10^4 PFU/ml) of administration through IP and oral route, respectively. The phage titer significantly decreased in the blood and other tissues, liver, kidneys, and spleen after 24 h and completely cleared after 72 h of administration. In the Kp56 infection model, the bacterial count significantly decreased in the blood and other organs by 4–7 $\log_{10}$ CFU/ml after 24 h of øKp_Pokalde_002 administration. Elimination half-life of øKp_Pokalde_002 was relatively shorter in the presence of host-bacteria Kp56 compared to phage only, suggesting rapid clearance of phage in the presence of susceptible host. Further, administration of the øKp_Pokalde_002 alone in healthy mice (*via* IP or oral) did not stimulate pro-inflammatory cytokines (TNF-α and IL-6). Also, treatment with øKp_Pokalde_002 resulted in a significant reduction of pro-inflammatory cytokines (TNF-α and IL-6) caused by bacterial infection, thereby reducing the tissue inflammation. In conclusion, the øKp_Pokalde_002 possess good PK/PD properties and can be considered as a potent therapeutic candidate for future phage therapy in carbapenem-resistant *K. pneumoniae* infections.

Keywords: bacteriophage, PK/PD, carbapenem-resistant infections, *Klebsiella pneumoniae*, phage therapy

INTRODUCTION

Antibiotic resistance has become one of the biggest challenges to the global public health. According to the World Health Organization (WHO), the world is heading towards a post-antibiotic era and it would force millions of people into extreme poverty and death by 2050 (WHO, 2017). The discovery of new class of antibiotics is often time consuming and requires tremendous investment, and as bacteria quickly become resistant to antibiotics, it will shortly be ineffective (Spellberg, 2014). As no new class of antibiotics has been discovered since the 1980s, researchers are warning about the imminent antibiotic resistance crisis of pandemic proportion if we fail to find effective alternative approaches to antibiotics in addition to development new classes of antibiotics. Recently, the ESKAPE (*Enterococcus faecium, Staphylococcus aureus, Klebsiella pneumoniae, Acinetobacter baumannii, Pseudomonas aeruginosa,* and *Enterobacter* species) pathogens are causing life-threatening infections throughout the world in both hospital and community settings with high morbidity and mortality (Paczosa and Mecsas, 2016). They are mostly multidrug-resistance (MDR) and acquire drug resistance potentially through different mechanisms such as drug inactivation, target modification, reduced permeability, or by increased efflux pump (Santajit and Indrawattana, 2016). Carbapenem-resistant *K. pneumoniae* is one of the ESKAPE pathogens categorized as critical by WHO, and research and development of new classes of antimicrobial agents is highly prioritized. A high prevalence of carbapenem-resistant *Enterobacteriaceae,* including *K. pneumoniae* infections, has also been reported in recent years in Southeast Asia including Nepal (Hsu et al., 2017; Nepal et al., 2017).

Bacteriophages (phages) are viruses that target specific bacterial species and has two distinct lifestyles: lytic and lysogenic, that dictate its role in bacterial biology. Recently, virulent phages (that strictly kill the host bacteria) have received heightened attention as a potent antimicrobial agent to treat bacterial infections, especially antibiotic resistant infections (Clokie et al., 2011). Phage therapy (using phage and its components as a therapeutic agent) has been known for more than 100 years and recently regained heightened interest as the modern understanding of phage biology, genetics, immunology, and pharmacology recognizes its use in mitigating the antibiotic resistance crisis (Young and Gill, 2015). Several studies have already demonstrated the safety and efficacy of phage therapy in systemic and tropical infections in both animal and human (Vinodkumar et al., 2008; Kumari et al., 2011; Pouillot et al., 2012; Furfaro et al., 2018; Wang et al., 2018). Phage therapy in humans is still routinely used in Georgia, Poland, and Russia, and Western countries like USA, UK, Belgium, France and Germany are using phages in therapeutics occasionally as personalized, magistral preparations and/or compassionate use to treat infections when all of the available antibiotics fail (Pirnay et al., 2018; Romero-Calle et al., 2019). Although there are more than 10 case reports published over last 10 years about phage therapy (Sybesma et al., 2018; Pirnay, 2020), and most of them showing encouraging results (Schooley et al., 2017; Dedrick et al., 2019; Petrovic Fabijan et al., 2020), it is yet to be adopted in mainstream medicine so far. Beside regulatory hurdles, one of the possible reasons for this is poor understanding of pharmacokinetics (PK) and pharmacodynamics (PD) of phages *in vivo*. Phages possess a unique tripartite dynamic relationship between their host bacteria and human immune system (Wahida et al., 2021) as they co-evolve and self-replicate within the human body in the presence of host bacteria (Payne and Jansen, 2003). As a result, the PK/PD of phages are distinct from those of classical antimicrobials. In addition, phages have ability to pass through body barriers, potentially eliciting an immune response (Barr et al., 2013; Dąbrowska and Abedon, 2019). It is necessary to understand the PK/PD of the phage in terms of biodistribution, bioavailability, clearance, and immune response *in vivo* (Caflisch et al., 2019). For successful phage therapy, route and dosage of phage administration must be assessed and standardized to each individual phage-bacteria combination (Payne and Jansen, 2003; Dąbrowska, 2019; Nilsson, 2019). In this study, we aimed to evaluate the PK/PD of a novel virulent (lytic) Klebsiella phage Kp_Pokalde_002 (GenBank ID: MT425185, hereafter referred as øKp_Pokalde_002) that infects carbapenem-resistant *K. pneumoniae* using oral and intraperitoneal (IP) route in a mouse model.

MATERIALS AND METHODS

Ethical Clearance and Animal Model

Ethical approval was obtained for the use of animal prior to the study (Ethical approval No.161/2018) from Nepal Health Research Council (NHRC), Kathmandu. The protocol was also approved by the Ethical Review Board, NHRC. Female Swiss albino mice (6–8 weeks old) weighing 23 ± 2.5 g were purchased from Natural Products Research Laboratory (NPRL), Kathmandu. The animals were housed in an animal room at Central Department of Biotechnology, Tribhuvan University and fed with normal antibiotic-free diet. Chloroform vapor was used to anesthetize the mice and then euthanized by cervical dislocation before any invasive procedures. Each experiment was performed in triplicates.

Bacterial Strain and Phage Amplification

A clinical isolate of *K. pneumoniae* (hereafter referred as Kp56) confirmed as a carbapenem-resistant strain (presence of gene *blaNDM1, blaKPC*) was obtained from the Microbiology Laboratory, Central Department of Biotechnology, Tribhuvan University (unpublished data). The bacteria were propagated in Luria-Bertani (LB) broth (HiMedia, India) at 37°C. A virulent øKp_Pokalde_002 (*Podoviridae,* C1 morphotype) isolated using Kp56 as a host was used in this study. The lytic-lifestyle and Gram-negative host of the phage was confirmed based on its physiochemical characteristics (Dhungana et al., 2021) and its genome analysis through PHACTS (https://edwards.sdsu.edu/PHACTS) (Mcnair et al., 2012).

The øKp_Pokalde_002 was amplified from glycerol stocks as described previously (Bourdin et al., 2014). Briefly, 1.0 ml overnight culture of the host bacteria (Kp56) was mixed with 100.0 ml LB broth and incubated at 37°C for 2.0 h with agitation

(100 rpm) to reach an exponential growth phase (OD_{600} = 0.3). The phage stock, acclimatized to room temperature, was then added at a multiplicity of infection (MOI) of 10, and the culture was further incubated at 37°C in a shaking incubator (250 rpm) for 5.0 h until the media was visually clear. The phage lysate was centrifuged at 3220xg (Centrifuge 5810 R, Eppendorf, Hamburg, Germany) for 15 min at 4°C, and the supernatant was filtered through a 0.22 µm pore-size Whatman™ syringe filter (Sigma-Aldrich, Missouri, United States). The phage lysate was further purified and concentrated by isopycnic cesium-chloride (CsCl) density-gradient ultracentrifugation as described elsewhere (Sambrook and Russell, 2001).

Phage/Bacteria Enumeration

Blood and homogenized tissue samples were serially diluted up to 10^{-6} in a 1.5 ml Eppendorf tubes. For bacterial count, 100 µl aliquot from each dilution was spread-plated on nutrient agar (NA) plates in duplicates and incubated at 37°C for 24 h. Similarly, for phage titer, the blood and homogenized tissue samples were centrifuged at 3220xg (Centrifuge 5810 R, Eppendorf, Hamburg, Germany) for 10 min at 4°C and filtered through a 0.22 µm pore size Whatman™ syringe filter (Sigma-Aldrich, Missouri, United States). The filtrate was serially diluted to up to 10^{-8} and phage titer was determined by Double Layer Agar (DLA) assay as described elsewhere. The phage and bacteria counts were corrected for tissue-fluid weights using following formula.

$$\frac{\text{\# plaques or colonies/ml plated} \times \text{dilution factor}}{\text{\# grams tissue/ml original homogenate}}$$

$$= \text{PFU or CFU/gm of tissue}$$

In Vivo Pharmacokinetics of øKp_Pokalde_002 Through Oral and IP Route

In vivo PK assessment was performed as described previously (Verma et al., 2009; Pouillot et al., 2012) with modifications. Seventy-two mice were divided into four groups [2 phage only and 2 vehicle (SM buffer) control, 18 mice in each group]. In a phage only control group, the first group of mice received 200 µl (1.2 x 10^8 PFU/ml) of the highly purified øKp_Pokalde_002 *via* oral route while the same dosage of phage preparation was injected *via* IP route in the second group. The vehicle control group (third and fourth) received 200 µl of SM buffer only *via* oral and IP route, respectively. Three mice from each group were euthanized by cervical dislocation at 1 h, 4 h, 8 h, 24 h, 48 h, and 72 h after phage administration. Blood samples were collected in tubes containing 0.05 M EDTA anticoagulant by cardiac puncture. Tissue samples from lungs, liver, spleen, and kidneys were collected aseptically from euthanized mice and further divided into two parts. One part of each tissue was immersed in 10% formalin for histopathological examinations. Another part of tissue was weighed and homogenized in 1.0 ml PBS aseptically. The homogenized tissue was centrifuged at 10,000 rpm for 10 min at 4°C, and supernatant was filtered through a

0.22 µm pore size Whatman™ syringe filter (Sigma-Aldrich, Missouri, United States). The phage titer was determined by standard DLA technique as described elsewhere (Dhungana et al., 2021).

Klebsiella pneumoniae Infection Model

In a separate study, 54 mice (3 groups, 18 in each group) were inoculated with 200 µl (1 x 10^8 CFU/ml) of exponentially growing Kp56 intraperitonially. Immediately after bacterial inoculation, 200 µl of SM buffer was injected to all mice in the first group (sepsis control) and 200 µl of øKp_Pokalde_002 (1.2 x 10^8 PFU/ml) was administered to all mice in second and third groups (treatment) through IP and oral routes, respectively. Three mice from each group were euthanized by cervical dislocation at 1 h, 4 h, 8 h, 24 h, 48 h, and 72 h post bacterial inoculation. Blood and tissue samples were collected and processed as described earlier to determine the phage titer and the levels of pro-inflammatory cytokines.

Histology

Histological examination of the lung tissue was done as described previously (Singla et al., 2015) with modifications. Briefly, tissues were fixed with 10% formalin and embedded in paraffin wax. Serial sections of 4–6 µm thickness were cut using microtome, de-paraffinized, rehydrated, and stained with Hematoxylin and Eosin (H&E stain). The tissue sections were examined under the light microscope for histological changes.

Cytokine Quantification

Pro-inflammatory cytokines: tumor necrosis factor alpha (TNF-α) and interleukin 6 (IL-6)] levels were measured in all Kp56 infected and øKp_Pokalde_002 treated mice. Total RNA was isolated from the blood samples using Direct-zol™ RNA MiniPrep Plus Kits (Zymo Research, USA), and cDNA was synthesized using iScript™ cDNA Synthesis Kit (Bio-Rad Laboratories, USA) following the manufacturer's instruction. DNAse I (6 U/µl) was used to digest any residual DNA. Total RNA concentration was measured using NanoDrop 8000 (Thermo Fisher Scientific, USA) by spectrophotometric optical density measurement at 260/280 nm. The mRNA levels of TNF-α and IL-6 were measured by two-step relative qRT-PCR. The β-actin housekeeping gene was amplified as an internal control. Gene expressions were normalized to the expression of β-actin gene. The sequences of primers of IL-6, TNF-α, and β-actin are listed in **Supplementary Table S1**. The real time PCR was performed using SYBR® Green Master Mix (2x) Kit in CFX Connect™ RT-PCR system (Bio-Rad Laboratories, USA). Melting curve analysis was performed after the amplification phase to eliminate the possibility of nonspecific amplification or primer-dimer formation. All samples were processed in duplicate, and the output level was reported as an average. The comparative CT method was used to calculate the relative expression ratio from the real time PCR efficiency and the CT (Livak and Schmittgen, 2001; Jain et al., 2006). mRNA expression level change was calculated using double delta Ct (DDCT) method, and the change in mRNA expression levels of cytokines was expressed as fold change.

$$\text{Fold change} = 2^{-\Delta\Delta Ct}$$

where 2-$\Delta\Delta$Ct = [(Ct of gene of interest – Ct of internal control) sample A - (Ct of gene of interest – Ct of internal control) sample B].

Data Interpretation and Statistical Analysis

Non-compartmental PK parameters: the peak plasma concentration (C_{max}) and the time to reach peak plasma concentration (T_{max}) were obtained by visual inspection of the data. The area under the plasma concentration-time curve (AUC) was calculated according to the linear trapezoidal rule up to the T_{last} phage concentration using GraphPad Prism 8 (Version 8.3.0). The half-life ($T_{1/2}$) was calculated from the one-phase exponential regression equation ($T_{1/2} = 0.693/K_{el}$) (Dufour et al., 2018; Chow et al., 2020). The elimination rate constant (K_{el}) was estimated from the slope of the elimination phase of the log transformed plasma concentration-time curve fitted by the method of least squares. All elimination phase data with associated variability were included in the estimation. Data were expressed as mean ± standard error of mean (SEM). Comparisons of phage count and cytokine levels were performed by one-way ANOVA with Tukey's multiple-comparison test and Student's t-test. Inter mice PD variability was expressed as coefficient of variation (%CV). All statistical analysis were performed using GraphPad Prism 8 (Version 8.3.0), and differences with $p < 0.05$ were considered statistically significant.

RESULTS

Pharmacokinetics

We examined the PK/PD of øKp_Pokalde_002 administered through IP and oral routes in mice model in the presence and absence of host bacteria Kp56 (**Figure 1**). Mice that received only øKp_Pokalde_002 through IP or oral routes did not show any sign of illness during the experimental period (72 h post phage inoculation), and øKp_Pokalde_002 was detected in blood and other body tissues within the first hour of both IP and/or oral route of administrations.

In an IP group and in the absence of host bacteria, maximum biodistribution of the øKp_Pokalde_002 was found at 4 h (43% of inoculated phage titer) post phage injection (**Figures 2A, B**). At 4 h, the phage titer was significantly higher in spleen (6.8 ± 0.10 $\log_{10}$ PFU/ml, 6.69 x 10^7 PFU/ml) compared to blood (5.3 ± 0.12 $\log_{10}$ PFU/ml, 2.22 x 10^5 PFU/ml), lungs (5.6 ± 0.4 $\log_{10}$ PFU/ml, 5.78 x 10^5 PFU/ml), liver (6.3 ± 0.05 $\log_{10}$ PFU/ml, 2.25 x 10^6 PFU/ml), and kidneys (5.8 ± 0.10 $\log_{10}$ PFU/ml, 6.04 x 10^5 PFU/ml) ($p < 0.0001$, two-way ANOVA with Tukey's multiple comparisons) (**Figure 2A** and **Supplementary Table S2**). After 4 h, there was a gradual decrease in phage titer in all organs and the phage was completely cleared within 48 h of phage inoculation except from spleen, where the complete clearance was seen at 72 h.

Similarly, in an oral route and in the absence of the host bacteria, maximum biodistribution of the øKp_Pokalde_002 was found at 8 h (28%) post phage administration (**Figures 2C, D**). At 8 h, the phage titer was significantly higher ($p < 0.0001$, two-way ANOVA with Tukey's multiple comparisons test) in spleen (6.7 ± 0.09 $\log_{10}$ PFU/ml, 5.21 x 10^6 PFU/ml) compared to blood (4.8 ± 0.1 $\log_{10}$ PFU/ml, 1.45 x 10^5 PFU/ml), lungs (5.1 ± 0.13 $\log_{10}$ PFU/ml, 1.44 x 10^5 PFU/ml), liver (5.9 ± 0.12 $\log_{10}$ PFU/ml, 8.10 x 10^5 PFU/ml), and kidneys (5.5 ± 0.35 $\log_{10}$ PFU/ml, 4.50 x 10^5 PFU/ml) (**Figure 2C**). After 8 h, the phage titer gradually decreased and completely cleared from all organs within 48 h of phage administration except spleen, where the complete clearance was seen at 72 h. As expected, we further observed that relative bioavailability was lower when phage was administered through oral route compared to IP (**Table 1**) in the absence of host bacteria Kp56. Although the results were similar in the presence of host Kp56, the relative bioavailability of phage was higher in blood and spleen when administered orally compared to IP.

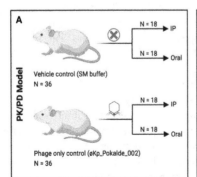 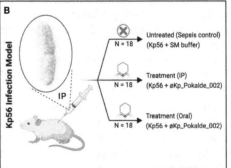

FIGURE 1 | Schematic representation of the experimental design. **(A)** In PK/PD model, SM buffer (vehicle control) and same dose of purified øKp_Pokalde_002 (phage only control) was administered *via* both IP and oral route. **(B)** In Kp56 infection model, bacteria (*K. pneumoniae*) were administered *via* IP route only, while treatment (øKp_Pokalde_002) was administered *via* both IP and oral route. Figure created in BioRender.com. PK, pharmacokinetics; PD, pharmacodynamics; SM, Sodium Magnesium; IP, intraperitoneal.

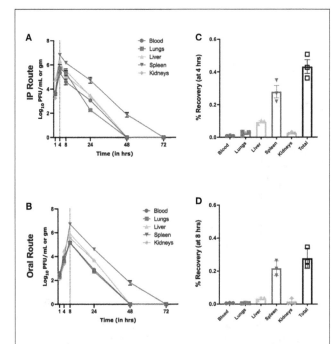

FIGURE 2 | Pharmacokinetics of øKp_Pokalde_002 *in vivo via* IP and oral route in the absence of host bacteria Kp56. The phage concentration in $\log_{10}$ PFU/ml in blood, lungs, liver, spleen, and kidney after 1, 4, 8, 24, 48, and 72 h of phage administration *via* IP **(A)** and oral **(C)** route (200 μl of ~1 × 10^8 PFU/ml). The result represents the mean from three independent experiments. Biodistribution of øKp_Pokalde_002 *via* IP **(B)** and oral **(D)** route at 4 h and 8 h, respectively. The dotted vertical line indicates T_{max}. Percentage recovery was calculated by dividing phage titer at the respective time-point by the administered dose (n = 3 mouse per time point).

In the presence of host bacteria Kp56, maximum titer of the øKp_Pokalde_002 was found at 8 h post phage injection (IP) and

24 h (oral) (**Figures 3A, B**) and gradually decreased after 24 h. In both group, maximum phage titer was found in the spleen at 24 h post phage injection. However, in contrast to phage inoculations without host, the phage did not clear from spleen until 72 h when inoculated with host Kp56.

We further report that mean elimination half-lives of øKp_Pokalde_002 in different organs were route independent [mean = 7.48 h, CV = 7.2% (IP) and mean = 7.6 h, CV = 10.5% (oral)] but the half-life was significantly lower [mean = 6.33 h, CV = 14.0% (IP) and mean = 5.3 h, CV = 4.0% (oral)] when susceptible host (Kp56) was present (**Table 1**) *via* both IP (p = 0.03, r^2 = 0.72, paired t-test) and oral (p = 0.0034, r^2 = 0.90, paired t-test) (**Figure 3C**) route possibly because of strong immune response from mice against bacteria and phage in the presence of Kp56 suggesting rapid clearance.

Pharmacodynamics

The groups of mice in PK/PD model (not infected by Kp56) that received øKp_Pokalde_002 *via* IP or oral route showed only mild to moderate alveolar wall thickening and remarkably reduced neutrophil infiltration in perivascular and peri bronchial areas (**Figure 4**). Moreover, they also did not show any significant histological changes compared to the vehicle control (SM buffer only) group at 24 h post phage inoculation. On the other hand, in the Kp56 infection model, bacterial count increased exponentially in the blood and lungs for up to 24 h when treated with SM buffer only (untreated group), while the bacterial count gradually decreased after 8 h when treated with øKp_Pokalde_002 (treatment group) *via* both IP and oral routes. The bacterial count significantly reduced by 4–7 $\log_{10}$ CFU/ml in the blood (p < 0.001) and lungs (p < 0.05) at 24 h of øKp_Pokalde_002 administration compared to untreated (Kp56 + SM buffer) group (**Supplementary Figure S3**, two-

TABLE 1 | Estimated pharmacokinetic parameters of virulent phage (øKp_Pokalde_002) in the absence and in the presence of host *K. pneumoniae* (Kp56).

Organ	Blood		Lungs		Liver		Spleen		Kidneys	
Route of administration	IP	Oral	IP	Oral	IP	Oral	IP	Oral	IP	Oral
Parameters										
				In the absence of host bacteria (Kp56)						
			Administered dose: 200 μl of 1.2 × 10^8 PFU/ml of øKp_Pokalde_002							
C_{max} (pfu/ml)	222778	72311	578611	14471	2258318	87056	6694839	521210	604444	45097
T_{max} (h)	4	8	4	8	4	8	4	8	4	8
Vd (L)	1.27	9.7	0.88	18.8	0.18	4.3	0.07	2.07	0.60	12.8
$T_{1/2}$ (h)	8.29	8.35	7.21	8.45	7.34	7.13	6.87	6.58	7.34	7.49
CL (L/h)	0.21	1.32	0.15	2.36	0.03	0.62	0.01	0.3	0.1	1.6
AUC_{0-t} (pfu/h/ml)	269539	155155	807450	149419	2407478	848459	8248503	5262198	948204	458160
Relative bioavailability (F)	58%		19%		35%		64%		48%	
				In the presence of host bacteria (Kp56)						
			Administered dose: 200 μl of 1.0 × 10^8 CFU/ml of Kp56 + 200 μl of 1.2 × 10^8 PFU/ml of øKp_Pokalde_002							
C_{max} (pfu/ml)	2923000	3315027	34693333	2107333	56589196	16643667	293940000	579333333	23068000	1695000
T_{max} (h)	8	24	8	24	24	24	24	24	24	24
Vd (L)	0.15	0.48	0.01	0.2	0.005	0.009	0.01	0.02	0.006	0.03
$T_{1/2}$ (h)	7.51	5.24	6.26	5.37	5.85	4.94	6.87	5.46	5.20	5.44
CL (L/h)	0.02	0.06	0.002	0.02	0.0009	0.001	0.001	0.002	0.001	0.005
AUC_{0-t} (pfu/h/ml)	3263704	4075882	43003899	2979558	97074444	25790850	399112587	626186433	190270651	3977100
Relative bioavailability (F)	125%		7%		27%		157%		2%	

C_{max}, maximum observed plasma concentration; T_{max}, time to the C_{max}; V_d, Volume of distribution; $T_{1/2}$, elimination half-time; CL, clearance; AUC_{0-t}, area under the concentration-time curve from time 1 h to the last quantifiable concentration. Relative bioavailability (F) was calculated using the following formula: F, AUC_{0-t} (oral)/AUC_{0-t} (IP)×100%.

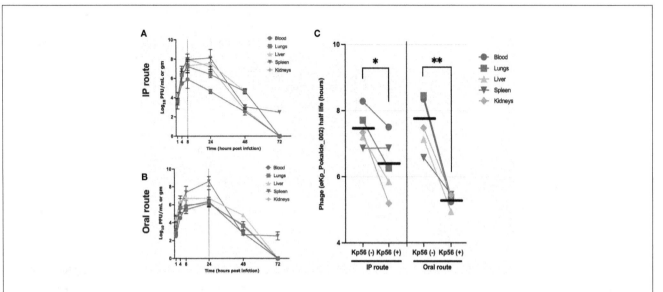

FIGURE 3 | Pharmacokinetics of øKp_Pokalde_002 *in vivo* and half-life of øKp_Pokalde_002 in the presence and absence of host bacteria Kp56 in mice when administered *via* IP and oral routes. The phage concentration in log10 PFU/ml in blood, lungs, liver, spleen, and kidneys after 1, 4, 8, 24, 48, and 72 h in Kp56 treatment group after administration of phage *via* IP **(A)** and oral **(B)** route (200 μl of ~1 x 10⁸ PFU/ml). The dotted vertical line indicates T_max. **(C)** The overall elimination half-life of øKp_Pokalde_002 is lower when host bacteria are present, signifying rapid clearance of phage from circulation in the presence of susceptible host. The individual data point represents an average from three replicates from three mouse. The horizontal line represents the grand mean.

way ANOVA with Tukey's multiple comparisons). Further, comparison of histological changes in the lung tissues from untreated group (Kp56 + SM buffer) and treatment group (Kp56 + øKp_Pokalde_002) revealed a noticeable interstitial infiltration by neutrophils and macrophages with severe thickening, congestion, and destruction of alveolar wall in the lungs of untreated group. Meanwhile, orally treated group showed relatively increased neutrophil infiltration in the alveoli (lung tissues) compared to the IP-treated group.

The expression level of two pro-inflammatory cytokine (TNF-α and IL-6) in blood was analyzed to evaluate the tissue inflammation either by øKp_Pokalde_002 or by Kp56. Cytokine expression levels in the control group (SM buffer only), phage administered group (øKp_Pokalde_002 only), Kp56 infected group (Kp56 + SM buffer), and phage-treated groups (Kp56 + øKp_Pokalde_002) were compared. A significant upregulation of both pro-inflammatory cytokines' TNF-α and IL-6 (p < 0.0001, Tukey's multiple comparisons test) was observed in the Kp56 infected (Kp56 + SM buffer) group compared to the control (SM buffer only) group, and at 24 h post infection, the increment in the TNF-α and IL-6 was 21.0-fold and 17.1-fold, respectively. Changes in TNF-α and IL-6 in phage-only administered group were 1.1-fold and 0.9-fold, respectively, compared to vehicle control (SM buffer only) arm. Interestingly, the levels of cytokine expressions in the phage-treated groups *via* both IP and oral route were significantly lower compared to Kp56 infected (Kp56 + SM buffer, untreated) arm (p < 0.05, Tukey's multiple comparisons test). The fold changes in cytokine TNF-α and IL-6 expression levels in phage-treated (Kp56 + øKp_Pokalde_002) groups compared to the uninfected control (phage only) arm are depicted in **Figure 5**.

DISCUSSION

Phage therapy is considered one of the promising alternatives to treat infections caused by MDR bacteria (Romero-Calle et al., 2019). PK/PD are fundamental parameters for better understanding the success of phage therapy and obtaining regulatory approval (Dąbrowska and Abedon, 2019). In this study, we focused on PK/PD of a novel øKp_Pokalde_002 that infects carbapenem-resistant *K. pneumoniae* using oral and IP routes of administration in a mouse model. Our results showed that øKp_Pokalde_002 rapidly distributed into the systemic circulation within an hour of administration *via* both oral and IP route. A relatively higher concentration of øKp_Pokalde_002 was recovered from plasma while injecting the phage through IP route compared to oral administration. When phage was administrated in mice through the IP route, highest phage titer in the blood reached after 4 h post administration, significantly decreased after 8 h, and negligible count was observed after 24 h. The result suggests that the phage net phage elimination is observed after 4 h if injected intraperitonially in the absence of host bacteria. The result is consistent with other studies where it is reported that the phages take 2–4 h to reach its maximum count in blood and is subsequently decreased after 12 h (Bogovazova et al., 1992; Capparelli et al., 2006; Kumari et al., 2010; Tiwari et al., 2011). Further, recovery of phages from blood and other tissue after oral administration shows that øKp_Pokalde_002 survived the gut environment and crossed the gut barrier to reach systemic circulation in mice subsequently reaching to different organs which is consistent with reports from other researchers (Cerveny et al., 2002; Gorski and Weber-Dabrowska, 2005). Several mechanisms have been proposed for phage absorption in the gastrointestinal tracts such as intestinal

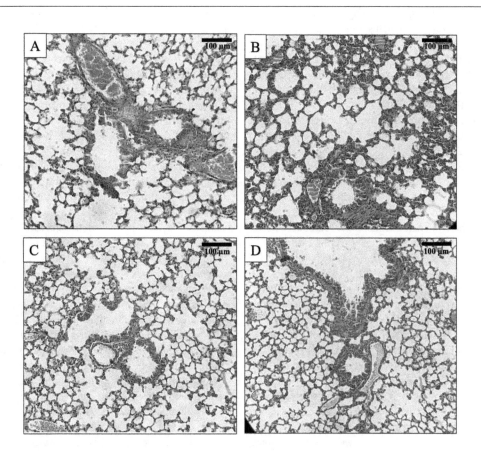

FIGURE 4 | Histology of mouse lung tissue sections after Hematoxylin and Eosin (H&E) staining at 200x magnification. **(A)** Lungs' tissue of a normal mouse. **(B)** Lungs' tissue of bacteria *K pneumoniae* (Kp56) infected mouse showing interstitial infiltration by neutrophils and macrophages with rupture of alveoli. **(C)** Lungs' tissue of mouse treated with øKp_Pokalde_002 *via* IP route. **(D)** Lungs' tissue of mouse treated with øKp_Pokalde_002 *via* oral route.

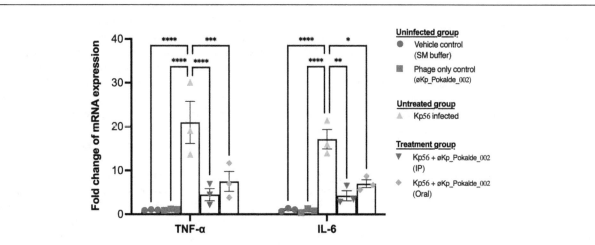

FIGURE 5 | Pro-inflammatory cytokine TNF-α and IL-6 levels in the plasma of mice (24 h post infection). Both TNF-α and IL-6 mRNA levels were significantly higher in Kp56 infected mice compared to uninfected and treated mice (p < 0.05) *via* both IP and oral routes. There was negligible fold increment of TNF-α and IL-6 mRNA level in vehicle control (SM buffer) and phage only control (øKp_Pokalde_002). Levels of TNF-α and IL-6 mRNA were normalized to β-actin mRNA levels and were expressed as n-fold ($2^{-\Delta\Delta Ct}$) increase with reference to the control groups. Results are shown as means ± SEM from triplicate experiments. The y-axis values represent the fold changes of mRNA relative to the β-actin mRNA in the same sample. The statistical comparison was done by two-way ANOVA. *p < 0.05, **p < 0.01, ***p < 0.001, ****p < 0.0001.

permeability and intestinal transport. Although the mechanism of controlling viral translocation remains unknown, researchers suggested that the phage passage is determined by various factors, including stomach acidity, phage concentration, and interactions with gut immune cells. Micropinocytosis may be a major endocytic pathway to translocate the phage from the intestinal wall into systemic circulation (Dąbrowska, 2019).

In our experiment, phages were recovered from blood, lungs, liver, and kidneys for up to 24 h and for up to 48 h in the spleen in the absence of host bacteria *via* both IP and oral route. However, there was significant difference in phage distribution, bioavailability, and elimination between IP and oral routes of administration. øKp_Pokalde_002 reached its maximum titer in blood at 4 h (2.3 x 10^5 PFU/ml) when administered through IP route which was relatively higher compared to administration *via* oral route (4.04 x 10^3 PFU/ml). Similar findings have been reported previously (Keller and Engley, 1958; Cerveny et al., 2002; Oliveira et al., 2009; Jun et al., 2014). Additionally, overall relative bioavailability of øKp_Pokalde_002 when administered *via* oral route (at 8 h) was lower compared to IP route (at 4 h) in both the absence and/or presence of host bacteria. The reason for reduced bioavailability *via* oral route compared to IP might be due to slow absorption of the phage in the gastrointestinal tract to reach into the systemic circulation. However, it must be noted that because of the low sampling resolution, the T_{max} could be higher than 4 h and 8 h in IP and oral administration respectively. As øKp_Pokalde_002 was stable within wide pH range (3–11) with minimal decrease in phage titer and did not show significant inactivation at 25°C and 37°C (Dhungana et al., 2021), the phage was well tolerated in mice gut with low acidity, making it a good candidate for oral phage therapy. It therefore appears that the øKp_Pokalde_002 is relatively stable in the mouse body when administered *via* the oral route but their availability is comparatively lower and slower. Similar findings have also been reported by Otero et al. (2019) and were able to recover orally administered encapsulated as well as non-encapsulated phages from various organs. Further, the inter mice PD variability [coefficient of variation (%CV)] was more pronounced in oral (7–78%) compared to IP (5–56%) route (**Supplementary Table S3**). The inter mice variability was profound in groups of Kp56 infection model. In addition to differential absorption of øKp_Pokalde_002 between animals and innate immunity, the higher variability between mice in the oral group may be because of the inconsistent neutralization of phages in the gut environment caused by gut acidity (feeding habit of mice). The phage absorption in the gastrointestinal tract is affected by various factors like gut acidity and gut permeability and is thus relatively slow. As such, lower phage particles reach into the blood stream through oral route compared to the IP route, which makes clinical application of phage *via* oral route for systemic infection unfavorable (Wolochow et al., 1966).

Further, the results suggest that liver and spleen are the most common organs of phage accumulation, suggesting phages are cleared by organs of the reticuloendothelial system such as the spleen, liver, and other filtering organs (Merril et al., 1996; Dąbrowska and Abedon, 2019). Similar results of non-homogenous biodistribution and preferential accumulation of

phages in organs like spleen and liver has also been observed in anti-pseudomonal phage in mice (Lin et al., 2020) and rabbit *in vivo* models (Uhr and Weissman, 1965). Further, phages are also reported in urine of human (Hildebrand and Wolochow, 1962) and animal models like rats (Wolochow et al., 1966) and rabbits (Schultz and Neva, 1965) after systemic injection which supports our finding that phage can pass through the renal filter. The role of the kidneys in the clearance of phages has also been observed in fish, where phages were detected in fish kidney a month after phage administration (Russell et al., 1976).

The PK of phages are fundamentally different from those of chemical drugs due to the self-replicative nature of phages in the presence of susceptible bacteria, its absorption rate, and clearance by host's immunity (Dąbrowska, 2019); thus, phage half-life cannot be estimated by conventional approach. Although researchers have demonstrated prolonged phage half-life *in vivo* with encapsulation of phage (Colom et al., 2015; Singla et al., 2016), the half-life of phage in the presence of a host is scarce. Using one phase decay model, our study showed that there was no significant difference in elimination half-life of øKp_Pokalde_002 when administered *via* IP and oral routes suggesting phage half-life to be route independent. However, the phage had a shorter elimination half-life in the blood and other organs when Kp56 was present, although phage titer was relatively higher in treatment groups compared to phage only control groups. This clearly suggests that phages can exponentially increase their number *in vivo* infecting and lysing the susceptible host bacteria and is cleared more rapidly by strong immune response developed against host bacteria (nonspecific) and phage itself (anti-phage). This may explain why multiple injections of phage is required for phage therapy, although theoretically phages are self-multiplying. However, a study on Klebsiella phage by Soleimani Sasani and Eftekhar (2020) found half-life in blood (4 h) when phages were administered intraperitoneally [100 µl of 10^{10} PFU/ml (*Myoviridae*)] and 8 h in lungs, whereas Kumari et al. (2010) reported maximum recovery from blood, peritoneal fluid, lungs, and skin at 6 h post IP injection [250 µl of 10^{10} PFU/ml (*Podoviridae*)]. Moreover, the half-life of phage seems to be comparable to that of antibiotics in animal models (Chang et al., 1991; Griffith et al., 2003) which ranges from 0.5 h to more than 7 h which makes it a good drug candidate against bacterial infections. However, more research is required in *in vivo* models to understand the half-life of different phages in the presence of susceptible host as this is important in designing the therapeutic dose of phage.

The histology results also revealed that the lung tissue of the øKp_Pokalde_002 administrated mice had a similar histological picture with reference to the wild-type and SM buffer only administrated mice group. Similar results of no detrimental histological effects were also observed by Gangwar et al. (2021) in various organs of Charles Foster rats when challenged by high (10^{15} and 10^{20} PFU/ml) of Klebsiella phage orally. Pro-inflammatory cytokines, TNF-α and IL-6, are useful markers of infection severity (Bozza et al., 2007). Present study revealed that there was negligible upregulation of pro-inflammatory cytokines (TNF-α, and IL-6) with the øKp_Pokalde_002 administrated *via* both IP and oral routes. In contrast, there was significant upregulation of the cytokines in the mice infected with the Kp56. Upon infection, pro-inflammatory cytokines are released by the macrophages to adhere the other inflammatory cells at the infection site (Liu et al., 2016). The expression of the cytokines was dropped after 24 h of the øKp_Pokalde_002 administration in both IP and oral routes signifying removal of Kp56. The result supports the findings of other researchers who have reported significant reduction in cytokines levels in phage-treated mice (Watanabe et al., 2007; Wang et al., 2016). Phage lysates that are prepared from the gram-negative bacteria may contain bacterial endotoxins. Endotoxins are highly immunogenic, which could trigger the inflammatory response. An overexpression of cytokines leads to a septic shock and consecutive death (Cavaillon, 2018). Phage preparation should be necessarily purified to ensure the low level of the endotoxin and other bacterial contamination. However, in our study, we did not measure the level of endotoxin in the phage lysate. Although researchers have highlighted that phage therapy causes lysis of the host bacteria within the body, thus releasing endotoxins/enterotoxins, which may induces higher levels of TNF-α and IL-6 causing septic shock (Hagens et al., 2004), the øKp_Pokalde_002 did not induce a significant inflammatory response in mice indicating a good PD efficiency. However, Chow et al. (2020) also reported that such upregulation of pro-inflammatory cytokines was transient and was diminished over time. Our results suggested that systemic inflammation of the tissues is lower in phage-treated mice as compared to the untreated. The histological findings of the lung tissue also support these findings.

In conclusion, PK/PD of øKp_Pokalde_002 *in vivo* were assessed. Inflammatory response, half-life, and biodistribution of the phage in blood, lungs, liver, kidneys, and spleen of mouse model were determined at different time interval *via* IP and oral routes of phage administration. The øKp_Pokalde_002 distributed more rapidly into the systemic circulation *via* the IP route compared to oral route. Importantly, the øKp_Pokalde_002 did not elicit any notable inflammation in lung tissues. Further, treatment by øKp_Pokalde_002 significantly reduced the inflammations caused by bacterial infection and downregulated the levels of the pro-inflammatory cytokine (TNF-α and IL-6) expression.

To the best of our knowledge, this is the first study that evaluates the PK/PD of a virulent Klebsiella phage that infects carbapenem-resistant clinical isolate of *K. pneumoniae via* IP and oral routes of administration. However, more work is necessary to better understand the PK/PD of the phage using different dose regimes and time of the phage exposure in *in vivo* model.

ETHICS STATEMENT

Ethical approval was obtained for the use of animal prior to the study from Nepal Health Research Council (NHRC), Nepal (Ethical approval No.161/2018). The protocol was also approved by the Ethical Review Board, NHRC.

AUTHOR CONTRIBUTIONS

GD and RM conceived the idea and designed the study. GD and MR performed the experiments. GD, MR, and RN analyzed the data. GD and RN drafted the manuscript. RM supervised the project. All authors contributed to the article and approved the submitted version.

ACKNOWLEDGMENTS

We gratefully acknowledge Prof. Dr. Krishna Das Manandhar, Head, Central Department of Biotechnology, Tribhuvan University, Nepal for providing consistent support in the study and members of Adhya's Laboratory, Laboratory of Molecular Biology, NCI, NIH, particularly Dr. Manoj Rajaure for guidance during the study. We also like to acknowledge Dr. Ashish Lakhey, Dr. Pooja Dhungana, Mr. Kapil Dev Neupane, Mr. Rajindra Napit, Ms. Apshara Parajuli, Ms. Elisha Upadhyay and Mr. Prashant Regmi for their valuable support during the study.

SUPPLEMENTARY MATERIAL

Supplementary Figure 1 | Analysis of øKp_Pokalde_002 genome for prediction of its lifestyle and host. The lytic-lifestyle and Gram-negative host of the phage was confirmed based on its physiochemical characters (Dhungana et al., 2021) and analysis of its amino acid sequences through PHACTS (https://edwards.sdsu.edu/PHACTS/index.php).

Supplementary Figure 2 | Area under the curve (AUC) from all groups of mice. **(A)** Phage pharmacokinetics and AUC after administration of phage *via* IP route in the absence of host Kp56. **(B)** Phage pharmacokinetics and AUC after administration of phage *via* oral route in the absence of host Kp56. **(C)** Phage pharmacokinetics and AUC after administration of phage *via* IP route in the presence of host Kp56. **(D)** Phage pharmacokinetics and AUC after administration of phage *via* oral route in the presence of host Kp56.

Supplementary Figure 3 | Quantification of bacterial burden in lungs and blood of mice from different group. Bacterial load was significantly decreased in phage treated group compared to group that only received SM buffer as treatment control. The bacterial burden in lungs **(A)** was similar to the bacterial burden in blood of phage treated group. Although the burden of bacterial significantly decreased, it appears that oral treatment is relatively less effective compared to IP and IP-one hour delay. The color-dotted line indicates the non-linear exponential growth fit (log population).

Supplementary Table 1 | Primers used in the study.

Supplementary Table 2 | P-values at 4 h (IP administration) and 8 h (oral administration) of øKp_Pokalde_002 in the absence of host bacteria Kp56.

REFERENCES

Barr, J. J., Auro, R., Furlan, M., Whiteson, K. L., Erb, M. L., Pogliano, J., et al. (2013). Bacteriophage Adhering to Mucus Provide a non-Host-Derived Immunity. *Proc. Natl. Acad. Sci. U.S.A.* 110 (26), 10771–10776. doi: 10.1073/pnas.1305923110

Bogovazova, G. G., Voroshilova, N. N., Bondarenko, V. M., Gorbatkova, G. A., Afanas'eva, E. V., Kazakova, T. B., et al. (1992). Immunobiological Properties and Therapeutic Effectiveness of Preparations From Klebsiella Bacteriophages. *Zh Mikrobiol Epidemiol. Immunobiol.* (3), 30–33.

Bourdin, G., Schmitt, B., Marvin Guy, L., Germond, J. E., Zuber, S., Michot, L., et al. (2014). Amplification and Purification of T4-Like Escherichia Coli Phages for Phage Therapy: From Laboratory to Pilot Scale. *Appl. Environ. Microbiol.* 80 (4), 1469–1476. doi: 10.1128/aem.03357-13

Bozza, F. A., Salluh, J. I., Japiassu, A. M., Soares, M., Assis, E. F., Gomes, R. N., et al. (2007). Cytokine Profiles as Markers of Disease Severity in Sepsis: A Multiplex Analysis. *Crit. Care* 11 (2), R49. doi: 10.1186/cc5783

Caflisch, K. M., Suh, G. A., and Patel, R. (2019). Biological Challenges of Phage Therapy and Proposed Solutions: A Literature Review. *Expert Rev. Anti Infect. Ther.* 17 (12), 1011–1041. doi: 10.1080/14787210.2019.1694905

Capparelli, R., Ventimiglia, I., Roperto, S., Fenizia, D., and Iannelli, D. (2006). Selection of an Escherichia Coli O157:H7 Bacteriophage for Persistence in the Circulatory System of Mice Infected Experimentally. *Clin. Microbiol. Infect.* 12 (3), 248–253. doi: 10.1111/j.1469-0691.2005.01340.x

Cavaillon, J. M. (2018). Exotoxins and Endotoxins: Inducers of Inflammatory Cytokines. *Toxicon.* 149, 45–53. doi: 10.1016/j.toxicon.2017.10.016

Cerveny, K. E., DePaola, A., Duckworth, D. H., and Gulig, P. A. (2002). Phage Therapy of Local and Systemic Disease Caused by Vibrio Vulnificus in Iron-Dextran-Treated Mice. *Infect. Immun.* 70 (11), 6251–6262. doi: 10.1128/iai.70.11.6251-6262.2002

Chang, H. R., Comte, R., Piguet, P. F., and Pechere, J. C. (1991). Activity of Minocycline Against Toxoplasma Gondii Infection in Mice. *J. Antimicrob. Chemother.* 27 (5), 639–645. doi: 10.1093/jac/27.5.639

Chow, M. Y. T., Chang, R. Y. K., Li, M., Wang, Y., Lin, Y., Morales, S., et al. (2020). Pharmacokinetics and Time-Kill Study of Inhaled Antipseudomonal Bacteriophage Therapy in Mice. *Antimicrob. Agents Chemother.* 65 (1), e01470–e01420. doi: 10.1128/aac.01470-20

Clokie, M. R., Millard, A. D., Letarov, A. V., and Heaphy, S. (2011). Phages in Nature. *Bacteriophage.* 1 (1), 31–45. doi: 10.4161/bact.1.1.14942

Colom, J., Cano-Sarabia, M., Otero, J., Cortes, P., Maspoch, D., and Llagostera, M. (2015). Liposome-Encapsulated Bacteriophages for Enhanced Oral Phage Therapy Against Salmonella Spp. *Appl. Environ. Microbiol.* 81 (14), 4841–4849. doi: 10.1128/aem.00812-15

Dąbrowska, K. (2019). Phage Therapy: What Factors Shape Phage Pharmacokinetics and Bioavailability? *Syst. Crit. Rev.* 39 (5), 2000–2025. doi: 10.1002/med.21572.

Dąbrowska, K., and Abedon, S. T. (2019). Pharmacologically Aware Phage Therapy: Pharmacodynamic and Pharmacokinetic Obstacles to Phage Antibacterial Action in Animal and Human Bodies. *Microbiol. Mol. Biol. Rev.* 83 (4), e00012–e00019. doi: 10.1128/mmbr.00012-19

Dedrick, R. M., Guerrero-Bustamante, C. A., Garlena, R. A., Russell, D. A., Ford, K., Harris, K., et al. (2019). Engineered Bacteriophages for Treatment of a Patient With a Disseminated Drug-Resistant Mycobacterium Abscessus. *Nat. Med.* 25 (5), 730–733. doi: 10.1038/s41591-019-0437-z

Dhungana, G., Regmi,, M., Paudel, P., Parajuli, A., Upadhyay, E., Indu, G., et al. (2021). Therapeutic Efficacy of Bacteriophage Therapy to Treat Carbapenem Resistant Klebsiella Pneumoniae in Mouse Model. *J. Nepal Health Res. Council* 19 (1), 76–82. doi: 10.33314/jnhrc.v19i1.3282

Dufour, N., Delattre, R., and Debarbieux, L. (2018). *In Vivo* Bacteriophage Biodistribution. *Methods Mol. Biol.* 123–137. doi: 10.1007/978-1-4939-7395-8_11

Furfaro, L. L., Payne, M. S., and Chang, B. J. (2018). Bacteriophage Therapy: Clinical Trials and Regulatory Hurdles. *Front. Cell. Infect Microbiol.* 8, 376. doi: 10.3389/fcimb.2018.00376

Gangwar, M., Rastogi, S., Singh, D., Shukla, A., Dhameja, N., Kumar, D., et al. (2021). Study on the Effect of Oral Administration of Bacteriophages in Charles Foster Rats With Special Reference to Immunological and Adverse Effects. *Front. Pharmacol.* 12, 615445. doi: 10.3389/fphar.2021.615445

Gorski, A., and Weber-Dabrowska, B. (2005). the Potential Role of Endogenous Bacteriophages in Controlling Invading Pathogens. *Cell Mol. Life Sci.* 62 (5), 511–519. doi: 10.1007/s00018-004-4403-6

Griffith, D. C., Harford, L., Williams, R., Lee, V. J., and Dudley, M. N. (2003). *In Vivo* Antibacterial Activity of RWJ-54428, a New Cephalosporin With Activity Against Gram-Positive Bacteria. *J. Antimicrob Agents Chemother.* 47 (1), 43–47. doi: 10.1128/AAC.47.1.43-47.2003%

Dhungana, G., Regmi,, M., Paudel, P., Parajuli, A., Upadhyay, E., Indu, G., et al. (2021). Therapeutic Efficacy of Bacteriophage Therapy to Treat Carbapenem Resistant Klebsiella Pneumoniae in Mouse Model. *J. Nepal Health Res. Council* 19 (1), 76–82. doi: 10.33314/jnhrc.v19i1.3282

Hagens, S., Habel, A., Von Ahsen, U., Von Gabain, A., and Bläsi, U. (2004). Therapy of Experimental Pseudomonas Infections With a Nonreplicating Genetically Modified Phage. *Antimicrob. Agents Chemother.* 48 (10), 3817–3822. doi: 10.1128/AAC.48.10.3817-3822.2004

Hildebrand, G. J., and Wolochow, H. (1962). Translocation of Bacteriophage Across the Intestinal Wall of the Rat. *Proc. Soc. Exp. Biol. Med.* 109, 183–185. doi: 10.3181/00379727-109-27146

Hsu, L. Y., Apisarnthanarak, A., Khan, E., Suwantarat, N., Ghafur, A., and Tambyah, P. A. (2017). Carbapenem-Resistant Acinetobacter Baumannii and Enterobacteriaceae in South and Southeast Asia. *Clin. Microbiol. Rev.* 30 (1), 1–22. doi: 10.1128/cmr.00042-16

Jain, M., Nijhawan, A., Tyagi, A. K., and Khurana, J. P. (2006). Validation of Housekeeping Genes as Internal Control for Studying Gene Expression in Rice by Quantitative Real-Time PCR. *Biochem. Biophys. Res. Commun.* 345 (2), 646–651. doi: 10.1016/j.bbrc.2006.04.140

Jun, J. W., Shin, T. H., Kim, J. H., Shin, S. P., Han, J. E., Heo, G. J., et al. (2014). Bacteriophage Therapy of a Vibrio Parahaemolyticus Infection Caused by a Multiple-Antibiotic-Resistant O3:K6 Pandemic Clinical Strain. *J. Infect. Dis.* 210 (1), 72–78. doi: 10.1093/infdis/jiu059

Keller, R., and Engley, F. B.Jr. (1958). Fate of Bacteriophage Particles Introduced Into Mice by Various Routes. *Proc. Soc. Exp. Biol. Med.* 98 (3), 577–580. doi: 10.3181/00379727-98-24112

Kumari, S., Harjai, K., and Chhibber, S. (2010). Isolation and Characterization of Klebsiella Pneumoniae Specific Bacteriophages From Sewage Samples. *Folia Microbiol.* 55 (3), 221–227. doi: 10.1007/s12223-010-0032-7

Kumari, S., Harjai, K., and Chhibber, S. (2011). Bacteriophage Versus Antimicrobial Agents for the Treatment of Murine Burn Wound Infection Caused by Klebsiella Pneumoniae B5055. *J. Med. Microbiol.* 60 (Pt 2), 205–210. doi: 10.1099/jmm.0.018580-0

Lin, Y. W., Chang, R. Y., Rao, G. G., Jermain, B., Han, M.-L., Zhao, J. X., et al. (2020). Pharmacokinetics/Pharmacodynamics of Antipseudomonal Bacteriophage Therapy in Rats: A Proof-of-Concept Study. *Clin. Microbiol. Infect* 26 (9), 1229–1235. doi: 10.1016/j.cmi.2020.04.039

Liu, K.-y., Yang, W.-h., Dong, X.-k., Cong, L.-m., Li, N., Li, Y., et al. (2016). Inhalation Study of Mycobacteriophage D29 Aerosol for Mice by Endotracheal Route and Nose-Only Exposure. *J. aerosol Med. Pulm Drug Delivery.* 29 (5), 393–405. doi: 10.1089/jamp.2015.1233

Livak, K. J., and Schmittgen, T. D. (2001). Analysis of Relative Gene Expression Data Using Real-Time Quantitative PCR and the 2(-Delta Delta C(T)) Method. *Methods.* 25 (4), 402–408. doi: 10.1006/meth.2001.1262

Mcnair, K., Bailey, B. A., and Edwards, R. A. (2012). PHACTS, a Computational Approach to Classifying the Lifestyle of Phages. *Bioinformatics* 28 (5), 614–618. doi: 10.1093/bioinformatics/bts014

Merril, C. R., Biswas, B., Carlton, R., Jensen, N. C., Creed, G. J., Zullo, S., et al. (1996). Long-Circulating Bacteriophage as Antibacterial Agents. *Proc. Natl. Acad. Sci. U.S.A.* 93 (8), 3188–3192. doi: 10.1073/pnas.93.8.3188

Nepal, K., Pant, N. D., Neupane, B., Belbase, A., Baidhya, R., Shrestha, R. K., et al. (2017). Extended Spectrum Beta-Lactamase and Metallo Beta-Lactamase Production Among Escherichia Coli and Klebsiella Pneumoniae Isolated From Different Clinical Samples in a Tertiary Care Hospital in Kathmandu, Nepal. *Ann. Clin. Microbiol. Antimicrob.* 16 (1), 62. doi: 10.1186/s12941-017-0236-7

Nilsson, A. S. (2019). Pharmacological Limitations of Phage Therapy. *Ups J. Med. Sci.* 124 (4), 218–227. doi: 10.1080/03009734.2019.1688433

Oliveira, A., Sereno, R., Nicolau, A., and Azeredo, J. (2009). the Influence of the Mode of Administration in the Dissemination of Three Coliphages in Chickens. *Poult Sci.* 88 (4), 728–733. doi: 10.3382/ps.2008-00378

Otero, J., García-Rodríguez, A., Cano-Sarabia, M., Maspoch, D., Marcos, R., Cortés, P., et al. (2019). Biodistribution of Liposome-Encapsulated Bacteriophages and Their Transcytosis During Oral Phage Therapy [Original Research]. *Front. Microbiol.* 10, 689. doi: 10.3389/fmicb.2019.00689

Paczosa, M. K., and Mecsas, J. (2016). Klebsiella Pneumoniae: Going on the Offense With a Strong Defense. *J. Microbiol. Mol. Biol. Rev.* 80 (3), 629–661. doi: 10.1128/MMBR.00078-15%

Payne, R. J., and Jansen, V. A. (2003). Pharmacokinetic Principles of Bacteriophage Therapy. *Clin. Pharmacokinet* 42 (4), 315–325. doi: 10.2165/00003088-200342040-00002

Petrovic Fabijan, A., Lin, R. C. Y., Ho, J., Maddocks, S., Ben Zakour, N. L., and Iredell, J. R. (2020). Safety of Bacteriophage Therapy in Severe Staphylococcus Aureus Infection. *Nat. Microbiol.* 5 (3), 465–472. doi: 10.1038/s41564-019-0634-z

Pirnay, J.-P. (2020). Phage Therapy in the Year 2035. *Front. Microbiol.* 11, 1171. doi: 10.3389/fmicb.2020.01171

Pirnay, J.-P., Verbeken, G., Ceyssens, P.-J., Huys, I., De Vos, D., Ameloot, C., et al. (2018). The Magistral Phage. *Viruses* 10 (2), 64. doi: 10.3390/v10020064

Pouillot, F., Chomton, M., Blois, H., Courroux, C., Noelig, J., Bidet, P., et al. (2012). Efficacy of Bacteriophage Therapy in Experimental Sepsis and Meningitis Caused by a Clone O25b:H4-ST131 Escherichia Coli Strain Producing CTX-M-15. *Antimicrob. Agents Chemother.* 56 (7), 3568–3575. doi: 10.1128/aac.06330-11

Romero-Calle, D., Guimaraes Benevides, R., Goes-Neto, A., and Billington, C. (2019). Bacteriophages as Alternatives to Antibiotics in Clinical Care. *Antibiot (Basel)* 8 (3), 138. doi: 10.3390/antibiotics8030138

Russell, W. J., Taylor, S. A., and Sigel, M. M. (1976). Clearance of Bacteriophage in Poikilothermic Vertebrates and the Effect of Temperature. *J. Reticuloendothel. Soc.* 19 (2), 91–96.

Sambrook, J., and Russell, D. J. P.NY (2001). *Molecular Cloning: A Laboratory Manual. 3rd Ed*, vol. 620. (Cold Spring Harbor Laboratory Press), 621.

Santajit, S., and Indrawattana, N. (2016). Mechanisms of Antimicrobial Resistance in ESKAPE Pathogens. *BioMed. Res. Int.* 2016, 2475067. doi: 10.1155/2016/2475067

Schooley, R. T., Biswas, B., Gill, J. J., Hernandez-Morales, A., Lancaster, J., Lessor, L., et al. (2017). Development and Use of Personalized Bacteriophage-Based Therapeutic Cocktails to Treat a Patient With a Disseminated Resistant Acinetobacter Baumannii Infection. *Antimicrob. Agents Chemother.* 61 (10), AAC.00954–00917. doi: 10.1128/aac.00954-17

Schultz, I., and Neva, F. A. (1965) *Relationship Between Blood Clearance and Viruria After Intravenous Injection of Mice and Rats With Bacteriophage and Polioviruses.* Available at: https://www.jimmunol.org/content/jimmunol/94/6/833.full.pdf.

Singla, S., Harjai, K., Katare, O. P., and Chhibber, S. (2015). Bacteriophage-Loaded Nanostructured Lipid Carrier: Improved Pharmacokinetics Mediates Effective Resolution of Klebsiella Pneumoniae–Induced Lobar Pneumonia. *J. Infect. Dis.* 212 (2), 325–334. doi: 10.1093/infdis/jiv029%

Singla, S., Harjai, K., Katare, O. P., and Chhibber, S. (2016). Encapsulation of Bacteriophage in Liposome Accentuates its Entry in to Macrophage and Shields it From Neutralizing Antibodies. *PloS One* 11 (4), e0153777. doi: 10.1371/journal.pone.0153777

Soleimani Sasani, M., and Eftekhar, F. (2020). Potential of a Bacteriophage Isolated From Wastewater in Treatment of Lobar Pneumonia Infection Induced by Klebsiella Pneumoniae in Mice. *Curr. Microbiol.* 77 (10), 2650–2655. doi: 10.1007/s00284-020-02041-z

Spellberg, B. (2014). The Future of Antibiotics. *Crit. Care* 18 (3), 228. doi: 10.1186/cc13948

Sybesma, W., Rohde, C., Bardy, P., Pirnay, J.-P., Cooper, I., Caplin, J., et al. (2018). Silk Route to the Acceptance and Re-Implementation of Bacteriophage Therapy—Part II. *Antibiotics* 7 (2), 35. doi: 10.3390/antibiotics7020035

Tiwari, B. R., Kim, S., Rahman, M., and Kim, J. (2011). Antibacterial Efficacy of Lytic Pseudomonas Bacteriophage in Normal and Neutropenic Mice Models. *J. Microbiol.* 49 (6), 994–999. doi: 10.1007/s12275-011-1512-4

Uhr, J. W., and Weissman, G. (1965). Intracellular Distribution and Degradation of Bacteriophage in Mammalian Tissues. *J. Immunol.* 94, 544–550.

Verma, V., Harjai, K., and Chhibber, S. (2009). Characterization of a T7-Like Lytic Bacteriophage of Klebsiella Pneumoniae B5055: A Potential Therapeutic Agent. *Curr. Microbiol.* 59 (3), 274–281. doi: 10.1007/s00284-009-9430-y

Vinodkumar, C. S., Kalsurmath, S., and Neelagund, Y. F. (2008). Utility of Lytic Bacteriophage in the Treatment of Multidrug-Resistant Pseudomonas Aeruginosa Septicemia in Mice. *Indian J. Pathol. Microbiol.* 51 (3), 360–366. doi: 10.4103/0377-4929.42511

Wahida, A., Tang, F., and Barr, J. J. (2021). Rethinking Phage-Bacteria-Eukaryotic Relationships and Their Influence on Human Health. *Cell Host Microbe.* 29 (5), 661–688. doi: 10.1016/j.chom.2021.02.007

Wang, J. L., Kuo, C. F., Yeh, C. M., Chen, J. R., Cheng, M. F., and Hung, C. H. (2018). Efficacy of Phikm18p Phage Therapy in a Murine Model of Extensively Drug-Resistant Acinetobacter Baumannii Infection. *Infect. Drug Resist.* 11, 2301–2310. doi: 10.2147/idr.S179701

Wang, Z., Zheng, P., Ji, W., Fu, Q., Wang, H., Yan, Y., et al. (2016). SLPW: A Virulent Bacteriophage Targeting Methicillin-Resistant Staphylococcus Aureus In Vitro and In Vivo. *Front. Microbiol.* 7, 934. doi: 10.3389/fmicb.2016.00934

Watanabe, R., Matsumoto, T., Sano, G., Ishii, Y., Tateda, K., Sumiyama, Y., et al. (2007). Efficacy of Bacteriophage Therapy Against Gut-Derived Sepsis Caused by Pseudomonas Aeruginosa in Mice. *J. Antimicrob Agents Chemother* 51 (2), 446 452. doi: 10.1128/AAC.00635-06%

WHO (2017). *Prioritization of Pathogens to Guide Discovery, Research and Development of New Antibiotics for Drug-Resistant Bacterial Infections, Including Tuberculosis* (Geneva: S. World Health Organization).

Wolochow, H., Hildebrand, G. J., and Lamanna, C. (1966). Translocation of Microorganisms Across the Intestinal Wall of the Rat: Effect of Microbial Size and Concentration. *J. Infect. Dis.* 116 (4), 523–528. doi: 10.1093/infdis/116.4.523

Young, R., and Gill, J. J. (2015). Phage Therapy Redux—What is to be Done? *J. Sci.* 350 (6265), 1163–1164. doi: 10.1126/science.aad6791%

16

The Type II Secretory System Mediates Phage Infection in *Vibrio cholerae*

Huihui Sun[1,2], Ming Liu[1], Fenxia Fan[1], Zhe Li[1], Yufeng Fan[1], Jingyun Zhang[1], Yuanming Huang[1], Zhenpeng Li[1], Jie Li[1], Jialiang Xu[3] and Biao Kan[1]*

[1] State Key Laboratory for Infectious Disease Prevention and Control, National Institute for Communicable Disease Control and Prevention, Chinese Center for Disease Control and Prevention, Beijing, China, [2] National Institute of Environment Health, Chinese Center for Disease Control and Prevention, Beijing, China, [3] School of Light Industry, Beijing Technology and Business University, Beijing, China

*Correspondence:
Biao Kan
kanbiao@icdc.cn

Attachment and specific binding to the receptor on the host cell surface is the first step in the process of bacteriophage infection. The lytic phage VP2 is used in phage subtyping of the *Vibrio cholerae* biotype El Tor of the O1 serogroup; however, its infection mechanism is poorly understood. In this study, we aimed to identify its receptor on *V. cholerae*. The outer membrane protein EpsD in the type II secretory system (T2SS) was found to be related to VP2-specific adsorption to *V. cholerae*, and the T2SS inner membrane protein EpsM had a role in successful VP2 infection, although it was not related to adsorption of VP2. The tail fiber protein gp20 of VP2 directly interacts with EpsD. Therefore, we found that in *V. cholerae*, in addition to the roles of the T2SS as the transport apparatus of cholera toxin secretion and filamentous phage release, the T2SS is also used as the receptor for phage infection and probably as the channel for phage DNA injection. Our study expands the understanding of the roles of the T2SS in bacteria.

Keywords: bacteriophage, type II secretory system, receptor, EpsD, *Vibrio cholerae*

INTRODUCTION

Cholera is a severe intestinal infectious disease caused by toxigenic *Vibrio cholerae*, which still seriously attacks human health in undeveloped countries. Cholera outbreaks and endemics occur mainly due to the ingestion of contaminated water and food (Sack et al., 2004; Weil and Ryan, 2018). Successfully colonized *V. cholerae* in the host small intestine may express a number of virulence factors in response to host signals, including cholera toxin (Reidl and Klose, 2002; Yang et al., 2013; Liu et al., 2016), thus causing vomiting and watery diarrhea symptoms. *V. cholerae* can be divided into more than 200 serogroups according to the diversity of surface O antigens; currently, only toxigenic O1 and O139 serogroup strains are believed to cause cholera epidemics or pandemics (Faruque et al., 1998), and O1 strains can be further classified into classical biotype and El Tor biotype.

Bacteriophage or phage is a general term for viruses that can infect bacteria, causing lysis or lysogenic conversion of the infected bacterial host according to the characteristics of virulent or lytic phages and temperate phages (Hatfull and Hendrix, 2011; Salmond and Fineran, 2015). Interactions between phages and bacteria result in the modulation and biodiversity of bacterial communities in the environment and host. In *V. cholerae*, phages may cause the proliferation and decline of the different clones in the environment and may contribute to the disappearance of epidemics or the appearance of new epidemics caused by new clones (Faruque et al., 2005; Jensen et al., 2006). Lytic phages can also be used in the subtyping of bacteria and even to eliminate drug-resistant pathogens in the clinic (Kazmierczak et al., 2014).

The first step for phages to infect the host bacteria is attachment to the specific receptors of the host cells. Tailed phages use a broad range of receptor-binding proteins to specifically interact with their cognate bacterial cell surface receptors. These receptors are diverse in different host cells, and most components are localized on the bacterial cell surface, such as many porins of the outer membrane, lipopolysaccharide (LPS) (Rakhuba et al., 2010; Bertozzi Silva et al., 2016), and flagella or pili, which can also act as phage receptors (Harvey et al., 2018; McCutcheon et al., 2018). Identifying the receptors of phages may facilitate understanding of the infection and host range of the phages and resistance mutations of the bacteria since a sensitive host may evolve resistance to phages by receptor mutation, for example, under infection pressure from phages.

In a phage typing scheme for the El Tor biotype of O1 serogroup *V. cholerae*, five *V. cholerae* lytic phages (named VP1 to VP5 in turn) are used for the subtyping of O1 El Tor strains (Zhang et al., 2009). Lipopolysaccharide and outer membrane proteins have been found to be receptors of some typing phages (Zhang et al., 2009). In this study, we aimed to identify the receptor of the phage VP2. We adopted the transposon library strategy to identify the genes related to VP2 infection in *V. cholerae* and found a type II secretion system (T2SS), which has been identified for its importance as an

extracellular protein transport apparatus for the secretion of cholera enterotoxin (CT) and release of the filamentous phage CTXΦ (Davis et al., 2000), also playing a vital role for VP2 adsorption and infection processes. Our study revealed a new role of T2SS, which is a common cross-membrane apparatus in many bacteria, and present a new insight for the function of this transporter.

MATERIALS AND METHODS

Phage, Bacterial Strains, Plasmids, and Media

VP2 was isolated from the river water of Wenzhou, Zhejiang Province, in 1962. The bacterial strains and plasmids used in this study are listed in **Table 1**. *V. cholerae* O1 El Tor 16017 is the host of VP2 and is used for VP2 propagation. The *V. cholerae* El Tor strain N16961 is sensitive to the phage VP2 and was used as the wild-type strain in this study. For *in vitro* growth experiments, the bacteria were cultured in LB medium unless otherwise noted. Antibiotics were used at the following concentrations: ampicillin (Amp), 100 µg/mL; streptomycin (Sm), 100 µg/mL; kanamycin (Kan), 50 µg/mL; gentamicin (Gm), 20 µg/mL; tetracycline (Tc), 2 µg/mL and chloramphenicol (Cm), 30 µg/mL for *Escherichia coli* but 2 µg/mL for *V. cholerae*.

Screening of VP2-Resistant Mutants

E. coli SM10λpir (Chiang and Mekalanos, 2000) bearing the plasmid pSC123 (Simon et al., 1983) named SM10-123, was used as the donor strain, and conjugation was performed by using the

TABLE 1 | Strains and plasmids used in this study.

Strains and plasmids	Relevant properties	Reference
V. cholerae		Laboratory
N16961	Spontaneous mutant of N16961, Inaba, Sm^r	collections
N-ΔepsM	epsM (VC2724) deletion of N16961, Sm^r	This study
N-ΔepsD	epsD (VC2733) deletion of N16961, Sm^r	This study
N-ΔepsM-C	N-ΔepsM strain complemented with pSRKTc-EpsM	This study
N-ΔepsD-C	N-ΔepsD strain complemented with pSRKGm-EpsD	This study
E. coli		
SM10λpir	Kan, thi thr leu tonA lacY supE recA::RP4-2-TC::Muλpir	
DH5αλpir	sup E44, ΔlacU169 (ΦlacZΔM15), recA1, endA1, hsdR17, thi-1, gyrA96, relA1	
XL1blue	endA1 gyrA96 thi-1 hsdR17 supE44 relA1 lac	
BTH101	F-, cya-99, araD139, galE15, galK16, rpsL1 (Strr), hsdR2, mcrA1, mcrB1	
Plasmids		
pSC123	Suicide plasmid carrying transposon; Kan^r Cm^r	
pWM91	Suicide plasmid; oriR oriT lacZ tetAR sacB	
pWM91-ΔepsM	pWM91 carrying upstream and downstream fragments flanking epsM	This study
pWM91-ΔepsD	pWM91 carrying upstream and downstream fragments flanking epsD	This study
pUT18C (abbreviated as pT18C)	pUT18C-derived vector, designed to create C-terminal heterologous protein fusion, Amp^r	
pKT25 (abbreviated as pT25)	lac promoter and the T25 fragment for C-terminal heterologous protein fusion. Kan^r	
pSRKTc	lac promoter and lacI^q, Tet^r	
pSRKTc-EpsM	pSRKTc-derived, VC2724 (epsM), Tet^r	This study
pSRKGm-EpsD	pSRKGm-derived, VC2733 (epsD), Tet^r	This study
pT25-EpsD	pKT25-derived, epsD, Kan^r	This study
pT18C-gp20	pUT18C-derived, gp20, Amp^r	This study
pGEX-4T-1-EpsD	pGEX-4T-1-derived, epsD, Amp^r	This study
pET30a-gp20	pET30a(+)-derived, gp20, Kan^r	This study

VP2-sensitive *V. cholerae* strain N16961 as the recipient to obtain a transposon insertion library. The transposon mutation pool was mixed with a VP2 suspension (10^8 PFU/mL) at a ratio of 1:5 and incubated for 10 min at 37°C. The resulting cultures were spread onto LB agar plates with Kan and Sm. The resistant strains were subsequently verified by double-layer plaque assay as described previously (Frost et al., 1999), and the confirmed nonlysed strains were selected as candidates for verifying transposon insertion location.

Arbitrary PCR (Judson and Mekalanos, 2000) was performed with two rounds to identify the transposon insertion site on the chromosome. In the first round, the chromosomal DNA of candidates was used as amplification templates, and the primers ARB-1, ARB-6, and 123-3 (**Table 2**) were used in amplification. PCR was performed under the following conditions: 95°C for 5 min; six cycles of 94°C for 30 s, 30°C for 30 s, and 72°C for 1 min; 30 cycles of 94°C for 30 s, 55°C for 30 s, and 72°C for 1 min; and 72°C for 5 min. The second round of PCR amplified the PCR product of the first round with the primers 123-4 and ARB-2 (**Table 2**). Amplification conditions were as follows: 30 cycles of 94°C for 30 s, 55°C for 30 s, and 72°C for 1 min, followed by 72°C for 5 min. The amplicons were sequenced using the primer 123-4. The transposon insertion sites were confirmed by comparing the sequencing results with the N16961 reference sequence.

Construction of Gene Deletions and Complementation

In-frame deletions were constructed by cloning the regions flanking target genes into the suicide vector pWM91 containing a *sacB* counterselectable marker (Metcalf et al., 1996). The recombinant plasmid was transformed into the strain SM10λ*pir* and introduced into *V. cholerae* N16961 by conjugation. Double-crossover recombination mutants were selected using 10% sucrose plates at 22°C and confirmed *via* PCR and sequencing. The plasmids overexpressing *epsM* and *epsD* were obtained by cloning the complete *epsM* into a pSRKTc plasmid and *epsD* genes into a pSRKGm plasmid (Khan et al., 2008).

The primers used for the construction are listed in **Table 2**.

VP2 Lysis Assay and Efficiency-of-Plating Assay

A double-agar overlay plaque assay (Korotkov and Sandkvist, 2019) was used to examine the lysis status of VP2 on *V. cholerae*. Briefly, 100 μL of exponential cultures of wild-type and *epsM* and *epsD* deletion mutant strains and their complements were mixed with 0.6% soft agar medium and poured on top of bottom agar. Ten microliters from a phage suspension containing approximately 10^8 PFU was spotted in the middle of the lawn of bacteria, incubated overnight at 37°C and imaged. Each strain experiment was repeated three times. Bacterial strains were considered sensitive to the phage if the degree of lysis was observed as complete clearing. In contrast, bacterial strains were considered resistant if there was no effect of the phage on bacterial growth. When indicated, 500 μM IPTG was included in the medium to induce gene expression.

The efficiency-of-plating (EOP) assay was also conducted to quantitate the lysis ability of VP2 as previously described with some modifications (Yang et al., 2020). In brief, the wild-type strain, *epsM* and *epsD* deletion mutant strains and their

TABLE 2 | Primers used in this study.

Primer	Sequence (5'–3')[a]	Destination
VC2724-UP-XhoI-5'	CCGCTCGAGAGTGGTACCGGTAGCGGTAG	pWM91-ΔepsM
VC2724-UP-3'	CAAGTAAGGAGAACAGCCGCGCGGCGAAATGAT	
VC2724-DOWN-5'	CGCCGCGCGGCTGTTCTCCTTACTTGGGCTTCA	
VC2724-DOWN-NotI-3'	AAGGAAAAAAGCGGCCGCCCAAGAGTGGCGTTATGAGC	
VC2733-UP-XhoI-5'	CCGCTCGAGTGGCCATCACTTTGACCCGT	
VC2733-UP-3'	GTTCCCAGTGAAACAACCAGCTCGCAAGTGGAA	
VC2733-DOWN-5'	TGCGAGCTGGTTGTTTCACTGGGAACTCCCTTG	pWM91-ΔepsD
VC2733-DOWN-NotI-3'	AAGGAAAAAAGCGGCCGCCGACTTGGAGCCCCACGTTA	
123-3	TCACCAACTGGTCCACCTAC	arbitrary PCR
123-4	CGCTCTTGAAGGGAACTATG	
ARB1	GGCCACGCGTCGACTAGTACNNNNNNNNNNGATAT	
ARB6	GGCCACGCGTCGACTAGTACNNNNNNNNNNNACGCC	
ARB2	GGCCACGCGTCGACTAGTAC	
EpsM- NdeI -F	GGAATTCCATATGATGAAAGAATTATTGGCTCCTGTG	pSRKTc-EpsM
EpsM- XbaI -R	GCTCTAGATCAGCCTCCACGCTTCAGTTG	
EpsD-XbaI-F	GCTCTAGACATTGCTTGGCTTCCATCTG	
EpsD-NdeI-R	GGAATTCCATATGAGGGAGTTCCCAGTGAAATA	EpsD
gp20-BamHI-F	CGCGGATCCCATGACTATCCAGAACAAAGAACC	pT18-gp20
gp20-KpnI-R	CGGGGTACCCGAACGTCCGTAAAATACAAGTT	
nT25-EpsD-BamHI-F	CGCGGATCCCAACGAGTTTAGCGCCAGCTTT	pT25-EpsD
nT25-EpsD-KpnI-R	CGGGGTACCCGTTGCTTGGCTTCCATCTGCTCAA	
EpsD-BamHI-F	CGCGGATCCCGCCGTGCGCAAGTGTTGA	pGEX-4T-1-EpsD
EpsD-XhoI-R	CCGCTCGAGTCATTGCTTGGCTTCCATCTGC	
gp20-BamHI-F	CGCGGATCCATGACTATCCAGAACAAAGAA	pET-30a-gp20
gp20-HindIIII-R	CCCAAGCTTTTAAACGTCCGTAAAATACAAG	

[a]Restriction sites are underlined.

complements (10^8 CFU/mL) were mixed with 10^6 PFU/mL concentrated VP2, incubated for 15 min, 10-fold dilutions of the mixtures were prepared with LB. For plating, 100 μl of diluents of the mixtures was add to 4 ml of 0.6% top agar and poured on the bottom agar, and the plate was incubated at 37°C overnight. The EOP value was calculated as the ratio of the number of lysis plaques produced on the bacterial lawn of the target to the number of plaques produced on the lawn of the host strain.

Phage Adsorption Assays

A titer of at least 10^6 PFU/mL concentrated VP2 was mixed separately with different *V. cholerae* variants (10^8 CFU/mL), incubated for 3 min, 5 min and 10 min at 37°C, and then centrifuged at 6,000 rpm for 8 min. The residual phage titers of the supernatant were counted in 10^{-3} dilutions and tested by double-layer plaque assay. Phage without N16961 treatment was used as a control.

Cloning, Expression and Purification of the VP2 Tail Filament Protein and T2SS EpsD

For a bacterial two-hybrid assay, the recombinant plasmids pKT25-*epsD* and pUT18C-gp20 were constructed as previously described (Fan et al., 2018). Briefly, two putative interacting proteins (EpsD and gp20) were genetically fused to two complementary fragments, T25 and T18, of the active domain of adenylate cyclase (CyaA) from *Bordetella pertussis* (Ladant, 1988). First, the *epsD* truncated sequence (lacking the signal peptide, encoding 25-674 aa) and gp20 complete sequence were amplified using the N16961 and VP2 genomes as templates, respectively. The PCR products of *epsD*$_{25-674}$ and gp20 were digested with the *Bam*HI and *Kpn*I restriction enzymes and ligated into the corresponding pKT25 and pUT18C vectors digested with the same enzymes. The resulting plasmids were cotransformed into the *E. coli* Δ*cya* mutant BTH101 for subsequent study. All primers used are included in **Table 2**.

For pull-down assays, the truncated EpsD and complete gp20 genes were subcloned into prokaryotic expression vectors to obtain the corresponding proteins. A gene fragment of *epsD* (encoding 340-675 aa) was cloned into the pGEX-4T-1 vector and introduced into the overexpression strain *E. coli* BL21 (DE3), and protein purification was performed as described previously (Howard et al., 2019). Full-length gp20 was inserted into the pET-30a vector and induced in *E. coli* strain BL21 (DE3). Cells containing the pET-30a-gp20 recombinant plasmid were grown in LB medium until the OD_{600} reached 0.5-0.6, and 0.5 mM IPTG was added to induce expression overnight at 16°C. Cells were harvested, and the pellets were resuspended in buffer A (20 mM Tris-HCl, pH 9.0, 300 mM NaCl, supplemented with protease inhibitors). The cells were lysed by sonication and centrifuged at 12,000 rpm for 30 min at 4°C. The His6-tagged protein gp20 was purified using Ni^{2+} resin (Invitrogen), and the elution samples were dialyzed in buffer B (20 mM Tris-HCl, pH 9.0, 300 mM NaCl) overnight and were used in interaction assays with GST-tagged EpsD. The protein concentration was determined using Pierce's BCA Protein Assay Reagent Kit. All primers and restriction enzymes used are listed in **Table 2**.

Binding Capacity of vp2 Tail Filament Protein With Wild-Type N16961 and N-ΔepsD

We fused gp20 to a His6 tag, mixed it with an Alexa Fluor 488-conjugated anti-His-tag monoclonal antibody, incubated it in the dark at room temperature and resuspended it in filter-sterilized phosphate-buffered saline (PBS). After the unbound antibodies were washed out fully with PBS, they were mixed with wild-type strains and the mutant strain N-Δ*epsD*. Antibodies and no antibodies were added to these two strains as controls. Samples were then analyzed using BD flow cytometry.

Bacterial Two-Hybrid System for Analysis of the EpsD and gp20 Interaction

The *cyaA* mutant *E. coli* BTH101 strain containing pKT25-*epsD* and pUT18C-gp20 was cultured overnight and then subcultured to log phase in LB medium with shaking at 220 rpm at 37°C. The β-galactosidase activities were measured in the presence of different concentrations of isopropyl-beta-D-thiogalactopyranoside (IPTG) as the inducer as previously described (Yang et al., 2013). The leucine zipper of GCN4 (Karimova et al., 1998) was used as a positive control.

Ni²⁺-Affinity Pull-Down of gp20 and EpsD

Mixtures of 0.3 mg of His6-tagged gp20 protein and 0.1 mg of GST-tagged EpsD protein were rotated at room temperature for 2 h, bound to Ni^{2+} resin and incubated for 1 h at 4°C. Mixtures of His6-tagged gp20 protein and GST protein were used as negative controls.

The Ni^{2+} resin was washed extensively to remove nonspecifically bound proteins, and then the bound proteins were eluted with elution buffer containing 300 mM imidazole, 10 mM Tris-HCl and 500 mM NaCl (pH 8.0). Five micrograms of each sample were submitted to 12% SDS-PAGE and Western blot analysis. Unless otherwise noted, all samples were boiled for 10 min in SDS loading buffer before separation. After electrophoresis, proteins on the gels were transferred to PVDF membranes (Immobilon-P, Millipore). Both mouse anti-GST and anti-His6 tag monoclonal antibodies (Tiangen Biotech, Beijing) were used in the Western blot analysis. An anti-mouse peroxidase-conjugated AffiniPure IgG (H+L) secondary antibody (Zhong Shan Jin Qiao, Beijing) was used for protein detection.

RESULTS AND DISCUSSION

Components of the Type II Secretion System Were Involved in VP2 Infection

To identify *V. cholerae* genes related to the resistance to VP2 infection phenotype, a selection strategy of phage-resistant mutants generated by transposon insertion was used. The pool of transposon mutants from the VP2-sensitive strain N16961 was generated by conjugation with SM10-123 carrying the plasmid pSC123. Then, the phage VP2 was added into this pool to lyse the mutant cells sensitive to VP2 infection, whereas the mutants resistant to VP2 survived. Possible resistant colonies were selected on agar and further confirmed for resistance to VP2 infection with double-layer agar. Eighteen candidates resistant to VP2 were collected. Each candidate was amplified through arbitrary PCR, and the amplicon was sequenced to verify the transposon location on the chromosome of the resistant strains. A total of six different insertion sites were identified, including in the coding sequences of the genes VCA0904 (H+/gluconate symporter and related permease), VC1936 (phosphatidate cytidylyltransferase), VC0718 (DNA recombination-dependent growth factor C), VC0420 (conserved hypothetical protein CHP02099), VCA0863 (lipase, Pla-1/cef, extracellular), and VC2724 (EpsM). Among these genes, VC2724 is located in the gene cluster of the T2SS, correspondingly coding for the inner membrane protein EpsM, which is located in the membrane (**Figure 1A**). For the phage receptor identification purpose of this study, we first selected the membrane-located protein EpsM as a candidate.

We further constructed the mutant strain N-ΔepsM with in-frame deletion of *epsM* from the wild-type strain N16961 and the complement strain N-ΔepsM-C carrying the intact *epsM* gene in the pSRKTc plasmid (**Table 2**). Phage lysis assays with both strains showed that N-ΔepsM was not lysed by VP2 (**Figure 1B**), whereas the strain N-ΔepsM-C carrying complementary *epsM* restored the sensitivity to VP2 (**Figure 1B**). EOP assay was consistent with the phage lysis assays (**Figure 1B**). Both assays showed that the *V. cholerae* T2SS protein EpsM is needed for VP2 infection.

The Outer Membrane-Localized Protein EpsD of T2SS Could Adsorb VP2

T2SS is a cell envelope-spanning macromolecular complex that is prevalent in gram-negative bacterial species and serves as the predominant virulence mechanism of many bacteria (Johnson et al., 2006). The system is composed of a core set of highly conserved proteins that assemble an inner membrane platform, a periplasmic pseudopilus and an outer membrane complex termed the secretin (Johnson et al., 2006). The model of the T2SS machine includes an outer membrane protein, the secretin EpsD, the first subdomain of which is related to domains in phage tail filament proteins and outer membrane TonB-dependent receptors (Johnson et al., 2006). We suspected that EpsD might be involved in the interaction of *V. cholerae* with the phage VP2. Subsequently, we constructed the *epsD* deletion strain N-ΔepsD and the complementary strain N-ΔepsD-C (containing intact *epsD* in the plasmid pSRK-Gm) to determine their sensitivities to phage VP2. VP2 infection assays showed that the *epsD* mutant strain could not be lysed by VP2, while the strain N-ΔepsD-C could be lysed (**Figure 1B**), showing the important role of EpsD in VP2 infection; therefore, it could be expected that EpsD possibly acts as the receptor for VP2.

The role of EpsD in VP2 infection was also determined by phage adsorption assays to detect the binding ability of the phage VP2 to the *epsD* and *epsM* mutant strains and their corresponding complementary strains. VP2 particles were mixed with the wild-type strain N16961 for 3 min, and after centrifugation, the remaining supernatant had a much lower phage titer than the control, which was determined by a PFU assay (**Figure 2**), showing that the sensitive strain N16961 had strong adsorption of VP2.

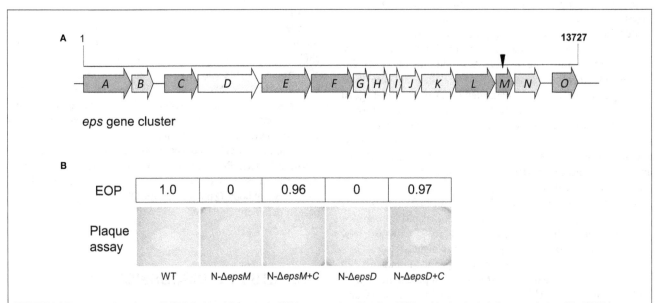

FIGURE 1 | Transposon insertion and VP2 infection of the mutants. **(A)** Transposon insertion site of VP2-resistant mutants in the gene cluster of the T2SS in N16961. The *eps* genes are colored according to the classification of functions and positions of the proteins in T2SS in *V. cholerae* (Korotkov et al., 2012), including inner-membrane plateform proteins (light blue), outer-membrane secretin (yellow), pseudopilin (light green), others (light brown) and unknown (grey). The black arrow represents the site where the transposon was inserted into the *epsM*. **(B)** Detection of VP2 infection in *V. cholerae* mutants by double-layer plaque assay and EOP assay. The wild-type *V. cholerae* El Tor strain N16961 was used as the control for plaque formation. N-ΔepsM showed VP2 resistance (no plaque formation). The strain ΔepsM-C, carrying the EpsM expression plasmid cloned into the strain N-ΔepsM, was sensitive to VP2. N-ΔepsD showed VP2 resistance (no plaque formation). The strain ΔepsD-C, carrying the EpsD expression plasmid cloned into the strain N-ΔepsD, was sensitive to VP2. The values of EOP were shown in the top half of the figure.

The Type II Secretory System Mediates Phage Infection in Vibrio cholerae

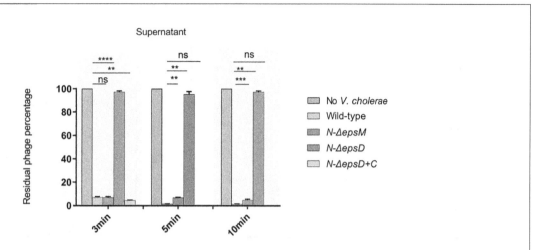

FIGURE 2 | VP2 adsorption by the wild-type strain N16961 and its mutants. The VP2 phage (10^6 CFU/mL) was mixed with fresh N16961 culture, N-$\Delta epsM$, N-$\Delta epsD$, N-$\Delta epsD$+C (10^8 CFU/mL) respectively for 3 min, 5min,10 min at 37°C, and then, each sample was centrifuged at 6000 rpm for 8 min. LB culture medium containing only VP2 phage was used as a negative control, and the phage titer in the control supernatant was set to 100%. The experiment was repeated three times. The mean of three independent assays was shown and error bars represent the standard deviation. **P =0.0026, ***P = 0.0001, ****P <0.0001, ns, no significance (Student's t test).

When VP2 was mixed with the strain N-$\Delta epsD$, its obvious VP2 titer difference in the supernatant was found when compared to the sensitive strain N16961 (**Figure 2**), indicating that VP2 did not bind to the *epsD* mutant. Such adsorption could be restored by complementing the plasmid carrying intact *epsD* into N-$\Delta epsD$ (strain N-$\Delta epsD$-C, **Figure 2**). The VP2 adsorption efficiency of the *epsM* deletion strain N-$\Delta epsM$ was similar to that of the wild-type strain N16961. These data suggested that EpsD could adsorb VP2 but EpsM could not, which could be explained by their different membrane locations in the T2SS apparatus in *V. cholerae*.

VP2 Adsorbed to EpsD of *V. cholerae* Through Its Tail Fiber Protein gp20

The genome of VP2 has been sequenced previously in our laboratory (GenBank accession number: NC_005879). Here, we submitted the VP2 genome sequence to RAST (http://rast.nmpdr.org/rast.cgi) for the prediction of open reading frames (ORFs). The ORF *gp20* was predicted as the phage tail fiber protein gene, and then we expressed this protein as the ligand to detect its interaction with *V. cholerae*. To observe the binding ability of gp20 to the wild-type strain N16961 and N-$\Delta epsD$, the expressed His6-tagged gp20 was labeled with an anti-His6 fluorescent antibody, mixed with the wild-type strain N16961 and mutant strain N-$\Delta epsD$, and then analyzed using flow cytometry to measure the geometric mean fluorescence intensity (MFI). The MFI in the tests of the His6-tagged gp20/N16961 mixture was much higher than that of the His6-tagged gp20/N-$\Delta epsD$, and the MFI of the latter was similar to that of the controls, representing the background fluorescence intensity, as shown in **Figure 3**, which indicated that no gp20 adsorbed to the *epsD* deletion mutant.

The VP2 Tail Protein gp20 Interacted Directly With EpsD

To determine the possible interaction between *V. cholerae* EpsD and gp20 of VP2, we performed mutual interaction assays

between these two proteins by using a bacterial two-hybrid (BACTH) approach (Karimova et al., 1998). In this study, the recombinant plasmids pKT25-*epsD* and pUT18C-gp20 were constructed and co-transformed into the *E. coli* Δcya mutant BTH101. The results showed that 0.5 mM IPTG could induce the maximum β-galactosidase activity, similar to that of 1.0 mM IPTG induction and the positive control (**Figure 4A**), suggesting that EpsD could interact with gp20.

In addition, pull-down assays were carried out to detect the interaction between gp20 and EpsD. His-tagged gp20 was immobilized on Ni2+ resin to capture GST-tagged EpsD. In the elution buffer, GST-tagged EpsD could be detected by Western blot (**Figure 4B**), further showing that gp20 can bind directly to EpsD.

Overall, we demonstrated that in *V. cholerae*, the outer membrane protein EpsD of T2SS acts as the receptor in phage VP2 infection. As an important secretion apparatus, T2SSs are widespread among gram-negative bacteria and contribute to pathogenesis in the host and environmental survival (Cianciotto and White, 2017; Korotkov and Sandkvist, 2019). The T2SS transports chitinase, lipase, hemagglutinin/protease and other proteases in some bacteria (Sandkvist, 2001; Evans et al., 2008; Sikora et al., 2011). *V. cholerae* may secrete cholera toxin (Sikora et al., 2011) and even mediate the release of the filamentous phage CTXΦ through EpsD (Davis et al., 2000). In *E. coli*, the membrane protein PulD of the T2SS contributes to phage extrusion across the membrane and assembly of phages (Genin and Boucher, 1994; Russel, 1998; Sandkvist, 2001). In our study, in addition to these roles of T2SS, we showed that it may mediate lytic phage infection by the specific adsorption of VP2 to the outer membrane component EpsD. EpsM is a part of the interface between the regulating part and the rest Eps proteins of the T2SS (Abendroth et al., 2004). Combined with the dot assays and the phage adsorption assays, the inner membrane protein

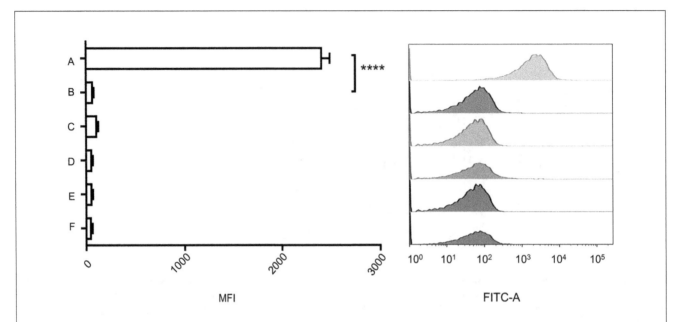

FIGURE 3 | Binding capacity of the vp2 tail filament protein with wild-type N16961 and N-Δ*epsD*. (A): Wild type+ His6-tagged gp20+anti-His6 tag antibody; (B): N-Δ*epsD* + His6-tagged gp20+anti-His6 tag antibody; (C): wild type +anti-His6 tag antibody; (D): N-Δ*epsD* +anti-His6 tag antibody; (E): wild type; (F): N-Δ*epsD*. Ten micrograms of His6-tagged gp20 protein and 10 μg of Alexa Fluor 488-conjugated anti-His-tag monoclonal antibody (product # MA1-21315-A488) were mixed and incubated for 30 min in the dark at room temperature and then transferred to the wild-type N16961 and N-Δ*epsD* strains, with OD600 = 1. After induction at 37°C, induced cultures were washed twice with 1 mL of filter-sterilized PBS. Antibodies and no antibodies were added to these two strains as controls. Samples were analyzed using BD flow cytometry. The data shown on the left represent the geometric MFI. The data shown on the right represent the fluorescence intensity distribution of the bacteria analyzed in the experiment shown on the left. The mean of three independent assays is shown and error bars represent the standard deviation. ****P <0.0001 (Student's *t* test).

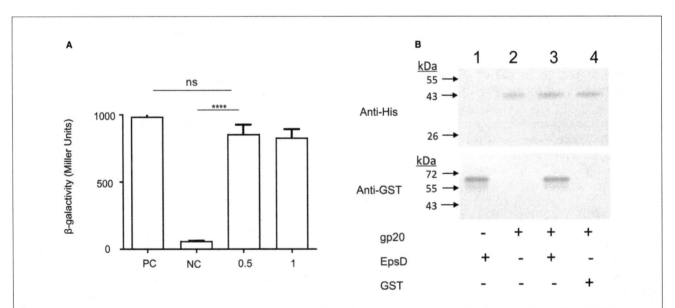

FIGURE 4 | Binding capacity of the VP2 tail filament protein with wild-type N16961 and N-Δ*epsD*, and analysis of the interactions of EpsD with gp20. **(A)** Analysis the gp20-EpsD interaction by BACTH. PC, positive control (leucine zipper of GCN4); NC, negative control (vector plasmid only). The resulting recombinant plasmid pair pT25-gp20/pT18C-EpsD was co-transformed into BTH101 cells, and the β-galactosidase activity was measured. ****P <0.0001. ns, no significance. (Student's *t* test). **(B)** Analysis of the interactions of EpsD with gp20 *in vitro*. Western blot analysis of His pull-down experiments was performed with GST-gp20 immobilized on Ni²⁺ resin, and the gp20 protein was incubated with GST for pull-down analysis as a negative control 0.3 mg of His6-tagged gp20 protein and 0.1 mg of GST-tagged EpsD protein were mixed, then the mixtures were rotated at room temperature for 2 h, bound to Ni2+ resin and incubated for 1 h at 4°C. Lane 1: His-gp20; 2: GST-EpsD; 3: Pull-down of His-gp20 and GST-EpsD; 4 Pull-down of His-gp20 + GST.

EpsM of T2SS plays a role in successful VP2 infection but does not affect VP2 binding to the host, suggesting that the intact T2SS structure probably acts as the phage DNA injection channel for crossing the outer and inner membranes of *V. cholerae*. The function of T2SS EpsD as a phage receptor has not been reported previously. Therefore, based on our study, the role of the T2SS in *V. cholerae* is expanded to the infection channel of the lytic phage, in addition to the transport of free proteins and release of filamentous phages.

REFERENCES

Abendroth, J., Rice, A. E., McLuskey, K., Bagdasarian, M., and Hol, W. G. (2004). The crystal structure of the periplasmic domain of the type II secretion system protein EpsM from Vibrio cholerae: the simplest version of the ferredoxin fold. *J. Mol. Biol.* 338 (3), 585–596. doi: 10.1016/j.jmb.2004.01.064

Bertozzi Silva, J., Storms, Z., and Sauvageau, D. (2016). Host receptors for bacteriophage adsorption. *FEMS Microbiol. Lett.* 363 (4), fnw002. doi: 10.1093/femsle/fnw002

Chiang, S. L., and Mekalanos, J. J. (2000). Construction of a *Vibrio cholerae* vaccine candidate using transposon delivery and FLP recombinase-mediated excision. *Infect. Immun.* 68 (11), 6391–6397. doi: 10.1128/iai.68.11.6391-6397.2000

Cianciotto, N. P., and White, R. C. (2017). Expanding Role of Type II Secretion in Bacterial Pathogenesis and Beyond. *Infect. Immun.* 85 (5), e00014–17. doi: 10.1128/IAI.00014-17

Davis, B. M., Lawson, E. H., Sandkvist, M., Ali, A., Sozhamannan, S., and Waldor, M. K. (2000). Convergence of the secretory pathways for cholera toxin and the filamentous phage, CTXphi. *Science* 288 (5464), 333–335. doi: 10.1126/science.288.5464.333

Evans, F. F., Egan, S., and Kjelleberg, S. (2008). Ecology of type II secretion in marine *gammaproteobacteria*. *Environ. Microbiol.* 10 (5), 1101–1107. doi: 10.1111/j.1462-2920.2007.01545.x

Fan, F. X., Li, X., Pang, B., Zhang, C., Li, Z., Zhang, L. J., et al. (2018). The outer-membrane protein TolC of Vibrio cholerae serves as a second cell-surface receptor for the VP3 phage. *J. Biol. Chem.* 293 (11), 4000–4013. doi: 10.1074/jbc.M117.805689

Faruque, S. M., Albert, M. J., and Mekalanos, J. J. (1998). Epidemiology, genetics, and ecology of toxigenic *Vibrio cholerae*. *Microbiol. Mol. Biol. Rev.* 62 (4), 1301–1314. doi: 10.1128/MMBR.62.4.1301-1314.1998

Faruque, S. M., Islam, M. J., Ahmad, Q. S., Faruque, A. S., Sack, D. A., Nair, G. B., et al. (2005). Self-limiting nature of seasonal cholera epidemics: Role of host-mediated amplification of phage. *Proc. Natl. Acad. Sci. U. S. A.* 102 (17), 6119–6124. doi: 10.1073/pnas.0502069102

Frost, J. A., Kramer, J. M., and Gillanders, S. A. (1999). Phage typing of *Campylobacter jejuni* and *Campylobacter coli* and its use as an adjunct to serotyping. *Epidemiol. Infect.* 123 (1), 47–55. doi: 10.1017/s095026889900254x

Genin, S., and Boucher, C. A. (1994). A superfamily of proteins involved in different secretion pathways in gram-negative bacteria: modular structure and specificity of the N-terminal domain. *Mol. Gen. Genet.* 243 (1), 112–118. doi: 10.1007/BF00283883

Harvey, H., Bondy-Denomy, J., Marquis, H., Sztanko, K. M., Davidson, A. R., and Burrows, L. L. (2018). *Pseudomonas aeruginosa* defends against phages through type IV pilus glycosylation. *Nat. Microbiol.* 3 (1), 47–52. doi: 10.1038/s41564-017-0061-y

Hatfull, G. F., and Hendrix, R. W. (2011). Bacteriophages and their genomes. *Curr. Opin. Virol.* 1 (4), 298–303. doi: 10.1016/j.coviro.2011.06.009

Howard, S. P., Estrozi, L. F., Bertrand, Q., Contreras-Martel, C., Strozen, T., Job, V., et al. (2019). Structure and assembly of pilotin-dependent and independent secretins of the type II secretion system. *PLoS Pathog.* 15 (5), e1007731. doi: 10.1371/journal.ppat.1007731

Jensen, M. A., Faruque, S. M., Mekalanos, J. J., and Levin, B. R. (2006). Modeling the role of bacteriophage in the control of cholera outbreaks. *Proc. Natl. Acad. Sci. U. S. A.* 103 (12), 4652–4657. doi: 10.1073/pnas.0600166103

AUTHOR CONTRIBUTIONS

BK, HS and ML designed the study and wrote the paper. FF, ZheL and YF purified protein and performed the experiments. JZ, ZheL, and JX provided technical assistance and contributed to the preparation of the figures. JL cryopreserved and saved the strains. YH contributed to diagram modification and protein purification in the process of article modification. All authors contributed to the article and approved the submitted version.

Johnson, T. L., Abendroth, J., Hol, W. G., and Sandkvist, M. (2006). Type II secretion: from structure to function. *FEMS Microbiol. Lett.* 255 (2), 175–186. doi: 10.1111/j.1574-6968.2006.00102.x

Judson, N., and Mekalanos, J. J. (2000). TnAraOut, a transposon-based approach to identify and characterize essential bacterial genes. *Nat. Biotechnol.* 18 (7), 740–745. doi: 10.1038/77305

Karimova, G., Pidoux, J., Ullmann, A., and Ladant, D. (1998). A bacterial two-hybrid system based on a reconstituted signal transduction pathway. *Proc. Natl. Acad. Sci. U. S. A.* 95 (10), 5752–5756. doi: 10.1073/pnas.95.10.5752

Kazmierczak, Z., Gorski, A., and Dabrowska, K. (2014). Facing antibiotic resistance: *Staphylococcus aureus* phages as a medical tool. *Viruses* 6 (7), 2551–2570. doi: 10.3390/v6072551

Khan, S. R., Gaines, J., Roop, R. M., and Farrand, S. K. (2008). Broad-host-range expression vectors with tightly regulated promoters and their use to examine the influence of TraR and TraM expression on Ti plasmid quorum sensing. *Appl. Environ. Microbiol.* 74 (16), 5053–5062. doi: 10.1128/Aem.01098-08

Korotkov, K. V., and Sandkvist, M. (2019). Architecture, Function, and Substrates of the Type II Secretion System. *EcoSal. Plus.* 8 (2). doi: 10.1128/ecosalplus.ESP-0034-2018

Korotkov, K. V., Sandkvist, M., and Hol, W. G. (2012). The type II secretion system: biogenesis, molecular architecture and mechanism. *Nat. Rev. Microbiol.* 10 (5), 336–351. doi: 10.1038/nrmicro2762

Ladant, D. (1988). Interaction of *Bordetella pertussis* adenylate cyclase with calmodulin. Identification of two separated calmodulin-binding domains. *J. Biol. Chem.* 263 (6), 2612–2618.

Liu, Z., Wang, H., Zhou, Z., Naseer, N., Xiang, F., Kan, B., et al. (2016). Differential Thiol-Based Switches Jump-Start *Vibrio cholerae* Pathogenesis. *Cell Rep.* 14 (2), 347–354. doi: 10.1016/j.celrep.2015.12.038

McCutcheon, J. G., Peters, D. L., and Dennis, J. J. (2018). Identification and Characterization of Type IV Pili as the Cellular Receptor of Broad Host Range *Stenotrophomonas maltophilia* Bacteriophages DLP1 and DLP2. *Viruses* 10 (6). doi: 10.3390/v10060338

Metcalf, W. W., Jiang, W., Daniels, L. L., Kim, S. K., Haldimann, A., and Wanner, B. L. (1996). Conditionally replicative and conjugative plasmids carrying lacZ alpha for cloning, mutagenesis, and allele replacement in bacteria. *Plasmid* 35 (1), 1–13. doi: 10.1006/plas.1996.0001

Rakhuba, D. V., Kolomiets, E. I., Dey, E. S., and Novik, G. I. (2010). Bacteriophage receptors, mechanisms of phage adsorption and penetration into host cell. *Pol. J. Microbiol.* 59 (3), 145–155. doi: 10.33073/pjm-2010-023

Reidl, J., and Klose, K. E. (2002). *Vibrio cholerae and* cholera: out of the water and into the host. *FEMS Microbiol. Rev.* 26 (2), 125–139. doi: 10.1111/j.1574-6976.2002.tb00605.x

Russel, M. (1998). Macromolecular assembly and secretion across the bacterial cell envelope: type II protein secretion systems. *J. Mol. Biol.* 279 (3), 485–499. doi: 10.1006/jmbi.1998.1791

Sack, D. A., Sack, R. B., Nair, G. B., and Siddique, A. K. (2004). Cholera. *Lancet* 363 (9404), 223–233. doi: 10.1016/s0140-6736(03)15328-7

Salmond, G. P., and Fineran, P. C. (2015). A century of the phage: past, present and future. *Nat. Rev. Microbiol.* 13 (12), 777–786. doi: 10.1038/nrmicro3564

Sandkvist, M. (2001). Type II secretion and pathogenesis. *Infect. Immun.* 69 (6), 3523–3535. doi: 10.1128/IAI.69.6.3523-3535.2001

Sikora, A. E., Zielke, R. A., Lawrence, D. A., Andrews, P. C., and Sandkvist, M. (2011). Proteomic analysis of the *Vibrio cholerae* type II secretome reveals new proteins, including three related serine proteases. *J. Biol. Chem.* 286 (19), 16555–16566. doi: 10.1074/jbc.M110.211078

Simon, R., Priefer, U., and Pühler, A. (1983). A broad host range mobilization system *for in vivo* genetic engineering: transposon mutagenesis in gramnegative bacteria. *Nat. Biotechnol.* 31 (5), 784–791. doi: 10.1038/nbt1183-784

Weil, A. A., and Ryan, E. T. (2018). Cholera: recent updates. *Curr. Opin. Infect. Dis.* 31 (5), 455–461. doi: 10.1097/QCO.0000000000000474

Yang, M., Liu, Z., Hughes, C., Stern, A. M., Wang, H., Zhong, Z., et al. (2013). Bile salt-induced intermolecular disulfide bond formation activates *Vibrio cholerae* virulence. *Proc. Natl. Acad. Sci. U. S. A.* 110 (6), 2348–2353. doi: 10.1073/pnas.1218039110

Yang, Y., Shen, W., Zhong, Q., Chen, Q., He, X., Baker, J. L., et al. (2020). Development of a Bacteriophage Cocktail to Constrain the Emergence of Phage-Resistant Pseudomonas aeruginosa. *Front. Microbiol.* 11, 327. doi: 10.3389/fmicb.2020.00327

Zhang, J., Li, W., Zhang, Q., Wang, H., Xu, X., Diao, B., et al. (2009). The core oligosaccharide and thioredoxin of *Vibrio cholerae* are necessary for binding and propagation of its typing phage VP3. *J. Bacteriol.* 191 (8), 2622–2629. doi: 10.1128/JB.01370-08

17

Inhalation of Immuno-Therapeutics/-Prophylactics to Fight Respiratory Tract Infections: An Appropriate Drug at the Right Place!

Thomas Sécher[1,2†], Alexie Mayor[1,2†] and Nathalie Heuzé-Vourc'h[1,2]*

[1] INSERM U1100, Centre d'Etude des Pathologies Respiratoires, Tours, France, [2] Centre d'Etude des Pathologies Respiratoires, Université de Tours, Tours, France

Keywords: respiratory infection, biopharmaceutics, immune-pharmaceutics, topical delivery, inhalation

Correspondence:
Nathalie Heuzé-Vourc'h
nathalie.vourch@med.univ-tours.fr

[†] *These authors have contributed equally to this work*

INTRODUCTION

Respiratory tract infections (RTIs) are the third leading cause of morbidity and mortality worldwide, accounting for ~4.25 million deaths in 2010, in either children, adults or the elderlies. RTIs encompass acute infections of the upper (rhinosinusitis, …) and lower airways (pneumonia, bronchiolitis, …) and are also inherently associated with chronic diseases such as chronic obstructive pulmonary disease (COPD) and cystic fibrosis (CF). In addition to premature mortality, RTIs result in a huge burden on the society considering quality-adjusted life year loss and additional pressure on the overwhelmed healthcare systems, thereby representing a major public health issue.

Antimicrobial chemotherapies (e.g., antibiotics, antivirals) are the standard interventions to prevent and to treat respiratory infections. However, their effectiveness is declining due to increased pathogen resistance, urging alternative or complementary strategies to reinforce the anti-infectious arsenal to fight RTIs. Among those under evaluation, immunomodulatory agents (immunopharmaceutics) like therapeutic antibodies (Ab) or other therapeutic proteins and vaccines may offer novel opportunities for the prevention and treatment of RTIs, by targeting pathogens and boosting the host immune system. When used in a preventive way in patients at risk, or therapeutically to stop or to limit the spread of infection, both immunopropylactics and immunotherapeutics are administered through parenteral routes (including intravenous, subcutaneous, and intramuscular) (**Table 1**). As demonstrated in preclinical studies, parenteral delivery may not be optimal for large molecular weight entities to treat respiratory diseases (1, 2) since they poorly reach the lung compartment. In contrast, inhalation, comprising the intranasal and oral respiratory routes, targets drugs into the respiratory tract. Currently, inhalation is used both for locally- and systemically-acting drugs as it allows a straight delivery to the diseased organ and a portal to the blood circulation, considering the extensive alveolus-capillary interface. By providing a better therapeutic index, inhalation is the gold standard for small molecules, delivered topically as an aerosol, like corticosteroids/steroids, decongestants or bronchodilators for the treatment of asthma, rhinosinusitis or COPD. Besides, it is also indicated for antibiotics (nasal and oral inhalation), a local-acting protein therapeutic—Dornase alpha (Pulmozyme®, oral inhalation), a mucolytic agent for patients with CF and an influenza live vaccine (FluMist® Quadrivalent, nasal inhalation).

LOCAL-ACTING IMMUNOPHARMACEUTICS DELIVERED BY INHALATION

There are accumulating evidences that administration of anti-infectious Abs, protein therapeutics (e.g., cytokines) and vaccines, to the upper and/or lower respiratory tract by inhalation, with the purpose of inducing a local action, is effective (3). Several preclinical studies showed the superiority of immunopharmaceutics administered topically to the respiratory tract in RTI models, in both therapeutic and prophylactic regimens. For instance, inhalation of anti-infectious Abs in models of pneumonia using *Pseudomonas aeruginosa* or influenza virus conferred higher protection and greater therapeutic response, respectively, compared to parenteral route administration (4, 5). Besides, other immunoprophylactics delivered through the respiratory route such as immunocytokines (e.g., IL-7 Fc) (6) and live-attenuated vaccines (7) showed superior performances over conventional routes against airborne viruses, in mice and non-human primates, respectively. Conversely, restricting the response to the site of action for pleiotropic molecules (e.g., IL-7 Fc), envisioned as adjuvant molecule, may reduce systemic side-effects. As reported for anti-infectious Abs, the inhaled route may also enable a higher efficacy with a lower dose (4). This means that the inhaled route may allow, in the future, to alleviate the financial burden of immunopharmaceutics (in particular Abs), which may exceed the ability of both individual patients and the healthcare systems to sustain them. Additional benefit of the inhaled route includes its non-invasiveness, offering a better comfort for patients, in particular those with chronic respiratory infections, and thus preventing additional healthcare costs. Besides, needle-free vaccination may prevent the risk of cross-contamination and facilitate mass vaccination efforts.

However, beyond clear preclinical proofs of concept and obvious theoretical advantages of the inhalation route for immunotherapeutics and -prophylactics, few of these benefits have materialized in the clinic (**Table 1**). Except for Flumist® Quadrivalent (Astrazeneca), an intranasal live attenuated influenza vaccine, other marketed immunoprophylactics vaccines (including those against *Streptococcus pneumoniae*, *Haemophilus influenza*, *Mycobacterium tuberculosis*, *Bordetella pertussis* or measles and Ab (anti-RSV Pavilizumab)—are administered systemically. Similarly, none of the protein therapeutics is given by inhalation. Recently, Ablynx developed an inhaled anti-RSV trimeric nanobody® (ALX-0171) for therapeutic purposes. Despite promising results in several animal models, the development has been interrupted due to insufficient evidences of efficacy during Phase 2 trial in children (in Japan). In 2019, only one phase 2 trial with an inhaled anti-infectious protein therapeutics is still ongoing (NCT03570359) assessing the efficacy of topical lung delivery of IFN-β1a (SNG001, Synairgen/Astrazeneca), as an immunostimulant to treat COPD exacerbations. Overall, this highlights the complexity of developing inhaled biopharmaceuticals and points out the persisting hurdles (**Figure 1**).

CHALLENGES FOR THE DEVELOPMENT OF INHALED IMMUNE-THERAPEUTICS/PROPHYLACTICS

The instability of immunopharmaceutics and vaccines often emerges as a challenge for inhalation delivery. Therapeutic

proteins and vaccines are sensitive to various conditions which may alter their structure, thereby decrease their activity. Delivering a drug through the inhalation route implies either spraying, drying or aerosolizing, which is associated with multiple stresses (shearing, temperature, air/liquid interface, ...) potentially deleterious as widely discussed elsewhere (8, 9). To deal with this, both the device used for the generation of the aerosol and the formulation must be adapted, as successfully reported for Ab-based therapeutics (3, 10). However, the excipients must be adapted for respiratory delivery. The choice of mucosal-licensed adjuvants, which should be exempt of intrinsic immune-toxicity, and the instability of the associated carrier [e.g., nanoparticles, liposomes, immune stimulating complexes (ISCOMs)] is particularly challenging for the inhalation delivery of vaccines, especially those of the latest generation (e.g., T, B-epitope-based vaccines). The drug and device combination yields proper aerodynamical properties (particle size, flow rate, ...) to achieve the anticipated deposition in the appropriate area of the respiratory tract. Indeed, appropriate deposition to the anatomical site is mandatory to ensure an optimal efficacy. On one hand, this depends on the drug formulation (e.g., surface tension and viscosity for liquid formulation) (11) and device performances to allow the therapeutic agent to reach the site of infection (**Figure 1**), by this means the microbe. For lung infections, most pneumonia consists of an aggregate of trachea-bronchitis and alveolar infections. Theoretically, this clinical condition may benefit from a uniform distribution all over the lungs, with a polydisperse aerosol (ranging 1–5 μm). However, several pathogens are associated with specific anatomic localization, like *S. pneumoniae,* which is mainly found in the alveolar spaces, thereby requiring low-size aerosols (<2–3 μm) to be targeted. On the other hand, delivery to the mucosal-associated lymphoid tissue (MALT), located in the tonsils, would be more adapted for vaccines to induce an adaptive immune response, since MALT plays a central role in the primary respiratory immune defense (**Figure 1**).

Biological barriers are additional hurdles to overcome and apply to all inhaled anti-infectious agents (12). First, a pathogen can "hide" itself inside host cells like *M. tuberculosis* in alveolar macrophages, thus being more difficult to be targeted by immunopharmaceutics. Other pathogens may produce extracellular barriers like the biofilm matrix produced by *P. aeruginosa* in the context of chronic lung infections. This biofilm acts as a diffusion barrier, preventing inhaled immunopharmaceutics from reaching their molecular target. Antibody-based fragments, such as fragment antigen-binding (Fab) and single-chain variable fragments (scFv) might be more efficient in crossing over the biofilm, like they penetrate better solid tumors (13), and eradicate *P. aeruginosa*. Secondly, the host physical defenses, which prevent foreign particles from penetrating into the respiratory tract, may limit the accessibility of inhaled immunopharmaceutics to their target. Among them, the mucus and the mucociliary escalator are highly efficient clearance mechanisms (14, 15). The development of mucoadhesive formulations may be helpful to enhance the bioavailability of inhaled drugs (16). In contrast, anti-adhesive molecules, such as polyethylene glycol may facilitate

TABLE 1 | Marketed immunotherapeutics and immunoprophylactics for infectious diseases.

Target	Product	Category	Sponsors	Administration route	Date of approval	Indication
RSV	Synagis	Monoclonal antibody	MedImmune	IM	1998	Prophylaxis
Influenza	Afluria	Inactivated vaccine Quadrivalent	Seqirus	IM	2007	Prophylaxis
	Fluad	Inactivated vaccine Trivalent	Seqirus	IM	2015	Prophylaxis
	Fluarix	Inactivated vaccine Quadrivalent	GSK	IM	2012	Prophylaxis
	Flublok	Recombinant vaccine Quadrivalent	Protein Sciences Corporation	IM	2013	Prophylaxis
	Flucelvax	Inactivated vaccine Quadrivalent	Seqirus	IM	2012	Prophylaxis
	Pandemic influenza vaccine H5N1	Recombinant vaccine	Medimmune	IN	2016	Prophylaxis
	FluLaval	Inactivated vaccine Quadrivalent	ID Biomedical Corporation of Quebec	IM	2013	Prophylaxis
	FluMist	Live-attenuated vaccine Quadrivalent	MedImmune	IN	2003	Prophylaxis
	Fluzone High Dose	Inactivated vaccine Quadrivalent	Sanofi Pasteur	IM	2014	Prophylaxis
	Fluzone	Inactivated vaccine Quadrivalent	Sanofi Pasteur	IM	2009	Prophylaxis
	Fluvirin	Inactivated vaccine Trivalent	Seqirus	IM	1988	Prophylaxis
Measle	Proquad	Subunit vaccine	Merck	SC	2005	Prophylaxis
	M-M-R II	Subunit vaccine	Merck	SC	2014	Prophylaxis
Smallpox	ACAM2000	Live vaccina virus	Emergent Product Development	Percutaneous	2007	Prophylaxis
Mycobacterium tuberculosis	BCG Vaccine	Live-attenuated vaccine	Organon	Percutaneous	2011	Prophylaxis
Streptococcus pneumoniae	Pneumovax 23	Subunit vaccine	Merck&Co	IM	1983	Prophylaxis
	Prevenar 13	Subunit vaccine	Wyeth Pharmaceuticals	IM	2010	Prophylaxis
Bordetella pertussis	Daptacel	Subunit vaccine	Sanofi Pasteur	IM	2008	Prophylaxis
	Pediarix	Subunit vaccine	GSK	IM	2002	Prophylaxis
	Kinrix	Subunit vaccine	GSK	IM	2008	Prophylaxis
	Quadracel	Subunit vaccine	Sanofi Pasteur	IM	2015	Prophylaxis
	Pentacel	Subunit vaccine	Sanofi Pasteur	IM	2008	Prophylaxis
Haemophilus influenzae	Hiberix	Subunit vaccine	GSK	IM	2009	Prophylaxis
	ActHIB	Subunit vaccine	Sanofi Pasteur	IM	1993	Prophylaxis
	PedvaxHIB	Subunit vaccine	Merck	IM	1989	Prophylaxis
Bordetella pertussis Haemophilus influenzae	Infanrix	Subunit vaccine	GSK	IM	1997	Prophylaxis
	Vaxelis	Subunit vaccine	MCM Vaccine	IM	2018	Prophylaxis
Bacillus anthracis	Anthim	Monoclonal antibody	Elusys Therapeutics	IV	2016	Prophylaxis/Therapy
	Abthrax	Monoclonal antibody	GSK	IV	2012	Prophylaxis/Therapy
	Biothrax	Subunit vaccine	Emergent BioSolutions	IM	2016	Prophylaxis

IM, intramuscular; IN, inhalation (nasal); SC, subcutaneous.

immunopharmaceutics translocation through the mucus blanket, as shown *in vitro* (17) and *in vivo* (18) for other applications. It is noteworthy that, in some pathological conditions (e.g., chronic sinusitis, CF and COPD), the mucus gets thicker. In CF, the mucus exhibited an increased density of disulfide cross-links, further tightening the mucus mesh space, thereby reinforcing its steric barrier potency to immunopharmaceutics (19). To date, overcoming this physical barrier has not been addressed in the design of inhaled immunopharmaceutics. Other biological barriers include alveolar macrophages and the pulmonary surfactant layer in the alveolar region. While the molecular interactions between inhaled particles and

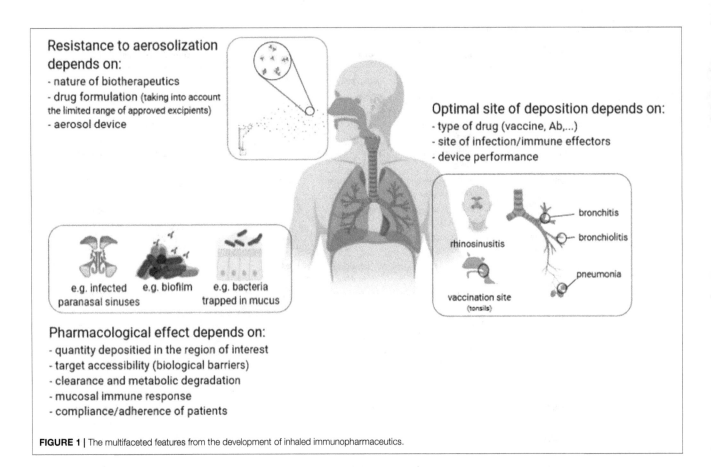

FIGURE 1 | The multifaceted features from the development of inhaled immunopharmaceutics.

the surfactant are largely unknown, some evidences indicate that surfactant proteins may facilitate the uptake of inhaled particles by alveolar macrophages (20). Alveolar macrophages patrol the airways and phagocytose inhaled organic (including pathogens) and inorganic particles ranging between 0.5 and 5μm (21). Interestingly, the size-discriminating property of their phagocytosis potency has led to the development of innovative approaches for inhaled drugs, in which carrier entrapped-particles of smaller or larger size are inhaled to escape the alveolar macrophage phagocytosis and to provide a better controlled drug release [(22, 23); **Figure 1**]. This strategy is investigated for mucosal vaccines to prevent the degradation or denaturation of the peptide/antigen, to sustain its release and favor delivery and adjuvancy (24).

The lung mucosa is a metabolic active environment (25). The presence of proteases [which is more prevalent in the nasal mucosa (26)] may degrade therapeutic proteins before they reach their targets. In addition to host enzymes, bacterial pathogens, like *P. aeruginosa*, release additional proteases, which may metabolize respiratory-delivered drugs (27). In this context, the presence of protease inhibitors in the formulation of inhaled protein therapeutics may improve their pharmacokinetics and efficacy, as previously demonstrated for inhaled peptides such as insulin and calcitonin (28). Furthermore, the encapsulation of protein therapeutics into liposomes may also improve stability and reduce the frequency of dosing (29). This strategy has already been clinically validated for the pulmonary

delivery of antibiotics (30). Of note, respiratory diseases are often associated with an impairment of the protease/anti-protease balance. In CF, high levels of proteases are a result of the chronic infection and inflammation induced by *P. aeruginosa* (31). This proteolytic environment self-perpetuates the intensity of inflammation, induces mucus hypersecretion and respiratory tissue damage, which may ultimately affect inhaled immunotherapeutics (**Figure 1**).

CONCLUSION

Compared to the expansion of biopharmaceutics (excluding non-recombinant vaccines) in all medical areas, the field of inhaled protein therapeutics/vaccines has stagnated, with only few drugs approved so far. Despite promising preclinical data and significant advances on macromolecule inhalation, a definitive demonstration that effective and intact inhaled immunopharmaceuticals could be delivered (topically) to humans is still lacking.

Although, we cannot rule out that the recent failures of inhaled biopharmaceutics (Exubera and ALX-0171) make it challenging, to our opinion, it may be time for thinking carefully where inhalation may have the edge over other routes: "finding the right use for this modality!" They may be many possibilities considering the unmet clinical needs for respiratory diseases and the growing market of immunopharmaceutics. But the inhalation route must be envisioned and integrated early taking into account the disease/population, the target, the drug and the device (**Figure 1**), rather than adapting an approved molecule for the inhalation route. RTIs are undoubtedly an appropriate clinical situation for inhalation, if we consider the importance of matching the delivery of immunoprophylatics or immunotherapeutics to their site of action. Anti-infectious macromolecules may certainly benefit from the success of inhaled antibiotics, but it is critical to remember their precise molecular nature associated with a unique pharmacokinetics

profile when considering their development for inhalation. Besides, the recent report of a universal flu vaccine, comprised of Ab-based therapeutics (VHH) produced by an adeno-associated virus delivered intranasally pushed further the boundaries of the potential of the inhalation route for immunoprophylactics (32).

AUTHOR CONTRIBUTIONS

TS, AM, and NH-V participated in the review of research. NH-V prepared figure. TS and AM prepared table. All authors contributed to the manuscript.

REFERENCES

Dall'Acqua WF, Kiener PA, Wu H. Properties of human IgG1s engineered for enhanced binding to the neonatal Fc receptor (FcRn). *J Biol Chem.* (2006) 281:23514–24. doi: 10.1074/jbc.M604292200

Labiris NR, Dolovich MB. Pulmonary drug delivery. Part I: physiological factors affecting therapeutic effectiveness of aerosolized medications. *Br J Clin Pharmacol.* (2003) 56:588–99. doi: 10.1046/j.1365-2125.2003.01892.x

Larios Mora A, Detalle L, Gallup JM, Van Geelen A, Stohr T, Duprez L, et al. Delivery of ALX-0171 by inhalation greatly reduces respiratory syncytial virus disease in newborn lambs. *mAbs.* (2018) 10:778–95. doi: 10.1080/19420862.2018.1470727

Leyva-Grado VH, Tan GS, Leon PE, Yondola M, Palese P. Direct administration in the respiratory tract improves efficacy of broadly neutralizing anti-influenza virus monoclonal antibodies. *Antimicrob Agents Chemother.* (2015) 59:4162–72. doi: 10.1128/AAC.00290-15

Secher T, Dalonneau E, Ferreira M, Parent C, Azzopardi N, Paintaud G, et al. In a murine model of acute lung infection, airway administration of a therapeutic antibody confers greater protection than parenteral administration. *J Control Release.* (2019) 303:24–33. doi: 10.1016/j.jconrel.2019.04.005

Kang MC, Choi DH, Choi YW, Park SJ, Namkoong H, Park KS, et al. Intranasal introduction of Fc-fused interleukin-7 provides long-lasting prophylaxis against lethal influenza virus infection. *J Virol.* (2015) 90:2273–84. doi: 10.1128/JVI.02768-15

de Swart RL, de Vries RD, Rennick LJ, van Amerongen G, McQuaid S, Verburgh RJ, et al. Needle-free delivery of measles virus vaccine to the lower respiratory tract of non-human primates elicits optimal immunity and protection. *NPJ vaccines.* (2017) 2:22. doi: 10.1038/s41541-017-0022-8

Bodier-Montagutelli E, Mayor A, Vecellio L, Respaud R, Heuze-Vourc'h N. Designing inhaled protein therapeutics for topical lung delivery: what are the next steps? *Exp Opin Drug Deliv.* (2018) 15:729–36. doi: 10.1080/17425247.2018.1503251

Respaud R, Vecellio L, Diot P, Heuze-Vourc'h N. Nebulization as a delivery method for mAbs in respiratory diseases. *Exp Opin Drug Deliv.* (2015) 12:1027–39. doi: 10.1517/17425247.2015.999039

Respaud R, Marchand D, Pelat T, Tchou-Wong KM, Roy CJ, Parent C, et al. Development of a drug delivery system for efficient alveolar delivery of a neutralizing monoclonal antibody to treat pulmonary intoxication to ricin. *J Control Release.* (2016) 234:21–32. doi: 10.1016/j.jconrel.2016. 05.018

Carvalho TC, McConville JT. The function and performance of aqueous aerosol devices for inhalation therapy. *J Pharm Pharmacol.* (2016) 68:556–78. doi: 10.1111/jphp.12541

Ho DK, Nichols BLB, Edgar KJ, Murgia X, Loretz B, Lehr CM. Challenges and strategies in drug delivery systems for treatment of pulmonary infections. *Eur J Pharm Biopharm.* (2019) 144:110–24. doi: 10.1016/j.ejpb.2019.09.002

Thurber GM, Schmidt MM, Wittrup KD. Antibody tumor penetration: transport opposed by systemic and antigen-mediated clearance. *Adv Drug Deliv Rev.* (2008) 60:1421–34. doi: 10.1016/j.addr.2008.04.012

Geiser M, Cruz-Orive LM, Im Hof V, Gehr P. Assessment of particle retention and clearance in the intrapulmonary conducting airways of hamster lungs with the fractionator. *J Microsc.* (1990) 160(Pt 1):75–88.

Gizurarson S. The effect of cilia and the mucociliary clearance on successful drug delivery. *Biol Pharm Bull.* (2015) 38:497–506. doi: 10.1248/bpb.b14-00398

Takeuchi H, Yamamoto H, Kawashima Y. Mucoadhesive nanoparticulate systems for peptide drug delivery. *Adv Drug Deliv Rev.* (2001) 47:39– 54. doi: 10.1016/s0169-409x(00)00120-4

Lai SK, O'Hanlon DE, Harrold S, Man ST, Wang YY, Cone R, et al. Rapid transport of large polymeric nanoparticles in fresh undiluted human mucus. *Proc Natl Acad Sci USA.* (2007) 104:1482–7. doi: 10.1073/pnas.0608611104

Muralidharan P, Mallory E, Malapit M, Hayes D Jr, Mansour HM. Inhalable PEGylated phospholipid nanocarriers and PEGylated therapeutics for respiratory delivery as aerosolized colloidal dispersions and dry powder inhalers. *Pharmaceutics.* (2014) 6:333–53. doi: 10.3390/pharmaceutics6020333

Yuan S, Hollinger M, Lachowicz-Scroggins ME, Kerr SC, Dunican EM, Daniel BM, et al. Oxidation increases mucin polymer cross- links to stiffen airway mucus gels. *Sci Transl Med.* (2015) 7:276ra27. doi: 10.1126/scitranslmed.3010525

Chroneos ZC, Sever-Chroneos Z, Shepherd VL. Pulmonary surfactant: an immunological perspective. *Cell Physiol Biochem.* (2010) 25:13–26. doi: 10.1159/000272047

Geiser M. Update on macrophage clearance of inhaled micro- and nanoparticles. *J Aerosol Med Pulm Drug Deliv.* (2010) 23:207–17. doi: 10.1089/jamp.2009.0797

Pudlarz AM, Czechowska E, Ranoszek-Soliwoda K, Tomaszewska E, Celichowski G, Grobelny J, et al. Immobilization of recombinant human catalase on gold and silver nanoparticles. *Appl Biochem Biotechnol.* (2018) 185:717–35. doi: 10.1007/s12010-017-2682-2

Tsapis N, Bennett D, Jackson B, Weitz DA, Edwards DA. Trojan particles: large porous carriers of nanoparticles for drug delivery. *Proc Natl Acad Sci USA.* (2002) 99:12001–5. doi: 10.1073/pnas.182233999

Osman N, Kaneko K, Carini V, Saleem I. Carriers for the targeted delivery of aerosolized macromolecules for pulmonary pathologies. *Exp Opin Drug Deliv.* (2018) 15:821–34. doi: 10.1080/17425247.2018.1502267

Candiano G, Bruschi M, Pedemonte N, Musante L, Ravazzolo R, Liberatori S, et al. Proteomic analysis of the airway surface liquid: modulation by proinflammatory cytokines. *Am J Physiol Lung Cell Mol Physiol.* (2007) 292:L185–98. doi: 10.1152/ajplung.00085.2006

Zhou XH. Overcoming enzymatic and absorption barriers to non-parenterally administered protein and peptide drugs. *J Control Release.* (1994) 29:239–52. doi: 10.1016/0168-3659(94)90071-X

Gellatly SL, Hancock RE. Pseudomonas aeruginosa: new insights into pathogenesis and host defenses. *Pathogens Dis.* (2013) 67:159–73. doi: 10.1111/2049-632X.12033

Hussain A, Arnold JJ, Khan MA, Ahsan F. Absorption enhancers in pulmonary protein delivery. *J Control Release.* (2004) 94:15–24. doi: 10.1016/j.jconrel.2003.10.001

Gibbons AM, McElvaney NG, Taggart CC, Cryan SA. Delivery of rSLPI in a liposomal carrier for inhalation provides protection against cathepsin L degradation. *J Microencapsul.* (2009) 26:513–22. doi:10.1080/02652040802466535

Haworth CS, Bilton D, Chalmers JD, Davis AM, Froehlich J, Gonda I, et al. Inhaled liposomal ciprofloxacin in patients with non-cystic fibrosis bronchiectasis and chronic lung infection with Pseudomonas aeruginosa (ORBIT-3 and ORBIT-4): two phase 3, randomised controlled trials. *Lancet Respir Med.* (2019) 7:213–26. doi: 10.1016/S2213-2600(18)30427-2

Twigg MS, Brockbank S, Lowry P, FitzGerald SP, Taggart C, Weldon S. The role of serine proteases and antiproteases in the cystic fibrosis lung. *Mediators Inflamm.* (2015) 2015:293053. doi: 10.1155/2015/2 93053

Laursen NS, Friesen RHE, Zhu X, Jongeneelen M, Blokland S, Vermond J, et al. Universal protection against influenza infection by a multidomain antibody to influenza hemagglutinin. *Science.* (2018) 362:598-602. doi:10.1126/science.aaq0620

18

Phage Endolysin LysP108 Showed Promising Antibacterial Potential Against Methicillin-Resistant *Staphylococcus aureus*

Yifei Lu[1†], Yingran Wang[2†], Jing Wang[3], Yan Zhao[3], Qiu Zhong[4], Gang Li[3], Zhifeng Fu[5*] and Shuguang Lu[3*]

[1] Institute of Burn Research, Southwest Hospital, State Key Lab of Trauma, Burn and Combined Injury, Army Medical University, Chongqing, China, [2] Department of Clinical Laboratory Medicine, Southwest Hospital, Army Medical University, Chongqing, China, [3] Department of Microbiology, College of Basic Medical Science, Army Medical University, Chongqing, China, [4] Department of Clinical Laboratory Medicine, Daping Hospital, Army Medical University, Chongqing, China, [5] College of Pharmaceutical Sciences, Southwest University, Chongqing, China

*Correspondence:
Zhifeng Fu
fuzf@swu.edu.cn
Shuguang Lu
shulang88@126.com

†These authors have contributed equally to this work

As a potential antibacterial agent, endolysin can directly lyse Gram-positive bacteria from the outside and does not lead to drug resistance. Considering that XN108 is the first reported methicillin-resistant *Staphylococcus aureus* (MRSA) strain in mainland China with a vancomycin MIC that exceeds 8 µg mL^{-1}, we conducted a systematic study on its phage-encoded endolysin LysP108. Standard plate counting method revealed that LysP108 could lyse *S. aureus* and *Pseudomonas aeruginosa* with damaged outer membrane, resulting in a significant reduction in the number of live bacteria. Scanning electron microscopy results showed that *S. aureus* cells could be lysed directly from the outside by LysP108. Live/dead bacteria staining results indicated that LysP108 possessed strong bactericidal ability, with an anti-bacterial rate of approximately 90%. Crystal violet staining results implied that LysP108 could also inhibit and destroy bacterial biofilms. *In vivo* animal experiments suggested that the area of subcutaneous abscess of mice infected with MRSA was significantly reduced after the combined injection of LysP108 and vancomycin in comparison with monotherapy. The synergistic antibacterial effects of LysP108 and vancomycin were confirmed. Therefore, the present data strongly support the idea that endolysin LysP108 exhibits promising antibacterial potential to be used as a candidate for the treatment of infections caused by MRSA.

Keywords: phage endolysin LysP108, antibacterial activity, drug-resistant bacteria infection treatment, vancomycin, methicillin-resistant *Staphylococcus aureus*

INTRODUCTION

The abuse of antibiotics has led to the frequent emergence of multidrug-resistant superbugs, which make the clinical treatment of infectious diseases difficult (Nathan and Cars, 2014; Blair et al., 2015). Moreover, due to the slow development of new antibiotics, drug-resistant bacteria have become one of the greatest threats to global public health (Woolhouse and Farrar, 2014; Marston et al., 2016).

Staphylococcus aureus is a common pathogen that causes various human infectious diseases (Suaifan et al., 2017). The emergence of methicillin-resistant *S. aureus* (MRSA) and its rapid development of drug resistance have made the clinical treatment of *S. aureus* infections very challenging (Rodvold and McConeghy, 2014). In recent years, some MRSA strains are reportedly able to resist vancomycin, which has long been considered as the last line of defense against MRSA (Staub and Sieber, 2009; McGuinness et al., 2017). Therefore, the development of new antimicrobial agents for the efficient prevention and treatment of MRSA infections is necessary.

As natural predators of bacteria, bacteriophages (phages) are used in the treatment of drug-resistant bacterial infections (Kutateladze and Adamia, 2010; Díez-Martínez et al., 2015). Besides the phage itself, phage-encoded endolysins can also selectively and quickly kill bacteria, and they showed great potential for application to the treatment of antibacterial infection (Huskins and Goldmann, 2005; Payne, 2008). Endolysin is a cell wall hydrolase that plays an important role in the later stage of phage infection (Gerstmans et al., 2018). It can lyse the cell wall from inside the bacteria and help release progeny phages outside the cell (Rodríguez-Rubio et al., 2013). Compared with phage, endolysin has many advantages, such as non-proliferation, easy-to-target drug delivery, wider host spectrum, and low bacterial resistance (Nelson et al., 2001; Nelson et al., 2012). As a biological macromolecule, its regulatory path is clearer than that of phages.

At present, the development of phage-related preparations that can lyse pathogens has become the focus of research. Since Gram-positive bacteria do not have an outer membrane, endolysin can directly lyse the cell wall from the outside, thereby providing a basis for the use of endolysin alone (Ahmed et al., 2014; Haddad Kashani et al., 2017; Chang, 2020). Considering the synergistic effect between the endolysin and antibiotics, the use of the endolysin in combination with antibiotics can expand the broad spectrum of the endolysin and avoid the development of resistance of target cells (Djurkovic et al., 2005; Schuch et al., 2014; Schmelcher et al., 2015). Some phage endolysin-related preparations are currently in clinical trials or already in the market (Jun et al., 2017; Totté et al., 2017). Therefore, endolysins bring new hope for the treatment of superbugs when antibiotics are ineffective against multidrug-resistant superbugs.

In this study, the endolysin LysP108 was derived from phage P108 of *S. aureus* strain XN108 and obtained by recombinant expression in *Escherichia coli* by molecular cloning. Considering that XN108 is the first MRSA strain in mainland China with vancomycin MIC that exceeds 8 µg mL^{-1} (Zhang et al., 2013; Wang et al., 2020), we conducted a systematic study on its phage-encoded endolysin LysP108. The lysozyme activity of endolysin LysP108 was analyzed by viable count method to determine the optimum conditions of LysP108. Afterward, its *in vitro* bactericidal capacity and its effect on bacterial biofilm were investigated by using live/dead bacteria and crystal violet staining experiments, respectively. To verify the antibacterial effect of LysP108 *in vivo*, a mouse model of subcutaneous MRSA

infection abscess was established. Then, LysP108 was used in combination with vancomycin to verify their synergistic effect and assess the possibility of using such a combination as a potential antimicrobial agent. In summary, we have validated the antibacterial effect of LysP108 *in vitro* and *in vivo* and explored its potential in combination with antibiotics, thereby providing a new way for solving the increasingly serious problem of bacterial drug resistance.

MATERIALS AND METHODS

Ethics Statement
All experiments were conducted with the approval of the Laboratory Animal Welfare and Ethics Committee of Third Military Medical University (NO. AMUWEC2020733) and in strict accordance with ethical principles. All participants were informed the purpose of this study and agreed to written consent.

Materials and Reagents
PCR primers with sequences were synthesized by Genomics institution (China). FastPfu DNA polymerase, *Escherichia coli* strains DH5α and BL21 (DE3) were purchased from TransGen Biotech (China). Quickcut restriction endonucleases NotI and NdeI were both purchased from Takara Bio (Japan). T4 DNA ligase was purchased from BioLab (U.S.A.). IPTG was purchased from Sangon (China). DNA marker, protein marker and live/dead bacteria staining kit were all purchased from Thermo Fisher Scientific (U.S.A.). LB broth and BHI broth were purchased from Oxoid (U.K.). Bicinchoninic acid assay kit was purchased from Beyotime Biotechnology (China). Vancomycin was purchased from Solarbio Life Sciences (China).

Apparatus
PCR experiments were conducted on a PCR instrument and a gel imager (Bio-Rad Laboratories, U.S.A.). Nickel affinity chromatography was conducted on an AKTA purifier equipped with a HisTrap FF column (GE Healthcare, U.S.A.). Scanning diagram of plate colony was conducted on an automatic colony counter (Shineso, China). Fluorescent micrographic imaging of stained bacteria was conducted on a NI–U fluorescent microscope (Nikon, Japan). OD$_{570}$ value was measured on a SpectraMAX M2e plate reader (Molecular Device, U.S.A.).

Bacterial Strains, Media, and Growth Conditions
MRSA strain XN108 was isolated from Southwest Hospital (Chongqing, China) (Zhang et al., 2013), and *Pseudomonas aeruginosa* strain PA1 (Lu et al., 2015; Li et al., 2016a; Li et al., 2016b) was isolated from Xinqiao Hospital (Chongqing, China), and they were both kept in our laboratory. Methicillin-sensitive *S. aureus* (MSSA) strain ATCC 25923, *P. aeruginosa* strain PAO1, and *Acinetobacter baumannii* strain AB1 were all purchased from China Center for Type Culture Collection.

All strains were grown in brain heart infusion (BHI) broth medium with constant shaking overnight at 37°C. Phage P108, which encodes the LysP108 endolysin, was isolated from hospital sewage using the MRSA strain XN108 as host bacterium. For transformation, *E. coli* strains DH5α and BL21 (DE3) were prepared for cloning and recombinant protein expression, respectively, and they were cultured in Luria-Bertani (LB) broth at 37°C.

Bioinformatics Analysis of LysP108

The phage P108 genome was sequenced and submitted to the GenBank database (accession number: NC025426). The amino acid sequence of LysP108 was analyzed using the Basic Local Alignment Search Tool (BLAST, http://www.ncbi.nlm.nih.gov/BLAST/) for comparison. Subsequently, based on the protein sequence, the 3D structure of LysP108 was predicted using the Swiss-Model tool (http://swissmodel.expasy.org). The amino acid sequences of LysGH15 (protein ID: ADG26756.1) (Zhang et al., 2018), LysK (protein ID: AAO47477.2) (Fujita et al., 2017), HydH5 (protein ID: ACJ64586.1) (Rodriguez et al., 2011), PlyGRCS (protein ID: AHJ10590.1) (Linden et al., 2015), CF-301 (protein ID: ZP_03625529.1) (Schuch et al., 2014), endolysin of *Listeria* phage vB_LmoS_293 (protein ID: AJE28090.1) (Pennone et al., 2019), PlyAB1 (protein ID: YP_008058242.1) (Huang et al., 2014), lysostaphin of *Nocardia seriolae* (protein ID: APB01676.1) (Jayakumar et al., 2020) were downloaded from the National Center for Biotechnology Information (NCBI) Protein Database (https://www.ncbi.nlm.nih.gov/protein). Sequence homology analysis of LysP108, LysGH15, LysK, HydH5, PlyGRCS, CF-301, endolysin of *Listeria* phage vB_LmoS_293, PlyAB1, and lysostaphin of *Nocardia seriolae* was performed using the software DNAMAN (https://www.lynnon.com/dnaman.html).

Cloning, Overexpression, and Purification of LysP108

Recombinant LysP108 was produced through the *E. coli* expression system. The gene fragment encoding LysP108 was amplified by PCR with a set of specific primers (forward: TAAG AAGGAGATATACATATGAAAAAAAAAGATAAACGTG GTAAGAAACC and reverse: TGGTGGTGCTCGAGTGCGG CCGCTTTGAATACTCCCCAAGCAA, with the NdeI/NotI restriction endonuclease sites underlined). The PCR amplification condition consisted of initial denaturation step at 95°C for 2 min, followed by 35 cycles of denaturation step at 95°C for 20 s, annealing at 52°C for 20 s, and elongation at 72°C for 30 s, and final extension step at 72°C for 5 min. After double enzyme digestion, the PCR product and pET21a vector were linked together by using Gibson Assembly at 50°C for 30 min to construct the recombinant plasmid pET21a-LysP108. DNA sequences were verified for the constructed plasmid. Next, C-terminal six-His-tagged LysP108 plasmid was transformed into *E. coli* BL21 (DE3) to screen the positive clones.

A single positive colony was cultured in LB broth added with 100 μg mL^{-1} ampicillin at 37°C under constant shaking at 180 rpm. When the OD$_{600}$ value of the bacterial fluid reached approximately 0.6, isopropyl β-D-1-thiogalactopyranoside (IPTG) was added to reach the working concentration of 0.1 mM. After incubation for 10 h at 23°C, the bacterial cells were collected by centrifugation and disrupted by ultrasonication, followed by centrifugation at 10,000 g for 30 min to remove the bacterial fragments. Then, the supernatant containing soluble protein was filtrated through a 0.4 μm filter membrane. The protein was purified with nickel affinity chromatography. The purity and size of the obtained protein were confirmed with sodium dodecyl sulfate-polyacryl amide gel electrophoresis (SDS-PAGE), in which the gel was stained by Coomassie brilliant blue. Then the protein concentration was detected by a bicinchoninic acid assay. The LysP108 solution was dialyzed against 10 mM PBS containing 20% glycerol and stored at -20°C.

Determination of LysP108 Antibacterial Activity

The antibacterial activity of LysP108 was determined by colony forming unit (CFU) reduction assay as previously described. (Dong et al., 2015) All bacteria strains were cultured to early log phase, harvested, and resuspended in the same volume of 20 mM Tris-HCl buffer (pH 7.5). For Gram-negative bacteria, early log phase cells were pelleted and resuspended in 20 mM Tris-HCl buffer supplemented with 0.1 M EDTA for 5 min at room temperature (RT). EDTA at high concentrations is toxic to the cells. Thus, the outer membrane was treated only for 5 min. Then, cells were pelleted and washed with 20 mM Tris-HCl buffer thrice to remove the remaining EDTA. Next, 20 μL of LysP108 (1 mg mL^{-1}) was added to 80 μL of resuspended bacteria and incubated for 30 min at 37°C. Afterward, the mixture was serially diluted by 10-fold and plated on BHI agar plates. The CFU was calculated after 24 h of incubation at 37°C to determine the number of viable cells. The above tests were repeated for three times, and the mean values were calculated. The final CFU was obtained by multiplying the average number of colonies on the plate by the dilution factor.

Factors affecting LysP108 lytic activity were analyzed using early log phase bacteria under different reaction conditions, as follows: LysP108 concentration of 0–1000 μg mL^{-1}; pH of 4.0–12.0; and temperature of 30°C–90°C. To assess the effect of LysP108 concentration on lytic activity, various concentrations (0–1000 μg mL^{-1}) of LysP108 and the MRSA strain XN108 cell suspensions were mixed thoroughly and incubated for 30 min at 37°C. To test the pH stability, 250 μg mL^{-1} of LysP108 was added to the bacterial cell suspension in the following buffers: 20 mM sodium acetate for pH 4.0–5.0; 20 mM Tris-HCl for pH 6.0–8.0; 20 mM glycine for pH 9.0–10.0; and 20 mM sodium carbonate for pH 11.0–12.0. Briefly, 80 μL bacterial resuspended solution at different pH was mixed with 20 μL LysP108 and incubated for 30 min at 37°C, while the control group was treated with bacterial resuspended solution at different pH and 20 μL PBS. To test the thermal stability, 250 μg mL^{-1} of LysP108 was incubated at different temperatures (30°C–90°C) for 10 min. After cooling to room temperature, 80 μL bacterial solution was mixed with 20 μL LysP108 treated at different temperatures and incubated at 37°C for 30 min, while the control group was treated with bacterial solution and 20 μL PBS without temperature treatment. All experiments were repeated thrice. The values were the means and standard deviations from triplicate assays.

Assessment of LysP108 Lytic Activity

The interactions between LysP108 and MRSA (XN108 and SCC*mec* V) strains were assessed *in vitro*. LysP108 and bacteria cells were suspended in 10 mM PBS (pH 7.4). Then, 200 μL of LysP108 (250 μg mL^{-1}) and 800 μL of the test bacteria (10^8 CFU mL^{-1}) were mixed together and incubated at 37°C for 5, 30, and 60 min, respectively. For the complete removal of free LysP108, the mixtures were then centrifuged at 5000 g for 5 min and washed thrice by PBS (10 mM; pH 7.4). Subsequently, the sediments comprising bacteria with LysP108 were suspended in PBS (10 mM; pH 7.4). The morphology of aggregated pellets were detected under a scanning electron microscope (SEM, Inspect F, Philips, The Netherlands).

In Vitro Live/dead Bacteria Staining Assay

Live/dead staining assay was performed by using a live/dead bacteria staining kit. The kit contained two fluorescent dyes, SYTO 9 and PI. The green SYTO 9 dye entered both intact bacteria and bacteria with damaged cell structure. However, the red PI dye only entered bacteria with the damaged cell membrane or wall. Briefly, 2 mL of MRSA strain XN108 was cultured to post log phase, harvested, and resuspended in 1 mL of 0.85% NaCl. Then, 200 μL of LysP108 (250 μg mL^{-1}) was added into 800 μL of resuspended bacteria and incubated for 1 h at 37°C with 100 rpm. The above mixture was centrifuged at 5000 g for 5 min and suspended in 0.85% NaCl. Next, the suspensions were stained with live/dead dye solution (1.5 μL of SYTO 9 and 1.5 μL of PI) simultaneously for 15 min in the dark. Then, the stained bacteria were washed with 0.85% NaCl twice and observed under a fluorescent microscope.

Crystal Violet Staining Assay

Crystal violet staining assay was performed as previously described with some modifications. (Wu et al., 2003) The MRSA strain XN108 was incubated overnight in BHI culture medium, after which it was prepared and sub-cultured in a 96-well polystyrene microplate with the same culture medium. After incubating the microplate for 24 h at 37°C, all wells were washed with 10 mM PBS (pH 7.4). Once the biofilm was formed, the experimental group wells were filled with 100 μL of LysP108 (250 μg mL^{-1}). PBS at 10 mM was used as the negative control. After incubation for 5 h at 37°C with 100 rpm, each well was washed once with 10 mM PBS and stained with 0.1% crystal violet for 10 min at RT. Washing with 10 mM PBS was repeated thrice, and solubilization with 33% acetic acid was performed. The absorbance of the obtained solution was detected with a plate reader and measured at 570 nm (OD$_{570}$).

Standard Checkerboard Broth Micro-Dilution Assay

A standard checkerboard broth micro-dilution assay was used to test whether there is a synergistic interaction between LysP108 and vancomycin. Briefly, different dilutions of vancomycin and LysP108 were incubated vertically and horizontally with a bacterial inoculum of 5×10^5 CFU per well in a final volume of 50 μL, respectively. MRSA strain XN108 was used to test the interaction between endolysin and vancomycin. The plates were incubated at 37°C with gentle shaking and the bacterial growth rate was determined by reading OD$_{600}$ for 20 h. The fractional inhibitory concentration of antibiotic and LysP108 was plotted as an isobologram.

In Vivo Animal Experiments

To study the antibacterial effect of LysP108 *in vivo*, a subcutaneous abscess model on male BALB/c mice (6–8 weeks old; 20–25 g in weight) was established. Mice were anesthetized with an intraperitoneal injection of 1% pentobarbital at a dose of 50 mg kg^{-1}, and the dorsal surface of mice was shaved and cleaned with 75% alcohol. Subsequently, 100 μL of MRSA suspension (1×10^8 CFU mL^{-1}) was injected subcutaneously into the right and left sides of the shaved back of each test mouse. After 24 h, a focal MRSA infection formed as a subcutaneous abscess.

For the endolysin group, the infected mice were injected subcutaneously with 100 μL of 250 μg ml^{-1} of LysP108, and for the vancomycin group, vancomycin solution was injected intravenously at a dose of 20 mg kg^{-1}. In addition, for the co-administration group, 100 μL of 250 μg ml^{-1} LysP108 was injected subcutaneously, and at the same time, the vancomycin solution was injected intravenously (20 mg kg^{-1}). PBS at 100 μL was injected subcutaneously as the control treatment. Except for vancomycin that was administered once every 12 h, LysP108 and PBS were administered once every 24 h for 10 days.

Using standard circular paper (blue) with a diameter of 6 mm as a reference, the mice were photographed, and observations were recorded daily. Meanwhile, the abscess area was calculated and analyzed through Image J (NIH) software to draw the abscess area curve of the skin infection on the back of the mice. After being treated with paraffin embedding, serial section, and hematoxylin and eosin (H&E) staining, the samples were histologically examined under an optical microscope.

Statistical Analysis

Data in line with normal distribution were presented as mean ± standard deviation (SD) of at least 3 or more independent measurements. Statistical analysis was performed by two-tailed Student's *t* test or one-way ANOVA using SPSS 18.0 (IBM, USA). Bonferroni *post hoc* test was used for multiple *post hoc* comparisons to determine statistical significance after one-way ANOVA. $P < 0.05$ was considered significant. Graph analysis was performed using GraphPad Prism 8.0 (GraphPad Software, USA).

RESULTS

LysP108 Sequence Analysis and Protein Purification

Genomic annotation revealed that the phage P108 encode a putative endolysin, which was named LysP108 (GenBank protein ID: YP_009099525.1). In silico analysis of LysP108 predicted a

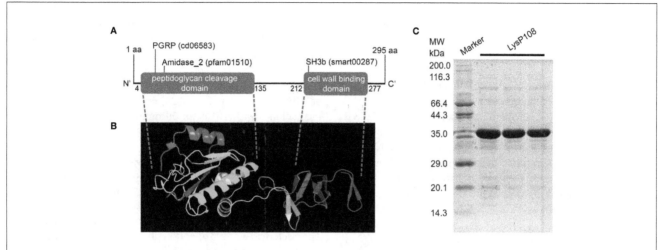

FIGURE 1 | Characterization and purification of endolysin LysP108. **(A)** Schematic illustration of structure of phage endolysin LysP108. **(B)** 3D structure of endolysin protein LysP108. **(C)** SDS-PAGE photograph of purified protein LysP108.

295-amino acid protein (~34 kDa) with two independent domains: the peptidoglycan cleavage domain (PCD) and cell wall binding domain (CBD) (**Figure 1A**). In general, PCD is responsible for cleaving specific peptidoglycan covalent bond structures, whereas CBD is responsible for adhering to the bacterial cell wall. The predicted sites of PCD ranged from 4 to 135 amino acids, and those of CBD ranged from 212 to 277 amino acids. To study the tertiary structure of endolysin LysP108, Swiss-Model homology modeling was used to construct a 3D structure. PCD and CBD were predicted to be folded independently, whereas amidase-2 was folded together with PCD, thereby enhancing the lytic activity of PCD (**Figure 1B**). Sequence homology analysis revealed that although LysP108 is homologous with several endolysins identified previously, it also has differences in the amino acid sequence and domain composition (**Figure S1**).

Sequences encoding LysP108 with His-tag at the C-terminus were successfully constructed into IPTG-inducible expression plasmid pET21a. Thus, the recombinant plasmid was named as pET21a-LysP108 (**Figure S2**). LysP108 was then expressed in *E. coli* cells bearing pET21a-LysP108 as a soluble form after it was induced by IPTG at 37°C (**Figure S3**). The purified protein showed the right mass and near homogeneity (~34 kDa), as revealed by SDS-PAGE (**Figure 1C**).

LysP108 Showed Lytic Activity to MRSA Strain XN108

The lytic activity of LysP108 was determined through a CFU reduction assay with MRSA strain XN108 as the target. LysP108 induced XN108 lysis, and the viable cell significantly decreased by approximately 2 log units after 30 min of treatment (**Figure 2A**). Meanwhile, through the automatic colony counter, the scanning diagram of plate colony directly reflected the significant decrease in the number of viable bacteria (**Figure 2B**). The above results demonstrated that endolysin LysP108 can directly lyse its host bacteria XN108 *in vitro*.

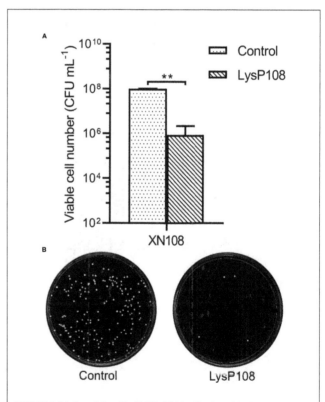

FIGURE 2 | Lytic activity of LysP108. **(A)** Identification of the lytic activity of endolysin LysP108 on XN108 by CFU reduction assay. **(B)** Scanning diagram of plate colony. (n=3). **$P < 0.01$.

Influence of Concentration, pH, and Temperature on LysP108 Antibacterial Activity

To assess the effect of concentration on the lytic activity of LysP108, different concentrations (0–1000 μg mL^{-1}) of LysP108 were tested. The addition of 250 μg mL^{-1} LysP108 reduced the viable numbers of XN108 by 2 log units, which was the most significant reduction. At a concentration greater than 250 μg mL^{-1}, the effect of LysP108 reached saturation, indicating that the optimal working concentration was 250 μg mL^{-1} (**Figure 3A**).

The result showed that LysP108 was highly active at the temperature range of 37°C–50°C, but its activity significantly decreased after heat treatment at 60°C (**Figure 3B**). Considering that the temperature of the human body is approximately 37 °C in practical applications, the optimum temperature of LysP108 is determined to be 37 °C.

Lytic activity analysis at different pH values demonstrated that the low pH of the reaction buffer significantly affected cell viability, whereas relatively high lytic activity was observed at pH 7.0, with a reduction of 2 log units of viable cells compared with the control (no LysP108 addition), as shown in **Figure 3C**. Thus, the optimum pH value of LysP108 was set at pH 7.0. All data further confirmed the antibacterial activity of LysP108.

The Antibacterial Spectrum of LysP108

Just like most of the reported phage derived endolysins, LysP108 could not lyse Gram-negative bacteria directly (data not shown), which was due to the protection of the outer membrane. EDTA

was used to treat *P. aeruginosa* strains PAO1 and PA1 and *A. baumannii* strain AB1 to remove the outer membrane before the addition of LysP108. As shown in **Figure 4**, LysP108 was able to lyse all three Gram-negative strains and reduced the viable cells by 1 log unit. Therefore, LysP108 was active against Gram-negative bacteria without outer membrane. Besides, the viability of *S. aureus* strain (ATCC 25923) was reduced by 2 log units after incubation with LysP108 for 30 min (**Figure 4**).

In Vitro Bactericidal Effect of LysP108

Supporting evidence for the lytic property of LysP108 was provided in the SEM analysis. As shown in **Figure 5**, after incubation with LysP108 for different durations, MRSA (XN108 and SCC*mec* V) cells were gradually lysed *in vitro*. The bactericidal effect of endolysin was further verified using a live/dead bacteria staining kit, and the results were observed using a fluorescent microscope. As shown in **Figure 6**, the green fluorescent channel showed all bacteria, whereas the red fluorescent channel only showed the dead bacteria. The two fluorescent signals were coincident, indicating that most bacteria

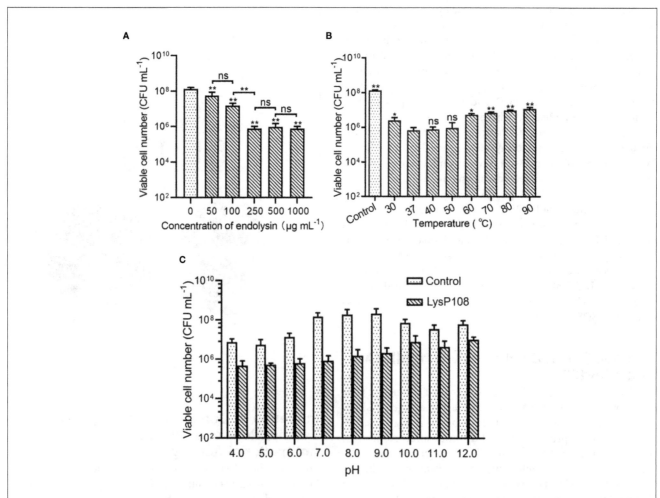

FIGURE 3 | Determination of the optimum conditions for the lytic activity of endolysin LysP108: **(A)** concentration (n=3), **(B)** temperature (n=3), and **(C)** pH (n=3). *$P < 0.05$, **$P < 0.01$, and ns, not significant.

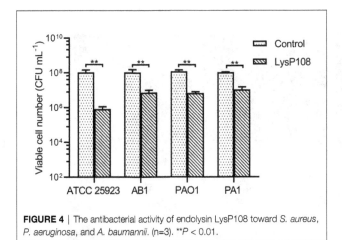

FIGURE 4 | The antibacterial activity of endolysin LysP108 toward *S. aureus*, *P. aeruginosa*, and *A. baumannii*. (n=3). **$P < 0.01$.

were killed under the effect of LysP108. The bactericidal rate was calculated as approximately 90%.

Biofilm Reduction Activity of LysP108

The biofilm matrix disruption by LysP108 was measured by plate reader at OD_{570} value and further verified by visual comparison in crystal violet-staining. As shown in **Figure 7**, the crystal violet-stained color was significantly reduced in the LysP108-treated group compared with the PBS-treated control group. Approximately 66% of the biofilm was successfully removed in the LysP108-treated group compared with the control, indicating that LysP108 had strong anti-biofilm activity.

Synergistic Antibacterial Activity of LysP108 and Vancomycin *In Vivo*

After abscesses formed on the subcutaneous tissues of mice, the subcutaneously infected abscesses were treated with vancomycin, LysP108, vancomycin combined with LysP108, and PBS. The mice were photographed, and observations were recorded daily. After 10 days of treatment, no obvious abscess was found in mice in the endolysin group and the co-administration group, whereas skin abscess still obviously existed and was accompanied by severe tissue ulceration in the vancomycin and control groups (**Figure 8A**). The poor therapeutic effect of vancomycin alone was due to the intermediate resistance of MRSA strain XN108 to vancomycin. A synergistic antibacterial effect existed between LysP108 and vancomycin, which indicated that the presence of endolysin may enhance the sensitivity of XN108 to vancomycin (**Figures 8B** and **S4**). Furthermore, H&E staining results suggested that obvious abscess and inflammatory reaction occurred in the vancomycin and control groups, but not in the combined therapy group (**Figure 8C**).

DISCUSSION

Over the recent years, resistance to antimicrobial drugs has become a growing global concern (Tornimbene et al., 2018). One of the most alarming antibiotic-resistant bacterial species is *S. aureus*. Specifically, MRSA are the group of *S. aureus* strains resistant to virtually all classes of antibiotics and lead to severe and life-threatening infections (Brown et al., 2021). Therefore, there is an urgent need to develop effective therapeutic agents against MRSA (Scallan et al., 2011). Among many antimicrobial agents against *S. aureus*, bacteriophage endolysins have been found promising because of their broad activity spectrum, rapid antibacterial activity, and low probability for developing resistance (Toyofuku et al., 2019). Several endolysins identified from genomes of bacteriophages have been applied exogenously

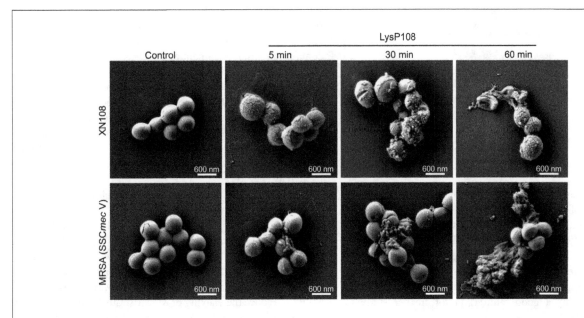

FIGURE 5 | SEM micrographs of MRSA strains (XN108 and SCC*mec* V) after incubation with LysP108 and PBS for different durations.

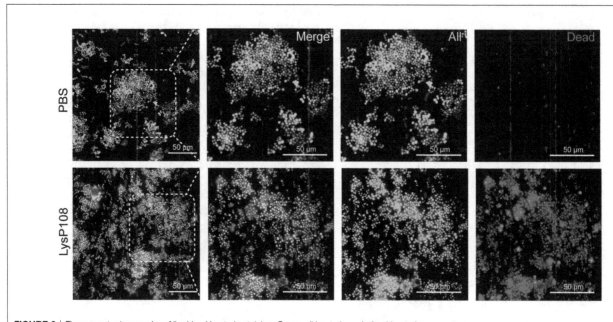

FIGURE 6 | Fluorescent micrographs of live/dead bacteria staining. Green, all bacteria; red, dead bacteria.

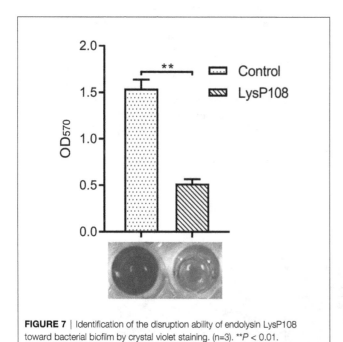

FIGURE 7 | Identification of the disruption ability of endolysin LysP108 toward bacterial biofilm by crystal violet staining. (n=3). **$P < 0.01$.

in the form of purified recombinant proteins, which can induce lysis and death of Gram-positive bacterial cells (Rodriguez et al., 2011; Schuch et al., 2014; Linden et al., 2015; Fujita et al., 2017; Zhang et al., 2018). However, these endolysins are still far from clinical applications, so more endolysins should be explored. In this study, both *in vitro* and *in vivo* assays revealed that LysP108 had potential application value to combat antibiotic-resistant bacteria, which lay a good foundation for further study to improve LysP108.

Generally, the structure of endolysins that act on Gram-positive cell walls consist of one or more PCDs with catalytic activity linked to CBD with binding activity. LysP108 employs a typical two-domain modular architecture consisting of an N-terminal PCD domain and a C-terminal CBD domain, encoding a 295-amino acid protein with a deduced molecular mass of 34 kDa (**Figure 1**). Phage derived endolysins can be classified in three groups based on their cleavage specificity: (1) endopeptidases – targeting peptide bonds, including L-alanoyl-D-glutamate endopeptidase and interpeptide bridge endopeptidase; (2) amidases – targeting amide bonds, including the N-acetylmuramoyl-L-alanine amidases; (3) glycosidases – targeting glyosidic bonds, including transglycosylases, N-acetyl-β-D-glucosaminidases, and N-acetyl-β-D-muramidases (Kashani et al., 2018). For LysP108, it contains an amidase domain at the N-terminal, which indicates that it belongs to the second group of N-acetylmuramoyl-L-alanine amidases. A number of studies have demonstrated the increased lytic activity of several enzymes upon deletion of their binding domains (Dunne et al., 2014; Singh et al., 2014). Hence, the results of this study can be served as the basis for the modification of LysP108, such as using only the catalytic domain instead of the full-length endolysin to enhance its activity.

Previous studies have shown that the stability of endolysin is critical to its application value (Kashani et al., 2018). LysP108 was highly active under a diverse range of pH and was tolerated to different temperatures. However, its optimal working concentration was 250 μg mL^{-1}, which was a disadvantage relative to the small dosage of most antibiotics (Wilm et al., 2021). The antibacterial activity of LysP108 was confirmed by its ability to reduce the viability of MRSA strain XN108 (**Figure 2**). As shown in **Figure 5**, LysP108 disintegrated the cell wall of

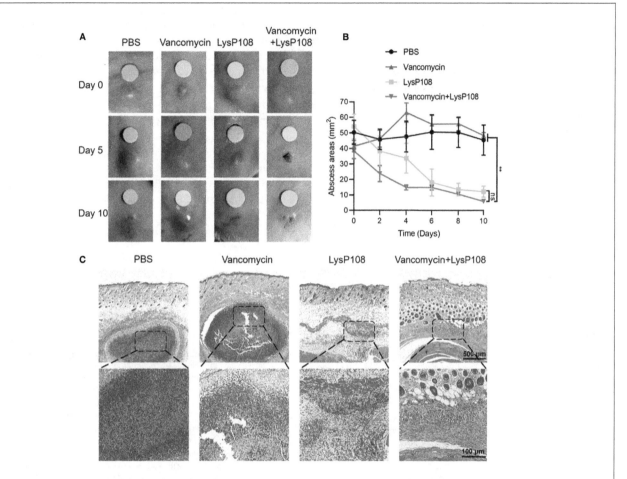

FIGURE 8 | Synergistic antibacterial effect of LysP108 and vancomycin *in vivo*. **(A)** Photographs of endolysin combined with vancomycin for the treatment of mice subcutaneous abscess. **(B)** Subcutaneous abscess area curve of MRSA infected on the back of mice. (n=6). **(C)** Representative H&E staining images of infected skin subjected to various treatments. The violet circles indicate the subcutaneous abscess. Scale bar: 100 μm. **P < 0.01; ns, not significant.

MRSA externally in a time-dependent manner, which eliminated the antibacterial activity of other pathways. This observation was quite similar with the typical phenomenon of osmotic-mediated cell lysis following the actions of phage lysins against Gram-positive bacteria reported elsewhere (Linden et al., 2015; Kashani et al., 2018).

Although LysP108 showed good antibacterial activity against other tested Gram-positive bacterial cells, including MSSA strain (ATCC 25923), it cannot directly destroy the cell wall of Gram-negative bacteria. For Gram-negative bacteria with outer membrane that prevents the entry of endolysin into the cell wall (Nikaido, 2003), EDTA was used as a pre-treatment to disrupt the outer membrane (Dong et al., 2015). Subsequently, LysP108 had antibacterial activity against the tested Gram-negative bacterial cells that have been pre-treated with EDTA, including *P. aeruginosa* strains PAO1 and PA1 and *A. baumannii* strain AB1 (**Figure 4**). However, the reagents used to treat the outer membrane are toxic and cannot be used in clinical treatment. Several reports have shown the feasibility of trans-membrane modification (Briers et al., 2014), so it is

expected that LysP108 could be modified in future study to act directly on Gram-negative bacteria.

Furthermore, LysP108 showed a 66% reduction in OD_{570} after crystal violet staining compared with the untreated control (**Figure 7**), thereby presenting a notable disrupting activity against biofilms formed by MRSA. LysP108 possibly lyses individual staphylococcal cells embedded in the extracellular matrix of the biofilm, resulting in destabilization of the biofilm and its detachment from the surface, as suggested by previous studies (Shen et al., 2013). Therefore, LysP108 could be used to treat infections, such as osteomyelitis, periodontitis, and chronic rhinosinusitis (Archer et al., 2011), which are caused by biofilm-forming *S. aureus* cells.

A considerable body of evidence has revealed that MRSA infection remains one of the main causes of hospital infections, leading to increasing rates of morbidity and mortality (Borg et al., 2021). Besides, community-acquired MRSA typically leads to superficial skin infections that can ultimately progress to induce severe invasive complications, such as necrotizing fasciitis (Takadama et al., 2020). Therefore, the selection of the skin abscess model of MRSA infection was representative. *In vivo* animal experiments revealed that the area of subcutaneous abscess of mice infected with MRSA was significantly reduced after the combined injection of LysP108 and vancomycin in comparison with monotherapy (**Figure 8**). Moreover, the standard checkerboard broth micro-dilution assay indicated that there is a synergistic interaction between LysP108 and vancomycin (**Figure S4**). When the concentration of vancomycin was 8 µg mL^{-1} and the concentration of LysP108 was greater than 100 µg mL^{-1}, the growth of bacteria could be inhibited (**Figure S4**). The standard broth microdilution method had been employed to measure susceptibility of MRSA strain XN108 toward vancomycin and the MIC of vancomycin was 16 µg mL^{-1} (Zhang et al., 2013; Wang et al., 2020). Likewise, the combination of endolysin CF-301 and daptomycin for the treatment of bacteremia caused by MRSA infection significantly improved the survival rate of mice compared with the individual application of these two antibacterial substances (Schuch et al., 2014). Thus, endolysin LysP108 is expected to be used in combined therapy, although more antibiotics should be tried in the future.

In conclusion, our present study demonstrated the antibacterial effect of endolysin LysP108 *in vitro* and *in vivo*, and showed the potential of LysP108 in combination with antibiotics, suggesting a new way for solving the increasingly serious problem of drug resistance in Gram-positive bacteria.

ETHICS STATEMENT

The animal study was reviewed and approved by Laboratory Animal Welfare and Ethics Committee of Third Military Medical University (Army Medical University), 30# Gaotanyan St., Shapingba District, Chongqing 400038, China.

AUTHOR CONTRIBUTIONS

ZF and SL conceived the study. YL and YW performed the experiments. JW, YZ, and QZ analyzed the data. YL, YW, and GL wrote the paper. All authors contributed to the article and approved the submitted version.

REFERENCES

Ahmed, A., Rushworth, J. V., Hirst, N. A., and Millner, P. A. (2014). Biosensors for whole-cell bacterial detection. *Clin. Microbiol. Rev.* 27, 631–646. doi: 10.1128/cmr.00120-13

Archer, N. K., Mazaitis, M. J., Costerton, J. W., Leid, J. G., Powers, M. E., and Shirtliff, M. E. (2011). *Staphylococcus aureus* biofilms: properties, regulation, and roles in human disease. *Virulence* 2, 445–459. doi: 10.4161/viru.2.5.17724

Blair, J. M., Webber, M. A., Baylay, A. J., Ogbolu, D. O., and Piddock, L. J. (2015). Molecular mechanisms of antibiotic resistance. *Nat. Rev. Microbiol.* 13, 42–51. doi: 10.1038/nrmicro3380

Borg, M. A., Monecke, S., Haider, J., Muller, E., Reissig, A., and Ehricht, R. (2021). MRSA improvement within a highly endemic hospital in Malta: infection control measures or clonal change? *J. Hosp. Infect.* 110, 201–202. doi: 10.1016/j.jhin.2021.02.003

Briers, Y., Walmagh, M., Van Puyenbroeck, V., Cornelissen, A., Cenens, W., Aertsen, A., et al. (2014). Engineered endolysin-based "Artilysins" to combat multidrug-resistant gram-negative pathogens. *mBio* 5, e01379–e01314. doi: 10.1128/mBio.01379-14

Brown, N. M., Brown, E. M., and Guideline Development, G. (2021). Treatment of methicillin-resistant *Staphylococcus aureus* (MRSA): updated guidelines from the UK. *J. Antimicrob. Chemother.* doi: 10.1093/jac/dkab036

Chang, Y. (2020). Bacteriophage-Derived Endolysins Applied as Potent Biocontrol Agents to Enhance Food Safety. *Microorganisms* 8, 724. doi: 10.3390/microorganisms8050724

Díez-Martínez, R., De Paz, H. D., García-Fernández, E., Bustamante, N., Euler, C. W., Fischetti, V. A., et al. (2015). A novel chimeric phage lysin with high in vitro and in vivo bactericidal activity against *Streptococcus pneumoniae*. *J. Antimicrob. Chemother.* 70, 1763–1773. doi: 10.1093/jac/dkv038

Djurkovic, S., Loeffler, J. M., and Fischetti, V. A. (2005). Synergistic killing of *Streptococcus pneumoniae* with the bacteriophage lytic enzyme Cpl-1 and penicillin or gentamicin depends on the level of penicillin resistance. *Antimicrob. Agents Chemother.* 49, 1225–1228. doi: 10.1128/aac.49.3.1225-1228.2005

Dong, H., Zhu, C., Chen, J., Ye, X., and Huang, Y. P. (2015). Antibacterial Activity of *Stenotrophomonas maltophilia* Endolysin P28 against both Gram-positive and Gram-negative Bacteria. *Front. Microbiol.* 6, 1299. doi: 10.3389/fmicb.2015.01299

Dunne, M., Mertens, H. D., Garefalaki, V., Jeffries, C. M., Thompson, A., Lemke, E. A., et al. (2014). The CD27L and CTP1L endolysins targeting *Clostridia* contain a built-in trigger and release factor. *PloS Pathog.* 10, e1004228. doi: 10.1371/journal.ppat.1004228

Fujita, S., Cho, S. H., Yoshida, A., Hasebe, F., Tomita, T., Kuzuyama, T., et al. (2017). Crystal structure of LysK, an enzyme catalyzing the last step of lysine biosynthesis in *Thermus thermophilus*, in complex with lysine: Insight into the mechanism for recognition of the amino-group carrier protein, LysW. *Biochem. Biophys. Res. Commun.* 491, 409–415. doi: 10.1016/j.bbrc.2017.07.088

Gerstmans, H., Criel, B., and Briers, Y. (2018). Synthetic biology of modular endolysins. *Biotechnol. Adv.* 36, 624–640. doi: 10.1016/j.biotechadv.2017.12.009

Haddad Kashani, H., Fahimi, H., Dasteh Goli, Y., and Moniri, R. (2017). A Novel Chimeric Endolysin with Antibacterial Activity against Methicillin-Resistant *Staphylococcus aureus*. *Front. Cell Infect. Microbiol.* 7, 290. doi: 10.3389/fcimb.2017.00290

Huang, G., Shen, X., Gong, Y., Dong, Z., Zhao, X., Shen, W., et al. (2014). Antibacterial properties of *Acinetobacter baumannii* phage Abp1 endolysin (PlyAB1). *BMC Infect. Dis.* 14, 681. doi: 10.1186/s12879-014-0681-2

Huskins, W. C., and Goldmann, D. A. (2005). Controlling meticillin-resistant *Staphylococcus aureus*, aka "Superbug". *Lancet* 365, 273–275. doi: 10.1016/s0140-6736(05)17799-x

Jayakumar, J., Kumar, V. A., Biswas, L., and Biswas, R. (2020). Therapeutic applications of lysostaphin against *Staphylococcus aureus*. *J. Appl. Microbiol.* doi: 10.1111/jam.14985

Jun, S. Y., Jang, I. J., Yoon, S., Jang, K., Yu, K. S., Cho, J. Y., et al. (2017). Pharmacokinetics and Tolerance of the Phage Endolysin-Based Candidate Drug SAL200 after a Single Intravenous Administration among Healthy Volunteers. *Antimicrob. Agents Chemother.* 61, e02629–16. doi: 10.1128/aac.02629-16

Kashani, H. H., Schmelcher, M., Sabzalipoor, H., Hosseini, E. S., and Moniri, R. (2018). Recombinant Endolysins as Potential Therapeutics against Antibiotic-Resistant *Staphylococcus aureus*: Current Status of Research and Novel Delivery Strategies. *Clin. Microbiol. Rev.* 31 (110), e00071–17. doi: 10.1128/CMR.00071-17

Kutateladze, M., and Adamia, R. (2010). Bacteriophages as potential new therapeutics to replace or supplement antibiotics. *Trends Biotechnol.* 28, 591–595. doi: 10.1016/j.tibtech.2010.08.001

Li, G., Shen, M., Le, S., Tan, Y., Li, M., Zhao, X., et al. (2016a). Genomic analyses of multidrug resistant *Pseudomonas aeruginosa* PA1 resequenced by single-molecule real-time sequencing. *Biosci. Rep.* 36, e00418. doi: 10.1042/bsr20160282

Li, G., Shen, M., Lu, S., Le, S., Tan, Y., Wang, J., et al. (2016b). Identification and Characterization of the HicAB Toxin-Antitoxin System in the Opportunistic Pathogen *Pseudomonas aeruginosa*. *Toxins (Basel)* 8, 113. doi: 10.3390/toxins8040113

Linden, S. B., Zhang, H., Heselpoth, R. D., Shen, Y., Schmelcher, M., Eichenseher, F., et al. (2015). Biochemical and biophysical characterization of PlyGRCS, a bacteriophage endolysin active against methicillin-resistant *Staphylococcus aureus*. *Appl. Microbiol. Biotechnol.* 99, 741–752. doi: 10.1007/s00253-014-5930-1

Lu, S., Le, S., Li, G., Shen, M., Tan, Y., Zhao, X., et al. (2015). Complete Genome Sequence of *Pseudomonas aeruginosa* PA1, Isolated from a Patient with a Respiratory Tract Infection. *Genome Announc.* 3, e01453-15. doi: 10.1128/genomeA.01453-15

Marston, H. D., Dixon, D. M., Knisely, J. M., Palmore, T. N., and Fauci, A. S. (2016). Antimicrobial Resistance. *Jama* 316, 1193–1204. doi: 10.1001/jama.2016.11764

McGuinness, W. A., Malachowa, N., and Deleo, F. R. (2017). Vancomycin Resistance in *Staphylococcus aureus*. *Yale J. Biol. Med.* 90, 269–281.

Nathan, C., and Cars, O. (2014). Antibiotic resistance–problems, progress, and prospects. *N. Engl. J. Med.* 371, 1761–1763. doi: 10.1056/NEJMp1408040

Nelson, D., Loomis, L., and Fischetti, V. A. (2001). Prevention and elimination of upper respiratory colonization of mice by group A *streptococci* by using a bacteriophage lytic enzyme. *Proc. Natl. Acad. Sci. U.S.A.* 98, 4107–4112. doi: 10.1073/pnas.061038398

Nelson, D. C., Schmelcher, M., Rodriguez-Rubio, L., Klumpp, J., Pritchard, D. G., Dong, S., et al. (2012). Endolysins as antimicrobials. *Adv. Virus Res.* 83, 299–365. doi: 10.1016/b978-0-12-394438-2.00007-4

Nikaido, H. (2003). Molecular basis of bacterial outer membrane permeability revisited. *Microbiol. Mol. Biol. Rev.* 67, 593–656. doi: 10.1128/mmbr.67.4.593-656.2003

Payne, D. J. (2008). Desperately seeking new antibiotics. *Science* 321, 1644–1645. doi: 10.1126/science.1164586

Pennone, V., Sanz-Gaitero, M., O'connor, P., Coffey, A., Jordan, K., Van Raaij, M. J., et al. (2019). Inhibition of *L. monocytogenes* Biofilm Formation by the Amidase Domain of the Phage vB_LmoS_293 Endolysin. *Viruses* 11, 722. doi: 10.3390/v11080722

Rodriguez, L., Martinez, B., Zhou, Y., Rodriguez, A., Donovan, D. M., and Garcia, P. (2011). Lytic activity of the virion-associated peptidoglycan hydrolase HydH5 of *Staphylococcus aureus* bacteriophage vB_SauS-phiIPLA88. *BMC Microbiol.* 11:138. doi: 10.1186/1471-2180-11-138

Rodríguez-Rubio, L., Martínez, B., Donovan, D. M., Rodríguez, A., and García, P. (2013). Bacteriophage virion-associated peptidoglycan hydrolases: potential new enzybiotics. *Crit. Rev. Microbiol.* 39, 427–434. doi: 10.3109/1040841x.2012.723675

Rodvold, K. A., and Mcconeghy, K. W. (2014). Methicillin-resistant *Staphylococcus aureus* therapy: past, present, and future. *Clin. Infect. Dis.* 58 Suppl 1, S20–S27. doi: 10.1093/cid/cit614

Scallan, E., Griffin, P. M., Angulo, F. J., Tauxe, R. V., and Hoekstra, R. M. (2011). Foodborne illness acquired in the United States–unspecified agents. *Emerg. Infect. Dis.* 17, 16–22. doi: 10.3201/eid1701.091101p2

Schmelcher, M., Powell, A. M., Camp, M. J., Pohl, C. S., and Donovan, D. M. (2015). Synergistic streptococcal phage λSA2 and B30 endolysins kill *streptococci* in cow milk and in a mouse model of mastitis. *Appl. Microbiol. Biotechnol.* 99, 8475–8486. doi: 10.1007/s00253-015-6579-0

Schuch, R., Lee, H. M., Schneider, B. C., Sauve, K. L., Law, C., Khan, B. K., et al. (2014). Combination therapy with lysin CF-301 and antibiotic is superior to antibiotic alone for treating methicillin-resistant *Staphylococcus aureus* induced murine bacteremia. *J. Infect. Dis.* 209, 1469–1478. doi: 10.1093/infdis/jit637

Shen, Y., Köller, T., Kreikemeyer, B., and Nelson, D. C. (2013). Rapid degradation of *Streptococcus pyogenes* biofilms by PlyC, a bacteriophage-encoded endolysin. *J. Antimicrob. Chemother.* 68, 1818–1824. doi: 10.1093/jac/dkt104

Singh, P. K., Donovan, D. M., and Kumar, A. (2014). Intravitreal injection of the chimeric phage endolysin Ply187 protects mice from *Staphylococcus aureus* endophthalmitis. *Antimicrob. Agents Chemother.* 58, 4621–4629. doi: 10.1128/AAC.00126-14

Staub, I., and Sieber, S. A. (2009). Beta-lactam probes as selective chemical-proteomic tools for the identification and functional characterization of resistance associated enzymes in MRSA. *J. Am. Chem. Soc.* 131, 6271–6276. doi: 10.1021/ja901304n

Suaifan, G. A., Alhogail, S., and Zourob, M. (2017). Rapid and low-cost biosensor for the detection of *Staphylococcus aureus*. *Biosens. Bioelectron.* 90, 230–237. doi: 10.1016/j.bios.2016.11.047

Takadama, S., Nakaminami, H., Kaneko, H., and Noguchi, N. (2020). A novel community-acquired MRSA clone, USA300-LV/J, uniquely evolved in Japan. *J. Antimicrob. Chemother.* 75, 3131–3134. doi: 10.1093/jac/dkaa313

Tornimbene, B., Eremin, S., Escher, M., Griskeviciene, J., Manglani, S., and Pessoa-Silva, C. L. (2018). WHO Global Antimicrobial Resistance Surveillance System early implementation 2016-17. *Lancet Infect. Dis.* 18, 241–242. doi: 10.1016/S1473-3099(18)30060-4

Totté, J. E. E., Van Doorn, M. B., and Pasmans, S. (2017). Successful Treatment of Chronic *Staphylococcus aureus*-Related Dermatoses with the Topical Endolysin Staphefekt SA.100: A Report of 3 Cases. *Case Rep. Dermatol.* 9, 19–25. doi: 10.1159/000473872

Toyofuku, M., Nomura, N., and Eberl, L. (2019). Types and origins of bacterial membrane vesicles. *Nat. Rev. Microbiol.* 17, 13–24. doi: 10.1038/s41579-018-0112-2

Wang, Y., He, Y., Bhattacharyya, S., Lu, S., and Fu, Z. (2020). Recombinant Bacteriophage Cell-Binding Domain Proteins for Broad-Spectrum Recognition of Methicillin-Resistant *Staphylococcus aureus* Strains. *Anal. Chem.* 92, 3340–3345. doi: 10.1021/acs.analchem.9b05295

Wilm, J., Svennesen, L., Ostergaard Eriksen, E., Halasa, T., and Kromker, V. (2021). Veterinary Treatment Approach and Antibiotic Usage for Clinical Mastitis in Danish Dairy Herds. *Antibiotics (Basel)* 10, 189. doi: 10.3390/antibiotics10020189

Woolhouse, M., and Farrar, J. (2014). Policy: An intergovernmental panel on antimicrobial resistance. *Nature* 509, 555–557. doi: 10.1038/509555a

Wu, J. A., Kusuma, C., Mond, J. J., and Kokai-Kun, J. F. (2003). Lysostaphin disrupts *Staphylococcus aureus* and *Staphylococcus epidermidis* biofilms on artificial surfaces. *Antimicrob. Agents Chemother.* 47, 3407–3414. doi: 10.1128/aac.47.11.3407-3414.2003

Zhang, X., Hu, Q., Yuan, W., Shang, W., Cheng, H., Yuan, J., et al. (2013). First report of a sequence type 239 vancomycin-intermediate *Staphylococcus aureus* isolate in Mainland China. *Diagn. Microbiol. Infect. Dis.* 77, 64–68. doi: 10.1016/j.diagmicrobio.2013.06.008

Zhang, Y., Cheng, M., Zhang, H., Dai, J., Guo, Z., Li, X., et al. (2018). Antibacterial Effects of Phage Lysin LysGH15 on Planktonic Cells and Biofilms of Diverse *Staphylococci*. *Appl. Environ. Microbiol.* 84, e00886-18. doi: 10.1128/AEM.00886-18

19

Antibody Epitopes of Pneumovirus Fusion Proteins

Jiachen Huang [1,2], Darren Diaz [1,2] and Jarrod J. Mousa [1,2]*

[1] Department of Infectious Diseases, College of Veterinary Medicine, University of Georgia, Athens, GA, United States,
[2] Center for Vaccines and Immunology, College of Veterinary Medicine, University of Georgia, Athens, GA, United States

*Correspondence:
Jarrod J. Mousa
jarrod.mousa@uga.edu

The pneumoviruses respiratory syncytial virus (RSV) and human metapneumovirus (hMPV) are two widespread human pathogens that can cause severe disease in the young, the elderly, and the immunocompromised. Despite the discovery of RSV over 60 years ago, and hMPV nearly 20 years ago, there are no approved vaccines for either virus. Antibody-mediated immunity is critical for protection from RSV and hMPV, and, until recently, knowledge of the antibody epitopes on the surface glycoproteins of RSV and hMPV was very limited. However, recent breakthroughs in the recombinant expression and stabilization of pneumovirus fusion proteins have facilitated in-depth characterization of antibody responses and structural epitopes, and have provided an enormous diversity of new monoclonal antibody candidates for therapeutic development. These new data have primarily focused on the RSV F protein, and have led to a wealth of new vaccine candidates in preclinical and clinical trials. In contrast, the major structural antibody epitopes remain unclear for the hMPV F protein. Overall, this review will cover recent advances in characterizing the antigenic sites on the RSV and hMPV F proteins.

Keywords: RSV, respiratory syncytial virus, human metapneumovirus, hMPV, antibody—antigen complex, X-ray crystallography, pneumovirus infections

INTRODUCTION

The recently reclassified *Pneumoviridae* virus family includes the human pathogens respiratory syncytial virus (RSV) and human metapneumovirus (hMPV) (1). These viruses are among the most common causes of childhood respiratory tract infection (2). Severe disease primarily occurs in young children, the elderly, and the immunocompromised, and reinfection can occur throughout childhood and adulthood, as sterilizing immunity is not acquired after infection. Both viruses exhibit genetic stability, with relatively few changes in viral sequences among circulating strains. Despite decades of research, there are no approved vaccines to prevent pneumovirus infection. Fortunately, a wave of new progress in recent years has led to the development of new vaccine candidates and therapeutics, largely due to breakthroughs in structural biology and immunological techniques. This review will cover recent findings on antigenic epitopes of RSV and hMPV fusion glycoproteins.

GLOBAL BURDEN OF PNEUMOVIRUSES

Respiratory Syncytial Virus

RSV is an enveloped, negative-sense, single stranded RNA virus, first isolated in 1955 from chimpanzees with respiratory illness (3), and subsequently isolated from infants with lower respiratory tract infection (4, 5). RSV is the leading cause of viral bronchiolitis and viral pneumonia in infants and children (6, 7), and nearly all children have been exposed to RSV before the age of 2 (8). RSV infection causes flu-like symptoms, bronchiolitis, and pneumonia that can be fatal to children. In addition, RSV infection poses a substantial threat to elderly populations and immunocompromised adults (9). RSV is highly contagious, and can be transmitted through direct contact or aerosol (10). Although numerous vaccines have undergone clinical trials (11), the monoclonal antibody (mAb) palivizumab remains the only approved therapeutic for RSV infection. Palivizumab has shown moderate efficacy at preventing RSV hospitalizations and intensive care unit admissions (12), however, the drug is only approved for prophylactic use, and in limited cases.

Human Metapneumovirus

hMPV was identified in 2001 in the Netherlands from samples collected from 28 children with respiratory tract infection (13). The clinical features of hMPV infection are virtually identical to RSV, and display as mid-to-upper respiratory tract infection, and can be severe enough to cause life-threatening bronchiolitis and pneumonia. Infants and the elderly are the major groups for which hMPV infection may require hospitalization (14–18). In addition, hMPV infection can be severe in immunocompromised patients such as lung transplant (19) and hematopoietic stem-cell transplant recipients (20–23), and can cause febrile respiratory illness in HIV-infected patients (24) as well as exacerbate chronic obstructive pulmonary disease (25). Nearly 100% of children are seropositive by 5 years of age. There are currently no vaccines to prevent hMPV infection, and unlike the related pathogen respiratory syncytial virus (RSV), for which the prophylactic treatment palivizumab (26) is available for high-risk infants, no treatment or prophylaxis is available for hMPV.

THE PNEUMOVIRUS FUSION PROTEIN

Pneumoviruses have three surface glycoproteins: the (F) fusion, (G) attachment, and small hydrophobic (SH) proteins, and the pneumovirus F protein is absolutely critical for viral infectivity. Antibodies are highly important for pneumovirus immunity (27, 28), and both RSV F and RSV G elicit neutralizing antibodies (29), while only antibodies to hMPV F are neutralizing (30). The pneumovirus F proteins belong to the family of class I viral fusion proteins that mediate the fusion of viral envelope and cell membrane during infection (31). The RSV F protein is first expressed as a F_0 precursor, which is then cleaved at two furin cleavage sites in the trans-Golgi network to become fusion competent, generating the N-terminal F_2 subunit and the C-terminal F_1 subunit, while the p27 fragment in between F_1 and F_2 is removed. In contrast, hMPV F is cleaved at one site by different intracellular enzymes than RSV (32). Cleaved pneumovirus F proteins are anchored on the viral envelope by the trans-membrane domain of F_1. The F_1 and F_2 fragments are covalently linked via two disulfide bonds, and the proteins form a trimeric structure consisting of three of the disulfide-linked fragments. The Pneumovirus F proteins fold into a pre-fusion conformation that contains a buried fusion peptide. Upon activation, the F protein undergoes a series of conformational changes leading to the post-fusion conformation

in concert with cell-virus membrane fusion (31). The pre-fusion conformation of the pneumovirus F protein is unstable, and refolding can occur spontaneously or under certain stimuli that irreversibly transform the globular pre-fusion F into the elongated post-fusion formation. During the process of the pre-to-post-fusion conformational change, the highly hydrophobic fusion peptide located at the N terminus of F2 will insert into host cell membrane, forming a hairpin structure that bridges the two membranes together before a refolding event causes membrane fusion.

Until recently, knowledge on the structural aspects of pneumovirus fusion proteins was severely lacking, primarily due to instability of the pre-fusion conformation when recombinantly expressed. An X-ray crystal structure of the post-fusion conformation of RSV F was determined in 2011 by removal of the fusion peptide in the construct used for crystallization (33, 34). A breakthrough in 2013 facilitated structural-determination of the RSV F protein in the pre-fusion conformation by co-expression of RSV F with the mAb Fab fragment D25 to trap the protein in the pre-fusion state (35). This subsequently led to stabilization of the RSV F protein in the pre-fusion conformation by locking the protein in the pre-fusion state via artificial disulfide-bond insertion in addition to cavity-filling mutations (the Ds-Cav1 construct) (36). Following this, an additional pre-fusion-stabilized protein was generated in an alternative approach using the substitution of proline residues in the refolding regions and expression of the protein as a single-chain through the introduction of a glycine-serine linker (the SC-TM construct) (37). For hMPV, a partial X-ray crystal structure of hMPV F in the pre-fusion conformation in complex with the neutralizing Fab DS7 was determined in 2012 (38). Following the success with stabilization of pre-fusion RSV F, crystal structures of trimeric hMPV pre-fusion and post-fusion hMPV F were determined (39, 40). Pre-fusion hMPV F was stabilized with proline-substitutions to prevent refolding to the post-fusion conformation, while post-fusion hMPV F required the addition of a trimerization domain. Both hMPV F constructs required cleavage-site modification and co-expression with furin in CV-1 cells to generate fully-cleaved trimeric proteins. In addition to the structures described above, similar strategies were utilized to stabilize the parainfluenza virus fusion proteins, and bovine RSV F in the pre-fusion state (41, 42).

ANTIGENIC DIFFERENCES BETWEEN RSV AND HMPV F

The RSV and hMPV F proteins share ~30% sequence identify, and among the antigenic sites on RSV F, at least two are shared with hMPV F (antigenic sites III and IV) as a result of this conservation (Figures 1A,B). Despite the shared sequence conservation, several distinct features influence the differing antibody response to these viruses. The majority of RSV neutralizing activity in human sera is mediated by pre-fusion-specific RSV F antibodies (43), while the majority of hMPV neutralizing activity is mediated by antibodies recognizing both pre-fusion and post-fusion conformations (40). In addition, vaccination with pre-fusion RSV F induces higher levels of neutralizing IgG than vaccination with post-fusion RSV F (36),

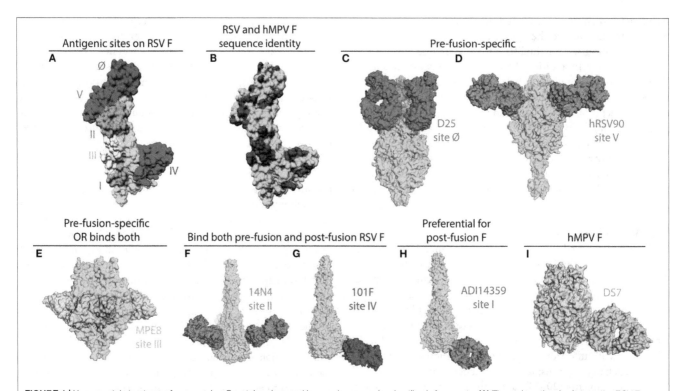

FIGURE 1 | X-ray crystal structures of pneumovirus F proteins alone and in complex monoclonal antibody fragments. **(A)** The main antigenic sites on the RSV F protein are depicted on a monomer of the F protein (PDB ID: 5C6B). **(B)** The same structure as in **(A)** is colored according to sequence conservation with hMPV F. Conserved residues are shown in maroon, and primarily reside within antigenic sites III, IV, and V. Sequences of RSV and hMPV F were derived from PDB IDs: 5C6B and 5WB0. **(C)** The pre-fusion specific antibody D25 binds at the apex of pre-fusion RSV F (PDB ID: 4JHW). **(D)** hRSV90 binds antigenic site V and is pre-fusion-specific (PDB ID: 5TPN). **(E)** MPE8 is pre-fusion-specific and cross-reactive with hMPV F (PDB ID: 5U68). **(F)** 14N4 is a human antibody that targets antigenic site II and binds both pre-fusion and post-fusion RSV F (PDB ID: 5J3D). **(G)** The humanized mouse mAb, 101F, binds at antigenic site IV. For this structure, the crystal structure of 101F binding the site IV peptide (PDB ID: 3O41) was aligned with antigenic site IV of the post-fusion RSV F protein (3RRR). **(H)** The non-neutralizing site I mAb ADI14359 was isolated from an RSV-infected infant, and is preferential for post-fusion RSV F (PDB ID: 6APB). **(I)** DS7 is a hMPV F-specific mAb that was co-crystallized with a fragment of pre-fusion hMPV F. The structure of the DS7-F complex (PDB ID: 4DAG) is overlaid onto the trimeric pre-fusion hMPV F structure (PDB ID: 5WB0). All antibodies are colored in accordance with the text label, the RSV F protein is shown in cyan, and the hMPV F protein is shown in wheat. All figures and alignments were prepared in PyMol and Chimera.

while vaccination with pre-fusion-stabilized hMPV F elicited similar neutralizing IgG titers as vaccination with post-fusion hMPV F (40). These data suggest that pre-fusion-specific RSV F antibodies are more prevalent in infected or vaccinated humans and mice, and pre-fusion-specific hMPV F antibodies are present at low levels as compared to antibodies that recognize both pre-fusion and post-fusion hMPV F. The low level of pre-fusion-specific hMPV F antibodies is likely due to a glycan shield near the corresponding RSV site Ø and site V regions on the head of hMPV F.

ANTIGENIC EPITOPES ON THE RSV F PROTEIN

mAbs binding to the RSV F protein could prevent F protein binding to host cell or hinder the conformational change from pre-fusion to post-fusion, and thus block viral entry into the cell. Due to its sequence conservation, and elicitation of potently neutralizing mAbs, the F protein has become the most popular target for vaccine development. As such, there has been a rapid increase in structural characterization of mAbs

in complex with the RSV F protein. Currently available solved structures of mAbs in complex with pneumovirus F proteins are summarized in **Table 1**. To date, multiple antigenic sites targeted by antibodies have been identified on the RSV F protein (**Figure 1**). Based on the secondary structure of the protein, six general regions have been designated as antigenic sites: Ø, I, II, III, IV, and V. Among them, antigenic sites I, II, and IV are quite similar between pre-fusion and post-fusion conformations due to their structural conservation upon transition from pre-fusion to post-fusion F. Antigenic sites Ø and V are only present in the pre-fusion conformation (58), while antigenic site III elicits mAbs that are pre-fusion-specific, such as MPE8, while also eliciting mAbs that bind both conformations, such as 25P13 (50). In addition, more than 60% of the most potent neutralizing mAbs bind to sites Ø and V (59), indicating these areas are crucial for immune system recognition and subsequent virus neutralization.

Antigenic Site Ø

Antigenic site Ø was the first pre-fusion-specific antigenic site identified on the RSV F protein. The methodology for isolating the first site Ø antibodies was crucial as the mAbs were isolated

TABLE 1 | List of structurally-characterized antibodies in complex with pneumovirus F proteins or fragments thereof.

mAb	PDB ID	Origin	Antigenic site	References
RSV F				
motavizumab	3IXT, 3QWO, 4JLR, 6OE5, 4ZYP	Mouse	II	(44)
101F	3O41, 3O45	Mouse	IV	(45)
hRSV90	5TPN	Human	V	(46)
D25	4JHW	Human	Ø	(36)
MEDI8897	5UDC, 5UDD	Human	Ø	(47)
AM22	6DC5, 6APD	Human	Ø	(48)
5C4	5W23	Mouse	Ø	(49)
MPE8	5U68	Human	III	(50)
ADI19425	6APD	Human	III	(51)
CR9501	6OE4/6OE5	Human	V	(52)
AM14	4ZYP	Human	IV, V	(53)
RSD5	6DC3	Human	Ø	(48)
14N4	5J3D	Human	II	(54)
ADI14359	6APD	Human	I	(51)
R4.C6	6CXC	Mouse	II, IV	(55)
RB1	6OUS	Human	IV	(56)
F-VHH-4	5TOJ	Llama	II, III, IV, V	(57)
F-VHH-L66	5TOK	Llama	II, III, IV, V	(57)
hMPV F				
DS7	4DAG	Human	DS7-site	(38)

on the basis of RSV neutralization rather than RSV F protein binding (60). This facilitated the isolation of pre-fusion-specific mAbs without the existence of a pre-fusion RSV F construct. Subsequently, one mAb, D25 (**Figure 1C**), was utilized to lock the RSV F protein in the pre-fusion conformation (35), which then facilitated stabilization of RSV F in the pre-fusion conformation (36). It is now clear that mAbs that target antigenic site Ø are a large portion of the human B cell repertoire (43, 46, 59). 5C4 is a mAb derived from mice immunized with gene-based vectors encoding the F protein, and is 50 times more potent than palivizumab. Human mAbs D25 and AM22, as well as the mouse mAb 5C4 bind to the apex of the pre-fusion F trimer (site Ø) (36). Importantly, a human mAb based on D25, MEDI-8897, is in clinical trials for prevention of RSV disease in infants (61).

Antigenic Site V

Antigenic site V was described recently, based on mAb isolation to new pre-fusion-stabilized constructs (46, 59). hRSV90 (**Figure 1D**) is a site V-targeting human mAb that was found to compete for binding with mAbs that target site II and site Ø. hRSV90 was co-crystallized with the RSV F protein and found to bind just below antigenic site Ø (46). In addition, several site V mAbs were isolated from both adults and infants (51, 59), suggesting these mAbs are prevalent in the human anti-RSV repertoire. CR9501 is a neutralizing mAb isolated from humans, and this mAb was used to demonstrate the dynamic motions of trimeric pre-fusion RSV F protein (52). An antibody that competes for site V of the RSV F protein, MC17, was also shown to cross-react with the hMPV F protein (56).

Antigenic Site III

The prototypical site III mAb MPE8 (**Figure 1E**) is unique as it cross-neutralizes multiple viruses in the *Pneumoviridae* family (62). This broad coverage is related to similar V gene usage and somatic mutations in the variable region based on the isolation of a highly similar human antibody 25P13 (50), as well as several other mAbs from a large panel of anti-RSV F human mAbs (59). In addition, site III-specific mAbs are elicited upon initial RSV infection in infants (51). One mAb, ADI19425, which was isolated from an RSV-infected infant, and is potently neutralizing despite lacking substantial somatic hypermutation, was co-crystallized with pre-fusion RSV F (51).

Antigenic Site II

Palivizumab and motavizumab are the prototypical mAbs to identify antigenic site II on the RSV F protein (26, 44, 63, 64). Targeting antigenic site II of RSV F protein (26), palivizumab is able to neutralize a broad panel of 57 RSV isolates from both subtypes A and B (65). This antigenic site primarily consists of the helix-loop-helix motif of residues 255-275 on the RSV F protein. Several human antibodies have been isolated that bind at antigenic site II (51, 54, 59). The human antibody 14N4 (**Figure 1F**) was co-crystallized in complex with post-fusion RSV F, and primarily focuses on the 255–275 motif. In the same study, a panel of non-neutralizing mAbs was identified that compete with antigenic site II mAbs on post-fusion RSV F, and suggest some limitations of the palivizumab competition assay used in some vaccine efficacy studies (54). The characterization of mAbs to this antigenic site has led to vaccine candidates focused on antigenic site II (66, 67). Furthermore, serum competition assays with palivizumab have been utilized to characterize vaccine candidates (68). In addition to the mAbs above, nanobodies targeting antigenic site II have been isolated (69, 70), and one nanobody, ALX-0171, has been evaluated as an antiviral therapy to treat RSV infection (71).

Antigenic Site IV

The site IV epitope is epitomized by the humanized mouse mAb 101F (**Figure 1G**) (72), and this epitope is structurally conserved between pre-fusion and post-fusion RSV F. The site IV epitope primarily consists of a linear region based on epitope mapping and structural data (45, 73). In addition, it was recently found that 101F cross-reacts with the hMPV F protein (39), presumably by binding to a conserved region at site IV that is similar between RSV and hMPV F (73). Several human mAbs targeting antigenic site IV have also been isolated (51, 59, 73), and human antibody cross-reactivity with hMPV F was correlated to a specific binding pose (73). In addition to the traditional site IV epitope, a mouse mAb, R4.C6, has been isolated that incorporates site IV as well as site II into its epitope (55). The structure of the R4.C6 Fab-post-fusion RSV F complex obtained by cryo-EM showed that the antibody binds to a cross-protomer area in between site II and IV. Recently, a site IV human antibody, RB1, was co-crystallized in complex with pre-fusion RSV F, and a half-life extended variant of this antibody is in clinical development (74).

Antigenic Site I

The site I epitope on the RSV F protein was identified by the prototypical mouse monoclonal antibody 131-2a (75). Recently, it was determined that human mAbs identified that bind at antigenic site I are weakly or non-neutralizing (51, 54), likely due to insufficient binding to pre-fusion RSV F, as many of these mAbs are post-fusion-specific. The crystal structure of an infant-derived non-neutralizing human mAb, ADI-14359 (**Figure 1H**), in complex with post-fusion RSV F was determined and defined the antigenic surface for site I (51).

Other Epitopes and Antibodies

In addition to the epitopes described above, there are several other antibodies isolated that bind unique regions on the RSV F protein. AM14 is a human mAb that recognizes a quaternary epitope spanning two protomers, suggesting the trimeric F protein has specific antigenic epitopes that are not found on the monomeric F protein (53). Single-domain antibody (VHH) or nanobodies from llama immunization were identified and co-crystallized with the RSV F protein (57). Both F-VHH-4 and F-VHH-L66 bind to a cavity in the intermediate area between antigenic site II of one protomer and antigenic site IV of the neighboring protomer. Intranasal administration of these VHHs significantly reduced viral replication in mice, which provides new therapeutic options for antiviral development.

MABS TARGETING THE HMPV F PROTEIN

The first hMPV F-specific neutralizing mAbs generated were derived from immunization of mice and hamsters with various strains of hMPV (76). Of the 12 mAbs in the study, murine mAbs 234 and 338 were effective as passive prophylaxis, protecting mice from hMPV challenge; mAb 338 was successful in reducing lung viral titers when given both prophylactically or therapeutically (77). By generating monoclonal antibody-resistant mutants of antibodies that neutralize hMPV, six antigenic sites of the hMPV F protein were identified (78). Since then, the terminology regarding pneumovirus antigenic sites for hMPV has followed that for RSV. Antigenic sites IV and III from the RSV F protein have been found to be conserved on hMPV F due to the isolation of cross-reactive mAbs discussed in the RSV section. hMPV F-specific mAbs have shown success in neutralizing hMPV both *in vitro* and *in vivo*.

The DS7-Antigenic Site

A human mAb isolated from a phage display library, termed DS7 (**Figure 1I**), was shown to reduce hMPV lung viral titers when administered therapeutically in cotton rats (79). mAb DS7 was co-crystallized in complex with a fragment of pre-fusion hMPV F (38), and has a unique molecular footprint in the bottom half of the hMPV F protein. Three additional human mAbs, which are naturally-occurring, termed MPV196, MPV201, and MPV314 were recently isolated and compete for binding with DS7, suggesting these mAbs target the same antigenic site (80).

Antigenic Site III

The first mAb identified to bind antigenic site III of hMPV F was the cross-reactive human mAb MPE8 (62). As discussed in the RSV section, MPE8 was co-crystallized with the RSV F protein, and the conserved regions at antigenic site III that facilitate cross-reactivity were also hypothesized (50). A similar mAb, 25P13, also discussed above, neutralized hMPV and RSV and competed for binding at antigenic site III (50). Recently, a human mAb, MPV364, was isolated and this mAb competes for binding at antigenic site III, yet does not cross-react with RSV F (80). MPV364 was shown to effectively limit viral replication in BALB/c mice (80). These data suggest antigenic site III can elicit both virus-specific and cross-reactive mAbs. However, the mechanism behind such mAb induction will require additional structural analysis.

Antigenic Site IV

As discussed earlier, the humanized mouse mAb 101F was identified to cross-react with hMPV F (39). Four human mAbs targeting antigenic site IV of the RSV F protein were isolated, and one mAb, termed 17E10, was identified to also cross-react with hMPV F. This mAb was subjected to peptide mapping and negative-stain microscopy. mAb 17E10 was found to bind a conserved GIIK motif on RSV and hMPV F (39). Furthermore, the binding angle of 17E10 and 101F were shown to be different than non-cross-reactive mAbs, suggesting an altered binding pose is required for cross-reactivity between RSV and hMPV F at antigenic site IV (73).

SUMMARY AND DISCUSSION

In recent years, several breakthroughs have facilitated new knowledge of pneumovirus antibody epitopes. Pre-fusion-stabilized constructs have allowed for isolation of mAbs with optimal neutralization potency, including those binding at antigenic site Ø and V on the RSV F protein. In addition, the use of mAbs to initially lock RSV in the pre-fusion conformation allowed for structure-based design of pre-fusion constructs. While hundreds of mAbs have now been isolated to the RSV F protein, the antigenic epitopes on the hMPV F protein, and related parainfluenza viruses remain unclear. Further studies into antigenic epitopes on these proteins will provide for new insights into pneumovirus immunity and vaccine design. In addition, pre-fusion-stabilized F constructs have now flooded the RSV vaccine field, and there is renewed excitement for the development of an effective RSV vaccine. The field is hopeful that future characterization of mAbs to other pneumovirus surface glycoproteins, as well as assessment of antibody responses to new vaccine candidates will lead to the first safe and effective pneumovirus vaccine.

AUTHOR CONTRIBUTIONS

JH, DD, and JM reviewed the literature, and wrote and edited the manuscript.

REFERENCES

Jones HG, Ritschel T, Pascual G, Brakenhoff JPJ, Keogh E, Furmanova- Hollenstein P, et al. Structural basis for recognition of the central conserved region of RSV G by neutralizing human antibodies. *PLoS Pathog.* (2018) 14:e1006935. doi: 10.1371/journal.ppat.1006935

Akhras N, Weinberg JB, Newton D. Human metapneumovirus and respiratory syncytial virus: subtle differences but comparable severity. *Infect Dis Rep.* (2010) 2:e12. doi: 10.4081/idr.2010.e12

Morris JA, Blount RE, Savage RE. Recovery of cytopathogenic agent from chimpanzees with goryza. *Proc Soc Exp Biol Med.* (1956) 92:544–9. doi: 10.3181/00379727-92-22538

Chanock R, Roizman B, Myers R. Recovery from infants with respiratory illness of a virus related to chimpanzee coryza agent (CCA): Isolation, properties and characterization. *Am J Epidemiol.* (1957) 66:291–300. doi: 10.1093/oxfordjournals.aje.a119902

Chanock R, Roizman B, Myers R. Recovery from infants with respiratory illness of a virus related to chimpanzee coryza agent (CCA): Isolation, properties and characterization. *Am J Epidemiol.* (1957) 66:281–290. doi: 10.1093/oxfordjournals.aje.a119901

Hall CB, Weinberg GA, Poehling KA, Erdman D, Grijalva CG, Zhu Y. The burden of respiratory synctial virus in young children. *N Engl J Med.* (2009) 360:588–98. doi: 10.1056/NEJMoa0804877

Shefali-Patel D, Paris MA, Watson F, Peacock JL, Campbell M, Greenough A. RSV hospitalisation and healthcare utilisation in moderately prematurely born infants. *Eur J Pediatr.* (2012) 171:1055–61. doi:10.1007/s00431-012-1673-0

Glezen WP, Taber LH, Frank AL, Kasel JA. Risk of primary infection and reinfection with respiratory syncytial virus. *Am J Dis Child.* (1986) 140:543–6. doi: 10.1001/archpedi.1986.02140200053026

Falsey AR, Walsh EE. Respiratory syncytial virus infection in adults. *Clin Microbiol Rev.* (2000) 13:371–84. doi: 10.1128/CMR.13.3.371

Grayson SA, Griffiths PS, Perez MK, Piedimonte G. Detection of airborne respiratory syncytial virus in a pediatric acute care clinic. *Pediatr Pulmonol.* (2017) 52:684–8. doi: 10.1002/ppul.23630

Higgins D, Trujillo C, Keech C. Advances in RSV vaccine research and development - A global agenda. *Vaccine.* (2016) 34:2870–5. doi:10.1016/j.vaccine.2016.03.109

Anderson EJ, Carosone-Link P, Yogev R, Yi J, Simões EAF. Effectiveness of palivizumab in high-risk infants and children: a propensity score weighted regression analysis. *Pediatr Infect Dis J.* (2017) 36:699–704. doi: 10.1097/INF.0000000000001533

van den Hoogen BG, de Jong JC, Groen J, Kuiken T, de Groot R, Fouchier RA, Osterhaus AD. A newly discovered human pneumovirus isolated from young children with respiratory tract disease. *Nat Med.* (2001) 7:719–24. doi: 10.1038/89098

Panda S, Mohakud NK, Pena L, Kumar S. Human metapneumovirus: review of an important respiratory pathogen. *Int J Infect Dis.* (2014) 25:45–52. doi:10.1016/j.ijid.2014.03.1394

Falsey AR, Erdman D, Anderson LJ, Walsh EE. Human metapneumovirus infections in young and elderly adults. *J Infect Dis.* (2003) 187:785–90. doi: 10.1086/367901

van den Hoogen BG, van Doornum GJ, Fockens JC, Cornelissen JJ, Beyer WE, de Groot R, et al. Prevalence and clinical symptoms of human metapneumovirus infection in hospitalized patients. *J Infect Dis.* (2003) 188:1571–7. doi:10.1086/379200

Madhi SA, Ludewick H, Abed Y, Klugman KP, Boivin G. Human metapneumovirus-associated lower respiratory tract infections among hospitalized human immunodeficiency virus type 1 (HIV-1)-infected and HIV-1-uninfected African infants. *Clin Infect Dis.* (2003) 37:1705–10. doi:10.1086/379771

Haas LEM, Thijsen SFT, van Elden L, Heemstra KA. Human metapneumovirus in adults. *Viruses.* (2013) 5:87–110. doi: 10.3390/v5010087

Larcher C, Geltner C, Fischer H, Nachbaur D, Müller LC, Huemer HP. Human metapneumovirus infection in lung transplant recipients: clinical presentation and epidemiology. *J Hear Lung Transpl.* (2005) 24:1891–901. doi: 10.1016/j.healun.2005.02.014

Cane PA, van den Hoogen BG, Chakrabarti S, Fegan CD, Osterhaus AD. Human metapneumovirus in a haematopoietic stem cell transplant recipient with fatal lower respiratory tract disease. *Bone Marrow Transplant.* (2003) 31:309–10. doi:10.1038/sj.bmt.1703849

Englund JA, Boeckh M, Kuypers J, Nichols WG, Hackman RC, Morrow RA, et al. Brief communication: fatal human metapneumovirus infection in stem-cell transplant recipients. *Ann Intern Med.* (2013) 144:344–9. doi: 10.7326/0003-4819-144-5-200603070-00010

Dokos C, Masjosthusmann K, Rellensmann G, Werner C, Schuler-Lüttmann S, Müller KM, et al. Fatal human metapneumovirus infection following allogeneic hematopoietic stem cell transplantation. *Transpl Infect Dis.* (2013) 15:97–101. doi:10.1111/tid.12074

Shah DP, Shah PK, Azzi JM, El Chaer F, Chemaly RF. Human metapneumovirus infections in hematopoietic cell transplant recipients and hematologic malignancy patients: a systematic review. *Cancer Lett.* (2016) 379:100–6. doi: 10.1016/j.canlet.2016.05.035

Klein MB, Yang H, DelBalso L, Carbonneau J, Frost E, Boivin G. Viral pathogens including human metapneumovirus are the primary cause of febrile respiratory illness in HIV-infected adults receiving antiretroviral therapy. *J Infect Dis.* (2010) 201:297–301. doi: 10.1086/ 649587

Kan-o K, Ramirez R, Macdonald MI, Rolph M, Rudd PA, Spann KM, et al. Human metapneumovirus infection in chronic obstructive pulmonary disease: impact of glucocorticosteroids and interferon. *J Infect Dis.* (2018) 215:1536–45. doi:10.1093/infdis/jix167

Group TIm-RS. Palivizumab, a humanized respiratory syncytial virus monoclonal antibody, reduces hospitalization from respiratory syncytial virus infection in high-risk infants. *Pediatrics.* (1998) 102:531–7. doi:10.1542/peds.102.3.531

Domachowske JB, Rosenberg HF. Respiratory syncytial virus infection: immune response, immunopathogenesis, and treatment. *Clin Microbiol Rev.* (1999) 12:298–309. doi: 10.1128/CMR.12.2.298

Falsey AR, Hennessey PA, Formica MA, Criddle MM, Biear JM, Walsh EE. Humoral immunity to human metapneumovirus infection in adults. *Vaccine.* (2010) 28:1477–80. doi: 10.1016/j.vaccine.2009.11.063

McLellan JS, Ray WC, Peeples ME. Structure and function of RSV surface glycoproteins. *Curr Top Microbiol Immunol.* (2013) 372:83–104. doi: 10.1007/978-3-642-38919-1_4

Skiadopoulos MH, Buchholz UJ, Surman SR, Collins PL, Murphy BR. Individual contributions of the human metapneumovirus F, G, and SH surface glycoproteins to the induction of neutralizing antibodies and protective immunity. *Virology.* (2006) 345:492–501. doi: 10.1016/j.virol.2005.10.016

White JM, Delos SE, Brecher M, Schornberg K. Structures and mechanisms of viral membrane fusion proteins: multiple variations on a common theme. *Crit Rev Biochem Mol Biol.* (2008) 43:189–219. doi: 10.1080/10409230802058320

Schowalter RM, Smith SE, Dutch RE. Characterization of human metapneumovirus F protein-promoted membrane fusion: critical roles for proteolytic processing and low pH. *J Virol.* (2006) 80:10931–41. doi:10.1128/JVI.01287-06

McLellan JS, Yang Y, Graham BS, Kwong PD. Structure of respiratory syncytial virus fusion glycoprotein in the postfusion conformation reveals preservation of neutralizing epitopes. *J Virol.* (2011) 85:7788–96. doi:10.1128/JVI.00555-11

Swanson KA, Settembre EC, Shaw CA, Dey AK, Rappuoli R, Mandl CW, et al. Structural basis for immunization with postfusion respiratory syncytial virus fusion F glycoprotein (RSV F) to elicit high neutralizing antibody titers. *Proc Natl Acad Sci USA.* (2011) 108:9619–24. doi:10.1073/pnas.1106536108

McLellan JS, Chen M, Leung S, Graepel KW, Du X, Yang Y, et al. Structure of RSV fusion glycoprotein trimer bound to a prefusion-specific neutralizing antibody. *Science.* (2013) 340:1113–7. doi:10.1126/science.1234914

McLellan JS, Chen M, Joyce MG, Sastry M, Stewart-Jones GBE, Yang Y, et al. Structure-based design of a fusion glycoprotein vaccine for respiratory syncytial virus. *Science.* (2013) 342:592–8. doi:10.1126/science.1243283

Krarup A, Truan D, Furmanova-Hollenstein P, Bogaert L, Bouchier P, Bisschop IJM, et al. A highly stable prefusion RSV F vaccine derived from structural analysis of the fusion mechanism. *Nat Commun.* (2015) 6:8143. doi:10.1038/ncomms9143

Wen X, Krause JC, Leser GP, Cox RG, Lamb R a, Williams J V, Crowe JE, Jardetzky TS. Structure of the human metapneumovirus fusion protein with neutralizing antibody identifies a pneumovirus antigenic site. *Nat Struc Mol Biol.* (2012) 19:461–3. doi:10.1038/nsmb.2250

Más V, Rodriguez L, Olmedillas E, Cano O, Palomo C, Terrón MC, et al. Engineering, structure and immunogenicity of the human metapneumovirus F protein in the postfusion conformation. *PLoS Pathog.* (2016) 12:e1005859. doi: 10.1371/journal.ppat.1005859

Battles MB, Más V, Olmedillas E, Cano O, Vázquez M, Rodríguez L, Melero JA, Mclellan JS. Structure and immunogenicity of pre-fusion-stabilized human metapneumovirus F glycoprotein. *Nat Commun.* (2017) 8:1528. doi:10.1038/s41467-017-01708-9

Stewart-Jones GBE, Chuang G-Y, Xu K, Zhou T, Acharya P, Tsybovsky Y, et al. Structure-based design of a quadrivalent fusion glycoprotein vaccine for human parainfluenza virus types 1–4. *Proc Natl Acad Sci USA.* (2018) 115:12265–70. doi:10.1073/pnas.1811980115

Zhang B, Chen L, Silacci C, Thom M, Boyington JC, Druz A, et al. Protection of calves by a prefusion-stabilized bovine RSV F vaccine. *Nat Struc Mol Biol.* (2017) 2:7. doi:10.1038/s41541-017-0005-9

Ngwuta JO, Chen M, Modjarrad K, Joyce MG, Kanekiyo M, Kumar A, et al. Prefusion F – specific antibodies determine the magnitude of RSV neutralizing activity in human sera. *Sci Transl Med.* (2015) 7:309ra162. doi: 10.1126/scitranslmed.aac4241

McLellan JS, Chen M, Kim A, Yang Y, Graham BS, Kwong PD. Structural basis of respiratory syncytial virus neutralization by motavizumab. *Nat Struc Mol Biol.* (2010) 17:248–50. doi:10.1038/nsmb.1723

McLellan JS, Chen M, Chang J-S, Yang Y, Kim A, Graham BS, et al. Structure of a major antigenic site on the respiratory syncytial virus fusion glycoprotein in complex with neutralizing antibody 101F. *J Virol.* (2010) 84:12236–44. doi:10.1128/JVI.01579-10

Mousa JJ, Kose N, Matta P, Gilchuk P, Crowe JE. A novel pre- fusion conformation-specific neutralizing epitope on the respiratory syncytial virus fusion protein. *Nat Microbiol.* (2017) 2:16271. doi:10.1038/nmicrobiol.2016.271

Zhu Q, McLellan JS, Kallewaard NL, Ulbrandt ND, Palaszynski S, Zhang J, et al. A highly potent extended half-life antibody as a potential RSV vaccine surrogate for all infants. *Sci Transl Med.* (2017) 9:1–12. doi:10.1126/scitranslmed.aaj1928

Jones HG, Battles MB, Lin C-C, Bianchi S, Corti D, McLellan JS. Alternative conformations of a major antigenic site on RSV F. *PLoS Pathog.* (2019) 15:e1007944. doi:10.1371/journal.ppat.1007944

Tian D, Battles MB, Moin SM, Chen M, Modjarrad K, Kumar A, et al. Structural basis of respiratory syncytial virus subtype-dependent neutralization by an antibody targeting the fusion glycoprotein. *Nat Commun.* (2017) 8:1877. doi: 10.1038/s41467-017-01858-w

Wen X, Mousa JJ, Bates JT, Lamb RA, Crowe JE, Jardetzky TS. Structural basis for antibody cross-neutralization of respiratory syncytial virus and human metapneumovirus. *Nat Microbiol.* (2017) 2:16272. doi:10.1038/nmicrobiol.2016.272

Goodwin E, Gilman MSA, Wrapp D, Graham BS, Mclellan JS, Walker LM. Infants infected with respiratory syncytial virus generate potent neutralizing antibodies that lack somatic hypermutation. *Immunity.* (2018) 48:339–49.e5. doi:10.1016/j.immuni.2018.01.005

Gilman MSA, Furmanova-Hollenstein P, Pascual G, van 't Wout BA, Langedijk JPM, McLellan JS. Transient opening of trimeric prefusion RSV F proteins. *Nat Commun.* (2019) 10:2105. doi:10.1038/s41467-019-09807-5

Gilman MSA, Moin SM, Mas V, Chen M, Patel NK, Kramer K, et al. Characterization of a prefusion-specific antibody that recognizes a quaternary, cleavage-dependent epitope on the RSV fusion glycoprotein. *PLoS Pathog.* (2015) 11:e1005035. doi:10.1371/journal.ppat.1005003

Mousa JJ, Sauer MF, Sevy AM, Finn JA, Bates JT, Alvarado G, et al. Structural basis for nonneutralizing antibody competition at antigenic site II of the respiratory syncytial virus fusion protein. *Proc Natl Acad Sci USA.* (2016) 113:E6849–58. doi:10.1073/pnas.1609449113

Xie Q, Wang Z, Ni F, Chen X, Ma J, Patel N, et al. Structure basis of neutralization by a novel site II/IV antibody against respiratory syncytial virus fusion protein. *PLoS ONE.* (2019) 14:e0210749. doi:10.1371/journal.pone.0210749

Xiao X, Tang A, Cox KS, Wen Z, Callahan C, Sullivan NL, et al. Characterization of potent RSV neutralizing antibodies isolated from human memory B cells and identification of diverse RSV/hMPV cross-neutralizing epitopes. *MAbs.* (2019) 11:1415–27. doi:10.1080/19420862.2019.1654304

Rossey I, Gilman MSA, Kabeche SC, Sedeyn K, Wrapp D, Melero A, et al. Potent single-domain antibodies that arrest respiratory syncytial virus fusion protein in its prefusion state. *Nat Commun.* (2017) 13:14158. doi:10.1038/ncomms16165

Melero JA, Mas V, McLellan JS. Structural, antigenic and immunogenic features of respiratory syncytial virus glycoproteins relevant for vaccine development. *Vaccine.* (2017) 35:461–8. doi:10.1016/j.vaccine.2016.09.045

Gilman MSA, Castellanos CA, Chen M, Ngwuta JO, Goodwin E, Moin SM, et al. Rapid profiling of RSV antibody repertoires from the memory B cells of naturally infected adult donors. *Sci Immunol.* (2016) 1:1–12. doi:10.1126/sciimmunol.aaj1879

Kwakkenbos MJ, Diehl SA, Yasuda E, Bakker AQ, van Geelen CMM, Lukens MV, et al. Generation of stable monoclonal antibody–producing B cell receptor-positive human memory B cells by genetic programming. *Nat Med.* (2010) 16:123–8. doi:10.1038/nm.2071

Domachowske JB, Khan AA, Esser MT, Jensen K, Takas T, Villafana T, et al. Safety, tolerability and pharmacokinetics of MEDI8897, an extended half- life single-dose respiratory syncytial virus prefusion F-targeting monoclonal antibody administered as a single dose to healthy preterm infants. *Pediatr Infect Dis J.* (2018) 37:886–92. doi:10.1097/INF.0000000000001916

Corti D, Bianchi S, Vanzetta F, Minola A, Perez L, Agatic G, et al. Cross-neutralization of four paramyxoviruses by a human monoclonal antibody. *Nature.* (2013) 501:439–43. doi:10.1038/nature12442

Bates JT, Keefer CJ, Slaughter JC, Kulp DW, Schief WR, Crowe JE. Escape from neutralization by the respiratory syncytial virus-specific neutralizing monoclonal antibody palivizumab is driven by changes in on- rate of binding to the fusion protein. *Virology.* (2014) 454–455:139–44. doi:10.1016/j.virol.2014.02.010

Wu H, Pfarr DS, Johnson S, Brewah YA, Woods RM, Patel NK, et al. Development of motavizumab, an ultra-potent antibody for the prevention of respiratory syncytial virus infection in the upper and lower respiratory tract. *J Mol Biol.* (2007) 368:652–65. doi:10.1016/j.jmb.2007.02.024

Johnson S, Oliver C, Prince GA, Hemming VG, Pfarr DS, Want S-C, et al. Development of a humanized monoclonal antibody (Medi-493) with potent *in vitro* and *in vivo* activity against respiratory syncytial virus. *J Infect Dis.* (1997) 17:1215–24. doi:10.1086/514115

Correia BE, Bates JT, Loomis RJ, Baneyx G, Carrico C, Jardine JG, et al. Proof of principle for epitope-focused vaccine design. *Nature.* (2014) 507:201–6. doi:10.1038/nature12966

Luo X, Liu T, Wang Y, Jia H, Zhang Y, Caballero D, et al. An epitope-specific respiratory syncytial virus vaccine based on an antibody scaffold. *Angew Chem Int Ed.* (2015) 54:14531–4. doi:10.1002/anie.201507928

Smith G, Raghunandan R, Wu Y, Liu Y, Massare M, Nathan M, et al. Respiratory syncytial virus fusion glycoprotein expressed in insect cells form protein nanoparticles that induce protective immunity in cotton rats. *PLoS ONE.* (2012) 7:e50852. doi:10.1371/journal.pone.0050852

Detalle L, Stohr T, Palomo C, Piedra PA, Gilbert BE, Mas V, et al. Generation and characterization of ALX-0171, a potent novel therapeutic nanobody for the treatment of respiratory syncytial virus infection. *Antimicrob Agents Chemother.* (2016) 60:6–13. doi:10.1128/AAC.01802-15

Hultberg A, Temperton NJ, Rosseels V, Koenders M, Gonzalez-Pajuelo M, Schepens B, et al. Llama-derived single domain antibodies to build multivalent, superpotent and broadened neutralizing anti-viral molecules. *PLoS ONE.* (2011) 6:e17665. doi:10.1371/journal.pone.0017665

Larios Mora A, Detalle L, Gallup JM, Van Geelen A, Stohr T, Duprez L, et al. Delivery of ALX-0171 by inhalation greatly reduces respiratory syncytial virus disease in newborn lambs. *MAbs.* (2018) 10:778–95. doi:10.1080/19420862.2018.1470727

Wu SJ, Albert Schmidt A, Beil EJ, Day ND, Branigan PJ, Liu C, et al. Characterization of the epitope for anti-human respiratory syncytial virus F protein monoclonal antibody 101F using synthetic peptides and genetic approaches. *J Gen Virol.* (2007) 88:2719–23. doi: 10.1099/vir.0.82753-0

Mousa JJ, Binshtein E, Human S, Fong RH, Alvarado G, Doranz BJ, et al. Human antibody recognition of antigenic site IV on Pneumovirus fusion proteins. *PLoS Pathog.* (2018) 14:e1006837. doi: 10.1371/journal.ppat. 1006837

Tang A, Chen Z, Cox KS, Su H, Callahan C, Fridman A, et al. A potent broadly neutralizing human RSV antibody targets conserved site IV of the fusion glycoprotein. *Nat Commun.* (2019) 10:4153. doi: 10.1038/s41467-019-12 137-1

Anderson LJ, Hierholzer JC, Stone Y, Tsou C, Fernie BF. Identification of epitopes on respiratory syncytial virus proteins by competitive binding immunoassay. *J Clin Microbiol.* (1986) 23:475–80.

Ulbrandt ND, Ji H, Patel NK, Riggs JM, Brewah YA, Ready S, et al. Isolation and characterization of monoclonal antibodies which neutralize human metapneumovirus *in vitro* and *in vivo. J Virol.* (2006) 80:7799–806. doi: 10.1128/JVI.00318-06

Hamelin ME, Gagnon C, Prince GA, Kiener P, Suzich J, Ulbrandt N, et al. Prophylactic and therapeutic benefits of a monoclonal antibody against the fusion protein of human metapneumovirus in a mouse model. *Antivir Res.* (2010) 88:31–7. doi: 10.1016/j.antiviral.2010.07.001

Ulbrandt ND, Ji H, Patel NK, Barnes AS, Wilson S, Kiener PA, et al. Identification of antibody neutralization epitopes on the fusion protein of human metapneumovirus. *J Gen Virol.* (2008) 89:3113–8. doi: 10.1099/vir.0.2008/005199-0

Williams JV, Chen Z, Cseke G, Wright DW, Keefer CJ, Tollefson SJ, et al. A recombinant human monoclonal antibody to human metapneumovirus fusion protein that neutralizes virus *in vitro* and is effective therapeutically *in vivo. J Virol.* (2007) 81:8315–24. doi: 10.1128/JVI.00106-07

Bar-Peled Y, Diaz D, Pena-Briseno A, Murray J, Huang J, Tripp RA, et al. A potent neutralizing site III-specific human antibody neutralizes human metapneumovirus *in vivo. J Virol.* (2019) 93:e00342-19. doi:10.1128/JVI.00342-19

20

Bacteriophage Cocktails Protect Dairy Cows Against Mastitis Caused By Drug Resistant *Escherichia coli* Infection

Mengting Guo, Ya Gao, Yibing Xue, Yuanping Liu, Xiaoyan Zeng, Yuqiang Cheng, Jingjiao Ma, Hengan Wang, Jianhe Sun, Zhaofei Wang[*] and Yaxian Yan[*]

School of Agriculture and Biology, Shanghai Jiao Tong University, Shanghai Key Laboratory of Veterinary Biotechnology, Shanghai, China

Correspondence:
Zhaofei Wang
wzfxlzjx@sjtu.edu.cn
Yaxian Yan
yanyaxian@sjtu.edu.cn

Mastitis caused by *Escherichia coli* (*E. coli*) remains a threat to dairy animals and impacts animal welfare and causes great economic loss. Furthermore, antibiotic resistance and the lagged development of novel antibacterial drugs greatly challenge the livestock industry. Phage therapy has regained attention. In this study, three lytic phages, termed vB_EcoM_SYGD1 (SYGD1), vB_EcoP_SYGE1 (SYGE1), and vB_EcoM_SYGMH1 (SYGMH1), were isolated from sewage of dairy farm. The three phages showed a broad host range and high bacteriolytic efficiency against *E. coli* from different sources. Genome sequence and transmission electron microscope analysis revealed that SYGD1 and SYGMH1 belong to the *Myoviridae*, and SYGE1 belong to the *Autographiviridae* of the order *Caudovirales*. All three phages remained stable under a wide range of temperatures or pH and were almost unaffected in chloroform. Specially, a mastitis infected cow model, which challenged by a drug resistant *E. coli*, was used to evaluate the efficacy of phages. The results showed that the cocktails consists of three phages significantly reduced the number of bacteria, somatic cells, and inflammatory factors, alleviated the symptoms of mastitis in cattle, and achieved the same effect as antibiotic treatment. Overall, our study demonstrated that phage cocktail may be a promising alternative therapy against mastitis caused by drug resistant *E. coli*.

Keywords: cow mastitis, *Escherichia coli*, phage cocktails, therapy, drug resistant

INTRODUCTION

Mastitis (intramammary inflammation) remains a devastating disease in dairy animals worldwide. It adversely threatens the health of udder, decreases the quality and production of milk, impedes the growth of bovine, increases rearing and prevention costs, and negatively impacts animal welfare (Khan et al., 2021). The incidence of clinical mastitis in China from 2015 to 2017 was estimated to range between 0.6% and 18.2% monthly among seven farms, which cost 12000 to 76000 USD/farm/month (He et al., 2020).

Mastitis usually caused by *Escherichia coli* (*E. coli*), *Streptococcus uberis*, *Staphylococcus aureus*, and *Klebsiella pneumonia* (Bar et al., 2008; Klaas and Zadoks, 2017; Machado and Bicalho, 2018).

Bacterial culture was done on milk samples from 161 large Chinese (>500 cows) dairy farms, the most frequently isolated pathogens were *Escherichia coli* (14.4%), *Klebsiella* spp. (13.0%), coagulase-negative staphylococci (11.3%), *Streptococcus dysgalactiae* (10.5%), and *Staphylococcus aureus* (10.2%) (Gao et al., 2017). Among the pathogens, *E. coli* is the most common Gram-negative bacteria causing acute clinical mastitis in dairy cows during early lactation (Cortinhas et al., 2016). During *E. coli* mastitis, the common visible symptoms of the affected part include the complete udder showing redness, swelling, pain upon touch, and the highest loss of milk or abnormal milk. Also, the cows become anorexic and pyrexial, thereby resulting in low production of milk (Khatun et al., 2013b). Additionally, *E.coli* mastitis incurs subclinical phenotypes, including an increase in somatic cell count (SCC) in milk (Abdi et al., 2021) and the production of proinflammatory cytokines in blood (Cobirka et al., 2020). Currently, several measures to control mastitis have been taken, such as antibiotic therapy (Mcdougall et al., 2019), antimicrobial peptides (Gurao et al., 2017), bacteriophage therapy (Ngassam-Tchamba et al., 2020), probiotics (Pellegrino et al., 2018), and nanoparticle-based therapy (Orellano et al., 2019). Among them, because of their remarkable effectiveness, antibiotics are the most common method (Gomes and Henriques, 2016). However, due to the abuse of antibiotics, multidrug-resistance bacteria have emerged which is projected to be the greatest challenges of the 21st century (Streicher, 2021).

Bacteriophages (referred to hereafter as phages) are a group of viruses that can infect and kill bacteria at the end of their lytic cycle (Rehman et al., 2019). Phages and their bacterial hosts coexist and coevolve in various environments, such as soil, oceans, freshwater, humans, and animals (Zalewska-Pitek and Pitek, 2020). Phages are the most abundant entities on earth, with approximately 10^{31} individual particles, which outnumber their hosts by 10 to 100 fold, depending on the environment, seemingly keeping an endless equilibrium state (Moelling et al., 2018; Zalewska-Pitek and Pitek, 2020). Further, interest in phage therapy began when a 'bacteriolytic agent' was discovered, and phage treatments were quickly applied to humans at the beginning of the 20th century (Chanishvili, 2012). Phage preparations remain in use and commercially available today in many countries, such as Georgia and Russia (Kutter et al., 2010). Although little progress has been made in phage research, phage therapy has been renewed due to the threat of multidrug-resistant bacterial infection and the advantages of phages, including specificity, efficacy, harmlessness to humans, and diversity (Clara, 2018; Aslam and Schooley, 2019). To increase efficacy, phages can be used alone, as cocktails, or synergistically with other antimicrobials *in vitro* or *in vivo* (Melo et al., 2020). Unprecedentedly, researchers have used a cocktail of three engineered phages to a 15-year-old patient who developed cystic fibrosis with *Mycobacterium abscess* infection, and the patient's clinical conditions improved without adverse reactions (Dedrick et al., 2019). A 63-year-old female patient suffering recurrent urinary tract infection (UTI) caused by drug-resistant *Klebsiella pneumoniae* (ERKp) was treated with antibiotic and phage cocktail. After treatment, the patient successfully combated UTI and was cured (Bao et al., 2020). Hence, phage therapy is an attractive approach for treating multidrug-resistant organisms.

To evaluate the efficiency and potential of the phage cocktail in treating cow mastitis, we isolated *E.coli* phages from dairy farm sewage. To learn more details, we further tested the spectra, efficiency of plating (EOP), and biological properties of three phages. We also identified their morphology and sequenced their genome. Finally, we evaluated their potential as phage therapy candidates in cows with mastitis caused by *E.coli* infection. This study expands our knowledge of the phage genome and highlights that phages have great potential as therapeutic adjuncts to relieve the embarrassing situation of antibiotic resistance.

MATERIALS AND METHODS

Ethics Statement
The animal experiments were carried out according to animal welfare standards and approved by the Ethical Committee for Animal Experiments of Shanghai Jiao Tong University, China. All animal experiments complied with the guidelines of the Animal Welfare Council of China.

Bacterial Strains and Culture Conditions
Eighteen *E. coli* (12 Food-borne strains and six strains isolated from the milk of dairy cows with mastitis) and two *E. coli* reference strains of MC1061 and MG1655 from the American Type Culture Collection (ATCC) were used in this study were stored in our laboratory (**Table 1**). Bacteria were cultured at 37°C in Luria-Bertani (LB) broth in a shaker at 200 rpm. The double-layer plate for purifying the phages was prepared by solid media containing LB and soft agar overlays, containing 0.75% agar into the LB broth agar (1.5%). Also, 5% sheep blood agar containing ampicillin (100 µg/mL) was used to determine the number of CFU/mL in milk sample.

Antibiotic Susceptibility Testing
All strains used in this study were subjected to antibiotic susceptibility testing against ampicillin, cefepime, gentamicin, kanamycin, ciprofloxacin, norfloxacin, and meropenem using the Kirby Bauer disc diffusion method. Briefly, bacteria were grown to an optical density at 600 nm (OD_{600}) of 0.4 to 0.6 in 3 mL LB, and 200 µL of each culture was swabbed on the surface of LB agar plates. Antibiotic discs (Beijing Pronade technology co., LTD, Beijing, China) were placed on the swabbed culture incubated for 16 to 18 h at 37°C, following which the inhibition zone was measured, and each strain was determined as resistant/intermediate/sensitive to each antibiotic tested following the chart provided by the manufacturer.

Isolation of Phages
Phages were isolated from the sewage of the different dairy farms in Shanghai using a traditional method, as described previously, with some modifications (Wang et al., 2016). Briefly, all samples

TABLE 1 | The host range and EOP of vB_EcoM_SYGD1, vB_EcoP_SYGE1, and vB_EcoM_SYGMH1.

Bacterial No.	Source[a]	vB_EcoM_SYGD1		vB_EcoM_SYGE1		vB_EcoM_SYGMH1	
		Spot test[b]	EOP[c]	Spot test	EOP	Spot test	EOP
MG1655	I	−	−	++	0.79 ± 0.03	−	−
MC1061	I	++	1.00	++	1.00	++	1.00
DG03512	II	++	0.66 ± 0.03	+	0.07 ± 0.00	++	0.20 ± 0.02
Min27	II	++	0.94 ± 0.02	++	0.40 ± 0.02	++	1.19 ± 0.02
ECS1	II	+	0.10 ± 0.01	+	0.11 ± 0.01	++	0.34 ± 0.02
ECS2	II	−	−	−	−	−	−
ECS3	II	++	0.36 ± 0.02	++	0.26 ± 0.01	+	0.09 ± 0.01
ECS4	II	−	−	−	−	−	−
ECS5	II	++	0.29 ± 0.02	++	0.29 ± 0.02	++	0.31 ± 0.02
ECS6	II	++	0.27 ± 0.03	++	0.30 ± 0.02	++	0.21 ± 0.02
ECS7	II	+	0.02 ± 0.00	+	0.21 ± 0.02	++	0.30 ± 0.02
ECS8	II	++	0.74 ± 0.03	++	0.41 ± 0.01	++	0.49 ± 0.03
ECS9	II	++	0.48 ± 0.04	++	0.28 ± 0.01	++	0.26 ± 0.00
ECS10	II	−	−	++	0.33 ± 0.02	−	−
ECD1	III	+	0.11 ± 0.02	+	0.19 ± 0.02	+	0.24 ± 0.02
ECD2	III	++	0.42 ± 0.02	++	0.49 ± 0.01	++	0.62 ± 0.06
ECD3	III	−	−	+	0.21 ± 0.02	−	−
ECD4	III	−	−	+	0.17 ± 0.01	−	−
ECD5	III	−	−	−	−	−	−
ECD6	III	−	−	−	−	−	−

[a]I, purchased from American Type Culture Collection; II, hospital-acquired strains; III, clinically-isolated strains from the milk of dairy cows with mastitis.
[b]++, clear plaque; +, hazy plaque, and -, no plaque.
[c]EOP, efficiency of plating (EOP = phage titre on test bacterium/phage titre on strains MC1061). The EOP values are shown as the mean of the three repeats ± SD. -, no plaque on target bacterium.

were centrifuged at 5,000 g for 20 min at 4°C, and the debris of supernatants was removed through the 0.22 μm microporous membrane and stored at 4°C. The pre-filtered samples were co-cultured with logarithmic phase DG03512, MG1655, and Min27 host strains for 12 h at 37°C before re-filtering through a 0.22 μm membrane filter to discard bacteria and their debris. The enriched phage suspensions were mixed with host strains (mid-log phase, OD_{600} = 0.4 to 0.6), and the mixture was added to 10 mL soft agar (0.75% agar) before pouring on top of an LB agar plate (1.5% agar). The plates were cultured at 37°C for 12 h until plaques were observed. To gain pure phage lysate, a single plaque was picked, and the above process was repeated following three successive times purification. Finally, phages were stored at 4°C or −80°C.

Phage particles were concentrated and purified by polyethylene glycol (PEG) precipitation and CsCl step gradients (Baker et al., 2006). Briefly, 200 mL of exponential-phase indicator bacteria was infected with phage stocks for 5 h at 37°C with shaking, and the supernatant lysates were collected by centrifuging at 10,000 g for 10 min before filtering through a 0.22 μM filter. To precipitate the phage particles, PEG 8000 was added at 10% final concentration to the supernatant, the mixture was incubated overnight at 4°C with constant shaking before centrifuging at 10000 g for 20 min, and the supernatant was removed. The resulting pellets were re-suspended in SM buffer (100 mM NaCl, 10 mM $MgSO_4 \cdot 7H_2O$, and 50 mM Tris·HCl pH 7.5). After the addition of 0.5 g/mL CsCl, the mixture was layered on top of CsCl step gradients (densities of 1.15 1.45, 1.50, and 1.70 g/mL) in Ultra-Clear centrifugation tubes and centrifuged at 28,000 × g for 2 h at 4°C, dialyzed in SM buffer. Phages were stored at 4°C or −80 °C for further experiments.

Determination of the Lytic Activity of the Phages Against Clinical Isolates of *E. coli*

The infection and lysis capacity of phages were determined using the spot test method, as previously described (Shahin et al., 2020). Briefly, 100 μL of 20 exponential growth strains were mixed evenly with 10 mL semisolid LB medium and overlaid on the LB Agar (1.5% agar). Also 5 μL of undiluted phage suspensions (~10^7 PFU/mL) were dropped on the culture surface. The plates were incubated at 37°C overnight, and a clear zone at the spot area indicated bacterial susceptibility to the phage. EOP, the ratio of the phage titer on the test strain to the phage titer obtained from the reference bacteria, was performed using the double-layer agar method. The reference strains for all isolated phages were MC1061. The experiment was performed in triplicate, and the results were recorded as the EOP mean ± standard deviation (SD). Finally, the EOP of each phage was classified as high (EOP ≥ 0.5), medium (0.1 ≤ EOP ≤ 0.5), low (0.001 < EOP < 0.1), and no lysis (EOP ≤ 0.001) (Shahin et al., 2021).

DNA Extraction and Sequencing

Phage DNA was extracted from 10 mL concentrated phage suspensions (10^{10} PFU mL^{-1}) using phenol-chloroform extraction and ethanol precipitation methods (Wang et al., 2016). Subsequently, Illumina MiSeq system was used for phages whole genome analysis. Sequence alignments were carried out using the Accelrys DS Gene software package of Accelrys Inc. (USA). Putative open reading frames were suggested using the algorithms of the software packages Accelrys Gene v2.5 (Accelrys Inc.) and ORF Finder (NCBI). Identity values were calculated using different BLAST algorithms (http://www.ncbi.nlm.nih.gov/BLAST/) at the NCBI homepage.

The sequences of phages were submitted to the NCBI. tRNA coding regions were searched using tRNAscan-SE 2.0 (Lowe and Chan, 2016).

Morphological Characterization
Purified phage particles (10^9 PFU/mL) were placed onto carbon-coated copper grids and negatively stained with 2% (w/v) uranyl acetate (pH 6.7) for 10 min. Finally, the purified viral particle morphology was examined using a FEI TEM Tecnai G2 Spirit Biotwin (FEI, Hillsboro, US) at an accelerating voltage of 120 kV.

One-Step Growth Curve
The one-step growth curves of phages were determined as previously reported (Yang Z. et al., 2019). Briefly, mid-exponential phase *E. coli* DG03512, MG1655, and Min27 were infected with vB_EcoM_SYGD1, vB_EcoP_SYGE1, and vB_EcoM_SYGMH1 at a multiplicity of infection (MOI) of 10, 1, 0.1, 0.01, 0.001, and 0.0001, respectively. After incubation for 4 h, the optimal MOIs of SYGD1, SYGE1, and SYGMH1 were determined using the double-layer agar method. For one-step growth experiments, host cells grew to an exponential phase and were infected with phages at the optimal MOI. After absorption for 10 min at 37°C, the cultures were centrifuged for 1 min at 13000 g to remove the unabsorbed phages. The pellets were washed with an LB medium, followed by resuspension in an equivalent LB medium. The cultures were grown at 37°C with shaking at 160 rpm. Samples were taken every 10 min (up to 120 min), and the number of phage particles was quantified using the method described above. The LB medium was only used as a control, and all experiments were conducted in triplicate.

Biological Characteristics of Phages
The procedures were performed as described previously, with modifications (Lu et al., 2017). To determine the thermostability of the three phages, phage suspensions at 10^8 PFU/mL were subjected to different temperatures (25°C, 37°C, 45°C, 50°C, 60°C, and 70°C) for 1 h. To evaluate the stability of the phage at different pH levels, phage suspensions were incubated in an LB broth adjusted to pH values ranging from 2 to 12 with HCl or NaOH for 1 h. Additionally, the ultraviolet (UV) sensitivity of phages was determined by exposing the phage suspensions at 35 cm under a UV light (30 w), and 100 μL aliquots were collected every 15 min until 75 min. The sensitivity of phages to chloroform was examined by mixing phage suspensions with different concentrations (5%, 25%, 50%, and 75%) of chloroform, respectively, and shaking vigorously, then incubated at 37°C for 30 min. The mixtures were centrifuged at 800 rpm for 15 min, and the hydrophilic layer was collected. The phage suspensions were diluted serially with $1 \times$ SM buffer, and phage titers were calculated using double-layer agar methods. All tests were performed in triplicate.

Determination of Endotoxins of Phage Cocktails
To improve the safety of the phage, an affinity matrix of modified polymyxin B (PMB) (GenScript, Nanjing, China) was used to remove phage cocktail endotoxins. Furthermore, the endotoxin

levels of the phage cocktails were evaluated by colorimetric method following the recommendations of the manufacturer (GenScript). The end-product was measured spectrophotometrically in a microplate reader.

The Treatment of Cow Mastitis Caused by *E. Coli* Using Phage Cocktails
The antibacterial activity of phage cocktails was evaluated in cows. We selected eight milk-secreting Holstein heifers (4–5 years old, 3–5 months after calving), and they were randomly divided into four groups, with two animals each. Three groups of cows were intramammary challenged with 60 CFU ECD2 suspended in 1 mL of pyrogen-free phosphate buffer saline PBS (Khatun et al., 2013a). After 24 h of inoculating *E. coli*, milk and blood samples were collected and analyzed immediately. Phage cocktails containing SYGD1, SYGE1, and SYGMH1 were prepared by mixing the three phages at a 1:1:1 ratio with a primary concentration of about 10^{10} PFU/mL, respectively. Finally, the mixture was diluted 100 times using (PBS) for therapy. One group was intramammary treated with 5 mL ceftiofur sodium (600 mg/mL). The second group was intramammary injected with 5 mL phage cocktails (1×10^8 PFU/mL). The third group was intramammary treated with 5 mL PBS alone. All treatments were administered once a day for three consecutive days. The fourth group, as a control group, was neither challenged nor treated. The eight animals were kept separately during the trial and monitored every day. After three-day treatment, milk and blood samples were collected and detected for three consecutive days.

Bacteriological Loading and Somatic Cell Count (SCC)
Milk samples were collected at 0 day before treatment and 4, 5, and 6 days after the beginning of the treatment from each individual quarter into 50 mL sterile tubes. Serial 10-fold dilutions of each milk sample were made under aseptic conditions by pipetting the sample into sterile PBS, and three 10 μL drops were plated on 5% sheep blood agar containing 100 μg/mL of ampicillin because of the resistance of ECD2 to ampicillin, and count colony was started after 24-hour incubation at 37°C. SCC of each milk sample was determined using a cell counter immediately after collection. Briefly, 10 μL of diluted fresh milk samples were thoroughly mixed with Trypan Blue and spread on a cell-counting plate.

Determination of Inflammatory Cytokine Levels in Serum
Blood samples were collected on the sixth day in 9 mL blood tubes stabilized with 50 to 200 IU of Na-heparin and immediately placed on ice for inflammatory biomarker analysis. A hot water bath (50°C) was used to evaporate the extracted solution. The blood tubes were centrifuged at 2,000 g at 4°C for 20 min. Serum was collected and stored at −20°C until used. Concentrations of inflammatory biomarker interleukin (IL)-1β and tumor necrosis factor (TNF)-α were measured *via* an enzyme-linked immunosorbent assay kit (ELISA kit) (Abcam, England) following the manufacturer's recommendations.

Statistical Analysis

All statistical analyses, unless otherwise stated, were executed using GraphPad Prism 8 (Graph Pad Software, Inc., La Jolla, CA). Error bars in graphs show the standard error of the mean (± SEM). The unpaired t-test was applied to compare the differences between each two groups. Most assays were performed in triplicate, and the data were expressed as the mean of three independent experiments. Statistical significance was considered as $p < 0.05$.

Data Availability

The whole-genome sequences of vB_EcoM_SYGD1, vB_EcoP_SYGE1, and vB_EcoM_SYGMH1 can be found in the GenBank Access Code MW883059, MW883060 and MW883061.

RESULTS

Phage Isolation and Host Range Determination

In this experiment, three samples from different dairy farms in Shanghai were detected to isolate the phages. Using DG03512, MG1655, and Min27 as host strains, we successfully isolated three phages that could form clear plaques in the lawn of their host cells, and phages were named vB_EcoM_SYGD1, vB_EcoP_SYGE1, and vB_EcoM_SYGMH1, respectively. Spot assay showed that SYGD1 and SYGMH1 had a wide host range with a similar spectrum (12 of 20, 60%), and SYGE1 could lyse more strains (16 of 20, 80%) (**Table 1**). In particular, 90% strains were resistant to two or more antibiotics (**Table 2**). EOPs assay

(**Table 1**) revealed that SYGE1 had higher production levels of progeny phages compared to SYGD1 and SYGMH1. The high and medium EOPs levels that is, the ratio of titers ≥ 0.1, of the former phage were observed in about 93.8% of tested strains; SYGD1 and SYGMH1 was 91.2% (11 out of 12 strains).

Phage Morphology and Characteristics of the Phage Genome

To determine the morphological characteristics of phages, the purified viral particles were stained, and TEM was performed. As shown in **Figure 1**, SYGD1 (**Figure 1A**) and SYGMH1 (**Figure 1C**) displayed a highly similar appearance with a prolate icosahedral head about 50–60 nm in diameter and a long tail with a length of nearly 100 nm and a width of about 10 nm surrounded by a helical sheath and long-tail fibers attached to the baseplates, similar to the *Myoviridae* family of the order *Caudovirales*. Phage SYGE1 (**Figure 1B**) was smaller than the other two phages with a short tail of about 10 nm, and had a head diameter of 30–40 nm which was typical for *Autographiviridae* phages. Genome sequencing analysis revealed that SYGD1, SYGE1, and SYGMH1 comprised 171.3 kb, 39.7 kb, and 137.4 kb, with G + C content of 35.33%, 48.69%, and 43.56%, as well as 271, 46, and 205 proposed open reading frames (ORFs), respectively. There were 8 and 6 tRNAs in the genome of SYGD1 and SYGMH1, respectively. No ORFs encoding tRNA were found in SYGE1 by analysis with tRNAscan-SE 2.0 (details were shown in **Supplementary Tables S4, S5**). The genome of phage SYGE1 were flanked with terminal repeats with a size of 170 bp. All of them comprised a typical modular format, including DNA replication and modification, structural components and DNA packaging, tail structural components

TABLE 2 | Antibiotic susceptibility profiles of *E. coli* strains used in this study.

Strains	AMP	FEP	GEN	KM	CIP	NOR	MEM
MG1655							
MC1061							
DG03512							
Min27							
ECS1							
ECS2							
ECS3							
ECS4							
ECS5							
ECS6							
ECS7							
ECS8							
ECS9							
ECS10							
ECD1							
ECD2							
ECD3							
ECD4							
ECD5							
ECD6							

▌Resistant.

Intermediate.

Sensitive.

AMP, Ampicillin; FEP, Cefepime; GEN, Gentamicin; KM, Kanamycin; CIP, Ciprofloxacin; NOR, Norfloxacin; MEM, Meropenem.

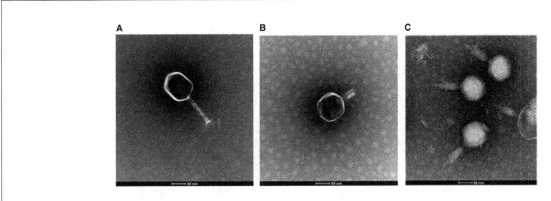

FIGURE 1 | Images of phage particles by transmission electron microscopy. **(A)** vB_EcoM_SYGD1. **(B)** vB_EcoP_SYGE1. **(C)** vB_EcoM_SYGMH1 (scale bar was 50 nm).

and host cell lysis (**Figure 2**). Furthermore, the BLAST analysis revealed that SYGD1 and SYGMH1 belonged to T4-like phage (**Table 2**), which showed relatively high homology (about 95%–97%) to NCBI database published T4-like phage (**Supplementary Tables S1, S3**). SYGE1 belonged to a T7-like phage, which showed partial homology (about 95%) to published T7-like phage (**Supplementary Table S2**). There are no homologs of known harmful genes, such as virulence, antibiotic resistance genes, or lysogenic genes, in the genome of phages. Thus, SYGD1, SYGE1, and SYGMH1 were considered lytic phages.

Determination of One-Step Growth Curve

From **Figure 3A**, SYGD1 and SYGE1 infected their host strains at an MOI of 0.01, generating the highest phage titer, while the

SYGMH1 optimal MOI was 10. From **Figure 3B**, the one-step growth curve of SYGD1 and SYGMH1 had similar characteristics, that both of them had latent period of about 20 min with almost no release of progeny phages and entered about 50 min and 70 min lysis period with a burst size of 52 and 58 PFU/cell, respectively. SYGE1 exhibited a relatively shorter latent period was about 10 min and the burst size was estimated as 129 PFU per infected cell.

Biological Characteristics of Phages

To examine the characteristics of the three phages, we analyzed their sensitivity to temperature, pH, UV, and chloroform. From **Figure 4A**, SYGD1, SYGE1, and SYGMH1 had similar thermostability under 25°C–37°C; with an increase in temperature, the activity of phage decreased gradually. When the

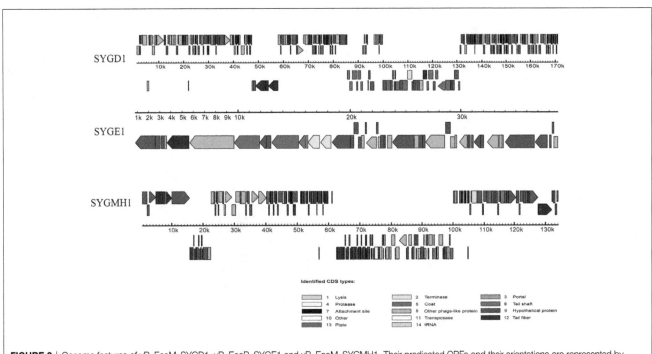

FIGURE 2 | Genome features of vB_EcoM_SYGD1, vB_EcoP_SYGE1 and vB_EcoM_SYGMH1. Their predicated ORFs and their orientations are represented by arrows. The function modules are shown in different colors.

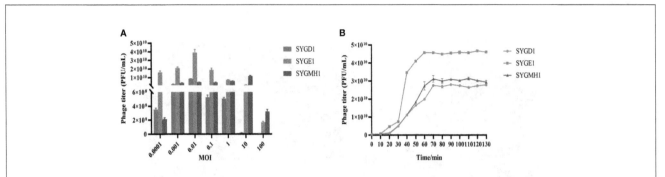

FIGURE 3 | The optimal MOI and one-step growth curve of phages. **(A)** vB_EcoM_SYGD1, vB_EcoP_SYGE1, and vB_EcoM_SYGMH1 infected their host strain at an MOI of 0.01 or 10, reaching their peak titer, indicating the most suitable concentration for lysing bacteria. **(B)** SYGD1, SYGE1, and SYGMH1 infected their host strains at the optimal MOI. The supernatants were harvested at 10 min intervals post-infection, and titers were determined using the double-layer method.

temperature reached 60°C, the phage titer decreased significantly, especially SYGD1, with only 3.4% survival. The activity of the three phages was completely lost after incubation at 70°C. Comparing, higher temperature inactivated the phages, but SYGMH1 had a relatively good resistance to temperature than other two phages. The pH sensitivity test showed that the three phages survived over a broad pH range (3–10), and pH 5–9 was their optimal growth condition, but became inactivated when pH was below 5 or above 10, indicating that the three phages were sensitive to strong acid or alkali (**Figure 4B**). From **Figure 4C**, all the phages were sensitive to UV radiation, and their activity decreased sharply after short exposure. Although the chloroform sensitivity test suggested that the activity of phages decreased with the prolongation of incubation time or the increase in chloroform concentration, it

was not significant, indicating that phages were tolerant of chloroform (**Figure 4D**).

Phage Therapy Alleviates CFU Loads and Inflammatory Response *In Vivo*

The lipopolysaccharide of Gram-negative bacteria is always recognized by host cell receptors (such as TLR-4), which is one of the induced factors of pathogenesis for mastitis (Griesbeck-Zilch et al., 2008; Bhattarai et al., 2018). The endotoxins of crude phages were higher up to 8 EUs/mL. After CsCl purification, the endotoxins were reduced the amounts to 0.48 EUs/mL (data not shown), which is a safe level for animal experiments (Bonilla and Barr, 2018; Luong et al., 2020). Cows were intramammary infused with phage cocktails or antibiotics

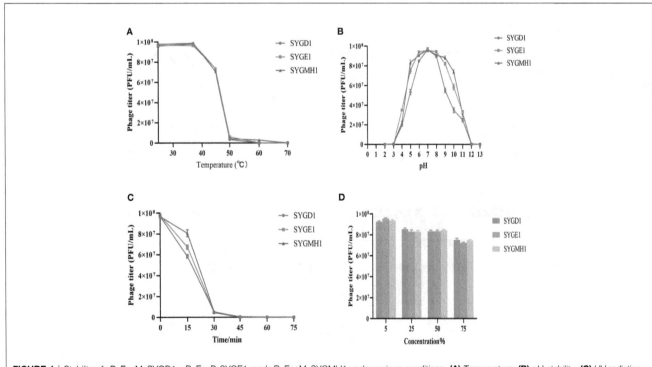

FIGURE 4 | Stability of vB_EcoM_SYGD1, vB_EcoP_SYGE1, and vB_EcoM_SYGMH1 under various conditions. **(A)** Temperature. **(B)** pH stability. **(C)** UV radiation stability. **(D)** Chloroform sensitivity. Survived phage particles were determined by double-layer tests. Error bars show the SEM among triplicate samples.

for three consecutive days after infection. From **Figure 5A**, PBS-treated group showed high bacterial loads at 4 day after infection, approximately 6×10^4 CFU/mL. However, compared to the untreated groups, both phage-treated and antibiotic-treated groups showed statistically significant decreases in CFU burden at all-time points. On the sixth day, the antibiotic or phage-treated groups almost could not detect bacteria. Milk SCCs were estimated once collected. High SCC values indicated a high prevalence of subclinical mastitis. From **Figure 5B**, cows treated with phage cocktails and antibiotics had lower SCC values than untreated cows. On the sixth day, the SCC values of the treated groups were basically the same as those of the healthy groups after three-day treatment. These results demonstrate that the quality of milk is efficiently enhanced through phage therapy. Analysis of cytokines showed that cows with mastitis significantly increased the levels of IL-1β and TNF-α. The cytokine in the phage and antibiotic-treated groups revealed a pattern of decreased proinflammatory markers after three-day treatment, indicating that phage therapy can alleviate inflammatory reaction (**Figures 5C, D**).

DISCUSSION

Recently, *E. coli* has become the most important pathogen inducing cow mastitis, mainly causing high fever or lower milk production, even resulting in lethal consequences (Fazel et al., 2019; Guerra et al., 2020). Also, *E. coli* is an important antibiotic-resistant priority pathogen and can disseminate

resistant genes in a process known as 'horizontal transfer' into other microbial communities (Jianying et al., 2008). Therefore, with the increase in antibacterial-resistant bacteria and discharge of antibiotics to the environment prompted scientists to explore alternative treatments.

Phage therapy is currently considered an efficient and suitable replacement for antibiotic therapy due to its specificity, safety, productive potential and lower economic burden (Mathieu et al., 2019; D'Accolti et al., 2021). Environmental source contains abundant phages which are able to lyse their target and the successful phage isolation is greatly facilitating the understanding of the ecology and the development of phage therapy (Gill and Hyman, 2010). In the present study, we isolated and characterized three phages, vB_EcoM_SYGD1, vB_EcoP_SYGE1, and vB_EcoM_SYGMH1, with broad host spectrum. The major advantages of phage therapy are specificity and strong bactericidal activity. However, Costa et al. have reported that *E. coli* can develop resistance to phage at a short time within 12 h (Costa et al., 2019). To overcome this disadvantage, phage cocktail comprising multiple phages may be considered an efficacy treatment modality (Costa et al., 2019; Pires et al., 2020). In our study, the three phages showed a high EOP against drug-resistant bacteria (EOP ≥ 0.1), which displayed the same or higher antibacterial efficacy as other reported lytic *E. coli* phage *in vitro* (Tolen et al., 2018; Montso et al., 2019). In addition, they had a broad host spectrum and could lysis *E.coli* strains with different degrees of antibiotic resistance. Compared with the other two phages, SYGE1 could lyse more strains (16 of 20, 80%), which indicated that phage

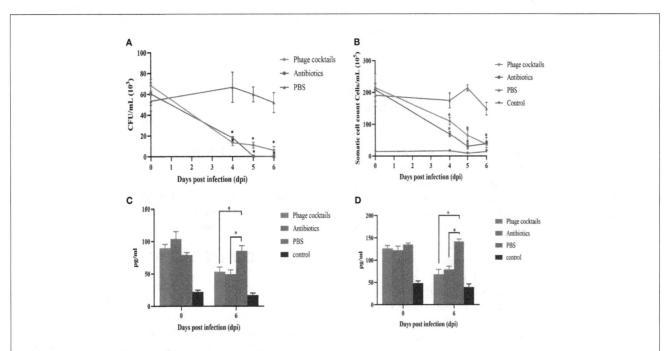

FIGURE 5 | Antibacterial efficacy of phage cocktails against mastitis induced by *E.coli*. Cows challenged by *E.coli*-induced mastitis were intramammarily infused with phage cocktails containing vB_EcoM_SYGD1, vB_EcoP_SYGE1, and vB_EcoM_SYGMH1, and the bacteria load **(A)** and SCC **(B)** of milk samples were detected after three-day treatment, every 24 h. Concentrations of IL-1β **(C)** and TNF-α **(D)** in the sera of cows before treatment (0 day) and on the sixth day after beginning of treatment were measured using indirect ELISA. Data were analyzed using GraphPad Prism v 8.0 software. *Indicate significant differences between phage cocktails or antibiotics and untreated groups, as calculated by *t*-tests ($p < 0.05$).

cocktails could lyse a wider range of hosts than a single phage. The phage multiplication stages in a life cycle were divided into attachment, adsorption, injection, biosynthesis, maturation, assembly, and lysis (Yang et al., 2019). The parameters of phage life cycle play a significant role in determining both *in vitro* and *in vivo* phage antibacterial activities, because phage multiplication is directly proportional to reduction in bacteria (Manohar et al., 2019). In this study, SYGD1 had a growth profile with the latent period of 20 min and burst size of 51.7 PFU/cell. SYGE1 and SYGMH1 had a latent period of 10 min which was shorter than earlier studies and also had a high burst size (Dalmasso et al., 2016; Manohar et al., 2019). The three phages had different latent period and higher productive potential indicates they could deliver sufficient infective phages where problematic bacteria appear and achieve the success of microbial control in the form of phage cocktail (Pires et al., 2020).

Understanding the genetic information of phage is essential for the safe and efficient clinical application (Shahin et al., 2020). All three isolated phages lacked harmful genes, such as lysogenic genes, antimicrobial resistance, and bacterial virulence, suggesting that they met the first criterion for phage therapy (Shahin et al., 2020). Moreover, the genomes of all the three phages showed 90% similarities to the already existing phage genomes in the database indicating that there is abundance of these phages in the environment and is valuable to study the interaction of phages and their host for therapeutic purpose (Manohar et al., 2019). Phages may be inactivated by various environmental stresses before reaching the target bacteria (Pires et al., 2020). The stability of phage preparations is a key requirement for successful treatment. In our study, SYGD1, SYGE1, and SYGMH1 were found to be relatively stable at various temperatures, pH values, and chloroform values, meaning that these three phages could be potential phage candidates for therapy.

Extensive clinical research and studies on bacteriophages and phage therapy could put forth phage therapy as one of the alternative treatment against 'superbug' infections (Manohar et al., 2019). However, a single phage therapy is easier to develop its resistance cells (Kaabi and Musafer, 2020). So, the phage mixtures could effective to solve this problem. As expected, our results, which was similar to most reported treatment effects of phage cocktails, exhibited that the symptoms of animals have improved significantly (Tanji et al., 2005b; Jin et al., 2020; Nale et al., 2021). Furthermore, the innate inflammatory response is the initial stage of infection and is a key factor in protecting the body from infectious pathogens (Khan et al., 2015). In numerous *in vitro* and *in vivo* studies, proinflammatory signals, such as TNF-α, IL-1β, and IL-6, have been implicated in deviating immune responses to infection with *S. aureus* and *E. coli* (Bannerman et al., 2004). In our study, the cows' blood had high concentrations of IL-1β and TNF-α when infected with *E. coli* which was consistent with early study (Bannerman et al., 2004), but the release of these proinflammatory mediators dropped to a lower level on the third day after three consecutive treatments with phages or antibiotics. Phage therapy achieved the similar therapeutic effect of antibiotics suggesting that phage cocktails could lysis bacteria effectively *in*

vivo and reduce the host inflammation. Moreover, the response of the immune system may be more important to the severity of the disease than the infection itself. The cell wall of lipopolysaccharides (LPS) in *E. coli* is a key virulence factor, which induces the upregulation of pro-inflammatory cytokines during the mastitis (Griesbeck-Zilch et al., 2008 and Guha and Mackman, 2001). Notably, *E. coli*, which makes use of LPS as a receptor of phage, generally evades phage infection by mutating genes involved in LPS biosynthesis (Labrie et al., 2010). This change in structure and function of LPS under the pressure of phage infection is usually accompanied by pleiotropic fitness costs which may have negative consequences (such as decrease in virulence) in pathogenic bacterial populations (Burmeister et al., 2020). Although, in this study, it was difficult to distinguish whether the effect is from bacteriolysis of phage or from decrease in pathogenic bacterial populations as mentioned above played the key role during phage therapy, the treatment with a phage cocktail significantly alleviates the symptoms of mastitis in cows. It is clear that SYGD1, SYGE1, and SYGMH1 in the form of phage cocktails could be the candidates of phage therapy.

CONCLUSION

Overall, antibiotic resistance and the transfer of resistant genes should be considered serious public health issues. Phages are a powerful option for the post-antibiotic era. This study described the isolation and characteristics of three phages of *E.coli* and evaluated their therapeutic effects in cow mastitis caused by drug resistant *E.coli*. We found that these three phages show promise as antimicrobial agents especially when used in a cocktail to significantly reduce the number of bacteria, somatic cells, and inflammatory factors, alleviates the symptoms of mastitis in cattle, and achieves the same effect as antibiotic treatment. It enhanced our knowledge about phage information and increased our confidence in using phage cocktails. Further research on the efficacy of phages in therapeutic applications will be significant.

ETHICS STATEMENT

The animal study was reviewed and approved by The Ethical Committee for Animal Experiments of Shanghai Jiao Tong University. Written informed consent was obtained from the owners for the participation of their animals in this study.

AUTHOR CONTRIBUTIONS

YY and ZW designed the experiments. ZW, MG, and YG performed the experiments and collected the data. MG, YX, YL, XZ, and YC collected and analyzed the data. JS, JM, and HW performed critical revision of the article. MG and ZW wrote the manuscript. All authors contributed to the article and approved the submitted version.

National Key Research and Development Program of China (2019YFA0904000), and the National Natural Science Foundation of China (31772744, 32072822, and 31902237).

REFERENCES

Abdi, R. D., Gillespie, B. E., Ivey, S., Pighetti, G. M., and Dego, O. K. (2021). Antimicrobial Resistance of Major Bacterial Pathogens From Dairy Cows With High Somatic Cell Count and Clinical Mastitis. *Anim. (Basel)* 11, 131. doi: 10.3390/ani11010131

Aslam, S., and Schooley, R. T. (2019). What's Old is New Again – Bacteriophage Therapy in the 21 St Century. *Antimicrob. Agents Chemother.* 64, e01987–e01919. doi: 10.1128/AAC.01987-19

Baker, A. C., Goddard, V. J., Davy, J., Schroeder, D. C., Adams, D. G., and Wilson, W. H. (2006). Identification of a Diagnostic Marker to Detect Freshwater Cyanophages of Filamentous Cyanobacteria. *Appl. Environ. Microbiol.* 72, 5713–5719. doi: 10.1128/AEM.00270-06

Bannerman, D. D., Paape, M. J., Lee, J. W., Zhao, X., and Rainard, P. (2004). *Escherichia Coli* and *Staphylococcus Aureus* Elicit Differential Innate Immune Responses Following Intramammary Infection. *Clin. Diagn. Lab. Immunol.* 11, 463–472. doi: 10.1128/CDLI.11.3.463-472.2004

Bao, J., Wu, N., Zeng, Y., Chen, L., Li, L., Yang, L., et al. (2020). Non-Active Antibiotic and Bacteriophage Synergism to Successfully Treat Recurrent Urinary Tract Infection Caused by Extensively Drug-Resistant *Klebsiella Pneumoniae*. *Emerg. Microbes Infect.* 9, 771–774. doi: 10.1080/22221751.2020.1747950

Bar, D., Tauer, L. W., Bennett, G., González, R. N., Hertl, J. A., Schukken, Y. H., et al. (2008). The Cost of Generic Clinical Mastitis in Dairy Cows as Estimated by Using Dynamic Programming. *J. Dairy. Sci.* 91, 2205–2214. doi: 10.3168/jds.2007-0573

Bhattarai, D., Worku, T., Dad, R., Rehman, Z. U., Gong, X., and Zhang, S. (2018). Mechanism of Pattern Recognition Receptors (Prrs) and Host Pathogen Interplay in Bovine Mastitis. *Microb. Pathog.* 120, 64–70. doi: 10.1016/j.micpath.2018.04.010

Bonilla, N., and Barr, J. J. (2018). Phage on Tap: A Quick and Efficient Protocol for the Preparation of Bacteriophage Laboratory Stocks. *Methods Mol. Biol.* 1838, 37–46. doi: 10.1007/978-1-4939-8682-8_4

Burmeister, A. R., Fortier, A., Roush, C., Lessing, A. J., Bender, R. G., Barahman, R., et al. (2020). Pleiotropy Complicates a Trade-Off Between Phage Resistance and Antibiotic Resistance. *Proc. Natl. Acad. Sci. U. S. A.* 21, 11207–11216. doi: 10.1073/pnas.1919888117

Chanishvili, N. (2012). Phage Therapy–History From Twort and D'herelle Through Soviet Experience to Current Approaches. *Adv. Virus Res.* 83, 3–40. doi: 10.1016/B978-0-12-394438-2.00001-3

Clara, T.-B. (2018). Phage Therapy Faces Evolutionary Challenges. *Viruses* 10, 323. doi: 10.3390/v10060323

Cobirka, M., Tancin, V., and Slama, P. (2020). Epidemiology and Classification of Mastitis. *Anim. (Basel)* 10, 2212. doi: 10.3390/ani10122212

Cortinhas, C. S., Tomazi, T., Zoni, M. S. F., Moro, E., and Santos, M. V. D. (2016). Randomized Clinical Trial Comparing Ceftiofur Hydrochloride With a Positive Control Protocol for Intramammary Treatment of Nonsevere Clinical Mastitis in Dairy Cows. *J. Dairy. Sci.* 99, 5619–5628. doi: 10.3168/jds.2016-10891

Costa, P., Pereira, C., Gomes, A., and Almeida, A. (2019). Efficiency of Single Phage Suspensions and Phage Cocktail in the Inactivation of *Escherichia Coli* and *Salmonella* Typhimurium: An *In Vitro* Preliminary Study. *Microorganisms* 7, 94. doi: 10.3390/microorganisms7040094

D'Accolti, M., Soffritti, I., Mazzacane, S., and Caselli, E. (2021). Bacteriophages as a Potential 360-Degree Pathogen Control Strategy. *Microorganisms* 9, 261. doi: 10.3390/microorganisms9020261

Dalmasso, M., Strain, R., Neve, H., Franz, C., and Hill, C. (2016). Three New *Escherichia Coli* Phages From the Human Gut Show Promising Potential for Phage Therapy. *PloS One* 11, e0156773. doi: 10.1371/journal.pone.0156773

Dedrick, R. M., Guerrero-Bustamante, C. A., Garlena, R. A., Russell, D. A., and Spencer, H. (2019). Engineered Bacteriophages for Treatment of a Patient With a Disseminated Drug-Resistant *Mycobacterium Abscessus*. *Nat. Med.* 25, 730–733. doi: 10.1038/s41591-019-0437-z

Fazel, F., Jamshidi, A., and Khoramian, B. (2019). Phenotypic and Genotypic Study on Antimicrobial Resistance Patterns of *E. Coli* Isolates From Bovine Mastitis. *Microb. Pathog.* 132, 355–361. doi: 10.1016/j.micpath.2019.05.018

Gao, J., Barkema, H. W., Zhang, L., Liu, G., Deng, Z., Cai, L., et al. (2017). Incidence of Clinical Mastitis and Distribution of Pathogens on Large Chinese Dairy Farms. *J. Dairy.* 6, 4797–4806. doi: 10.3168/jds.2016-12334

Gill, J. J., and Hyman, P. (2010). Phage Choice, Isolation, and Preparation for Phage Therapy. Cybernetics and Systems Analysis. *Curr. Pharm. Biotechnol.* 11, 2–14. doi: 10.2174/138920110790725311

Gomes, F., and Henriques, M. (2016). Control of Bovine Mastitis: Old and Recent Therapeutic Approaches. *Curr. Microbiol.* 72, 377–382. doi: 10.1007/s00284-015-0958-8

Griesbeck-Zilch, B., Meyer, H. H. D., Kühn, C., Schwerin, M., and Wellnitz, O. (2008). *Staphylococcus Aureus* and *Escherichia Coli* Cause Deviating Expression Profiles of Cytokines and Lactoferrin Messenger Ribonucleic Acid in Mammary Epithelial Cells. *J. Dairy. Sci.* 91, 2215–2224. doi: 10.3168/jds.2007-0752

Guerra, S. T., Orsi, H., Joaquim, S. F., Guimaraes, F. F., Lopes, B. C., Dalanezi, F. M., et al. (2020). Short Communication: Investigation of Extra-Intestinal Pathogenic *Escherichia Coli* Virulence Genes, Bacterial Motility, and Multidrug Resistance Pattern of Strains Isolated From Dairy Cows With Different Severity Scores of Clinical Mastitis. *J. Dairy. Sci.* 103, 3606–3614. doi: 10.3168/jds.2019-17477

Guha, M., and Mackman, N. (2001). LPS Induction of Gene Expression in Human Monocytes. *Cell. Signal.* 13, 85–94. doi: 10.1016/S0898-6568(00)00149-2

Gurao, A., Kashyap, S. K., and Singh, R. (2017). β-Defensins: An Innate Defense for Bovine Mastitis. *Vet. World* 10, 990–998. doi: 10.14202/vetworld.2017.990-998

He, W., Ma, S., Lei, L., He, J., Li, X., Tao, J., et al. (2020). Prevalence, Etiology, and Economic Impact of Clinical Mastitis on Large Dairy Farms in China. *Vet. Microbiol.* 242, 108570. doi: 10.1016/j.vetmic.2019.108570

Jianying, H. U., Shi, J., Chang, H., Dong, L. I., Yang, M., and Kamagata, Y. (2008). Phenotyping and Genotyping of Antibiotic-Resistant *Escherichia Coli* Isolated From a Natural River Basin. *Environ. Sci. Technol.* 42, 3415–3420. doi: 10.1021/es7026746

Jin, H. K., Kim, H. J., Jung, S. J., Mizan, M. R., Si, H. P., and Ha, S. (2020). Characterization of Salmonella Spp.-Specific Bacteriophages and Their Biocontrol Application in Chicken Breast Meat. *J. Food. Sci.* 85, 526–534. doi: 10.1111/1750-3841.15042

Kaabi, S., and Musafer, H. K. (2020). New Phage Cocktail Against Infantile Sepsis Bacteria. *Microb. Pathog.* 148, 104447. doi: 10.1016/j.micpath.2020.104447

Khan, S., Dhama, K., Tiwari, R., Bashir, M., and Chaicumpa, W. (2021). Advances in Therapeutic and Managemental Approaches of Bovine Mastitis: A Comprehensive Review. *Vet. Q.* 41, 107–136. doi: 10.1080/01652176.2021.1882713

Khan, F. A., Pandupuspitasari, N. S., Huang, C. J., Hao, X., and Zhang, S. J. (2015). Sumoylation: A Link to Future Therapeutics. *Curr. Issues Mol. Biol.* 18, 49–56.

Khatun, M., Sørensen, P., Ingvartsen, K. L., Bjerring, M., and Røntved, C. M. (2013a). Effects of Combined Liver and Udder Biopsying on the Acute Phase Response of Dairy Cows With Experimentally Induced *E. Coli* Mastitis. *Animal* 7, 1721–1730. doi: 10.1017/S1751731113001353

Khatun, M., Sorensen, P., Jorgensen, H. B. H., Sahana, G., Sorensen, L. P., Lund, M. S., et al. (2013b). Effects of *Bos Taurus* Autosome 9-Located Quantitative Trait Loci Haplotypes on the Disease Phenotypes of Dairy Cows With Experimentally Induced *Escherichia Coli* Mastitis. *J. Dairy. Sci.* 96, 1820–1833. doi: 10.3168/jds.2012-5528

Klaas, I. C., and Zadoks, R. N. (2017). An Update on Environmental Mastitis: Challenging Perceptions. *Transbound Emerg. Dis.* 65, 166–185. doi: 10.1111/tbed.12704

Kutter, E., De Vos, D., Gvasalia, G., Alavidze, Z., Gogokhia, L., Kuhl, S., et al. (2010). Phage Therapy in Clinical Practice: Treatment of Human Infections. *Curr. Pharm. Biotechnol.* 11, 69–86. doi: 10.2174/138920110790725401

Labrie, S. J., Samson, J. E., and Moineau, S. (2010). Bacteriophage Resistance Mechanisms. *Nat. Rev. Microbiol.* 5, 317–327. doi: 10.1038/nrmicro2315

Lowe, T. M., and Chan, P. P. (2016). tRNAscan-SE on-Line: Integrating Search and Context for Analysis of Transfer RNA Genes. *Nucleic Acids Res.* W1, W54–W57. doi: 10.1093/nar/gkw413

Lu, L., Cai, L., Jiao, N., and Zhang, R. (2017). Isolation and Characterization of the First Phage Infecting Ecologically Important Marine Bacteria *Erythrobacter*. *Virol. J.* 14, 104. doi: 10.1186/s12985-017-0773-x

Luong, T., Salabarria, A. C., Edwards, R. A., and Roach, D. R. (2020). Standardized Bacteriophage Purification for Personalized Phage Therapy. *Nat. Protoc.* 9, 2867–2890. doi: 10.1038/s41596-020-0346-0

Machado, V. S., and Bicalho, R. C. (2018). Prepartum Application of Internal Teat Sealant or Intramammary Amoxicillin on Dairy Heifers: Effect on Udder Health, Survival, and Performanc. *J. Dairy. Sci.* 101, 1388–1402. doi: 10.3168/jds.2017-13415

Manohar, P., Tamhankar, A. J., Lundborg, C. S., and Nachimuthu, R. (2019). Therapeutic Characterization and Efficacy of Bacteriophage Cocktails Infecting *Escherichia Coli*, *Klebsiella Pneumoniae*, and *Enterobacter* Species. *Front. Microbiol.* 10, 574. doi: 10.3389/fmicb.2019.00574

Mathieu, J., Yu, P., Zuo, P., Da Silva, M. L. B., and Alvarez, P. J. J. (2019). Going Viral: Emerging Opportunities for Phage-Based Bacterial Control in Water Treatment and Reuse. *Acc. Chem. Res.* 52, 849–857. doi: 10.1021/acs.accounts.8b00576

Mcdougall, S., Clausen, L., Hintukainen, J., and Hunnam, J. (2019). Randomized, Controlled, Superiority Study of Extended Duration of Therapy With an Intramammary Antibiotic for Treatment of Clinical Mastitis. *J. Dairy. Sci.* 102, 4376–4386. doi: 10.3168/jds.2018-15141

Melo, L. D. R., Oliveira, H., Pires, D. P., Dabrowska, K., and Azeredo, J. (2020). Phage Therapy Efficacy: A Review of the Last 10 Years of Preclinical Studies. *Crit. Rev. Microbiol.* 46, 78–99. doi: 10.1080/1040841X.2020.1729695

Moelling, K., Broecker, F., and Willy, C. (2018). A Wake-Up Call: We Need Phage Therapy Now. *Viruses* 10, 688. doi: 10.3390/v10120688

Montso, P. K., Mlambo, V., and Ateba, C. N. (2019). Characterization of Lytic Bacteriophages Infecting Multidrug-Resistant Shiga Toxigenic Atypical *Escherichia Coli* O177 Strains Isolated From Cattle Feces. *Front. Public Health* 7, 355. doi: 10.3389/fpubh.2019.00355

Nale, J. Y., Vinner, G. K., Lopez, V. C., Thanki, A. M., Phothaworn, P., Thiennimitr, P., et al. (2021). An Optimized Bacteriophage Cocktail can Effectively Control *Salmonella In Vitro* and in *Galleria Mellonella*. *Front. Microbiol.* 11, 609955. doi: 10.3389/fmicb.2020.609955

Ngassam-Tchamba, C., Duprez, J. N., Fergestad, M., Visscher, A. D., and Thiry, D. (2020). In Vitro and In Vivo Assessment of Phage Therapy Against *Staphylococcus Aureus* Causing Bovine Mastitis. *J. Glob. Antimicrob. Resist.* 22, 762–770. doi: 10.1016/j.jgar.2020.06.020

Orellano, M. S., Isaac, P., Breser, M. L., Bohl, L. P., Conesa, A., Falcone, R. D., et al. (2019). Chitosan Nanoparticles Enhance the Antibacterial Activity of the Native Polymer Against Bovine Mastitis Pathogens. *Carbohydr. Polym.* 213, 1–9. doi: 10.1016/j.carbpol.2019.02.016

Pellegrino, M. S., Frola, I. D., Natanael, B., Gobelli, D., Nader-Macias, M., and Bogni, C. I. (2018). In Vitro Characterization of Lactic Acid Bacteria Isolated From Bovine Milk as Potential Probiotic Strains to Prevent Bovine Mastitis. *Probiotics Antimicrob. Proteins* 11, 74–84. doi: 10.1007/s12602-017-9383-6

Pires, D. P., Rita, C. A., Graça, P., Luciana, M., and Joana, A. (2020). Current Challenges and Future Opportunities of Phage Therapy. *FEMS Microbiol. Rev.* 44, 684–700. doi: 10.1093/femsre/fuaa017

Rehman, S., Ali, Z., Khan, M., Bostan, N., and Naseem, S. (2019). The Dawn of Phage Therapy. *Rev. Med. Virol.* 29, e2041. doi: 10.1002/rmv.2041

Shahin, K., Barazandeh, M., Zhang, L., Hedayatkhah, A., and Wang, R. (2021). Biodiversity of New Lytic Bacteriophages Infecting Shigella Spp. In Freshwater Environment. *Front. Microbiol.* 12, 619323. doi: 10.3389/fmicb.2021.619323

Shahin, K., Bouzari, M., Komijani, M., and Wang, R. (2020). A New Phage Cocktail Against Multidrug, ESBL-producer Isolates of *Shigella Sonnei* and *Shigella Flexneri* With Highly Efficient Bacteriolytic Activity. *Microb. Drug Resist.* 26, 831–841. doi: 10.1089/mdr.2019.0235

Streicher, L. M. (2021). Exploring the Future of Infectious Disease Treatment in a Post-Antibiotic Era: A Comparative Review of Alternative Therapeutics. *J. Glob. Antimicrob. Resist.* 24, 285–295. doi: 10.1016/j.jgar.2020.12.025

Tanji, Y., Shimada, T., Fukudomi, H., Miyanaga, K., Nakai, Y., and Unno, H. (2005). Therapeutic Use of Phage Cocktail for Controlling *Escherichia Coli* O157:H7 in Gastrointestinal Tract of Mice. *J. Biosci. Bioeng.* 100, 280–287. doi: 10.1263/jbb.100.280

Tolen, T. N., Xie, Y., Hairgrove, T. B., Gill, J. J., and Taylor, T. M. (2018). Evaluation of Commercial Prototype Bacteriophage Intervention Designed for Reducing O157 and Non-O157 Shiga-Toxigenic *Escherichia Coli* (STEC) on Beef Cattle Hide. *Foods* 7, 114. doi: 10.3390/foods7070114

Wang, Z., Zheng, P., Ji, W., Fu, Q., Wang, H., Yan, Y., et al. (2016). SLPW: A Virulent Bacteriophage Targeting Methicillin-Resistant *Staphylococcus Aureus In Vitro* and *In Vivo*. *Front. Microbiol.* 7, 934. doi: 10.3389/fmicb.2016.00934

Yang, Z., Yin, S., Li, G., Wang, J., Huang, G., Jiang, B., et al. (2019). Global Transcriptomic Analysis of the Interactions Between Phage φabp1 and Extensively Drug-Resistant *Acinetobacter Baumannii*. *mSystems* 4, e00068–e00019. doi: 10.1128/mSystems.00068-19

Zalewska-Pitek, B., and Pitek, R. (2020). Phage Therapy as a Novel Strategy in the Treatment of Urinary Tract Infections Caused by E. Coli. *Antibiotics (Basel)* 9, 304. doi: 10.3390/antibiotics9060304

21

Prospects of Inhaled Phage Therapy for Combatting Pulmonary Infections

Xiang Wang, Zuozhou Xie, Jinhong Zhao, Zhenghua Zhu, Chen Yang and Yi Liu *

Department of Pulmonary and Critical Care Medicine, The Second People's Hospital of Kunming, Kunming, China

*Correspondence:
Yi Liu
icu_huxike@163.com

With respiratory infections accounting for significant morbidity and mortality, the issue of antibiotic resistance has added to the gravity of the situation. Treatment of pulmonary infections (bacterial pneumonia, cystic fibrosis-associated bacterial infections, tuberculosis) is more challenging with the involvement of multi-drug resistant bacterial strains, which act as etiological agents. Furthermore, with the dearth of new antibiotics available and old antibiotics losing efficacy, it is prudent to switch to non-antibiotic approaches to fight this battle. Phage therapy represents one such approach that has proven effective against a range of bacterial pathogens including drug resistant strains. Inhaled phage therapy encompasses the use of stable phage preparations given *via* aerosol delivery. This therapy can be used as an adjunct treatment option in both prophylactic and therapeutic modes. In the present review, we first highlight the role and action of phages against pulmonary pathogens, followed by delineating the different methods of delivery of inhaled phage therapy with evidence of success. The review aims to focus on recent advances and developments in improving the final success and outcome of pulmonary phage therapy. It details the use of electrospray for targeted delivery, advances in nebulization techniques, individualized controlled inhalation with software control, and liposome-encapsulated nebulized phages to take pulmonary phage delivery to the next level. The review expands knowledge on the pulmonary delivery of phages and the advances that have been made for improved outcomes in the treatment of respiratory infections.

Keywords: inhaled phage therapy, nebulizer, pulmonary infection, antimicrobial resistance, multi-drug resistance

1 INTRODUCTION

Respiratory tract infections (RTIs) represent a leading cause of suffering and death worldwide. Respiratory diseases are the third major cause of mortality and sickness globally and account for more than 10% of all disability-adjusted life-years (DALYs) (GBD, 2016; Bodier-Montagutelli et al., 2017; WHO-Global Respiratory Burden, 2017). According to the World Lung Foundation's Acute Respiratory Infections Atlas, acute RTIs cause more than four million deaths each year. A range of pulmonary infections develop into life-threatening and difficult to treat conditions with many leading to chronic conditions. Pneumonia is one such complication, which accounts for the highest number of juvenile deaths. As per data, a total of 9 million children under 5 years die annually, with pneumonia the leading killer among patients (WHO Pneumonia factsheet, 2019). Moreover, nosocomial cases of ventilator-associated pneumonia (VAP) refractory to traditional antibiotics are on the rise. This intensive care unit (ICU) acquired infection has a high incidence rate, ranging from 5%-40% in patients with mortality as high as 50% (Forel et al., 2012; Papazian et al., 2020).

Deaths due to tuberculosis (TB) are another similar eye-opener. Annually, a total of 1.4 million people die from TB in 2019, making it the leading cause of death from a single infectious agent, ranking above HIV/AIDS as declared by WHO (Global tuberculosis report WHO, 2018). Although TB is fully curable, the treatment is complicated due to the development of multi-drug resistance TB (MDR-TB) (Seung et al., 2015). The condition is still worse in the developing and third world nations and more than two-thirds of the active cases of TB reported globally come from these countries (WHO, Tuberculosis Factsheet, 2021).

Many other pulmonary conditions such as chronic obstructive pulmonary disease (COPD) and cystic fibrosis (CF) are easily associated and complicated with opportunistic bacterial pathogens (e.g *Pseudomonas aeruginosa* and *Burkholderia cepacia* complex-BCC) making the treatment and management a challenge adding significant financial burden, with poor clinical success achieved. It has been reported that the total healthcare cost for treating CF patients ranges to as high as 50,000 USD per patient per year and this is largely due to repeated hospital stays and treatment costs to manage the bacterial infections associated with such conditions (Sansgiry et al., 2012; Angelis et al., 2015; Trend et al., 2017).

This scenario is made worse by the decline in the effectiveness of current antibiotic therapies due to the rapid spread of resistant bacterial infections, which do not respond to traditional treatment protocols. The spread of antimicrobial resistance (AMR) is a global emergency and is very much prevalent and emerging in the pulmonary setting. Nosocomial outbreaks caused by resistant bacterial strains have been increasingly reported worldwide, creating significant therapeutic challenges for the treatment of lung infections (Rice, 2010; Santajit and Indrawattana, 2016). Moreover, there exists a dearth of new alternatives and with the present attrition rate in new antibiotic molecule developments by pharma companies, the situation is not encouraging, posing a serious threat and indicating that we are entering a post-antibiotic era (Nelson, 2003; Gupta and Nayak, 2014). This emphasizes the urgent necessity to promote and explore alternative approaches other than antibiotics that can be used either singly or better as an adjunct therapy for improved clinical outcomes and reduced mortality rates.

Among the approaches that are worth exploring is 'Phage Therapy'. Phage therapy or the use of phages against bacterial pathogens is not a new concept. There has been a renewed interest in this field in recent years due to the rising resistance menace. Phage therapy represents a safe yet potent antibacterial strategy, with numerous reviews and data supporting and strongly advocating its further use (Carlton, 1999; Weber-Dabrowska et al., 2000; Sulakvelidze et al., 2001; Capparelli et al., 2007; Chanishvili, 2012). However, major roadblocks and challenges in this field need to be investigated.

The present review discusses the prospects of pulmonary phage therapy and its efficacy in treating various RTIs considering antimicrobial resistance. It later details the major challenges and new advances made in delivering phages to the infection site for improved outcome and availability, with major recent studies supporting these developments. This review aims to give a complete insight into the latest developments in inhaled phage therapy and how we can address the gaps and further improve it, which is essential for the clinical success of this new era of treatment.

2 INHALED PHAGE THERAPY: A NEW ERA OF THERAPEUTICS

Phage therapy represents the use of obligatory lytic phages to kill specific host bacteria. The issue of growing multidrug resistance represents a potent and safe alternative. Phage therapy has shown both preclinical and clinical efficacy against a range of bacterial pathogens and data suggests that it also works well against pulmonary pathogens (Soothill, 1992; Biswas et al., 2002; Mathur et al., 2003; Wang et al., 2006; Watanabe et al., 2007; Chang et al., 2018; Chhibber et al., 2008). Inhaled phage therapy has long been used and is still in use in Eastern European countries i.e Georgia, Russia, and Poland. Studies focused on inhaled phage therapy in humans executed in these countries have been reviewed and compiled by Abedon (2015). There have been studies dating as early as 1936 wherein phages have been mostly delivered through inhalation route against a range of pulmonary pathogens such as *E. coli*, *Klebsiella*, Streptococci, Staphylococci, Pseudomonas, and the results of many studies have shown efficacy as high as 80-100% although some studies resulted in treatment failure owing to a lack of a better understanding of phage specificity, quality control, and stability issues (Hoe et al., 2013; Abedon, 2015; Chang et al., 2018). Modern phage therapy has come a long way and improved inhalation and aerosolization techniques have also helped to fill these gaps in knowledge about pulmonary phage therapy.

2.1 Major Pulmonary Pathogens: An Overview

VAP is a major nosocomial infection in which the causative agents can form biofilms on the surface of endotracheal tubes. These biofilms are mostly polymicrobial, with multiple organisms isolated (Hall-Stoodley and Stoodley, 2009; Rodrigues et al., 2017). This may not just include members of the oral flora (e.g., *Streptococcus and Prevotella* species), but also ESKAPE organisms (*Enterococcus faecium, Staphylococcus aureus, Klebsiella pneumoniae, Acinetobacter baumannii, P. aeruginosa, Enterobacter* spp) (Penes et al., 2017; Vadivoo and Usha, 2018). A hallmark of biofilms is the inherent resistance to killing and recalcitrance to antimicrobials and immune attack, outer environmental stress, enabling them to survive well within the body, leading to difficulty to treat chronic and relapsing infections (Romling and Balsalobre, 2012; Sharma et al., 2019). Biofilm cells can survive 100 to 1,000 higher concentrations of antimicrobials and biocides than planktonic cells (Gilbert et al., 2002; Høiby et al., 2010). Methicillin-resistant *S. aureus* (MRSA) is the second most frequently isolated pathogen from patients who die from HAP and is commonly associated with many cases of ICU acquired VAP (Rubinstein et al., 2008; Jean et al., 2020). It secretes a range of virulence factors, toxins, and biofilm-promoting adhesins that favor its colonization on medical devices and catheter tubings. Similarly, a major chronic lung disease i.e Cystic Fibrosis (CF) has gained much attention as its management and outcome are always complicated by persistent bacterial infections of the airways and destructive lung inflammation (Gibson et al., 2003; Pragman et al., 2016). With *P. aeruginosa* as the major pathogen isolated in most CF patients, this bacterium poses the greatest challenge, with treatment failures owing to its potent biofilm-forming ability and recalcitrant nature (Burns et al., 2001; Folkesson et al., 2012; Malhotra et al., 2019). Biofilm-like aggregates are commonly seen within the sputum in CF airways and such biofilms do not respond to courses of conventional antibiotics. Moreover, *P. aeruginosa* exhibits significant changes in gene expression, with up-regulation of exopolysaccharide production, excessive alginate production, and activated secretion of various quorum sensing molecules, multiple mechanisms of antibiotic resistance e.g overexpression of efflux pumps and beta-lactamases which further aid in the formation and survival of bacteria within the biofilm shelters (Lister et al., 2009; Harmsen et al., 2010; Poole, 2011). Another major pulmonary pathogen is the *B. cepacian* complex (Bcc) which consists of 18 closely related species that have been known to persist in the airways of people with CF although they are less common colonizers than *P. aeruginosa* (Lipuma, 2005; Drevinek and Mahenthiralingam, 2010; Kenna et al., 2017). These Bcc bacteria are associated with worst prognosis, high rates of morbidity and mortality amongst sufferers (Jones et al., 2004; Sousa et al., 2011; Hassan et al., 2019), owing to bacteria-induced acute-onset lung deterioration with associated septic bacteremia, termed 'cepacia syndrome'. Apart from this, most members of this complex exhibit multidrug resistance and can form biofilms while evading immune attack (Tomlin et al., 2001; Mahenthiralingam et al., 2005; Van Acker et al., 2013).

Besides bacteria, one of the major pulmonary pathogens accounting for a large number of deaths annually showing a high degree of multidrug resistance is *Mycobacterium tuberculosis* (Mtb). The success of this intracellular pathogen is due to the ability of Mtb to remain hidden from the immune system, associated with relapse or frequent recurrence of active TB, which is often seen in patients despite anti-TB treatment (McCune et al., 1966; Jasmer et al., 2004; Ackart et al., 2014). Whether Mtb forms biofilms during infection remains unknown but notably, Mtb has a natural tendency to adhere to surfaces and forms cords in the culture medium and this cording behavior is associated with virulence and pathogenicity of Mtb (Esteban and García-Coca, 2018; Chakraborty et al., 2021). There have been recent studies reporting the formation of biofilm-like aggregates by this bacteria and the role of glycolipids, shorter-chain free mycolic acids, GroE-1 chaperone in the formation of these biofilms that play a detrimental role in causing caseous necrosis and cavity formation in lung tissue and treatment failures (Ojha et al., 2008; Sambhadan et al., 2013; Trivedi et al., 2016; Esteban and Garcia-Coca, 2018).

2.2 Phage Against Pulmonary Pathogens: Attack at Multiple Fronts

With this scenario, an ideal agent attacking the respiratory pathogens needs to exhibit remarkable anti-biofilm ability and phages completely fit into this class. Phage therapy works on multiple fronts to combat the course of pulmonary bacterial infections. Lytic phages work as killing machines. Lytic phages first bind to their target bacterium through specific receptors, injecting the genetic material and later taking over the host machinery for progeny phage production. The phage progeny are released from the host *via* cell lysis and the cycle restarts for many such rounds, leading to secondary infection. This property of self-replication or auto-doing enables phage titer build-up, which is essential for containment of the bacterial population.

Besides this conventional mode of killing, phages also exhibit anti-biofilm activity (Azeredo and Sutherland, 2008; Sillankorva and Azeredo, 2014; Morris et al., 2019). This is particularly important as biofilms play an important role in many pulmonary infections (Pintucci et al., 2010; Boisvert et al., 2016). They work on two fronts i.e they are capable of both preventing the onset and initiation of biofilm formation as well as disruption of fully formed biofilms, which they do in multiple manners. The successful eradication of an established biofilm requires the chemical or drug to have the ability to penetrate the EPS matrix and then kill the biofilm-embedded cells. Phages possess both these properties (Fu et al., 2010; Harper et al., 2014). Phages are naturally equipped with virion-associated de-polymerases and endolysins, phage-borne enzymes released at the later stages of the phage replication cycle, which degrade bacterial peptidoglycan and help in bacterial cell lysis and phage progeny release. These phage enzymes play an important role in dissolving the tough outer biofilm matrix (Roach and Donovan, 2015; Maciejewska et al., 2018). This allows the phages and progeny population to penetrate the deeper areas within the biofilm and kill the host bacterium through their classical killing mechanism Although phage diffusion may be slow in such layers, phages still retain their ability to bind and lysis the metabolically dormant or the slow-growing persister cells (unlike antibiotics) through receptor-mediated binding and killing. Apart from this, the phage-encoded de-polymerase enzyme degrades the EPS matrix, which not only facilitates the entry of phages but also makes way for the antibiotic molecule to gain entry into the biofilm structure and reach bacterial cells, thus leading to augmentation through the clearance and treatment outcome in a combination or co-therapy approach (Bedi et al., 2009; Ryan et al., 2012; Akturk et al., 2019). This phage-antibiotic synergy has been reported in past studies wherein phage enables the augmentation of antibiotics, making them ideal for use in combination mode with different antibiotics. This approach also decreases the development of resistant mutants (Bedi et al., 2009; Ryan et al., 2012; Tagliaferri et al., 2019).

Another major mechanism through which phages help to ameliorate the course of pulmonary infection is their ability to modulate the immune system towards a more subtle state, discouraging tissue damage. Studies report that phages administered for therapeutic purposes are able to regulate and reduce the heightened levels of inflammation. Phages have been shown to down-regulate the TLR expression which is the key molecule that leads to activation of NF-κB, leading to cytokine production, cell infiltration, phagocytosis. Many studies indicate a decrease in pro-inflammatory cytokine levels post-treatment (TNF-α, IL-1, IL-8, MIP-1) (Górski et al., 2012; Pabary et al., 2015; Kaur et al., 2016; Zhang L. et al., 2018; Cafora et al., 2020). Phages lead to inhibition of excessive reactive oxygen free radical production and also induce the production of anti-inflammatory cytokines, maintaining homeostasis while limiting cell and tissue injury (Przerwa et al., 2006; Borysowski et al., 2010; Van Belleghem et al., 2017). Phage ISP specific for S. aureus phage showed induction of anti-inflammatory IL-1 receptor antagonist (IL-1RA) synthesis by human monocytes, thus leading to the repression of pro-inflammatory cytokines (Van Belleghem et al., 2017). Two-way cooperation exists between phages and the immune system called "Immunophage Synergy", whereby both complement each other towards faster resolution of infections and minimal tissue damage, as seen in neutrophil-phage cooperation, reported by Roach et al. (2017) against *P. aeruginosa*. In a similar study, Cafora et al. (2020) showed the anti-inflammatory role of the phage cocktail in terms of reduction of pro-inflammatory markers in *P. aeruginosa* infection using the zebrafish model. Phage cocktail injections significantly reduced neutrophil migration and heightened pro-inflammatory cytokine levels highlighting the molecular interaction between phages and the cells of the vertebrate immune system in CF disease and the anti-inflammatory role of phages. Similar animal studies have shown the anti-inflammatory ability of phages in downregulating the exaggerated immune response by decreasing the levels of pro-inflammatory cytokines during the infection process against a range of pulmonary pathogens (Chhibber et al., 2008; Kumari et al., 2019). The immune-modulating ability of phages is a unique field and requires further investigation. Another important point worth mentioning is the fact that phages may themselves also evoke an immune response and thus phage preparation needs to ensure high purity (Boratyński et al., 2004; Liu et al., 2021) as it becomes an extremely important parameter in determining whether phage therapy will reduce or promote inflammation and antibody response.

Free phages have limited ability to enter the human eukaryotic cells and reach intracellular pathogens (Sulakvelidze et al., 2001; Drulis-Kawa et al., 2012; Doss et al., 2017). Despite this, a few studies indicate that phages can penetrate eukaryotic cells and attack the intracellular populations of pathogens by adopting a different strategy to invade the eukaryotic cells. Kaur et al. (2014) evaluated the intracellular killing potential of macrophages in the presence of free phage MR-5 as well as phage adsorbed onto host MRSA strain. Results depicted that free phage did not influence intracellular killing of engulfed

S. aureus by macrophages while phage adsorbed onto its host bacterial cells showed a time-dependent and titer-dependent significant reduction in the number of viable intracellular cocci. This means that phages utilized host bacteria as a vehicle to shuttle inside the macrophage and kill the intracellular cocci. In another study, the use of a novel delivery Trojan Horse approach i.e *Mycobacterium smegmatis* as a carrier for delivering phages to the intracellular bacteria (Broxmeyer et al., 2002) was reported. Another strategy to deliver phages intracellularly is *via* the use of liposomes, which is detailed in later sections of this review. The multiple fronts at which phages attack respiratory bacterial pathogens and thus ameliorating the disease outcome are compiled in **Figure 1**.

2.3 Pulmonary Phage Delivery

Having studied the multiple mechanisms of phage therapy, we now focus on the different methods that have been adopted in the delivery of phages to pulmonary sites along with proof of data against the clinically relevant pathogens causing RTIs. In later sections, we focus on the challenges and advances made in this direction.

2.3.1 Nebulizer Based Inhalation

Nebulization is the process of creating of converting liquid into a fine mist of active ingredient solution through the special nozzle. It is the first choice for delivering drugs through the pulmonary route, owing to its high efficiency and ability to deliver high volumes of the agent due to liquid-based preparations (Ali, 2010; Haddrell et al., 2014; Martin and Finlay, 2015).To deliver a drug by nebulization, the drug must first be dispersed in a liquid (usually aqueous) medium. After the application of a dispersing force (either a jet of gas or ultrasonic waves), the drug particles are contained within the aerosol droplets, which are then inhaled (Javadzadeh and Yaqoubi, 2017). There are many types of nebulization-based methods that use different mechanisms to produce aerosols. In jet nebulization, which worked on Venturi Principle, compressed air is passed through a narrow orifice with a force that leads to a pressure gradient, and this enables to draw/ suck the drug suspension up into the feed tube. The liquid gets atomized into micron size droplets *via* viscosity-induced instability whereas the larger droplets are trapped and filtered by the baffle (Finlay, 2001; Hickey, 2004). The smaller droplets leave the nebulizer to reach the target sites, but the bigger droplets are returned to the reservoir for re-nebulization. In vibrating mesh nebulization, the generation of droplets occurs either by a piezoelectric crystal that vibrates at high frequency and then these vibrations are transferred to a transducer that pushes the liquid suspension upward and downward through a mesh plate to extrude the liquid and generate aerosol droplets or in active arrangement, the crystal directly vibrates the mesh plate (Vecellio, 2006; Ali, 2010). Ultrasonic nebulizers also work on the principle of converse piezoelectric effect, whereby the piezoelectric crystal vibrates high frequency acoustic energy waves (no mesh plate is required here), which leads to aerosol creation (Flament et al., 2001; Rau, 2002). The vibrations are transmitted to the drug solution *via* a buffer medium. Droplets

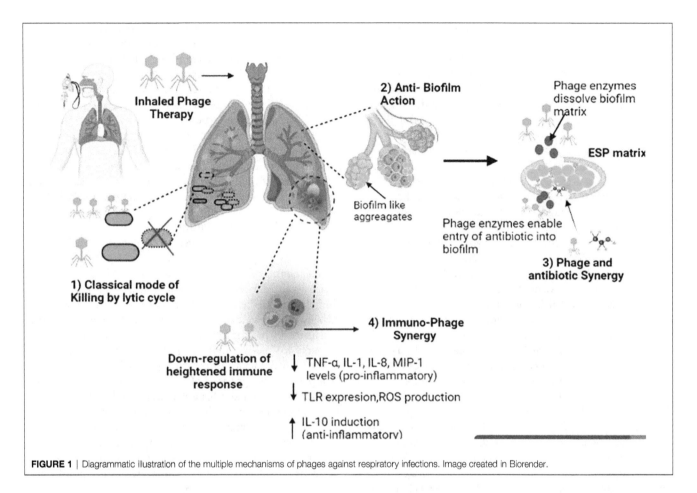

FIGURE 1 | Diagrammatic illustration of the multiple mechanisms of phages against respiratory infections. Image created in Biorender.

are formed either by the breakup of surface capillaries or by the collapse of cavitation bubbles within the liquid. Ultrasonic nebulizers produce a more uniform particle size than jet nebulizers but are less widely used due to high pricing (Flament et al., 2001; Rau, 2002; Javadzadeh and Yaqoubi, 2017). To date, many drugs have been nebulized and given through this technique to reach the lungs and show their desired action. Phage-based nebulization has been reported by past studies using different types of nebulizers. However, one major disadvantage is that each of the nebulization processes is associated with the mechanical stress produced during the formation of high-frequency vibrations, passing of compressed air, heat stress during the generation of high-frequency acoustic energy, re-nebulization process, shear stress during impaction. These physical stresses can have potentially damaging effects on the phage structure leading to a reduction in phage viability and infectivity. A study by Turgeon et al. (2014) reported that aerosolization produced by nebulizers led to reduced infectivity of five tail-less phages while 1000-fold more genome copies were found in the nebulized product as compared with low PFU values suggesting that nebulizers damaged the structural integrity of phages required for infection. Air jet nebulizers and, to a lesser extent, vibrating mesh nebulizers, cause tail detachment leading to broken phages that are incapable of initiating the phage infection process. Another change in phage morphology is the production of phages with empty capsids and

mesh-type nebulizers, which produce a higher fraction of such phages (Astudillo et al., 2018). The stress of liquid breakup, large hydrodynamic stress with high-speed nozzle, and impaction on primary and secondary baffles contribute to the damaging effect on phage structure leading to loss of tails and nucleic acid ejection (Carrigy et al., 2017; Leung et al., 2019). Hence, the selection of the nebulization mechanism that best suits a particular phage may vary, and thus detailed post-nebulization studies on phage titer and viability need to be carried out for each nebulization technique.

In a study, the effect of three types of nebulizers i.e air-jet, vibrating-mesh, and static-mesh nebulizers, on the structural stability of a *Myoviridae* phage, PEV44, active against *P. aeruginosa* was visualized by TEM. Results indicated that the fraction of "broken" phages (capsid separated from the tail) was significantly increased after the process of nebulization and maximum was obtained with the air-jet nebulizer (83%) while with mesh- nebulizers it was 50 - 60% (Astudillo et al., 2018). In a study by Leung et al. (2019), the team examined the susceptibility of phage from different morphological classes against the same type of jet-nebulizer with transmission electron microscopy (TEM). Results showed that phage degradation was closely associated with phage tail length. Phage PEV2, a podovirus characterized by a short, stubby, non-contractile tail showed negligible effect with a similar fraction of intact and viable phages (with filled capsids) post-nebulization in parent stock solution.

However, in the case of PEV40 (a myovirus characterized by a long, straight, contractile tail) and D29 (a siphovirus characterized by a long, flexible, non-contractile tail), the fraction of intact structures seen after nebulization were considerably reduced from 50% to ~27% for PEV40 and from 15% to ~2% for D29 respectively. This suggested that the long-tailed phages were highly susceptible to the stress of the jet nebulization process compared to phages with stubby short tails and for these long tail phages, the tail detachment was the most common type of damage. This damaging effect can be minimized by the presence of organic fluid in the nebulization buffer, which exhibits a protecting effect on phage morphology in the case of some phages (e.g phages PR772 and Φ6) throughout the aerosolization, as observed by Turgeon et al. (2014).

In another in vitro study, Golshahi et al. (2008) investigated the suitability of respiratory phage administration by nebulization method against B. cepacia complex. Phage KS4-M at titers with mean value (standard deviation) of 2.15x10^8 (1.63 x 10^8) PFU/ml was aerosolized with Pari LC star and eFlow nebulizers and the breathing pattern of an adult was simulated using a pulmonary waveform generator. The size distributions of the nebulized aerosol and the overall efficiency of nebulizer delivery were measured. The aerosol was collected on low resistance filters (at the exit of the nebulizer mouthpiece) and the phage counts were determined termed as the "phage inhaled count." The data was then used in a mathematical lung deposition model to predict the regional deposition of phages in the lung. Results based on a mathematical model suggested that LCstar and eFlow both appear suitable for BCC phage therapy with good inhaled and deposition titers. Phages (post nebulization) showed high phage inhaled counts i.e 1.06 x10^8 and 1.15x10^8 PFU for the LC star and eFlow, respectively, more than that effective dose required in mice (10^7 PFU). The alveolar deposition predicted was also high i.e 3.02 x 107 PFU (LCstar) and 2.96 x 107 PFU (eFlow). Thus, respiratory phage delivery via nebulization has potential in resolving BCC infection in cystic fibrosis patients, and further in vivo work in this direction is warranted.

Other factors such as relative humidity and temperature may also effect the final selection of the most suitable method of nebulization. Liu et al. (2012) showed that relative humidity has a strong effect on the cultivability of the mycobacteriophage D29 and it was best seen in a low-humidity condition (25%) than medium to high (55-85%). They also assessed the aerosolization (by collision jet nebulizer) process in the presence of three different spray liquids—deionized water, phosphate buffered saline (PBS), and normal saline. The results indicated that significantly more D29 aerosol particles were generated when the spray fluid was deionized water than PBS or normal saline. Phage particles generated by deionized water retained better viability (30-300 fold more) than those prepared in PBS and normal saline, hinting toward the fact that both high salt concentration and high ionic strength have negative effects on the bioaerosol generation process. The aerosols generated with deionized water had a median mass aerodynamic diameter (MMAD) of 2.4 μm, which is well within the range (1-3 μm) required for reaching and depositing within deeper lung pockets (Thomas, 2013).

The above studies indicate that for morphologically stable phages (that can tolerate the sheer stress produced), both jet and vibrating mesh nebulization represent ideal choices for aerosolized delivery, achieving high rates of deep lung deposition that are essential for the effective resolution of respiratory infection. However, this may not be the case for all phages, and multiple factors such as phage-type, its sensitivity, temperature and humidity conditions, method of nebulization all impact the outcome. These need to be optimized for the best phage-inhalation technique combination and to get the least phage titer loss and highest lung delivery. Some major efficacy studies using different nebulization methods are outlined in **Table 1**.

2.3.2 Dry Powder Inhalation

Although nebulization is the preferred method for phage delivery, other areas of delivery via inhalation include solid phage formulations or dry powder inhalation-based methods. Since phage essentially consists of coat proteins, the protein-based formulations are better suited, as proteins tend to show higher stability in a dry state than in solution form (Cicerone et al., 2015) and hence dry powder formulation show enhanced shelf-life. This accounts for the main advantage favoring this method, which stems from the high degree of phage stability seen during the transport and storage period of such formulations, which is always preferred and required (Chang et al., 2018). Unlike the mechanical stresses associated with nebulizers (ultrasonic, vibrating mesh, or jet type), which may have a detrimental effect on phage morphology, physical stresses are not encountered during the preparation of dry powder aerosols. DPIs are breath-actuated, and the patient's inhalation helps to disaggregate the powder into smaller particles (Geller, 2005). Apart from this, the ease of handling, fast delivery time, no need for electricity for operation, and no regular disinfection make it worth exploring as an ideal delivery platform (Zhou et al., 2014; Respaud et al., 2015).

There are primarily three main ways of producing phage-based dry powders for use which include a) spray drying (SD) b) freeze-drying (FD) and c) spray freeze drying (SFD). Briefly, SD is a single-step method for producing dry powders from liquid suspensions using a gaseous hot drying medium. This occurs in a phased manner whereby the liquid solution upon entering the atomizer gets broken into a spray of fine droplets followed by the droplets being ejected into the drying gas medium, allowing moisture vaporization to form dry particles and final particle collections (Mujumdar, 2007; Vehring, 2008). However, in the SD method, drying occurs when a continuous liquid film is converted into droplets followed by exposure to a hot, dry airflow. The increase in heat exchange area with a high-temperature difference enables to speed up the drying process (Moreira et al., 2021). However, the heat exchange process can have a direct damaging effect on thermosensitive phages affecting their viability. FD addresses this issue of preserving heat-labile components, as it involves a low-temperature dehydration method whereby the solvent (mostly water) is first frozen into ice and later removed by sublimation (direct transition from solid to vapor state) obtained under low pressures in a vacuum chamber (Schwegman et al., 2005; Liu, 2006). The long drying times, drying cycles, and the high vacuum used

TABLE 1 | Treatment outcomes of recent *in vivo* efficacy studies and clinical case studies in which different inhalation delivery methods were used in animal models.

Delivered as:	Bacteria	Phage involved	Study highlights	Main Findings	Reference
Liquid Aerosol (LC-star jet nebulizer)	*B. cenocepacia* K56-2 and C6433	• Phages KS4-M, KS5, and KS12 against *B. cenocepacia* K56-2 • Phages DC1 and KS14 against *B. cenocepacia* C6433	• Experimental *B. cenocepacia* (BCC) respiratory infections were established in mice and post-infection, animals received treatment with one of five bacteriophages specific to this bacterial species, administered as an aerosol or intraperitoneal injection. • Bacterial and bacteriophage titers were determined in the animals' lungs after 2 days	• BCC-infected mice treated with aerosolized phage treatments showed a significant decline in bacterial load in affected lung tissue • Phage KS12 given at an MOI of 131 produced a 2.5-log mean reduction in *B. cenocepacia* K56-2 counts two days post-infection. • Phage KS5 given at MOI of 32 produced a 3-log mean reduction in *B. cenocepacia* K56-2 in the lungs one day post-treatment and further high reduction of 4-log were observed 3 days post-treatment. • Nebulization is a more effective way in delivering phage particles to the lung than other methods	Semler et al., 2014
Liquid Aerosol (Penn-century aerosolizer, Collison 6-jet, and Spinning top aerosol nebulizers)	*M. tuberculosis*	D29 mycobacteriophage	• Deposition and distribution of aerosolized phage D29 particles in naive BALB/C mice were studied. • Phage D29 aerosols were given to animals by endotracheal route using Penn-century aerosolizer; Collison 6-jet and spinning top aerosol nebulizers (STAG) and also compared with nose only route. • Post-exposure, the deposited amounts of phage D29 particles in respiratory tracts and deposition efficiencies were calculated.	• 10% of D29 phage could reach the lung of mice after nebulization and complete phage elimination was noted in 72 h, whereas only 0.1% of the phage could reach the lung by IP injection and no phage was detected after 12 h. Also, no inflammation was observed in the lungs of mice receiving phage aerosols as per the BALF analysis • Aerosol delivery of phage D29 is an effective way of treating pulmonary infections caused by *M. tuberculosis*.	Liu et al., 2016
Powder Aerosol (DPI)	*P. aeruginosa*	Phage PEV20	• Phage PEV20 spray dried inhalable powder with lactose and leucine produced. • Multidrug-resistant (MDR) strain *P. aeruginosa* FADDI-PA001 was established in a mouse lung infection model. • At 2 h after the bacterial challenge, mice were treated with 2 mg of phage dry powder using a dry-powder insufflator.	• Bacterial load got reduced by ~0.5 log in mice received phage *via* ip route while 2-log bacterial reduction was observed in the group treated with inhaled phage. • Nebulization is a more effective way in delivering phage particles to the lung than intranasal instillation	Chang et al., 2018
Liquid Aerosol (Vibrating mesh nebulizer)	*M. tuberculosis*	D29 phage	• Prophylactic pulmonary delivery of active aerosolized phage D29 was studied in female C57BL/6 mice. • An average phage conc. of 1 PFU/alveolus was delivered *via* nose-only inhalation device using a dose simulation technique and then adapted for use with vibrating mesh nebulizer. • Post 30 min, mice were given either a low dose (~50-100 CFU) or an ultra-low dose (~5-10 CFU), of bacteria aerosols. • Bacterial burden of Mtb was evaluated 24 hours and 21 days post-challenge for the low dose model and at 24 hours for the ultra-low dose model.	• A prophylactic effect was observed with phage aerosol pre-treatment significantly decreasing *M. tuberculosis* burden in mouse lungs 24 hours and 3 weeks post-challenge. • This represents a valuable prophylactic approach for the healthcare professional and staff that are at high risk of exposure to *M. tuberculosis*.	Carrigy et al., 2019a; Carrigy et al., 2019b
Spray dried Powder Aerosol (DPI)	*P. aeruginosa*	Phage PEV20 and ciprofloxacin	• Inhalable powder of Pseudomonas phage PEV20 with ciprofloxacin by co-spray drying was developed. • Mouse model of neutropenic mouse model of acute lung infection was established. • Post-infection, different mice groups were given spray-dried single PEV20	• Significant reduction in lung bacterial load (as high as by 5.9 $\log_{10}$) was obtained with PEV20 and ciprofloxacin combination powder along with reduced inflammation in the lung unlike when either phage or ciprofloxacin were given singly.	Lin et al., 2021

(Continued)

TABLE 1 | Continued

Delivered as:	Bacteria	Phage involved	Study highlights	Main Findings	Reference
			(10^6 PFU/mg), single ciprofloxacin (0.33 mg/mg), or combined PEV20-ciprofloxacin treatment using a dry powder insufflator.		
pMDI	*P. aeruginosa*	FKZ/D3 and KS4-M phages	• Aqueous FKZ/D3 and KS4-M phage solutions were formulated in a reverse emulsion with Tyloxapol surfactant and filled into hydrofluoroalkane 134a pMDI canisters (50-μl metering valve). The canisters were shaken well, and five actuations were collected. • The phage titer loss post-actuation was measured. • Storage stability was not tested.	• Phage titer loss was less than one log PFU thus maintaining good viability of both the phages. • Phage delivery from a pMDI showed an acceptable titer loss for the two myoviridae phages post actuation.	Hoe et al., 2014
Liquid Aerosol (Modified Vibrating mesh nebulizer)	Methicillin-resistant *S. aureus* (MRSA) clinical isolate AW7	Phage cocktail of four phages (2003, 2002, 3A, and phage K)	• Male Wistar rats were divided into different groups and ventilated for four hours and after ventilation, rats were inoculated *via* the endotracheal tube with MRSA then extubated. • Different animal groups received: aerophages; intravenous (IV) phages; a combination of IV and aerophages; a combination of IV linezolid and aerophages. • Aerophages were delivered using a modified vibrating mesh aerosol drug delivery system (1.5×10^{10} PFU] • The primary outcome was survival at 96 hours.	• The inhaled phage cocktails given with IV, and delivered phages given alone could each rescue 50% of test animals from death due to MRSA pneumonia. • In combination mode of aerophages and IV phages, 91% of animals were saved from death. • But when aerophages were given along with linezolid no synergistic effect was seen and there was a 55% survival. • Aerosolized phage therapy showed potential for the treatment of MRSA pneumonia.	Prazak et al., 2020

Case studies of Pulmonary Phage therapy in humans

Delivered as:	Bacteria	Phage involved	Study highlights	Main Findings	Reference
Liquid Aerosol (Collision-jet nebulizer)	MDR-*Achromobacter xylosoxidans*	Cocktail of two *Achromobacter* phages (Siphoviridae) prepared at Eliava Institute, Tbilisi)	• A case of 17 year old female with cystic fibrosis and chronic infection with *A. xylosoxidans* (starting at age of 12) not responding to many rounds of antibiotics. • Phage was administered *via* inhalation using a compression nebulizer once daily (3×10^8 PFU/ml) and phages were also given orally twice daily for 20 days. • The same treatment course (inhaled plus oral) was repeated four times (at 1 month, 3 months, 6 months, and 12 months).	• After the initial round of phage treatment, the patient's conditions significantly improved, dyspnea resolved, and cough reduced. • Her lung function measured as Forced expiratory volume (FEV1) increased from an initial 1.83 L (54%) to 1.88 L (62%) in 3 months post treatment. • After the final treatment t round of *Achromobacter* phages, there was a significant improvement in lung function reaching to a final FEV1 value of 3.33 L (84%).	Hoyle et al., 2018
Liquid Aerosol (Vibrating mesh nebulizer)	Carbapenem-resistant *A. baumannii* (CRAB)	Personalized lytic pathogen-specific single-phage (Unnamed)	• A case of an 88-year-old man already suffering from chronic obstructive pulmonary disease developed hospital acquired pneumonia (HAP) with carbapenem-resistant *A. baumannii* as the etiological agent. • A personalized single-phage preparation was nebulized to the patient continuously for 16 days in combination with tigecycline and polymyxin E.	• The treatment was well tolerated and resulted in clearance of the infection from patient's lung with clinical improvement in lung function.	Tan et al., 2021
Liquid Aerosol (Vibrating mesh nebulizer)	*Achromobacter xylosoxidans*	Cocktail of three lytic phages ((JW Delta, JWT, and 2-1)- APC 1.1 And another cocktail mix (APC	• A 12-year-old lung-transplanted cystic fibrosis patient with persistent lung infection with pandrug-resistant *A. xylosoxidans* • Patient received two rounds of phage therapy. In first round 3	• Clinical tolerance was perfect after each round of therapy with no observed side effects. • However, the culture was positive with bronchoalveolar lavage (BAL) showing low densities of *A. xylosoxidans*.	Lebeaux et al., 2021

(Continued)

TABLE 1 | Continued

Delivered as:	Bacteria	Phage involved	Study highlights	Main Findings	Reference
		2.1) with phage JWalpha was added to the above three phage cocktail.	nebulizations/day of 5 mL (10^{10} PFU/ml) of APC 1.1 phage cocktail. In the second round, APC 2.1 was given (phage JWalpha added to the previous cocktail mix) and given. • Initially, 30 mL of APC 2.1, tenfold diluted was instilled in each pulmonary lobe, and later on, discharge, continued phage nebulization at home: three times a day 5 mL of preparation for 14 days.	• But, overall there was a constant improvement in the respiratory condition, and oxygen therapy was stopped. • Low-grade counts of *A. xylosoxidans* (10^3 CFU/ml) persisted for months and finally turned negative although it took almost 10-12 months. • No re-colonization occurred more than two years after phage therapy was stopped.	

may cause additional damage, leading to a loss in phage titers during the lyophilization process itself (Lopez-Quiroga et al., 2012; Ishwarya et al., 2014). The more recent non-conventional SFD method uses a combination of a series of steps i.e droplet formation, freezing, and sublimation, producing uniquely powdered products. SFD is a unique drying technique, as it is a combination of both spray drying and freeze-drying. Furthermore, the unique aerodynamic qualities of the porous particles produced during SFD make it attractive for use in pulmonary delivery (Wang et al., 2006; Filkova et al., 2007). SFD has proven benefits with improved structural integrity, superior quality, and better shelf stability than existing drying techniques (Ishwarya et al., 2014; Fukushige et al., 2020).

Having been used for a long time, FD is a common method for reducing the dry powders of different drugs with high storage stability. One necessary parameter is the use of excipients for effective phage lyophilization and also for protecting their viability (Malenovská, 2014; Manohar and Ramesh, 2019). The type and concentration of excipients and stabilizing agents used need to be optimized. Using the traditional FD method, Puapermpoonsiri et al. (2009) developed inhalable dry powders of *S. aureus* and *P. aeruginosa* phages. The phage-loaded poly (lactic-co-glycolic acid) (PLGA) microspheres were first optimized and later lyophilized to form powders. This system although showed a desirable release profile i.e a burst release phase followed by a sustained release till 6h, but encapsulated phage got deactivated within 7 days either stored at 4°C or 22°C. Similarly, a study by Merabishvilli et al. (2013) focused on evaluating the choice of different stabilizers on *S. aureus* phage ISP free dried preparation over 37 months at 4°C. This study showed that sucrose and trehalose were the best-stabilizing additives, causing a decrease of only 1 log immediately after the lyophilization procedure with high stability over the test period. These sugars act as water substitutes and have a stabilizing effect on phage titers over the storage period.

As freeze-dried powders are not respirable, after their production an extra milling step is required to reduce the particle size to <5 μm, which is ideal for pulmonary delivery. However, this milling process may cause loss of phage due to the mechanical stress produced (Yan et al., 2021). Golshahi et al. (2011) prepared endotoxin-free lyophilized formulations of KS4-M and ΦKZ phages with 60% lactose and 40% lactoferrin as the selected cryo-protectant and stabilizers and then de-agglomerated in a mixer mill (without beads)

to formulate respirable powders and aerosolized using an Aerolizer® capsule inhaler. Post-lyophilization, there was a titer loss in the range of 1-2 $\log_{10}$ for both phages and the size of the phage powder was within the inhalable range (< 5 μm). The freeze-dried phage powders showed good stability with negligible titer reduction within 3 months when stored either at 4°C or 22 C in controlled relative humidity (RH of 21 ± 2%). *In vitro* aerosol testing showed that the phage titers collected downstream of the mouth throat were within the range of 10^6-10^7 PFU with a slight titer drop from capsule dose to respirable dose (titer loss of 1.2 $\log_{10}$ for KS4-M, and 0.84 $\log_{10}$ for ΦKZ phages), which was acceptable.

The SD method produces fine drug particles for pulmonary delivery as a single-step method and is less expensive than FD. SD method works well to maintain the stability and activity of phages and this work was initiated by Matinkhoo and co-workers (2011) produced dry powder inhalable formulation of bacteriophages KS4-M, KS14, and cocktails of phages ΦKZ/D3 and ΦKZ/D3/KS4-M using a low-temperature spray-drying process due to thermal sensitivity of phages. In the formulation, trehalose was used to protect phage against dehydration, while leucine added helped to enhance the dispersibility of powders. The aerosol performance of the resulting dry powders was measured by determining their median mass aerodynamic diameter (MMAD). MMAD represents the aerodynamic diameter at which half of the aerosolized drug mass lies below the stated diameter. It is the average size of particles constituting the dose that reaches the impactor. Particles with an aerodynamic diameter of between 0.5 to 5 μm show a high probability of reaching and depositing in the lung and small ones can penetrate deeper lung tissues (Sheth et al., 2015). However, aerosol particles with a diameter larger than 5 μm tend to remain deposited in the throat or oropharyngeal cavity and fail to reach the lungs. In this study, the SD phage powders had an MMAD diameter of 2.5–2.8 μm suitable for pulmonary delivery of phages to reach the lungs. The actual phage dose reaching lungs released from a single actuation of the inhaler ranged from 10^7 to 10^8 PFU. According to past studies, this phage dose is likely to be effective at containing infection, with phage being effective at these PFU values (Wright et al., 2009; Morello et al., 2011).

Another important parameter that is crucial for determining drug efficacy in the case of pulmonary delivery is pulmonary deposition (highest dose fraction deposition in the lower airways i.e deep lung areas rather than lost in the oropharyngeal sphere), which not only depends on the inhalation device used but also on the ability of the dry powder to be dispersed in the air i.e powder dispersibility (Labiris and Dolovich, 2003; Newman, 2017). The fine particle fraction (FPF) represents the proportion of emitted particles that have a lower particle size than the diameter of the upper airway, which is fixed at 5 μm (Guo et al., 2013; Sibum et al., 2018). To enhance the FPF value, higher dispersibility is essential. This is a delicate process, as micron-sized particles are generally very cohesive and adhesive. The use of excipients needs to be optimized for each formulation. Amino acid, i.e leucine and trileucine, are often used as excipients to SD powders as enhancers of dispersibility and to provide moisture protection (Lechanteur and Evrard, 2020; Zhang Y. et al., 2018). SD powder is mostly amorphous and tends to gain moisture leading to agglomeration. These amino acids exhibit surface-active properties and form a hydrophobic shell that protects spray-dried particles from moisture (Matinkhoo et al., 2011; Mah et al., 2019). For example, with the addition of 20% (w/w) l-leucine to a range of formulations, there was a significant increase i.e 17.3–41.5% for FPFs (Momin et al., 2019; Stewart et al., 2019; Lu et al., 2020). Similarly, when 37.5% (w/w) leucine was added to a spray-dried formulation of budesonide, FPP values increased by 28% (Simková et al., 2020). Next, we have different sugars (lactose, mannitol, trehalose, sucrose), which act as a diluent and flow enhancer, improving aerosolization properties. Further sugars act as stabilizers and protect the active drug during drying and subsequent storage (Zhang Y. et al., 2018; Zillen et al., 2021). However, in the case of sugars, another important parameter to be investigated is the value of glass transition temperature (Tg) of the chosen sugars, which is the temperature at which an amorphous system changes from the brittle glassy state to a viscous rubbery state. Sugars with low Tg tend to crystallize easily, such as mannitol, which has a very low Tg value (Pyne et al., 2002), while Trehalose has a relatively high Tg i.e 106°C and hence is a suitable stabilizer, as it forms a glassy sugar matrix (Buitink et al., 2000).

In addition to these factors, the choice of excipients has a significant impact on maintaining phage stability and phage titers in the final formulation. Chang R. Y. K. et al. (2017) focused their study on evaluating the effect of excipients on the stabilization of spray-dried powders against anti-pseudomonal phages of different morphologies. Both podovirus and myovirus phages showed high stability with trehalose or lactose and leucine as excipients with a negligible loss of less than one log titer. Still, lactose showed superior phage protection over trehalose. Lactose has also been only approved by the FDA as a stabilizing excipient for use, while others may need more safety and regulatory approvals. On similar grounds, the same team then evaluated the storage stability of inhalable phage powders with lactose and leucine as excipients at 20°C/60% RH for 12 months. Results indicated that 90% lactose was able to maintain the viability of phage over the 12 months storage period while ~1.2 $\log_{10}$ titer reduction was observed in formulations with less lactose. The spray-dried anti-pseudomonal phage powders were also shown to be non-toxic to lung alveolar macrophage and epithelial cells *in vitro* (Chang et al., 2019). Thus, leucine not only helps to minimize recrystallization of trehalose/lactose during the powder production process, preventing particle merging and enhancing powder flow but also showing a stabilizing

effect on maintaining phage titers. Similarly, trileucine has also been shown to maintain high phage stability when used as excipients in phage-based formulations. In one such study, Carrigy and the team (Carrigy et al., 2019a, 2019b, 2020) evaluated the stability of engineered spray-dried microparticle based phage formulations of anti-Campylobacter bacteriophage CP30A. They produced amorphous spray-dried powder with excipient formulations containing trehalose and a high glass transition temperature amorphous shell former, either trileucine or pullulan. Results showed the high stability of phage titers with a combination of trileucine and trehalose, with titer reduction of only 0.6 ± 0.1 $\log_{10}$ (PFU/ml) over a 30 day period of storage. Such SD formulations can thus be safely transported a long-distance without the need for maintaining a cold chain system, thus cutting the cost by significant margins. Besides the choice of excipients, the temperature and relative humidity during the storage of SD preparations are equally crucial. Studies on RH show that formulations stored at high humidity conditions (RH > 50%) showed recrystallization of the amorphous content and hence SD powders need to be stored at low humidity conditions (RH ≤ 20%) (Vandenheuvel et al., 2014; Leung et al., 2016). It is also generally recommended to store phage drug powder at a temperature at least 50°C below the glass transition temperature (Tg) of the powders (Chang et al., 2020).

More recently, an SFD method of producing dry phage powders has been developed. This method shows enhanced structural integrity and stability over other drying methods. SFD yields particles of sizes and densities that show higher stability in the lungs and nasal mucosa (Vishali et al., 2019). SFD has also been shown to produce powders with particles larger and more porous than spray drying (Maa et al., 1999). Leung et al. (2016) compared both SD and SFD methods of procuring inhalable phage powders of *Pseudomonas* podoviridae phage, PEV2. Their results showed a loss of 2 log titers in the SFD method owing to the use of ultrasonic nozzle but the *in vitro* aerosol performance showed that the SFD powders showed significantly higher phage recovery (~80% phage recovery) compared with the SD counterparts (~20% phage recovery). This needs to be taken into consideration while using the SFD based method due to phage sensitivity to the mechanical stress. The frozen powders in SFD are also dried under vacuum pressure, adding to the long drying times (Shoyele and Cawthorne, 2006) that may cause more titer loss. While addressing this issue, Ly and their team (2019) studied a new technique of atmospheric spray freeze drying (ASFD) in developing a solid dry formulation of mycobacterium phage D29. In this process, phage D29 (in presence of varying concentrations of trehalose and mannitol) was sprayed and then frozen in a cold chamber followed by the passing of cold drying gas through the chamber resulting in the sublimation of ice forming a free-flowing powder. The result showed that this technique of AFSD showed a minimal titer reduction of ~0.6 log in presence of trehalose-mannitol at a mass ratio of 7:3 thus advocating the further exploration of ASFD as an attractive alternative method over conventional freeze-drying processes providing similar biological preservative in a shorter time. **Table 1** provides a useful insight into recent *in vitro* and *in vivo* studies (2014 onwards), wherein different inhalation delivery methods (nebulizers, DPI, pMDI) have been used.

The major conclusions summarized from the studies of **Table 1** include that pulmonary delivery *via* nebulization and dry powder inhalation both represent a favorable and safe route (effective than other methods) for phage administration, enabling phage to reach the affected lung tissue and target respiratory pathogens. This is indicated by the significant reductions in lung bacterial counts as well as low inflammation seen in various animal studies. Secondly, although human studies using aerosolized, phage preparations are limited, results indicate good clinical tolerance with no side effects and complete resolution of infection over time. Pulmonary delivery may be used in combination with *i.v* administered phages or antibiotics. Combined administration of phage and antibiotics also showed higher reductions in bacterial burden and needs to be advocated further. The co-therapy mode (Phage and antibiotic) is an attractive approach over the traditional treatment protocols due to the proven synergistic antimicrobial effect (Torres-Barcelo et al., 2014; Kamal and Dennis, 2015; Oechslin et al., 2017]. The synergistic effect of phage PEV20 along with ciprofloxacin against the drug-resistant strain of *P. aeruginosa* administered *via* both air-jet and vibrating mesh nebulizers has been reported and studied in detail by Lin et al. (2018). Apart from the use of the nebulization method, Lin et al. (2019) also tested the SD-based inhalable powders of PEV20 and ciprofloxacin as dry powders for inhalation, which tend to show better patient compliance. Results showed that inhalable combination powder formulations of phage PEV20 and ciprofloxacin were stable and exhibited a strong synergistic antimicrobial killing effect against *P. aeruginosa* strains isolated from CF patients. Such findings advocate further research into the development of phage-antibiotic inhalable formulations for pulmonary delivery with improved and faster containment of infection. However, given the limited studies conducted to date on humans, more clinical research with a high sample size is required to understand the efficacy and safety of this approach. Finally, complete optimization studies need to be done for each phage (i.e which type of nebulization as well as the dry powder inhalation technique to be used, the choice of stabilizers, effect on phage morphology, stability and viability, lung deposition percentage, testing phage-antibiotic synergism, etc.) to ensure the greatest clinical benefits.

2.3.3 Metered-Dose or Propellant Based Inhalation

Pressurized Metered-dose inhalation (pMDI) is based on a specifically designed device that delivers a minute and fixed amount of medication as a short burst of aerosolized form taken by the patient through their mouth (Ibrahim et al., 2015; Martin and Finlay, 2015). It contains three major parts, which include a) canister which holds the formulation b) metering valve, that allows a metered quantity of the formulation to be dispensed, and c) an actuator (or mouthpiece) allowing the patient to operate the device and it is attached to a nozzle which enables to spread the component in the mouth of the person using it. Metered-dose inhalers are mostly and more commonly used by asthmatics or people with COPD (Boyd, 1995; Brand et al., 2008). The drug formulation present in the canister is mixed with liquefied gas propellant and stabilizing chemicals. Such a metered-dose inhalation method offers the advantages of allowing the delivery of metered and specific amounts of

medication, with no pre-drug preparation required and multi-dose capability available, while also being portable and comparatively inexpensive (Carrie, 2009; Javadzadeh and Yaqoubi, 2017). However, very little work has been reported on the use of this type of inhaler to deliver phage against RTIs. In a study by Hoe et al. (2014), phage suspension of two *myoviridae* phage (FKZ/D3 and KS4-M) was prepared using a reverse emulsion process with Tyloxapol as surfactant and filled into hydrofluoroalkane 134a pMDI canisters. The phages were actuated from the device and there was a negligible loss in titers, showing successful delivery to the lungs. Despite this, more dedicated studies on the different aspects of this inhaler for phage delivery are required. Moreover, one drawback is that just 10%–20% of the expelled dose reaches the lung (Liu et al., 2012; Chaturvedi and Solanki, 2013; Liang et al., 2020), which needs to be developed and improved.

2.3.4 Soft–Mist Inhalation

A new class of propellant-free inhalers known as Soft Mist Inhalers (SMIs) have also been developed in recent years, also known as respimat inhalers. These inhalers release medication in a fine mist that comes out slowly. Hochrainer et al. (2005) showed that the velocity and spray duration of aerosols clouds released from SMI inhaler moved much slower and has a prolonged spray duration as well as compared to pMDIs and this will account for improved lung and reduced oropharyngeal deposition essential for moving outcome. SMIs come with a dose counter built-in, which enables us to see how many doses of medication are remaining and a lock itself system after the medication is all used up, but to date, there is limited data regarding this method. One study by Carrigy et al. (2017) compared the efficiency of phage delivery using vibrating mesh nebulizer, jet nebulizer, and soft mist inhalation (SMI) methods. The results showed that the SMI was able to deliver the mycophage D29 more quickly with high titers ($\sim 5 \times 10^8$ PFU/actuation). There was a minimal titer reduction ($0.6 \log_{10}$ PFU/ml) and a higher lung delivery was achieved (3.2×10^6 PFU/actuation of inhalable active phage). Similar to MDIs, this device again needs more exploration in phage delivery.

3 ADVANCES IN DELIVERY AND FORMULATIONS-INHALED PHAGE THERAPY

3.1 Surface Acoustic Waves Nebulization and High-Frequency Acoustic Nebulization For Improved Pulmonary Delivery

The nebulization process and the hydrodynamic stress it generates (as in the case of ultrasonic nebulizer and cavitational process for aerosol formation) have been shown to have a detrimental effect on phage morphology and overall viability in past studies (Astudillo et al., 2018; Leung et al., 2018). One approach is the use of surface acoustic wave (SAW) nebulizers. SAWs operate at considerably higher (>10 MHz) frequencies than the ultrasonic nebulizers and essentially comprise surface waves and do not drive cavitation. In the absence of large cavitational pressures, high surface vibrational acceleration is produced and the acoustic energy produced causes the drop interface to rapidly destabilize and break up to form aerosol droplets containing the therapeutic molecule (Rajapaksa et al., 2014). The entire process occurs within such a short period that it is not sufficient to degrade biomolecules and thus represents a much gentler way of procuring aerosol particles (Qi et al., 2008; Collins et al., 2012). With its ability to generate aerosols within the 1–5 μm aerodynamic diameter range required for maximizing deep lung deposition (Qi et al., 2009), particularly in the smaller bronchioles that are common sites of pulmonary infection, SAW nebulization is an ideal and efficient platform for pulmonary administration of various biomolecules (Rajapaksa et al., 2014; Alhasan et al., 2016; Wang et al., 2016). However, one drawback of most nebulizers including SAW nebulizers is the long administration time taken for adequate dosing to reach deeper areas.

One approach of potential interest is the novel acoustic wave platform (HYDRA) for advanced levels for nebulization. HYDRA nebulizers exploit the combined effects of both bulk wave nebulization and surface waves i.e SAW nebulization enjoying an advantage for higher output and improved efficiency and efficacy with better preservation of molecular structure and function (Cortez-Jugo et al., 2015; Kwok et al., 2020).In a recent study by Marqus et al. (2020), the authors assessed the capability of this low-cost and portable hybrid surface and bulk acoustic wave platform (HYDRA) to nebulize a phage K and lytic enzyme (lysostaphin). Results showed that the HYDRA platform was able to produce monodispersed phage aerosol particles within a defined size range (1-5 μm) ideal to be delivered to the lower respiratory airways and deep pockets. There was a minimal loss in the phage viability (negligible titer loss of 0.1 $\log_{10}$ (PFU/ml) with a high viable respirable fraction (90%) reaching the active site. This indicates that the HYDRA nebulization process does not result in appreciable denaturation of phages or even proteins (as seen with lysostaphin results) preserving function and structure. This calls for further exploration of this novel HYDRA nebulization platform for improved delivery of mono-disperse aerosol down to the lower airways, especially targeting chronic deep-seated infections.

3.2 Electrospray for Controlled and Targeted Drug Delivery *via* Inhalation

Although nebulization remains the preferred method of drug delivery *via* the inhalation route, it suffers from common pitfalls. Nebulization typically generates contaminant particles in the ultrafine size range from dried solutes and biological fragments in the nebulizer suspension. These contaminants can mask the size distribution of virus particles that are of comparable size (Hogan et al., 2004; Hogan et al., 2005), reducing the overall efficacy of the process. Another drawback observed is that some portion of the nebulized solution may flow back to the nebulizer reservoir, and fraction will evaporate over time causing the solution to become more concentrated (Chen and John, 2001) and again changing the aerosolized particle size distribution function which is not desirable (Eninger et al., 2009). In addition, with these traditional inhalation techniques including

nebulizers, DPIs, and pMDIs, high deposition efficiency is often a problem with less than 20% of the spray reaching the target area of the lungs as most of the drug particles get deposited in the upper airway. Moreover, they tend to produce more of a polydisperse type of particle with varying diameters. The bigger diameter particle tends to deposit in upper airways rather than reaching lungs with less than the actual administered dose (or phage titers) reaching the actual site for action thus decreasing the desired outcome (Tena and Clarà, 2012; Cheng, 2014). Electrospray (ES) or electrohydrodynamic atomization (EHDA) is a promising atomization process due to its ability to produce a spray with monodisperse droplet size. It is an atomization technique that uses electro-hydrodynamic forces to disperse a liquid into fine droplets thus forming micro and nano-sized mono-dispersed droplets of the same and uniform size (Jaworek, 2007; Ryan et al., 2012). With the use of the electrospray process, the production of a relatively uniform narrow aerosol size distribution is achievable. The aerosolized formulation produced is comparatively without aggregates and free of generated contaminants from dried solutes i.e a cleaner and stable preparation (Thomas et al., 2004). There have been few dedicated studies focusing on this aspect.

Jung et al. (2009) investigated the characteristics of airborne MS2 bacteriophage particles <30 nm in size, using a charge-reduced electrospray technique. For this, the suspension of phage was sprayed cone-jet mode using a specially designed electrospray system in a cone-jet mode. Results indicated that the electro-sprayed MS2 particles so formed showed excellent monodisperse size distribution, high stability, and uniformity which was not seen with nebulized particles. Thus, the authors reported the electrospray method being able to produce non-agglomerated particles, resulting in a narrow size range of uniform size. In another study reported by Eninger et al. (2009), the aerosolization of bacteriophage MS2 virions by nebulization and charge-reduced electrospray were compared during testing of three filter media. Results depicted that although both aerosolization methods generated culturable MS2 virions electrospray method produced an airborne concentration of phages that was 20-fold higher than the nebulizer. The electrospray produced cleaner, more stable, and higher viable phages in the aerosolized particles as compared to the classical nebulization process. The nebulized aerosol particle count was 2.8 times more variable than the electro-sprayed aerosol particle count. This indicates that the nebulizer produced a poly-disperse aerosol, unlike the electrospray protocol, which also produced a more desirable and relatively mono-disperse aerosol and a better way of filter testing the delivery method. These findings encourage exploration of this mode of generating aerosolized phages and the possible effect of the electrospray technique on the viability of phage titers.

3.3 Liposome Encapsulated Phage Preparation for Improved Pulmonary Delivery

Liposomes are one of the lipid-based nano-vesicles that self-assemble, forming lipid nano-spheres that act as an ideal drug delivery approach for encapsulating and protecting phages, showing bio-compatibility with various phage preparations (Singla et al., 2015; Chadha et al., 2017; Chhibber et al., 2018; Otero et al., 2019). Liposome-loaded phages are protected from outer stress such as the action of body fluids, enzymes, clearance from the reticuloendothelial system (RES), the action of neutralizing antibodies (Colom et al., 2015; Singla et al., 2016; Chhibber et al., 2018; Leung et al., 2018). They are also capable of undergoing conformational transitions as they mimic biological membranes and this allows them to reach and penetrate the deeper areas crossing the host tissue barriers. This is especially important in the case of penetrating the biofilm-affected areas. Liposome encapsulation may enable phages to gain access into the eukaryotic cell to target intracellular pathogens, as free phages have limited ability to penetrate eukaryotic cells (Nieth et al., 2015). The use of liposome encapsulation technology in the delivery of phages and various antibiotics has been successfully reported by recent studies against a range of pulmonary pathogens. Singla et al. (2015) reported the successful encapsulation of phage KPO1K2, specific for *K. pneumoniae in* cationic liposomes with high efficiency of 92% and significant structural and biological stability for nine weeks at 4°C and room temperature. The liposomal preparation was able to protect all tested mice from pneumonia-induced death even when the therapy was delayed by 3 days after induction of infection by *K. pneumoniae* with complete clearance of organisms from the lungs within 72 hours after treatment. Liposomal encapsulated phage treatment also led to a higher reduction in inflammatory cytokines levels. Although the result shows the enhanced persistence of encapsulated phages in lung tissue and higher therapeutic effect against pneumonia, the liposomal phage preparation was here given intra-peritoneal and not tested *via* the inhalation route.

The biggest advantage of inhaled antibacterial therapy would be its ability to target intracellular respiratory pathogens such as *M. tuberculosis*. While studying liposome-mediated intracellular delivery, Nieth et al. (2015) reported the successful encapsulation of mycobacteriophages in giant unilamellar liposomes (≥ 5 µm) by two different techniques i.e gel assisted GUV formation and inversion emulsion technique. These liposome-associated bacteriophages were able to enter THP-1 cultured eukaryotic cells significantly more efficiently than free bacteriophages and co-localize with early- and recycling endosomes. Similarly, in a recent study by Vladimirsky et al. (2019), macrophage cell culture (RAW 264-7-ATCC) was first infected for 24 hours with *M. tuberculosis* strain i.e H37RV MTB at a concentration of 10^7 CFU/ml and then incubated with free phage and liposome-encapsulated phage D29 to study the decline in bacterial counts post 24 h of co-incubation. The results of counting of MTB colonies showed 62 colonies in control (no treatment), 17 ± 1 in free mycobacteriophage treated and only 7 MTB colonies in the liposomal mycobacteriophage treated, showing significantly high bactericidal effect with liposomal phage preparation. These results indicate new opportunities for treating mycobacterial infections.

Besides the above studies, no major studies have directly focused on the preparation of inhalable liposome-encapsulated phage formulations and their delivery through liquid or dry powder aerosolization and their efficacy testing, although inhalable liposome loaded antibiotics against respiratory pathogens have been accessed in many studies (Waters and Ratjen, 2014; Grifth et al., 2018; Bassetti et al., 2020). Liposome encapsulated phage delivery *via* aerosolization may be associated with its own challenges. Firstly, during liposome formation following the conventional thin-film hydration and extrusion method, phages are exposed to the heat used during hydration and high mechanical stress generated upon extrusion, which may account for significant losses and low encapsulation efficiency (Colom et al., 2015). Even with an improved method such as gel assisted formation followed by extrusion and inversed emulsion, the liposome that are formed are large in size ≥ 5 (Nieth et al., 2015), which is not ideal for pulmonary delivery, as most of them may fail to reach deeper lung areas. Secondly, the major challenge is the stability of liposome vesicles during the nebulization process. The shearing stress of the nebulization process to convert liposome dispersions into fine aerosol droplets may result in vesicle fragmentation and loss of the encapsulated phage. Vesicles may also undergo marked size reduction during jet nebulization, as reported by Saari et al. (1999). These physical changes highlight that applying a mild nebulization technology to minimize the process of fragmentation and shear degradation of lipid nanovesicles. The inclusion of stabilizers such as cholesterol or high-phase transition phospholipids in the liposome formulations has been shown to exhibit a protective effect (Elhissi et al., 2007; Clancy, 2013).

Keeping the challenges in mind, these lipid-based nanocarriers represent an ideal platform for successful encapsulation and pulmonary delivery of the sensitive phages, phage cocktails, and even phage endolysins, while maintaining their viability and infectivity intact and thus, more research and future studies are required to explore this direction.

3.4 Individualized Controlled Inhalation Technology: Integrated Software Control

ICI technology is one of the most promising novel approaches for the improvement of pulmonary aerosol deposition, offering higher drug targeting, reduced lung dose variability with unique integrated software control (Chandel et al., 2019; Longest et al., 2019). The AKITA® technology is the most advanced ICI technology-based aerosol delivery technology as it controls the entire inhalation maneuver of the patient resulting in more precise drug targeting. This is accomplished by positive air pressure delivered by a computer-controlled processor, which is made to program as per the patient's individual lung function data, which is tested prior to use (Fischer et al., 2009; Kesser and Geller, 2009; Tashkin, 2016).

AKITA® works well with ultrasonic mesh nebulizers and the latest versions are fully compatible with vibrating mesh nebulizers, delivering as high as 99% of the filled dose nebulized into aerosol particles with Median mass aerodynamic diameter (MMAD) of < 4 µm (Kesser and Geller, 2009; Fischer et al., 2009). Such ICI-based technology is associated with clear advantages of minimal dose variability and maximum efficiency as this technology enables better control over aerosol flow rates, delivery volumes, dosing timings giving higher compliance to the treatment protocol. In a cross-over study on inhaled tobramycin done in healthy individuals (Brand et al., 2005), it was observed that individuals using conventional jet nebulizer system achieved lung deposition of a total of 40.78 mg with as high as 30% variation in total lung dose while AKITA® system showed deposition of 42.81 mg with less than 11% as the dose variation seen.

The integrated software controls provided with these technologies further allow the physician to have more control over the therapy and when to change the controls as per the constant monitoring of parameters and observed adverse effects which are possible with such latest systems (Bennett, 2005; Ibrahim et al., 2015). For example, past studies have shown that lung deposition of lipopolysaccharide, an endotoxin if present in drug formulations leads to triggering of airway inflammation and adverse effects in patients with COPD, CF (Thorn and Rylander, 1998; Muhlebach and Noah, 2002). However, this can be well controlled and managed by the use of such ICT systems with advanced features such as constant scanning of information about nebulized drug dose, treatment time, adverse effects if any. This feature is particularly useful in the case of phage preparations wherein endotoxin may contaminate the formulation owing to gaps during high titer phage production and purification if any. On similar grounds, there is another technology i.e the I-Neb®, which consists of high-level software control integrated with mesh nebulizer as a single device (Geller and Kesser, 2010; Tashkin, 2016). This system works on either of the two modes i.e a tidal breathing mode and a targeted-inhalation mode. In tidal breathing mode, the device aerosolization process is adapted as per the patient's tidal breathing pattern. However, in the targeted inhalation mode, a vibrating feedback system guides the patient towards an optimal breathing pattern to enhance and further improve the aerosol deposition and final efficacy (Zhou et al., 2014).

Many studies on these ICT-based nebulizers and phage therapy have not seen the light yet. However, in the case of personalized pulmonary phage therapy, such software integrated systems (with better control over dosing volumes, dosing times, aerosolization rates, higher physician monitoring) that are optimized as per individual patients' needs and lung function will help to further enhance the success and outcome of phage treatment (with more phages dose reaching the lower and deeper lung pockets). This is especially important while treating patients with recurrent chronic bacterial infections.

4 CONCLUSION

Inhaled phage therapy has the potential to transform the prevention and treatment of bacterial respiratory infections, including those caused by antibiotic-resistant bacteria. The results of various studies advocate that inhaled phage therapy is a safe and potent antibacterial option with no reported adverse events. There is a long way to go before clinical approval of inhaled phage therapy. Robust randomized clinical trials, a deeper understanding of the pharmacological studies of the inhalable formulations, and further research on the stability of phage in various formulations need attention for moving this therapy closer to final approval and use. However, the use of inhaled phage therapy on compassionate grounds needs to be looked at as a priority. Despite the concerns outlined here, inhaled phage therapy holds strong potential and represents a new era of inhalable phages that act on multiple fronts to resolve respiratory infection working well even against drug-resistant strains.

AUTHOR CONTRIBUTIONS

Literature search, data extraction, writing-review, and final editing: XW, ZX, JZ, ZZ, CY, and YL. All authors have reviewed and approved the final version of the article, including the authorship list.

REFERENCES

Abedon, S. T. (2015). Phage Therapy of Pulmonary Infections. *Bacteriophage* 5 (1), e1020260. doi: 10.1080/21597081.2015.1020260

Ackart, D. F., Hascall-Dove, L., Caceres, S. M., Kirk, N. M., Podell, B. K., Melander, C., et al. (2014). Expression of Antimicrobial Drug Tolerance by Attached Communities of Mycobacterium Tuberculosis. *Pathog. Dis.* 70, 359–369. doi: 10.1111/2049-632X.12144

Akturk, E., Oliveira, H., Santos, S. B., Costa, S., Kuyumcu, S., Melo, L. D. R., et al. (2019). Synergistic Action of Phage and Antibiotics: Parameters to Enhance the Killing Efficacy Against Mono and Dual-Species Biofilms. *Antibiotics (Basel)* 8 (3):103. doi: 10.3390/antibiotics8030103

Alhasan, L., Qi, A., Rezk, A. R., Yeo, L. Y., and Chan, P. P. (2016). Assessment of the Potential of a High Frequency Acoustomicrofluidic Nebulisation Platform for Inhaled Stem Cell Therapy. *Integr. Biol. (Camb)* 8 (1), 12–20. doi: 10.1039/c5ib00206k

Ali, M. (2010). "Pulmonary Drug Delivery," in *Personal Care & Cosmetic Technology, Handbook of Non-Invasive Drug Delivery Systems* (Elsevier Science, USA: William Andrew Publishing), 209–246. Available at: https://doi.org/10.1016/B978-0-8155-2025-2.10009-5.

Angelis, A., Kanavos, P., López-Bastida, J., Linertová, R., Nicod, E., Serrano-Aguilar, P., et al. (2015). Social and Economic Costs and Health-Related Quality of Life

in Non-Institutionalised Patients With Cystic Fibrosis in the United Kingdom. *BMC Health Serv. Res.* 15, 428. doi: 10.1186/s12913-015-1061-3

Astudillo, A., Leung, S. S. Y., Kutter, E., Morales, S., and Chan, H.-K. (2018). Nebulization Effects on Structural Stability of Bacteriophage PEV 44. *Eur. J. Pharm. Biopharm.* 125, 124–130. doi: 10.1016/j.ejpb.2018.01.010

Azeredo, J., and Sutherland, I. W. (2008). The Use of Phages for the Removal of Infectious Biofilms. *Curr. Pharm. Biotechnol.* 9 (4), 261–266. doi: 10.2174/138920108785161604

Bassetti, M., Vena, A., Russo, A., and Peghin, M. (2020). Inhaled Liposomal Antimicrobial Delivery in Lung Infections. *Drugs* 80 (13), 1309–1318. doi: 10.1007/s40265-020-01359-z

Bedi, M., Verma, V., and Chhibber, S. (2009). Amoxicillin and Specific Bacteriophage Can Be Used Together for Eradication of Biofilm of Klebsiella Pneumoniae B5055. *World J. Microbiol. Biotechnol.* 25, 1145-1151. doi: 10.1007/s11274-009-9991-8

Bennett, W. D. (2005). Controlled Inhalation of Aerosolised Therapeutics. *Expert Opin. Drug Deliv.* 2 (4), 763–767. doi: 10.1517/17425247.2.4.763

Biswas, B., Adhya, S., Washart, P., Paul, B., Trostel, A. N., Powell, B., et al. (2002). Bacteriophage Therapy Rescues Mice Bacteremic From a Clinical Isolate of Vancomycin-Resistant Enterococcus Faecium. *Infect. Immun.* 70, 204–210. doi: 10.1128/IAI.70.1.204-210.2002

Bodier-Montagutelli, E., Morello, E., L'Hostis, G., Guillon, A., Dalloneau, E., Respaud, R., et al. (2017). Inhaled Phage Therapy: A Promising and Challenging Approach to Treat Bacterial Respiratory Infections. *Expert Opin. Drug Deliv.* 14 (8), 959–972. doi: 10.1080/17425247.2017.1252329

Boisvert, A. A., Cheng, M. P., Sheppard, D. C., and Nguyen, D. (2016). Microbial Biofilms in Pulmonary and Critical Care Diseases. *Ann. Am. Thorac. Soc* 13 (9), 1615–1623. doi: 10.1513/AnnalsATS.201603-194FR

Boratyński, J., Syper, D., Weber-Dabrowska, B., Łusiak-Szelachowska, M., Poźniak, G., and Górski, A. (2004). Preparation of Endotoxin-Free Bacteriophages. *Cell. Mol. Biol. Lett.* 9 (2), 253–259.

Borysowski, J., Wierzbicki, P., Kłosowska, D., Korczak-Kowalska, G., Weber-Dabrowska, B., and Górski, A. (2010). The Effects of T4 and A3/R Phage Preparations on Whole-Blood Monocyte and Neutrophil Respiratory Burst. *Viral Immunol.* 23 (5), 541–544. doi: 10.1089/vim.2010.0001

Boyd, G. (1995). The Continued Need for Metered Dose Inhalers. *J. Aerosol Med.* 8 Suppl 1, S9–12. doi: 10.1089/jam.1995.8.suppl_1.s-9

Brand, P., Häußermann, S., Müllinger, B., Fischer, A., Wachall, B., and Stegemann, J. (2005). Intra-Pulmonal Deposition of Two Different Tobramycin Formulations. *J. Cyst. Fibros.* 4, S34–S58.

Brand, P., Hederer, B., Austen, G., Dewberry, H., and Meyer, T. (2008). Higher Lung Deposition With Respimat Soft Mist Inhaler Than HFA-MDI in COPD Patients With Poor Technique. *Int. J. Chron. Obstruct. Pulmon. Dis.* 3 (4), 763–770.

Broxmeyer, L., Sosnowska, D., Miltner, E., Chacón, O., Wagner, D., McGarvey, J., et al. (2002). Killing of *Mycobacterium Avium* and *Mycobacterium Tuberculosis* by a Mycobacteriophage Delivered by a Nonvirulent Mycobacterium: A Model for Phage Therapy of Intracellular Bacterial Pathogens. *J. Infect. Dis.* 186 (8), 1155–1160. doi: 10.1086/343812

Buitink, J., van den Dries, I. J., Hoekstra, F. A., Alberda, M., and Hemminga, M. A. High Critical Temperature Above T(g) May Contribute to the Stability of Biological Systems. *Biophys J.* (2000) 79(2):1119-28. doi: 10.1016/S0006-3495(00)76365-X

Burns, J. L., Gibson, R. L., McNamara, S., Yim, D., Emerson, J., Rosenfeld, M., et al. (2001). Longitudinal Assessment of *Pseudomonas Aeruginosa* in Young Children With Cystic Fibrosis. *J. Infect. Dis.* 183 (3), 444–452. doi: 10.1086/318075

Cafora, M., Brix, A., Forti, F., Loberto, N., Aureli, M., Briani, F., et al. (2020). Phages as Immunomodulators and Their Promising Use as Anti-Inflammatory Agents in a CFTR Loss-of-Function Zebrafish Model. *J. Cyst. Fibros.* S1569-1993 (20), 30927–9. doi: 10.1016/j.jcf.2020.11.017.

Capparelli, R., Parlato, M., Borriello, G., Salvatore, P., and Iannelli, D. (2007). Experimental Phage Therapy Against *Staphylococcus Aureus* in Mice. *Antimicrob. Agents Chemother.* 51, 2765–2773. doi: 10.1128/AAC.01513-06

Carlton, R. M. (1999). Phage Therapy: Past History and Future Prospects. *Arch. Immunol. Ther. Exp. (Warsz)* 47, 267–274.

Carrie, J. M. (2009). "Aerosolized Medications," in *Small Animal Critical Care Medicine*. Eds. D. C. Silverstein and K. Hopper (USA: WB Saunders), 814–817, ISBN: . doi: 10.1016/B978-1-4160-2591-7.10192-4

Carrigy, N. B., Chang, R. Y., Leung, S. S. Y., Harrison, M., Petrova, Z., Pope, W. H., et al. (2017). Anti-Tuberculosis Bacteriophage D29 Delivery With a Vibrating Mesh Nebulizer, Jet Nebulizer, and Soft Mist Inhaler. *Pharm. Res.* 34, 2084–2096. doi: 10.1007/s11095-017-2213-4

Carrigy, N. B., Larsen, S. E., Reese, V., Pecor, T., Harrison, M., Kuehl, P. J., et al. (2019a). Prophylaxis of *Mycobacterium Tuberculosis* H37Rv Infection in a Preclinical Mouse Model *via* Inhalation of Nebulized Bacteriophage D29 *Antimicrob. Agents Chemother.* 63 (12), e00871–e00819. doi: 10.1128/AAC.00871-19

Carrigy, N. B., Liang, L., Wang, H., Kariuki, S., Nagel, T. E., Connerton, I. F., et al. (2019b). Spray-Dried Anti-Campylobacter Bacteriophage CP30A Powder Suitable for Global Distribution Without Cold Chain Infrastructure. *Int. J. Pharm.* 569, 118601. doi: 10.1016/j.ijpharm.2019.118601

Carrigy, N. B., Liang, L., Wang, H., Kariuki, S., Nagel, T. E., Connerton, I. F., et al. (2020). Trileucine and Pullulan Improve Anti-Campylobacter Bacteriophage Stability in Engineered Spray-Dried Microparticles. *Ann. BioMed. Eng.* 48, 1169–1180. doi: 10.1007/s10439-019-02435-6

Chadha, P., Katare, O. P., and Chhibber, S. (2017). Liposome Loaded Phage Cocktail: Enhanced Therapeutic Potential in Resolving *Klebsiella Pneumoniae* Mediated Burn Wound Infections. *Burns* 43 (7), 1532–1543. doi: 10.1016/j.burns.2017.03.029

Chakraborty, P., Bajeli, S., Kaushal, D., Radotra, B. D., and Kumar, A. (2021). Biofilm Formation in the Lung Contributes to Virulence and Drug Tolerance of Mycobacterium Tuberculosis. *Nat. Commun.* 12, 1606. doi: 10.1038/s41467-021-21748-6

Chandel, A., Goyal, A. K., Ghosh, G., and Rath, G. (2019). Recent Advances in Aerosolised Drug Delivery. *BioMed. Pharmacother.* 112, 108601. doi: 10.1016/j.biopha.2019.108601

Chang, R. Y. K., Chen, K., Wang, J., Wallin, M., Britton, W., Morales, S., et al. (2017). Anti-Pseudomonal Activity of Phage PEV20 in a Dry Powder Formulation — A Proof-of-Principle Study in a Murine Lung Infection Model. *Antimicrob. Agents Chemother.* 62 (2), e01714–17. doi: 10.1128/AAC.01714-17

Chang, R. Y. K., Kwok, P. C. L., Khanal, D., Morales, S., Kutter, E., Li, J., et al. (2020). Inhalable Bacteriophage Powders: Glass Transition Temperature and Bioactivity Stabilization. *Bioeng. Transl. Med.* 5 (2), e10159. doi: 10.1002/btm2.10159

Chang, R. Y. K., Wallin, M., Kutter, E., Morales, S., Britton, W., Li, J., et al. (2019). Storage Stability of Inhalable Phage Powders Containing Lactose at Ambient Conditions. *Int. J. Pharm.* 560, 11–18. doi: 10.1016/j.ijpharm.2019.01.050

Chang, R. Y. K., Wallin, M., Lin, Y., Leung, S. S. Y., Wang, H., Morales, S., et al. (2018). Phage Therapy for Respiratory Infections. *Adv. Drug Deliv. Rev.* 133, 76–86. doi: 10.1016/j.addr.2018.08.001

Chanishvili, N. (2012). Phage Therapy–History From Twort and D'Herelle Through Soviet Experience to Current Approaches. *Adv. Virus Res.* 83, 3–40. doi: 10.1016/B978-0-12-394438-2.00001-3

Chaturvedi, N. P., and Solanki, H. (2013). Pulmonary Drug Delivery System: Review. *Int. J. Appl. Pharm.* 5, 7–10.

Cheng, Y. S. (2014). Mechanisms of Pharmaceutical Aerosol Deposition in the Respiratory Tract. *AAPS PharmSciTech* 15 (3), 630–640. doi: 10.1208/s12249-014-0092-0

Chen, B. T., and John, W. (2001). "Instrument Calibration, in Aerosol Measurement," in *Principles, Techniques and Applications*. Eds. P. A. Baron and K. Willeke (New York: Wiley-Interscience), 627–666.

Chhibber, S., Kaur, J., and Kaur, S. (2018). Liposome Entrapment of Bacteriophages Improves Wound Healing in a Diabetic Mouse MRSA Infection. *Front. Microbiol.* 9:561. doi: 10.3389/fmicb.2018.00561

Chhibber, S., Kaur, S., and Kumari, S. (2008). Therapeutic Potential of Bacteriophage in Treating *Klebsiella Pneumoniae* B5055-Mediated Lobar Pneumonia in Mice. *J. Med. Microbiol.* 57, 1508–1513. doi: 10.1099/jmm.0.2008/002873-0

Cicerone, M. T., Pikal, M. J., and Qian, K. K. (2015). Stabilization of Proteins in Solid Form. *Adv. Drug Deliv. Rev.* 93, 14–24. doi: 10.1016/j.addr.2015.05.006

Clancy, J. P., Dupont, L., Konstan, M. W., Billings, J., Fustik, S., Goss, C. H., et al. (2013). Phase II Studies of Nebulised Arikace in CF Patients With Pseudomonas Aeruginosa Infection. *Thorax* 68 (9), 818–825. doi: 10.1136/thoraxjnl-2012-202230

Collins, D. J., Manor, O., Winkler, A., Schmidt, H., Friend, J. R., and Yeo, L. Y. (2012). Atomization Off Thin Water Films Generated by High-Frequency Substrate Wave Vibrations. *Phys. Rev. E* 86:56312. doi: 10.1103/PhysRevE.86.056312

Colom, J., Cano-Sarabia, M., Otero, J., Cortés, P., Maspoch, D., and Llagostera, M. (2015). Liposome-Encapsulated Bacteriophages for Enhanced Oral Phage Therapy Against Salmonella Spp. *Appl. Environ. Microbiol.* 81 (14), 4841–4849. doi: 10.1128/AEM.00812-15

Cortez-Jugo, C., Qi, A., Rajapaksa, A., Friend, J. R., and Yeo, L. Y. (2015). Pulmonary Monoclonal Antibody Delivery *via* a Portable Microfluidic Nebulization Platform. *Biomicrofluidics* 89 (5), 052603. doi: 10.1063/1.4917181

Doss, J., Culbertson, K., Hahn, D., Camacho, J., and Barekzi, N. (2017). A Review of Phage Therapy Against Bacterial Pathogens of Aquatic and Terrestrial Organisms. *Viruses* 9 (3), 50. doi: 10.3390/v9030050

Drevinek, P., and Mahenthiralingam, E. (2010). *Burkholderia Cenocepacia* in Cystic Fibrosis: Epidemiology and Molecular Mechanisms of Virulence. *Clin. Microbiol. Infect.* 16 (7), 821–830. doi: 10.1111/j.1469-0691.2010.03237.x

Drulis-Kawa, Z., Majkowska-Skrobek, G., Maciejewska, B., Delattre, A. S., and Lavigne, R. (2012). Learning From Bacteriophages - Advantages and Limitations of Phage and Phage-Encoded Protein Applications. *Curr. Protein Pept. Sci.* 13 (8), 699–722. doi: 10.2174/138920312804871193

Elhissi, A. M., Faizi, M., Naji, W. F., Gill, H. S., and Taylor, K. M. (2007). Physical Stability and Aerosol Properties of Liposomes Delivered Using an Air-Jet Nebulizer and a Novel Micropump Device With Large Mesh Apertures. *Int. J. Pharm.* 334 (1-2), 62–70. doi: 10.1016/j.ijpharm.2006.10.022

Eninger, R., Hogan, C., Biswas, P., Adhikari, A., Reponen, T., and Grinshpun, S. (2009). Electrospray Versus Nebulization for Aerosolization and Filter Testing With Bacteriophage Particles. *Aerosol Sci. Technol.* 43, 298–304. doi: 10.1080/02786820802626355

Esteban, J., and García-Coca, M. (2018). Mycobacterium Biofilms. *Front. Microbiol.* 8:2651. doi: 10.3389/fmicb.2017.02651

Filkova, I., Huang, L. X., and Mujumdar, A. S. (2007). "Industrial Spray Drying Systems," in *Hankbook of Industrial Drying, 3rd edn.* Ed. A. S. Mujumdar (New York: CRC Press), pp 215–pp 254.

Finlay, W. H. (2001). *The Mechanics of Inhaled Pharmaceutical Aerosols: An Introduction* Vol. 13 (UK: Published by Academic Press), 9780123994844.

Fischer, A., Stegemann, J., Scheuch, G., and Siekmeier, R. (2009). Novel Devices for Individualized Controlled Inhalation Can Optimize Aerosol Therapy in Efficacy, Patient Care and Power of Clinical Trials. *Eur. J. Med. Res.* 14 Suppl 4 (Suppl 4), 71–77. doi: 10.1186/2047-783x-14-s4-71

Flament, M.-P., Leterme, P., and Gayot, A. (2001). Study of the Technological Parameters of Ultrasonic Nebulization. *Drug Dev. Ind. Pharm.* 27, 643–649. doi: 10.1081/DDC-100107320

Folkesson, A., Jelsbak, L., Yang, L., Johansen, H. K., Ciofu, O., Høiby, N., et al. (2012). Adaptation of *Pseudomonas Aeruginosa* to the Cystic Fibrosis Airway: An Evolutionary Perspective. *Nat. Rev. Microbiol.* 10 (12), 841–851. doi: 10.1038/nrmicro2907

Forel, J. M., Voillet, F., Pulina, D., Gacouin, A., Perrin, G., Barrau, K., et al. (2012). Ventilator-Associated Pneumonia and ICU Mortality in Severe ARDS Patients Ventilated According to a Lung-Protective Strategy. *Crit. Care* 16 (2), R65. doi: 10.1186/cc11312

Fu, W., Forster, T., Mayer, O., Curtin, J. J., Lehman, S. M., and Donlan, R. M. (2010). Bacteriophage Cocktail for the Prevention of Biofilm Formation by *Pseudomonas Aeruginosa* on Catheters in an *In Vitro* Model System. *Antimicrob. Agents Chemother.* 54 (1), 397–404. doi: 10.1128/AAC.00669-09

Fukushige, K., Tagami, T., Naito, M., Goto, E., Hirai, S., Hatayama, N., et al. (2020). Developing Spray-Freeze-Dried Particles Containing a Hyaluronic Acid-Coated Liposome-Protamine-DNA Complex for Pulmonary Inhalation. *Int. J. Pharm.* 583, 119338. doi: 10.1016/j.ijpharm.2020.119338

GBD 2016 Lower Respiratory Infections Collaborators (2018). Estimates of the Global, Regional, and National Morbidity, Mortality, and Aetiologies of Lower Respiratory Infections in 195 Countries 1990-2016: A Systematic Analysis for the Global Burden of Disease Study 2016. *Lancet Infect. Dis.* 18 (11), 1191–1210. doi: 10.1016/S1473-3099(18)30310-4

Geller, D. (2010). Comparing Clinical Features of the Nebulizer, Metered-Dose Inhaler, and Dry Powder Inhaler. *Respir. Care* 50, 1313–1321.

Geller, D. E., and Kesser, K. C. (2020). The I-Neb Adaptive Aerosol Delivery System Enhances Delivery of Alpha1-Antitrypsin With Controlled Inhalation. *J. Aerosol Med. Pulm. Drug Deliv.* 23 Suppl 1 (Suppl 1), S55–S59. doi: 10.1089/jamp.2009.0793

Gibson, R. L., Burns, J. L., and Ramsey, B. W. (2003). Pathophysiology and Management of Pulmonary Infections in Cystic Fibrosis. *Am. J. Respir. Crit. Care Med.* 168 (8), 918–951. doi: 10.1164/rccm.200304-505SO

Gilbert, P., Maira-Litran, T., McBain, A. J., Rickard, A. H., and Whyte, F. W. (2002). The Physiology and Collective Recalcitrance of Microbial Biofilm Communities. *Adv. Microb. Physiol.* 46, 202–256. doi: 10.1016/S0065-2911(02)46005-5

Golshahi, L., Lynch, K. H., Dennis, J. J., and Finlay, W. H. (2011). *In Vitro* Lung Delivery of Bacteriophages KS4-M and ΦKZ Using Dry Powder Inhalers for Treatment of *Burkholderia Cepacia* Complex and *Pseudomonas Aeruginosa* Infections in Cystic Fibrosis. *J. Appl. Microbiol.* 110, 106–117. doi: 10.1111/j.1365-2672.2010.04863.x

Golshahi, L., Seed, K. D., Dennis, J. J., and Finlay, W. H. (2008). Toward Modern Inhalational Bacteriophage Therapy: Nebulization of Bacteriophages of *Burkholderia Cepacia* Complex. *J. Aerosol Med. Pulm. Drug Deliv.* 21, 351–360. doi: 10.1089/jamp.2008.0701

Górski, A., Międzybrodzki, R., Borysowski, J., Dąbrowska, K., Wierzbicki, P., Ohams, M., et al. (2012). Phage as a Modulator of Immune Responses: Practical Implications for Phage Therapy. *Adv. Virus Res.* 83, 41–71. doi: 10.1016/B978-0-12-394438-1.00002-5

Griffith, D. E., Eagle, G., Thomson, R., Aksamit, T. R., Hasegawa, N., Morimoto, K., et al. (2018). Amikacin Liposome Inhalation Suspension for Treatment-Refractory Lung Disease Caused by Mycobacterium Avium Complex (CONVERT). A Prospective, Open-Label, Randomized Study. *Am. J. Respir. Crit. Care Med.* 198 (12), 1559–1569. doi: 10.1164/rccm.201807-1318OC

Guo, C., Ngo, D., Ahadi, S., and Doub, W. H. (2013). Evaluation of an Abbreviated Impactor for Fine Particle Fraction (FPF) Determination of Metered Dose Inhalers (MDI). *AAPS PharmSciTech* 14 (3), 1004–1011. doi: 10.1208/s12249-013-9984-7

Gupta, S. K., and Nayak, R. P. (2014). Dry Antibiotic Pipeline: Regulatory Bottlenecks and Regulatory Reforms. *J. Pharmacol. Pharmacother.* 5, 4–7. doi: 10.4103/0976-500X.124405

Høiby, N., Bjarnsholt, T., Givskov, M., Molin, S., and Ciofu, O. (2010). Antibiotic Resistance of Bacterial Biofilms. *Int. J. Antimicrob. Agents* 35 (4), 322–332. doi: 10.1016/j.ijantimicag.2009.12.011

Haddrell, A. E., Davies, J. F., Miles, R. E., Reid, J. P., Dailey, L. A., and Murnane, D. (2014). Dynamics of Aerosol Size During Inhalation: Hygroscopic Growth of Commercial Nebulizer Formulations. *Int. J. Pharm.* 463 (1), 50–61. doi: 10.1016/j.ijpharm.2013.12.048

Hall-Stoodley, L., and Stoodley, P. (2009). Evolving Concepts in Biofilm Infections. *Cell Microbiol.* 11 (7), 1034–1043. doi: 10.1111/j.1462-5822.2009.01323.x

Harmsen, M., Yang, L., Pamp, S. J., and Tolker-Nielsen, T. (2010). An Update on *Pseudomonas Aeruginosa* Biofilm Formation, Tolerance, and Dispersal. *FEMS Immunol. Med. Microbiol.* 59 (3), 253–268. doi: 10.1111/j.1574-695X.2010.00690.x

Harper, D. R., Parracho, H. M. R. T., Walker, J., Sharp, R., Hughes, G., Werthén, M., et al. (2014). Bacteriophages and Biofilms. *Antibiotics (Basel)* 3 (3), 270–284. doi: 10.3390/antibiotics3030270

Hassan, A. A., Coutinho, C. P., and Sá-Correia, I. (2019). *Burkholderia Cepacia* Complex Species Differ in the Frequency of Variation of the Lipopolysaccharide O-Antigen Expression During Cystic Fibrosis Chronic Respiratory Infection. *Front. Cell Infect. Microbiol.* 9:273. doi: 10.3389/fcimb.2019.00273

Hickey, A. J. (2004). *Pharmaceutical Inhalation Aerosol Technology. 2nd ed* (New York: Marcel Dekker).

Hochrainer, D., Hölz, H., Kreher, C., Scaffidi, L., Spallek, M., and Wachtel, H. (2005). Comparison of the Aerosol Velocity and Spray Duration of Respimat Soft Mist Inhaler and Pressurized Metered Dose Inhalers. *J. Aerosol Med.* 18 (3), 273–282. doi: 10.1089/jam.2005.18.273

Hoe, S., Boraey, M. A., Ivey, J. W., Finlay, W. H., and Vehring, R. (2014). Manufacturing and Device Options for the Delivery of Biotherapeutics. *J. Aerosol. Med. Pulm. Drug Deliv.* 27 (5), 315–328. doi: 10.1089/jamp.2013.1090

Hoe, S., Semler, D. D., Goudie, A. D., Lynch, K. H., Matinkhoo, S., Finlay, W. H., et al. (2013). Respirable Bacteriophages for the Treatment of Bacterial Lung Infections. *J. Aerosol Med. Pulm. Drug Deliv.* 26, 317–335. doi: 10.1089/jamp.2012.1001

Hogan, C. J. Jr, Kettleson, E. M., Lee, M. H., Ramaswami, B., Angenent, L. T., and Biswas, P. (2005). Sampling Methodologies and Dosage Assessment Techniques for Submicrometre and Ultrafine Virus Aerosol Particles. *J. Appl. Microbiol.* 99 (6), 1422–1434. doi: 10.1111/j.1365-2672.2005.02720.x

Hogan, C. J., Lee, M. H., and Biswas, P. (2004). Capture of Viral Particles in Soft X-Ray-Enhanced Corona Systems: Charge Distribution and Transport Characteristics. *Aerosol Sci. Technol.* 38 (5), 475–486. doi: 10.1080/02786820490462183

Hoyle, N., Zhvaniya, P., Balarjishvili, N., Bolkvadze, D., Nadareishvili, L., Nizharadze, D., et al. (2018). Phage Therapy Against Achromobacter Xylosoxidans Lung Infection in a Patient With Cystic Fibrosis: A Case Report. *Res. Microbiol.* 169 (9), 540–542. doi: 10.1016/j.resmic.2018.05.001

Ibrahim, M., Verma, R., and Garcia-Contreras, L. (2015). Inhalation Drug Delivery Devices: Technology Update. *Med. Devices (Auckl)* 8, 131–139. doi: 10.2147/MDER.S48888

Ishwarya, P. S., Anandharamakrishnanab, C., and Stapley, A. G. F. (2014). Spray Freeze Drying: A Novel Process for the Drying of Foods and Bioproducts. *Trends Food Sci. Technol.* 41. doi: 10.1016/j.tifs.2014.10.008

Jasmer, R. M., Bozeman, L., Schwartzman, K., Cave, M. D., Saukkonen, J. J., Metchock, B., et al. (2004). Recurrent Tuberculosis in the United States and

Canada: Relapse or Reinfection? *Am. J. Respir. Crit. Care Med.* 170, 1360–1366. doi: 10.1164/rccm.200408-1081OC

Javadzadeh, Y., and Yaqoubi, S. (2017). "Therapeutic Nanostructures for Pulmonary Drug Delivery," in *Micro and Nano Technologies, Nanostructures for Drug Delivery* (Amsterdam, The Netherlands: Elsevier), 619–638, ISBN: . doi: 10.1016/B978-0-323-46143-6.00020-8

Jaworek, A. (2007). Electrospray Droplet Sources for Thin Film Deposition. *J. Mater. Sci.* 42, 266–297. doi: 10.1007/s10853-006-0842-9

Jean, S. S., Chang, Y. C., Lin, W. C., Lee, W. S., Hsueh, P. R., and Hsu, C. W. (2020). Epidemiology, Treatment, and Prevention of Nosocomial Bacterial Pneumonia. *J. Clin. Med.* 9 (1):275. doi: 10.3390/jcm9010275

Jones, A. M., Dodd, M. E., Govan, J. R., Barcus, V., Doherty, C. J., Morris, J., et al. (2004). Burkholderia Cenocepacia and Burkholderia Multivorans: Influence on Survival in Cystic Fibrosis. *Thorax* 59 (11), 948–951. doi: 10.1136/thx.2003.017210

Jung, J. H., Lee, J. E., and Kim, S. S. (2009). Generation of Nonagglomerated Airborne Bacteriophage Particles Using an Electrospray Technique. *Anal. Chem.* 81 (8), 2985–2990. doi: 10.1021/ac802584z

Kamal, F., and Dennis, J. J. (2015). Burkholderia Cepacia Complex Phage-Antibiotic Synergy (PAS): Antibiotics Stimulate Lytic Phage Activity. *Appl. Environ. Microbiol.* 81 (3), 1132–1138. doi: 10.1128/AEM.02850-14

Kaur, S., Harjai, K., and Chhibber, S. (2014). Bacteriophage-Aided Intracellular Killing of Engulfed Methicillin-Resistant *Staphylococcus Aureus* (MRSA) by Murine Macrophages. *Appl. Microbiol. Biotechnol.* 98 (10), 4653–4661. doi: 10.1007/s00253-014-5643-5

Kaur, S., Harjai, K., and Chhibber, S. (2016). *In Vivo* Assessment of Phage and Linezolid Based Implant Coatings for Treatment of Methicillin Resistant S. Aureus (MRSA) Mediated Orthopaedic Device Related Infections. *PloS One* 11 (6), e0157626. doi: 10.1371/journal.pone.0157626

Kenna, D. T. D., Lilley, D., Coward, A., Martin, K., Perry, C., Pike, R., et al. (2017). Prevalence of Burkholderia Species, Including Members of *Burkholderia Cepacia* Complex, Among UK Cystic and non-Cystic Fibrosis Patients. *J. Med. Microbiol.* 66 (4), 490–501. doi: 10.1099/jmm.0.000458

Kesser, K. C., and Geller, D. E. (2009). New Aerosol Delivery Devices for Cystic Fibrosis. *Respir. Care* 54 (6), 754–67; discussion 767-8. doi: 10.4187/002013209790983250

Kumari, S., Harjai, K., and Chhibber, S. (2009). Efficacy of Bacteriophage Treatment in Murine Burn Wound Infection Induced by Klebsiella Pneumoniae. *J. Microbiol. Biotechnol.* 19 (6), 622–628. doi: 10.4014/jmb.0808.493

Kwok, P. C. L., McDonnell, A., Tang, P., Knight, C., McKay, E., Butler, S. P., et al. (2020). *In Vivo* Deposition Study of a New Generation Nebuliser Utilising Hybrid Resonant Acoustic (HYDRA) Technology. *Int. J. Pharm.* 580, 119196. doi: 10.1016/j.ijpharm.2020.119196

Labiris, N. R., and Dolovich, M. B. (2003). Pulmonary Drug Delivery. Part I: Physiological Factors Affecting Therapeutic Effectiveness of Aerosolized Medications. *Br. J. Clin. Pharmacol.* 56 (6), 588–899. doi: 10.1046/j.1365-2125.2003.01892.x

Lebeaux, D., Merabishvili, M., Caudron, E., Lannoy, D., Van Simaey, L., Duyvejonck, H., et al. (2021). A Case of Phage Therapy Against Pandrug-Resistant Achromobacter Xylosoxidans in a 12-Year-Old Lung-Transplanted Cystic Fibrosis Patient. *Viruses* 13 (1):60. doi: 10.3390/v13010060

Lechanteur, A., and Evrard, B. (2020). Influence of Composition and Spray-Drying Process Parameters on Carrier-Free DPI Properties and Behaviors in the Lung: A Review. *Pharmaceutics* 12 (1), 55. doi: 10.3390/pharmaceutics12010055

Leung, S. S. Y., Carrigy, N. B., Vehring, R., Finlay, W. H., Morales, S., Carter, E. A., et al. (2019). Jet Nebulization of Bacteriophages With Different Tail Morphologies - Structural Effects. *Int. J. Pharm.* 554, 322–326. doi: 10.1016/j.ijpharm.2018.11.026

Leung, S. S. Y., Parumasivam, T., Gao, F. G., Carrigy, N. B., Vehring, R., Finlay, W. H., et al. (2016). Production of Inhalation Phage Powders Using Spray Freeze Drying and Spray Drying Techniques for Treatment of Respiratory Infections. *Pharm. Res.* 33, 1486–1496. doi: 10.1007/s11095-016-1892-6

Leung, S. S. Y., Parumasivam, T., Nguyen, A., Gengenbach, T., Carter, E. A., Carrigy, N. B., et al. (2018). Effect of Storage Temperature on the Stability of Spray Dried Bacteriophage Powders. *Eur. J. Pharm. Biopharm.* 127, 213–222. doi: 10.1016/j.ejpb.2018.02.033

Liang, W., Pan, H. W., Vllasaliu, D., and Lam, J. K. W. (2020). Pulmonary Delivery of Biological Drugs. *Pharmaceutics* 12 (11), 1025. doi: 10.3390/pharmaceutics12111025

Lin, Y., Chang, R. Y. K., Britton, W. J., Morales, S., Kutter, E., and Chan, H. K. (2018). Synergy of Nebulized Phage PEV20 and Ciprofloxacin Combination Against Pseudomonas aeruginosa. *Int. J. Pharm.* 551 (1-2), 158–165. doi: 10.1016/j.ijpharm.2018.09.024

Lin, Y., Chang, R. Y. K., Britton, W. J., Morales, S., Kutter, E., Li, J., et al. (2019). Inhalable Combination Powder Formulations of Phage and Ciprofloxacin for P. aeruginosa Respiratory Infections. *Eur. J. Pharm. Biopharm* 142, 543–552. doi: 10.1016/j.ejpb.2019.08.004

Lin, Y., Quan, D., Chang, R. Y. K., Chow, M. Y. T., Wang, Y., Li, M., et al. (2021). Synergistic Activity of Phage PEV20-Ciprofloxacin Combination Powder Formulation-A Proof-of-Principle Study in a P. Aeruginosa Lung Infection Model. *Eur. J. Pharm. Biopharm.* 158, 166–171. doi: 10.1016/j.ejpb.2020.11.019

Lipuma, J. J. (2005). Update on the Burkholderia Cepacia Complex. *Curr. Opin. Pulm. Med.* 11 (6), 528–533. doi: 10.1097/01.mcp.0000181475.85187.ed

Lister, P. D., Wolter, D. J., and Hanson, N. D. (2009). Antibacterial-Resistant *Pseudomonas Aeruginosa*: Clinical Impact and Complex Regulation of Chromosomally Encoded Resistance Mechanisms. *Clin. Microbiol. Rev.* 22 (4), 582–610. doi: 10.1128/CMR.00040-09

Liu, J. (2006). Physical Characterization of Pharmaceutical Formulations in Frozen and Freeze-Dried Solid States: Techniques and Applications in Freeze-Drying Development. *Pharm. Dev. Technol.* 11 (1), 3–28. doi: 10.1080/10837450500463729

Liu, D., Van Belleghem, J. D., de Vries, C. R., Burgener, E., Chen, Q., Manasherob, R., et al. (2021). The Safety and Toxicity of Phage Therapy: A Review of Animal and Clinical Studies. *Viruses* 13 (7), 1268. doi: 10.3390/v13071268

Liu, K., Wen, Z., Li, N., Yang, W., Wang, J., Hu, L., et al. (2012). Impact of Relative Humidity and Collection Media on Mycobacteriophage D29 Aerosol. *Appl. Environ. Microbiol.* 78, 1466–1472. doi: 10.1128/AEM.06610-11

Liu, K. Y., Yang, W. H., Dong, X. K., Cong, L. M., Li, N., Li, Y., et al. (2016). Inhalation Study of Mycobacteriophage D29 Aerosol for Mice by Endotracheal Route and Nose-Only Exposure. *J. Aerosol Med. Pulm. Drug Deliv.* 29, 393–405. doi: 10.1089/jamp.2015.1233

Longest, W., Spence, B., and Hindle, M. (2019). Devices for Improved Delivery of Nebulized Pharmaceutical Aerosols to the Lungs. *J. Aerosol Med. Pulm Drug Deliv.* 32 (5), 317–339. doi: 10.1089/jamp.2018.1508

Lopez Quiroga, E., Antelo, L. T., and Antonio, A. A. (2012). Time-Scale Modelling and Optimal Control of Freeze-Drying. *J. Food Eng.* 111, 655–666. doi: 10.1016/j.jfoodeng.2012.03.001

Lu, P., Xing, Y., Peng, H., Liu, Z., Zhou, Q. T., Xue, Z., et al. (2020). Physicochemical and Pharmacokinetic Evaluation of Spray-Dried Coformulation of Salvia Miltiorrhiza Polyphenolic Acid and L-Leucine With Improved Bioavailability. *J. Aerosol Med. Pulm Drug Deliv.* 33 (2), 73–82. doi: 10.1089/jamp.2019.1538

Ly, A., Carrigy, N. B., Wang, H., Harrison, M., Sauvageau, D., Martin, A. R., et al. (2019). Atmospheric Spray Freeze Drying of Sugar Solution With Phage D29. *Front. Microbiol.* 10:488. doi: 10.3389/fmicb.2019.00488

Maa, Y. F., Nguyen, P. A., Sweeney, T., Shire, S. J., and Hsu, C. C. (1999). Protein Inhalation Powders: Spray Drying vs Spray Freeze Drying. *Pharm. Res.* 16 (2), 249–254. doi: 10.1023/a:1018828425184

Maciejewska, B., Olszak, T., and Drulis-Kawa, Z. (2018). Applications of Bacteriophages Versus Phage Enzymes to Combat and Cure Bacterial Infections: An Ambitious and Also a Realistic Application? *Appl. Microbiol. Biotechnol.* 102 (6), 2563–2581. doi: 10.1007/s00253-018-8811-1

Mah, P. T., O'Connell, P., Focaroli, S., Lundy, R., O'Mahony, T. F., Hastedt, J. E., et al. (2019). The Use of Hydrophobic Amino Acids in Protecting Spray Dried Trehalose Formulations Against Moisture-Induced Changes. *Eur. J. Pharm. Biopharm* 144, 139–153. doi: 10.1016/j.ejpb.2019.09.014

Mahenthiralingam, E., Urban, T. A., and Goldberg, J. B. (2005). The Multifarious, Multireplicon *Burkholderia Cepacia* Complex. *Nat. Rev. Microbiol.* 3 (2), 144–156. doi: 10.1038/nrmicro1085

Malenovská, H. (2014). The Influence of Stabilizers and Rates of Freezing on Preserving of Structurally Different Animal Viruses During Lyophilization and Subsequent Storage. *J. Appl. Microbiol.* 117 (6), 1810–1819. doi: 10.1111/jam.12654

Malhotra, S., Hayes, D.Jr, and Wozniak, D. J. (2019). Cystic Fibrosis and *Pseudomonas Aeruginosa*: The Host-Microbe Interface. *Clin. Microbiol. Rev.* 32 (3), e00138-e00118. doi: 10.1128/CMR.00138-18

Manohar, P., and Ramesh, N. (2019). Improved Lyophilization Conditions for Long-Term Storage of Bacteriophages. *Sci. Rep.* 9 (1), 15242. doi: 10.1038/s41598-019-51742-4

Marqus, S., Lee, L., Istivan, T., Kyung Chang, R. Y., Dekiwadia, C., Chan, H. K., et al. (2020). High Frequency Acoustic Nebulization for Pulmonary Delivery of Antibiotic Alternatives Against *Staphylococcus Aureus*. *Eur. J. Pharm. Biopharm.* 151, 181–188. doi: 10.1016/j.ejpb.2020.04.003

Martin, A. R., and Finlay, W. H. (2015). Nebulizers for Drug Delivery to the Lungs. *Expert Opin. Drug Deliv.* 12 (6), 889–900. doi: 10.1517/17425247.2015.995087

Mathur, M. D., Vidhani, S., and Mehndiratta, P. L. (2003). Bacteriophage Therapy: An Alternative to Conventional Antibiotics. *J. Assoc. Physicians India* 51, 593–596.

Matinkhoo, S., Lynch, K. H., Dennis, J. J., Finlay, W. H., and Vehring, R. (2011). Spray-Dried Respirable Powders Containing Bacteriophages for the Treatment of Pulmonary Infections. *J. Pharm. Sci.* 100 (12), 5197–5205. doi: 10.1002/jps.22715

McCune, R. M., Feldmann, F. M., Lambert, H. P., and McDermott, W. (1966). Microbial Persistence. I. The Capacity of Tubercle Bacilli to Survive Sterilization in Mouse Tissues. *J. Exp. Med.* 123, 445–468. doi: 10.1084/jem.123.3.445

Merabishvili, M., Vervaet, C., Pirnay, J. P., De Vos, D., Verbeken, G., Mast, J., et al. (2013). Stability of *Staphylococcus Aureus* Phage ISP After Freeze-Drying (Lyophilization). *PloS One* 8 (7), e68797. doi: 10.1371/journal.pone.0068797

Momin, M. A. M., Sinha, S., Tucker, I. G., and Das, S. C. (2019). Carrier-Free Combination Dry Powder Inhaler Formulation of Ethionamide and Moxifloxacin for Treating Drug-Resistant Tuberculosis. *Drug Dev. Ind. Pharm.* 45 (8), 1321–1331. doi: 10.1080/03639045.2019.1609494

Moreira, M. T. C., Martins, E., Perrone, ÍT, de Freitas, R., Queiroz, L. S., and de Carvalho, A. F. (2021). Challenges Associated With Spray Drying of Lactic Acid Bacteria: Understanding Cell Viability Loss. *Compr. Rev. Food Sci. Food Saf.* 20 (4), 3267–3283. doi: 10.1111/1541-4337.12774

Morello, E., Saussereau, E., Maura, D., Huerre, M., Touqui, L., and Debarbieux, L. (2011). Pulmonary Bacteriophage Therapy on Pseudomonas Aeruginosa Cystic Fibrosis Strains: First Steps Towards Treatment and Prevention. *PloS One* 6 (2), e16963. doi: 10.1371/journal.pone.0016963

Morris, J., Kelly, N., Elliott, L., Grant, A., Wilkinson, M., Hazratwala, K., et al. (2019). Evaluation of Bacteriophage Anti-Biofilm Activity for Potential Control of Orthopedic Implant-Related Infections Caused by Staphylococcus Aureus. *Surg. Infect. (Larchmt)* 20 (1), 16–24. doi: 10.1089/sur.2018.135

Muhlebach, M. S., and Noah, T. L. (2002). Endotoxin Activity and Inflammatory Markers in the Airways of Young Patients With Cystic Fibrosis. *Am. J. Respir. Crit. Care Med.* 165 (7), 911–915. doi: 10.1164/ajrccm.165.7.2107114

Mujumdar, A. S. (2007). *Handbook of Industrial Drying* (Boca Raton: CRC Press), 710. UK.

Nelson, R. (2003). Antibiotic Development Pipeline Runs Dry. New Drugs to Fight Resistant Organisms Are Not Being Developed, Experts Say. *Lancet* 362 (9397), 1726–1727. doi: 10.1016/s0140-6736(03)14885-4

Newman, S. P. (2017). Drug Delivery to the Lungs: Challenges and Opportunities. *Ther. Deliv.* 8 (8), 647–661. doi: 10.4155/tde-2017-0037

Nieth, A., Verseux, C., Barnert, S., Süss, R., and Römer, W. (2015). A First Step Toward Liposome-Mediated Intracellular Bacteriophage Therapy. *Expert Opin. Drug Deliv.* 12 (9), 1411–1424. doi: 10.1517/17425247.2015.1043125

Oechslin, F., Piccardi, P., Mancini, S., Gabard, J., Moreillon, P., Entenza, J. M., et al. (2017). Synergistic Interaction Between Phage Therapy and Antibiotics Clears Pseudomonas Aeruginosa Infection in Endocarditis and Reduces Virulence. *J. Infect. Dis.* 215 (5), 703–712. doi: 10.1093/infdis/jiw632

Ojha, AK, Baughn, AD, Sambandan, D, Hsu, T, Trivelli, X, Guerardel, Y, et al. (2008). Growth of Mycobacterium Tuberculosis Biofilms Containing Free Mycolic Acids and Harbouring Drug-Tolerant Bacteria. *Mol. Microbiol.* 69 (1), 164–174. doi: 10.1111/j.1365-2958.2008.06274.x

Otero, J., García-Rodríguez, A., Cano-Sarabia, M., Maspoch, D., Marcos, R., Cortés, P., et al. (2019). Biodistribution of Liposome-Encapsulated Bacteriophages and Their Transcytosis During Oral Phage Therapy. *Front. Microbiol.* 10:689. doi: 10.3389/fmicb.2019.00689

Pabary, R., Singh, C., Morales, S., Bush, A., Alshafi, K., Bilton, D., et al. (2015). Antipseudomonal Bacteriophage Reduces Infective Burden and Inflammatory Response in Murine Lung. *Antimicrob. Agents Chemother.* 60 (2), 744–751. doi: 10.1128/AAC.01426-15

Papazian, L., Klompas, M., and Luyt, C. E. (2020). Ventilator-Associated Pneumonia in Adults: A Narrative Review. *Intensive Care Med.* 46 (5), 888–906. doi: 10.1007/s00134-020-05980-0

Penes, N. O., Muntean, A. A., Moisoiu, A., Muntean, M. M., Chirca, A., Bogdan, M. A., et al. (2017). An Overview of Resistance Profiles ESKAPE Pathogens From 2010-2015 in a Tertiary Respiratory Center in Romania. *Rom. J. Morphol. Embryol.* 58 (3), 909–922.

Pintucci, J. P., Corno, S., and Garotta, M. (2010). Biofilms and Infections of the Upper Respiratory Tract. *Eur. Rev. Med. Pharmacol. Sci.* 14 (8), 683–690.

Poole, K. (2011). Pseudomonas Aeruginosa: Resistance to the Max. *Front. Microbiol.* 2, 65. doi: 10.3389/fmicb.2011.00065

Pragman, A. A., Berger, J. P., and Williams, B. J. (2016). Understanding Persistent Bacterial Lung Infections: Clinical Implications Informed by the Biology of the Microbiota and Biofilms. *Clin. Pulm. Med.* 23 (2), 57–66. doi: 10.1097/CPM.0000000000000108

Prazak, J., Valente, L., Iten, M., Grandgirard, D., Leib, S. L., Jakob, S. M., et al. (2020). Nebulized Bacteriophages for Prophylaxis of Experimental Ventilator-Associated Pneumonia Due to Methicillin-Resistant *Staphylococcus Aureus*. *Crit. Care Med.* 48 (7), 1042–1046. doi: 10.1097/CCM.0000000000004352

Przerwa, A., Zimecki, M., Switała-Jeleń, K., Dabrowska, K., Krawczyk, E., Łuczak, M., et al. (2006). Effects of Bacteriophages on Free Radical Production and Phagocytic Functions. *Med. Microbiol. Immunol.* 195 (3), 143–150. doi: 10.1007/s00430-006-0011-4

Puapermpoonsiri, U., Spencer, J., and van der Walle, C. F. (2009). A Freeze-Dried Formulation of Bacteriophage Encapsulated in Biodegradable Microspheres. *Eur. J. Pharm. Biopharm.* 72 (1), 26–33. doi: 10.1016/j.ejpb.2008.12.001

Pyne, A., Surana, R., and Suryanarayanan, R. (2002). Crystallization of Mannitol Below Tg' During Freeze-Drying in Binary and Ternary Aqueous Systems. *Pharm. Res.* 19 (6), 901–908. doi: 10.1023/a:1016129521485

Qi, A., Friend, J. R., Yeo, L. Y., and Friend, J. R. (2008). Interfacial Destabilization and Atomization Driven by Surface Acoustic Waves. *Phys. Fluids* 20, 074103. doi: 10.1063/1.2953537

Qi, A., Friend, J. R., Yeo, L. Y., Morton, D. A., McIntosh, M. P., and Spiccia, L. (2009). Miniature Inhalation Therapy Platform Using Surface Acoustic Wave Microfluidic Atomization. *Lab. Chip.* 9 (15), 2184–2193. doi: 10.1039/b903575c

Rajapaksa, A. E., Ho, J. J., Qi, A., Bischof, R., Nguyen, T. H., Tate, M., et al. (2014). Effective Pulmonary Delivery of an Aerosolized Plasmid DNA Vaccine *via* Surface Acoustic Wave Nebulization. *Respir. Res.* 15 (1):60. doi: 10.1186/1465-9921-15-60

Rau, J. L. (2002). Design Principles of Liquid Nebulization Devices Currently in Use. *Respir. Care* 47 (11), 1257–75; discussion 1275-8.

Respaud, R., Vecellio, L., Diot, P., and Heuzé-Vourc'h, N. (2015). Nebulization as a Delivery Method for Mabs in Respiratory Diseases. *Expert Opin. Drug Deliv.* 12 (6), 1027–1039. doi: 10.1517/17425247.2015.999039

Rice, L. B. (2010). Progress and Challenges in Implementing the Research on ESKAPE Pathogens. *Infect. Control Hosp. Epidemiol.* 31 Suppl 1, S7–10. doi: 10.1086/655995

Roach, D. R., and Donovan, D. M. (2015). Antimicrobial Bacteriophage-Derived Proteins and Therapeutic Applications. *Bacteriophage* D5 (3), e1062590. doi: 10.1080/21597081.2015.1062590

Roach, D. R., Leung, C. Y., Henry, M., Morello, E., Singh, D., Di Santo, J. P., et al. (2017). Synergy Between the Host Immune System and Bacteriophage Is Essential for Successful Phage Therapy Against an Acute Respiratory Pathogen. *Cell Host Microbe* 22 (1), 38–47.e4. doi: 10.1016/j.chom.2017.06.018

Rodrigues, M. E., Lopes, S. P., Pereira, C. R., Azevedo, N. F., Lourenço, A., Henriques, M., et al. (2017). Polymicrobial Ventilator-Associated Pneumonia: Fighting *In Vitro Candida Albicans-Pseudomonas Aeruginosa* Biofilms With Antifungal-Antibacterial Combination Therapy. *PloS One* 12 (1), e0170433. doi: 10.1371/journal.pone.0170433

Romling, U., and Balsalobre, C. (2012). Biofilm Infections, Their Resilience to Therapy and Innovative Treatment Strategies. *J. Intern. Med.* 272 (6), 541–561. doi: 10.1111/joim.12004

Rubinstein, E., Kollef, M. H., and Nathwani, D. (2008). Pneumonia Caused by Methicillin-Resistant Staphylococcus Aureus. *Clin. Infect. Dis.* 46 (Suppl 5), S378–S385. doi: 10.1086/533594

Ryan, E. M., Alkawareek, M. Y., Donnelly, R. F., and Gilmore, B. F. (2012). Synergistic Phage-Antibiotic Combinations for the Control of Escherichia Coli

Biofilms *In Vitro. FEMS Immunol. Med. Microbiol.* 65 (2), 395–398. doi: 10.1111/j.1574-695X.2012.00977.x

Saari, M., Vidgren, M. T., Koskinen, M. O., Turjanmaa, V. M., and Nieminen, M. M. (1999). Pulmonary Distribution and Clearance of Two Beclomethasone Liposome Formulations in Healthy Volunteers. *Int. J. Pharm.* 181 (1), 1–9. doi: 10.1016/s0378-5173(98)00398-6

Sambandan, D., Dao, D. N., Weinrick, B. C., Vilchèze, C., Gurcha, S. S., Ojha, A., et al. (2013). Keto-Mycolic Acid-Dependent Pellicle Formation Confers Tolerance to Drug-Sensitive Mycobacterium Tuberculosis. *mBio* 4, e00222-e00213. doi: 10.1128/mBio.00222-13

Sansgiry, S. S., Joish, V. N., Boklage, S., Goyal, R. K., Chopra, P., and Sethi, S. (2012). Economic Burden of *Pseudomonas Aeruginosa* Infection in Patients With Cystic Fibrosis. *J. Med. Econ.* 15 (2), 219–224. doi: 10.3111/13696998.2011.638954

Santajit, S., and Indrawattana, N. (2016). Mechanisms of Antimicrobial Resistance in ESKAPE Pathogens. *BioMed. Res. Int.* 2, 2475067. doi: 10.1155/2016/2475067

Schwegman, J. J., Hardwick, L. M., and Akers, M. J. (2005). Practical Formulation and Process Development of Freeze-Dried Products. *Pharm. Dev. Technol.* 10 (2), 151–173. doi: 10.1081/pdt-56308

Semler, D. D., Goudie, A. D., Finlay, W. H., and Dennis, J. J. (2014). Aerosol Phage Therapy Efficacy in *Burkholderia Cepacia* Complex Respiratory Infections. *Antimicrob. Agents Chemother.* 58 (7), 4005–4013. doi: 10.1128/AAC.02388-13

Seung, K. J., Keshavjee, S., and Rich, M. L. (2015). Multidrug-Resistant Tuberculosis and Extensively Drug-Resistant Tuberculosis. *Cold Spring Harb. Perspect. Med.* 5 (9):a017863. doi: 10.1101/cshperspect.a017863

Sharma, D., Misba, L., and Khan, A. U. (2019). Antibiotics Versus Biofilm: An Emerging Battleground in Microbial Communities. *Antimicrob. Resist. Infect. Control* 8, 76. doi: 10.1186/s13756-019-0533-3

Sheth, P., Stein, S. W., and Myrdal, P. B. (2015). Factors Influencing Aerodynamic Particle Size Distribution of Suspension Pressurized Metered Dose Inhalers. *AAPS PharmSciTech.* 16 (1), 192–201. doi: 10.1208/s12249-014-0210-z

Shoyele, S. A., and Cawthorne, S. (2006). Particle Engineering Techniques for Inhaled Biopharmaceuticals. *Adv. Drug Deliv. Rev.* 58 (9-10), 1009–1029. doi: 10.1016/j.addr.2006.07.010

Sibum, I., Hagedoorn, P., de Boer, A. H., Frijlink, H. W., and Grasmeijer, F. (2018). Challenges for Pulmonary Delivery of High Powder Doses. *Int. J. Pharm.* 548 (1), 325–336. doi: 10.1016/j.ijpharm.2018.07.008

Sillankorva, S., and Azeredo, J. (2014). Bacteriophage Attack as an Anti-Biofilm Strategy. *Methods Mol. Biol.* 1147, 277–285. doi: 10.1007/978-1-4939-0467-9_20

Singla, S., Harjai, K., Katare, O. P., and Chhibber, S. (2015). Bacteriophage-Loaded Nanostructured Lipid Carrier: Improved Pharmacokinetics Mediates Effective Resolution of *Klebsiella Pneumoniae*-Induced Lobar Pneumonia. *J. Infect. Dis.* 212, 325–334. doi: 10.1093/infdis/jiv029

Singla, S., Harjai, K., Katare, O. P., and Chhibber, S. (2016). Encapsulation of Bacteriophage in Liposome Accentuates its Entry in to Macrophage and Shields it From Neutralizing Antibodies. *PloS One* 11, e0153777. doi: 10.1371/journal.pone.0153777

Šimková, K., Joost, B., and Imanidis, G. (2020). Production of Fast-Dissolving Low-Density Powders for Improved Lung Deposition by Spray Drying of a Nanosuspension. *Eur. J. Pharm. Biopharm* 146, 19–31. doi: 10.1016/j.ejpb.2019.11.003

Soothill, J. S. (1992). Treatment of Experimental Infections of Mice With Bacteriophages. *J. Med. Microbiol.* 37, 258–261. doi: 10.1099/00222615-37-4-258

Sousa, S. A., Ramos, C. G., and Leitão, J. H. (2011). *Burkholderia Cepacia* Complex: Emerging Multihost Pathogens Equipped With a Wide Range of Virulence Factors and Determinants. *Int. J. Microbiol.* 2011, 607575. doi: 10.1155/2011/607575

Sulakvelidze, A., Alavidze, Z., and Morris, J. G. (2001). Bacteriophage Therapy. *Antimicrob. Agents Chemother.* 45, 649–659. doi: 10.1128/AAC.45.3.649-659.2001

Stewart, I. E., Lukka, P. B., Liu, J., Meibohm, B., Gonzalez-Juarrero, M., Braunstein, M. S., et al. (2019). Development and Characterization of a Dry Powder Formulation for Anti-Tuberculosis Drug Spectinamide 1599. *Pharm. Res.* 36 (9), 136. doi: 10.1007/s11095-019-2666-8

Tagliaferri, T. L., Jansen, M., and Horz, H. P. (2019). Fighting Pathogenic Bacteria on Two Fronts: Phages and Antibiotics as Combined Strategy. *Front. Cell. Infect. Microbiol.* 9, 22. doi: 10.3389/fcimb.2019.00022

Tan, X., Chen, H., Zhang, M., Zhao, Y., Jiang, Y., Liu, X., et al. (2021). Clinical Experience of Personalized Phage Therapy Against Carbapenem-Resistant *Acinetobacter Baumannii* Lung Infection in a Patient With Chronic Obstructive Pulmonary Disease. *Front. Cell Infect. Microbiol.* 11:631585. doi: 10.3389/fcimb.2021.631585

Tashkin, D. P. (2016). A Review of Nebulized Drug Delivery in COPD. *Int. J. Chron. Obstruct. Pulmon. Dis.* 11, 2585–2596. doi: 10.2147/COPD.S114034

Thomas, J., Bothner, B., Traina, J., Benner, H., and Siuzdak, G. (2004). Electrospray Ion Mobility Spectrometry of Intact Viruses. *J. Spectrosc.* 18. doi: 10.1155/2004/376572

Thomas, R. J. (2013). Particle Size and Pathogenicity in the Respiratory Tract. *Virulence* 4 (8), 847–858. doi: 10.4161/viru.27172

Thorn, J., and Rylander, R. (1998). Inflammatory Response After Inhalation of Bacterial Endotoxin Assessed by the Induced Sputum Technique. *Thorax* 53 (12), 1047–1052. doi: 10.1136/thx.53.12.1047

Tena, F. A., and Clarà, C. P. (2012). Deposition of Inhaled Particles in the Lungs. *Arch. Bronconeumol.* 48 (7), 240–246. doi: 10.1016/j.arbres.2012.02.003

Tomlin, K. L., Coll, O. P., and Ceri, H. (2001). Interspecies Biofilms of *Pseudomonas Aeruginosa* and Burkholderia Cepacia. *Can. J. Microbiol.* 47 (10), 949–954. doi: 10.1139/w01-095

Torres-Barceló, C., Arias-Sánchez, F. I., Vasse, M., Ramsayer, J., Kaltz, O., and Hochberg, M. E. (2014). A Window of Opportunity to Control the Bacterial Pathogen Pseudomonas Aeruginosa Combining Antibiotics and Phages. *PloS One* 9 (9), e106628. doi: 10.1371/journal.pone.0106628

Trend, S., Fonceca, A. M., Ditcham, W. G., Kicic, A., and Cf, A. (2017). The Potential of Phage Therapy in Cystic Fibrosis: Essential Human-Bacterial-Phage Interactions and Delivery Considerations for Use in Pseudomonas Aeruginosa-Infected Airways. *J. Cyst. Fibros.* 16 (6), 663–670. doi: 10.1016/j.jcf.2017.06.012

Trivedi, A., Mavi, P. S., Bhatt, D., and Kumar, A. (2016). Thiol Reductive Stress Induces Cellulose-Anchored Biofilm Formation in Mycobacterium Tuberculosis. *Nat. Commun.* 7, 11392. doi: 10.1038/ncomms11392

Turgeon, N., Toulouse, M. J., Martel, B., Moineau, S., and Duchaine, C. (2014). Comparison of Five Bacteriophages as Models for Viral Aerosol Studies. *Appl. Environ. Microbiol.* 80 (14), 4242–4250. doi: 10.1128/AEM.00767-14

Van Acker, H., Sass, A., Bazzini, S., De Roy, K., Udine, C., Messiaen, T., et al. (2013). Biofilm-Grown *Burkholderia Cepacia* Complex Cells Survive Antibiotic Treatment by Avoiding Production of Reactive Oxygen Species. *PloS One* 8 (3), e58943. doi: 10.1371/journal.pone.0058943

Van Belleghem, J. D., Merabishvili, M., Vergauwen, B., Lavigne, R., and Vaneechoutte, M. (2017). A Comparative Study of Different Strategies for Removal of Endotoxins From Bacteriophage Preparations. *J. Microbiol. Methods* 132, 153–159. doi: 10.1016/j.mimet.2016.11.020

Vandenheuvel, D., Meeus, J., Lavigne, R., and Van den Mooter, G. (2014). Instability of Bacteriophages in Spray-Dried Trehalose Powders Is Caused by Crystallization of the Matrix. *Int. J. Pharm.* 472 (1-2), 202–205. doi: 10.1016/j.ijpharm.2014.06.026

Vadivoo, N. S., and Usha, B. (2018). ESKAPE Pathogens: Trends in Antibiotic Resistance Pattern. *MedPulse Int. J. Microbiol.* 7 (3), 26–32. doi: 10.26611/1008732

Vecellio, L. (2006). The Mesh Nebuliser: A Recent Technical Innovation for Aerosol Delivery. *Breathe* 2, 252. doi: 10.1183/18106838.0203.252

Vehring, R. (2008). Pharmaceutical Particle Engineering via Spray Drying. *Pharm. Res.* 25 (5), 999–1022. doi: 10.1007/s11095-007-9475-1

Vishali, D. A., Monisha, J., Sivakamasundari, S. K., Moses, J. A., and Anandharamakrishnan, C. (2019). Spray Freeze Drying: Emerging Applications in Drug Delivery. *J. Control Release* 300, 93–101. doi: 10.1016/j.jconrel.2019.02.044

Vladimirsky, M., Lapenkova, M., Alyapkina, Y., and Vasilyeva, I. (2019). Efficiency of Bactericidal Activity of Liposomal Mycobacteriophages Against Intracellular Mycobacteria Tuberculosis in the Model of Macrophages RAW 264. *Eur. Respir. J.* 54 (suppl 63):PA4607. doi: 10.1183/13993003.congress-2019.PA4607

Wang, J., Hu, B., Xu, M., Yan, Q., Liu, S., Zhu, X., et al. (2006). Use of Bacteriophage in the Treatment of Experimental Animal Bacteremia From Imipenem-Resistant Pseudomonas Aeruginosa. *Int. J. Mol. Med.* 17, 309–317. doi: 10.3892/ijmm.17.2.309

Wang, J. X., Hu, H., Ye, A., Chen, J., and Zhang, P. (2016). Experimental Investigation of Surface Acoustic Wave Atomization. *Sens. Actuators A Phys.* 238, 1–7. doi: 10.1016/j.sna.2015.11.027

Watanabe, R., Matsumoto, T., Sano, G., Ishii, Y., Tateda, K., Sumiyama, Y., et al. (2007). Efficacy of Bacteriophage Therapy Against Gut-Derived Sepsis Caused by *Pseudomonas Aeruginosa* in Mice. *Antimicrob. Agents Chemother.* 51, 446–452. doi: 10.1128/AAC.00635-06

Waters, V., and Ratjen, F. (2014). Inhaled Liposomal Amikacin. *Expert Rev. Respir. Med.* 8 (4), 401–409. doi: 10.1586/17476348.2014.918507

Weber-Dabrowska, B., Mulczyk, M., and Górski, A. (2000). Bacteriophage Therapy of Bacterial Infections: An Update of Our Institute's Experience. *Arch. Immunol. Ther. Exp. (Warsz)* 48, 547–551.

WHO-Global Respiratory Burden (2017). *The Global Impact of Respiratory Disease – WHO. 2nd ed.* (Sheffi eld, European Respiratory Society).

WHO Pneumonia Factsheet 2019. Available at: https://www.who.int/news-room/fact-sheets/detail/pneumonia.

WHO *Tuberculosis: Multidrug-Resistant Tuberculosis (MDR-Tb).* Available at: https://www.who.int/news-room/q-a-detail/tuberculosis-multidrug-resistant-tuberculosis-(mdr-tb).

WHO Tuberculosis Factsheet (2021) Available at: https://www.who.int/news-room/fact-sheets/detail/tuberculosis.

World Health Organization (2018). *Global Tuberculosis Report 2018* (France: World Health Organization). Available at: https://apps.who.int/iris/handle/10665/274453. License: CC BY-NC-SA 3.0 IGO.

Wright, A., Hawkins, C. H., Anggård, E. E., and Harper, D. R. (2009). A Controlled Clinical Trial of a Therapeutic Bacteriophage Preparation in Chronic Otitis Due to Antibiotic-Resistant Pseudomonas Aeruginosa; A Preliminary Report of Efficacy. *Clin. Otolaryngol.* 34 (4), 349–357. doi: 10.1111/j.1749-4486.2009.01973.x

Yan, W., Mukhopadhyay, S., To, K. K. W., and Leung, S. S. Y. (2021). Potential of Inhaled Bacteriophage Therapy for Bacterial Lung Infection [Online First]. *IntechOpen.* doi: 10.5772/intechopen.96660

Zhang, L., Hou, X., Sun, L., He, T., Wei, R., Pang, M., et al. (2018). Staphylococcus Aureus Bacteriophage Suppresses LPS-Induced Inflammation in MAC-T Bovine Mammary Epithelial Cells. *Front. Microbiol.* J9:1614. doi: 10.3389/fmicb.2018.01614

Zhang, Y., Peng, X., Zhang, H., Watts, A. B., and Ghosh, D. (2018). Manufacturing and Ambient Stability of Shelf Freeze Dried Bacteriophage Powder Formulations. *Int. J. Pharm.* 542 (1-2), 1–7. doi: 10.1016/j.ijpharm.2018.02.023

Zhou, Q. T., Tang, P., Leung, S. S., Chan, J. G., and Chan, H. K. (2014). Emerging Inhalation Aerosol Devices and Strategies: Where are We Headed? *Adv. Drug Deliv. Rev.* 75, 3–17. doi: 10.1016/j.addr.2014.03.006

Zillen, D., Beugeling, M., Hinrichs, W. L. J., Frijlink, H. W., and Grasmeijer, F. (2021). Natural and Bioinspired Excipients for Dry Powder Inhalation Formulations. *Curr. Opin. Colloid Interface Sci.* 56, 101497. doi: 10.1016/j.cocis.2021.101497

22

Phage vB_PaeS-PAJD-1 Rescues Murine Mastitis Infected with Multidrug-Resistant *Pseudomonas aeruginosa*

*Zhaofei Wang, Yibing Xue, Ya Gao, Mengting Guo, Yuanping Liu, Xinwei Zou, Yuqiang Cheng, Jingjiao Ma, Hengan Wang, Jianhe Sun and Yaxian Yan**

School of Agriculture and Biology, Shanghai Jiao Tong University, Shanghai Key Laboratory of Veterinary Biotechnology, Shanghai, China

Correspondence:
Yaxian Yan
yanyaxian@sjtu.edu.cn

Pseudomonas aeruginosa is a Gram-negative pathogen that causes a variety of infections in humans and animals. Due to the inappropriate use of antibiotics, multi-drug resistant (MDR) *P. aeruginosa* strains have emerged and are prevailing. In recent years, cow mastitis caused by MDR *P. aeruginosa* has attracted attention. In this study, a microbial community analysis revealed that *P. aeruginosa* could be a cause of pathogen-induced cow mastitis. Five MDR *P. aeruginosa* strains were isolated from milk diagnosed as mastitis positive. To seek an alternative antibacterial agent against MDR, *P. aeruginosa*, a lytic phage, designated vB_PaeS_PAJD-1 (PAJD-1), was isolated from dairy farm sewage. PAJD-1 was morphologically classified as *Siphoviridae* and was estimated to be about 57.9 kb. Phage PAJD-1 showed broad host ranges and a strong lytic ability. A one-step growth curve analysis showed a relatively short latency period (20 min) and a relatively high burst size (223 PFU per infected cell). Phage PAJD-1 remained stable over wide temperature and pH ranges. Intramammary-administered PAJD-1 reduced bacterial concentrations and repaired mammary glands in mice with mastitis induced by MDR *P. aeruginosa*. Furthermore, the cell wall hydrolase (termed endolysin) from phage PAJD-1 exhibited a strong bacteriolytic and a wide antibacterial spectrum against MDR *P. aeruginosa*. These findings present phage PAJD-1 as a candidate for phagotherapy against MDR *P. aeruginosa* infection.

Keywords: *Pseudomonas aeruginosa*, MDR, phage PAJD-1, mastitis, lysin

INTRODUCTION

Mastitis, one of the most prevalent diseases in the dairy cattle industry, leads to great economic losses for farmers caused by reduced milk production, early culling, veterinary services, and labour costs (Klaas and Zadoks, 2018). Usually, mastitis is caused by Gram-positive pathogens, such as *Staphylococcus* and *Streptococcus* (Keane, 2019). As the prevalence of udder infections due to Gram-positive pathogens is reduced to very low levels in dairy herds by the implementation of advanced mastitis control systems, the relative significance of mastitis due to Gram-negative bacterial pathogens, such as *Escherichia coli* and *P. aeruginosa*, is expected to increase (Kawai et al., 2017; Keane, 2019; El Garch et al., 2020).

P. aeruginosa is widely present in nature and in the intestines and skin of humans and animals (Otto, 2014; Bachta et al., 2020). In clinical treatment, the increasing resistance of *P. aeruginosa* strains to different antibiotics has led to an increase in the emergence of multi-drug resistant (MDR) *P. aeruginosa* (Javed et al., 2020; Maslova et al., 2020). Traditional antibiotics are almost ineffective against MDR *P. aeruginosa* (Tummler, 2019). In recent years, cow mastitis caused by MDR *P. aeruginosa* has attracted increasing attention and has led to significant economic losses for farmers (Kawai et al., 2017; Klaas and Zadoks, 2018). In view of this, exploring alternative treatments has tremendous value.

In the last 15 years, a marked increase in the number of identified *P. aeruginosa* bacteriophages (termed phages) has been reported, as has great progress in the phage treatment of infections caused by *P. aeruginosa* (Dzuliashvili et al., 2007; Chegini et al., 2020). Phages are the most common organism found on earth and, as such, represent great diversity in their overall host range (Khalid et al., 2020). The bacteriolysis of phages is mainly dependent on endolysin (termed lysin), which is a kind of bacterial cell wall hydrolase synthesized by phages in the late stages of infection (Wang et al., 2018; Gutierrez and Briers, 2020). Compared to traditional antibiotics, bacteriophage agents have obvious advantages, such as being simple, cheap, highly effective in killing their target bacteria and especially available in inhibiting drug-resistant bacteria, as well as causing no serious side effects (Hesse and Adhya, 2019; Principi et al., 2019). Moreover, phages are unable to infect human or animal cells because phages recognise and bind to unique bacterial receptors. Thus, the side effects associated with phage therapy in humans and animals are thought to be minimal (Rios et al., 2016).

Numerous studies have revealed that phages are able to treat various human or animal diseases caused by *P. aeruginosa*, including lung, skin, eye and other infections (Fukuda et al., 2012; Raz et al., 2019; Ng et al., 2020). However, there is no research focused on using phages to overcome mastitis caused by *P. aeruginosa*. In this study, we investigated potential pathogen diversity in cows with mastitis in Shanghai, China using microbial community analysis. A novel lytic phage, vB_PaeS_PAJD-1 (PAJD-1), was isolated from sewage in dairy farms, and its antibacterial spectrum, stability and bacteriolytic activity of its endolysin were assessed. Specifically, we evaluated the therapeutic effect of using PAJD-1 in mice with mastitis infected by MDR *P. aeruginosa*.

MATERIALS AND METHODS

Ethics Statement

The animal experiments were carried out in accordance with animal welfare standards and approved by the Ethical Committee for Animal Experiments of Shanghai Jiao Tong University, China (Approval no. 20190103). All animal experiments complied with the guidelines of the Animal Welfare Council of China.

Bacterial Strains and Culture Conditions

In this study, 18 clinical isolates of *P. aeruginosa* (13 hospital-acquired strains and 5 strains isolated from the milk of dairy cows with mastitis) and 2 reference strains of *P. aeruginosa* PA01 and PA14 from the American Type Culture Collection (ATCC) were used (**Table 1**). All strains were grown in Luria–Bertani broth (LB) or in a 1.5% agar medium at 37°C. Also, 5% sheep blood agar was used to isolate bacteria from milk samples. *P. aeruginosa* ATCC 27853 was used as a reference strain for identification utilising the VITEK 2 system (BioMerieux, France). Antimicrobial susceptibility testing of the isolates was performed using the Kirby–Bauer disk diffusion method as described by Fathizadeh et al. with seven antimicrobials: meropenem (MEM), ampicillin (AMP), gentamicin (GN), amikacin (AK), piperacillin/tazobactam (TZP), ciprofloxacin (CIP) and cefepime (FEP) (Fathizadeh et al., 2020). Antibiotic discs (Beijing Pronade technology co., LTD, Beijing, China) were placed on the swabbed culture and incubated for 16 to 18 h at 37°C, after which the inhibition zone was measured and each strain was determined as resistant (R)/intermediate (I)/sensitive (S) to each antibiotic tested following the instruction of the experiment provided by the manufacturer.

Sample Analysis of Microbial Community Composition and Diversity From a Dairy Farm

The udder surfaces of cows with mastitis from three dairy farms (at least three samples per dairy farm) in Shanghai were sampled using sterile cotton swabs. These samples were then suspended in sterilised phosphate-buffered saline (PBS) buffer and placed in sterilised, RNase-free tubes. After homogeneous mixing, centrifugation, and filtration, 2 mL of the filtrate was stored at -80°C. The total microbial RNA samples were extracted using an RNA Mini Kit (Bio-Rad, Hercules, CA, USA). RNA samples were reverse-transcribed to complementary DNA (cDNA) using the iScript cDNA Synthesis Kit (Bio-Rad). The quantity and quality of the extracted cDNA were measured using a NanoDrop ND-1000 spectrophotometer (Thermo, Waltham, MA, USA) and agarose gel electrophoresis, respectively. 16S rRNA gene amplicon sequencing and analysis were performed as described previously (Morella et al., 2018). The cDNA was amplified using the primer sets 515F and 806R, which targeted the V4 region of the bacterial 16S rDNA, with the reverse primer containing a 6-bp error-correcting barcode unique to each sample (Caporaso et al., 2012). Sequencing by synthesis was performed on an Illumina HiSeq MiSeq platform (Shanghai Personal Biotechnology Co., Ltd., Shanghai, China).

The Quantitative Insights into Microbial Ecology (QIIME, v1.8.0) pipeline was employed to process the sequencing data, as previously described (Caporaso et al., 2010). Briefly, the high-quality sequences were clustered into operational taxonomic units (OTUs) at 97% sequence identity by UCLUST (Edgar, 2010). A representative sequence was selected from each OTU using default

TABLE 1 | Drug resistance of strain and lytic activity of phage PAJD-1.

No. of strains	[a]Source	[b]EOP	Antibiotic susceptibility						
			MEM	AMP	GN	AK	TZP	CIP	FEP
PA01	I	-[c]	S	R	S	S	S	S	S
PA14	I	1	S	R	I	S	S	S	I
PAmas1	II	0.28	S	R	I	I	S	S	R
PAmas2	II	0.26	S	R	S	S	S	S	S
PAmas3	II	0.44	I	R	I	S	S	S	S
PAmas4	II	0.27	S	R	S	S	S	S	S
PAmas5	II	0.84	S	R	S	I	S	S	S
PA8094	III	–	S	R	I	S	S	S	I
PA8299	III	0.32	S	R	S	S	R	S	R
PA8243	III	–	S	R	S	S	S	S	S
PA7959	III	0.41×10^{-3}	S	R	S	S	S	S	I
PA8070	III	0.68×10^{-2}	S	S	I	S	S	R	I
PA7978	III	0.38	S	R	I	I	S	S	S
PA8244	III	0.64	S	R	S	S	S	S	S
PA8408	III	0.21×10^{-3}	S	R	S	S	R	S	R
PA8362	III	0.71	S	R	R	S	R	R	R
PA7979	III	0.91	S	R	S	S	S	S	I
PA8177	III	–	S	R	S	S	S	S	S
PA8333	III	0.21	S	R	S	S	S	S	I
PA8218	III	0.27	S	R	S	S	R	S	R

[a]I, purchased from American Type Culture Collection; II, clinically-isolated strains from the milk of dairy cows with mastitis; III, hospital-acquired strains.
[b]EOP, efficiency of plating (EOP = phage titre on test bacterium/phage titre on strains PA14). Assays were conducted at least three times. The data shown are means from three independent experiments.
[c]no plaque on target bacterium.
R, resistant; I, intermediate; S, sensitive.

parameters. The OTU taxonomic classification was conducted by BLAST, searching the representative sequences set against the Greengenes Database (Desantis et al., 2006) using the best hit (Altschul et al., 1997). An OTU table was further generated to record the abundance of each OTU in each sample and the taxonomy of these OTUs. OTUs containing less than 0.001% of the total sequences across all samples were discarded. To minimize the difference in sequencing depth across samples, an averaged, rounded, rarefied OTU table was generated by averaging 100 evenly resampled OTU subsets under 90% of the minimum sequencing depth for further analysis. Taxonomy assignment of OTUs was performed by comparing sequences to the Greengenes database. The Mann–Whitney U test was used to test for the significance of alpha diversity. A two-sided Student's t-test was conducted to determine the significance of beta diversity between sample groups. Linear discriminant analysis coupled with effect size (LEfSe) was performed to identify the bacterial taxa represented between groups at the genus or higher taxonomic levels (Segata et al., 2011).

Phage Isolation, Purification and Host Range Determination

The isolation method described by Wang et al. was applied for the isolation of *P. aeruginosa* phages, with some modifications (Wang et al., 2016). Sewage from dairy farms was centrifuged at $5,000 \times g$ (centrifuging radius = 17.6 cm) for 20 min at 4°C. The supernatants were passed through 0.22-μm pore size membrane filters. *P. aeruginosa* PA14 of the logarithmic phase was cultured overnight together with sewage samples in LB broth at 37°C with shaking at 180 rpm. The culture was centrifuged at $5,000 \times g$ for

20 min at 4°C; the supernatant was then filtered through 0.22-μm pore size membrane filters and checked for the presence of lytic phages by *P. aeruginosa* PA14 using the double-layer agar plate method as previously described (Wang et al., 2016). After overnight incubation, the formation of obvious zones suggested the presence of a lytic phage, which was purified by three rounds of single-plaque isolation.

For purification, single-phage plaques were precipitated in the presence of 10% (wt/vol) polyethylene glycol (PEG) 8000 and 1 M NaCl at 4°C for at least 1 h. The precipitate was collected by centrifugation at $10,000 \times g$ for 10 min at 4°C and suspended in SM buffer (100 mM NaCl, 10 mM $MgSO_4 \cdot 7H_2O$ and 50 mM Tris·HCl pH 7.5). After the addition of 0.5 g/mL CsCl, the mixture was layered on top of CsCl step gradients (densities of 1.15, 1.45, 1.50 and 1.70 g/mL) in Ultra-Clear centrifugation tubes and centrifuged at $28,000 \times g$ for 2 h at 4°C, dialysed in SM buffer. Phages were stored at 4°C for further experiments.

The PAJD-1 phage was screened against *S. aureus* strains using the efficiency of the plating method (EOP = phage titre on test bacterium/phage titre on strains PA14) to determine the effectiveness and host range against a variety of target bacteria. Ten-fold serial dilutions of phage suspensions (100 μL) were mixed with 100 μL of bacteria (1×10^8 CFU/mL), incubated for 5 min at room temperature (25°C) and plated as double layers on LB to determine phage titres.

Transmission Electron Microscopy (TEM) of Phage Particles

The purified phage was loaded onto a copper grid for 10 min, negatively stained with 2% (v/v) phosphotungstic acid (pH 6.7)

and dried. The morphology of the phage was observed using a FEI TEM Tecnai G2 Spirit Biotwin (FEI, Hillsboro, US) at an accelerating voltage of 120 kV.

Genome Sequencing and Annotation

Purified PAJD-1 phage genomic DNA was prepared using phenol–chloroform extraction and ethanol precipitation methods, as described previously (Wang et al., 2016). The Illumina MiSeq system was used for the PAJD-1 phage whole genome analysis. Sequence alignments were carried out using the Accelrys DS Gene software package of Accelrys Inc. (USA). Putative open reading frames were suggested using the algorithms of the software packages Accelrys Gene v2.5 (Accelrys Inc.) and ORF Finder (NCBI). Identity values were calculated using different BLAST algorithms (http://www.ncbi.nlm.nih.gov/BLAST/) on the NCBI homepage. The sequence of the PAJD-1 phage was submitted to the NCBI (GenBank accession number: MW835180).

One-Step Growth Analysis of Phages

To determine the one-step growth of PAJD-1, *P. aeruginosa* PA14 was used as the indicator strain. One-step growth experiments were performed with a modification to the methods described previously (Pajunen et al., 2000). Briefly, PAJD-1 phage (1×10^6 PFU) was added at a MOI of 0.1 to the cells of *P. aeruginosa* (1×10^7 CFU) and allowed to adsorb for 10 min at 37°C. The mixture was then centrifuged at 4°C for 1 min at a speed of $12,000 \times g$. After the supernatants were removed, the pellets containing the phage-infected bacterial cells were suspended in fresh LB and incubated with shaking at 180 rpm and 37°C. Partial samples were taken at 10 min intervals, and the titrations from the aliquots were immediately determined using the double-layer agar plate method. Burst size was calculated as the ratio between the number of total released phages and the number of infected bacterial cells. This assay was performed in triplicate.

Adsorption Analyses of Phages

The adsorption rate of PAJD-1 was performed as previously described, with some modifications (Ong et al., 2020). Briefly, *P. aeruginosa* PA14 (1×10^7 CFU/mL) was mixed with phage (1×10^6 PFU/mL) incubated at 37°C. Samples of the mixture (100 μL) were taken at 5, 10, 15, and 20 min, and filtered (0.22-μm pore size membrane) immediately. The filtered supernatants (unadsorbed phages) were determined using the double-layer agar plate method. The adsorption rate of PAJD-1 (%) = (1 unadsorbed phages/initial concentration of phage) × 100%.

Phage Stability Assay

To determine phage stability at different temperatures (25°C, 37°C, 45°C, 50°C, 55°C, 60°C, 65°C and 70°C), an aliquot of the PAJD-1 phage was taken after 1 h of incubation, and the titres of the phage were assayed using the double-layer agar plate method. To determine the optimum storage temperature of the PAJD-1, phages were stored at 4°C, -20°C and -80°C for 6 months, after which their bactericidal activity (titres of the phage) were determined by the double-layer agar plate method and compared with initial titres. To test for phage stability at the different pH values, titres were determined after the phage lysates were diluted (1:100) in SM buffer at different pH values and kept at 37°C for 3 h using the double-layer agar plate method.

Phage Bacteriolytic Assay *In Vivo*

To improve the safety of the phage used in animals, an affinity matrix of modified polymyxin B (PMB) (GenScript, Piscataway, Nanjing, China) was used to remove phage endotoxins. Furthermore, the endotoxin levels of the phage were evaluated by the colorimetric method following the recommendations of the manufacturer (GenScript). The end-product was measured spectrophotometrically in a microplate reader. Female lactating BALB/c specific-pathogen-free (SPF) mice (10–14 days after the birth of their offspring) were purchased from the Experimental Animal Center, Shanghai Jiao Tong University. A mixture of ketamine 100 mg/kg (Imalgene, Merial Laboratorios, S.A) and xylacine 10 mg/kg (Rompun, Bayer Health Care) were administered intraperitoneally as anaesthesia for the mice. A syringe with a 33-gauge blunt-end needle was used to inoculate both the L4 (on the left) and R4 (on the right) of the fourth abdominal mammary gland pair with 1×10^5 CFU/gland (50 μL) of *P. aeruginosa* PAmas5. After 6 h, the phage-treated groups ($n = 5$) received an intramammary dose of 1×10^6 PFU/gland (50 μL). After 6 h, PAmas5-infected mice were treated through intramammary injection of 20 μg/gland ceftiofur sodium (50 μL) and 50 μL/gland PBS as the antibiotic-treated ($n = 5$) and PBS control ($n = 5$) groups, respectively. After a 24-h period, the mammary glands of the mice were photographed. The L4 mammary glands were aseptically removed, individually weighed, serially diluted in PBS (1:9) and plated in agar containing ampicillin (50 μg/mL) to determine the number of CFU/gland. The R4 mammary glands were gently removed and immediately placed in 4% formalin. Formalin-fixed tissues were processed and stained with hematoxylin and eosin (H&E) and toluidine blue using a routine staining procedure and were subsequently analysed using microscopy. (Note that the mammary glands removed from healthy lactating mice served as positive controls for histopathology).

The alteration of mammary gland histology was measured semi-quantitatively as described previously with slight modifications (Camperio et al., 2017). A scale from 0 to 3 was applied to the following alterations: 0 = normal healthy lactating alveoli without pathological changes; 1 = a minimal degree of necrotic acinar epithelial cells and/or interstitial inflammation and relatively normal mammary glands; 2 = a moderate degree of necrotic acinar epithelial cells and/or interstitial inflammation and relatively normal mammary glands; 3 = severe tissue damage, a very large number of interstitial inflammatory cells and extensive necrotic areas. All slides were assessed by three blinded observers (ZW, MG and YY) using a light microscope, and the discordant cases were reviewed at a multi-head microscope until a consensus was reached.

Cloning, Expression and Purification of the Lysin of the PAJD-1 Phage (PlyPAJD-1)

The PlyPAJD-1-encoding region was PCR-amplified with primers 5' *Bam*HI_JDlys (CGC<u>GGATCC</u>ATGAAC

GGTGCGACATAC, where the *Bam*HI site is underlined) and 3' *Xho*I_JDlys (CCG<u>CTCGAG</u>TTATCGCCAATCCACTTTCTT, where the *Xho*I site is underlined), using the genomic DNA of the PAJD-1 phage as a template for PlyPAJD-1. The PCR product was digested with *Bam*HI/*Xho*I and cloned into the pET-28a vector. Constituted plasmids were expressed in *E. coli* BL21 (DE3) grown to an optical density of 0.6 at 600 nm (OD_{600}) at 37°C, induced with 1 mM isopropyl-β-D-thiogalactoside (IPTG) and expressed for 14 h at 16°C. Cells were disrupted by sonication and purified with a Ni Sepharose 6 Fast Flow resin gravity column (GE Healthcare BioSciences, Pittsburgh, USA), as described previously (Zhang et al., 2016).

Bactericidal Activity and Lytic Spectrum of PlyPAJD-1

To determine the bactericidal activity of PlyPAJD-1 against *P. aeruginosa* PA14, 20 mL of early log-phase bacteria cells (5×10^8 CFU/mL) were pelleted and resuspended in 20 mM Tris–HCl buffer (pH 7.5) supplemented with 0.1 M EDTA for 5 min at room temperature. Then, cells were pelleted and thrice washed with PBS to remove the remaining EDTA. Next, the washed cells were mixed with 10 mL semisolid TSB medium at 42°C and then spotted on a plate. After solidification, 100 μL of PlyPAJD-1 protein (1mg/mL) was put into a punched hole. PBS was spotted into the other hole as a negative control. The plates were incubated for 12 h at 37°C, and the inhibition zone was used to check the lytic activity of PlyPAJD-1. The assay was performed at least three times in biological repeats.

To verify the lytic spectrum of PlyPAJD-1, a 96-well plate was used, as described by Wang et al. with minor modifications (Wang et al., 2018). Briefly, fresh bacterial cells (1×10^9 CFU/mL)

were pelleted and resuspended in 20 mM Tris–HCl buffer (pH 7.5) supplemented with 0.1 M EDTA for 5 min at room temperature. Then, cells (5×10^8 CFU/mL) were pelleted and thrice washed with PBS to remove the remaining EDTA. The lytic effect was monitored by blending 100 μL of bacterial suspension with 100 μL (1 mg/mL) of PlyPAJD-1 in a 96-well microtiter plate. The OD_{600} values were monitored after 2h. The decrease in bacterial turbidity was calculated by the OD_{600} after 2 h/original OD_{600} of the mixture. The assay was performed at least three times in biological repeats.

Statistical Analysis

In all experiments, the data were plotted using GraphPad Prism 6.01 (GraphPad Software, Inc., San Diego, CA, USA). The statistical significance of changes between groups was assessed with an unpaired Student's *t*-test. The *p*-values are indicated in the figure legends.

RESULTS

P. aeruginosa Could Cause Pathogen-Induced Cow Mastitis

To evaluate the microbes from three dairy farms in Shanghai, microbial community analysis of the udder surface of cows with mastitis was carried out, as shown in **Figure 1**. The results revealed that the predominant genera for cows with mastitis mainly included *Pseudomonas* (22.12%, 22.71% and 50.16%), *Flavobacterium* (1.15%, 2.21% and 22.06%), *Brachybacterium* (8.97%, 9.46% and 0.075%), and *Staphylococcus* (2.97%, 2.16% and 0.36%). Furthermore, five *P. aeruginosa* strains identified by

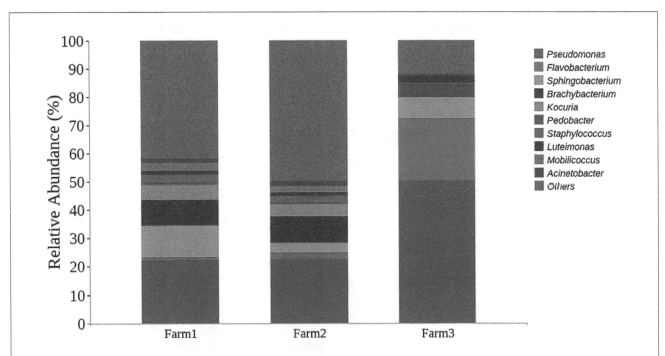

FIGURE 1 | Representation of the top bacterial genus in cows with mastitis by microbial community analysis. Bar graphs show the relative abundance of the top 10 bacterial genera from three dairy farms in Shanghai, China.

the VITEK 2 system were isolated from milk obtained from cows diagnosed with mastitis (**Tables S1–S5**). In particular, these strains were multidrug resistant (**Table 1**). These findings suggest that *Pseudomonas*, especially *P. aeruginosa*, could be a potential pathogen in dairy farms in Shanghai.

Isolation, Identification and Host Range Determination of *Pseudomonas* Phage PAJD-1

In this study, we isolated a lytic *Pseudomonas* phage, PAJD-1, from faecal sewage in dairy farms in Shanghai, China. Using *P. aeruginosa* PA14 as the host strain, the phage formed plaques 1 to 2 mm in diameter (**Figure 2A**). Among 20 *P. aeruginosa* strains, 80% (16/20) of the isolates were lysed by PAJD-1. In particular, PAJD-1 could effectively lyse five MDR *P. aeruginosa* strains isolated from dairy farms (**Table 1**).

The morphology of the isolated phage PAJD-1 was further characterised. TEM showed that the PAJD-1 particle had an isometric head of approximately 50 nm and a long, noncontractile tail with a length of approximately 200 nm (**Figure 2B**). Thus, it was morphologically similar to phages of the family *Siphoviridae* according to the classification of the International Committee on Taxonomy of Viruses (ICTV).

General Features of the PAJD-1 Genome

The PAJD-1 genome comprised 57.9 kb, double-stranded DNA and an average G+C content of 58.32%. Analysis *via* BLAST showed that the genome sequence of PAJD-1 belonged to a NP1-like phage (**Table 2**), which showed partial homology to phage NP1 (94%), phage Quinobequin (93%), phage PaMx25 (93%), phage PaMx25 (93%), phage PaMx25 (93%) and phage PaMx25 (93%). As shown in the whole-genome arrangement map (**Figure 3**), 72 open reading frames (ORFs) were defined as potential genes of PAJD-1. The genes of PAJD-1 were categorized into six modules: morphogenesis (purple), such as head or tail structural proteins and some putative virion synthetic

proteins; DNA replication (light green), such as DNA topoisomerase, DNA ligase and ribonuclease; nucleotide metabolism (blue), such as thymidylate synthase, ribonucleotide reductase glutamine amidotransferases and GTP cyclohydrolase; lysis modules (lysozyme-like transglycosylase, red); DNA packaging (pink), including terminase large subunit and terminase small subunit; and hypothetical proteins (bottle green). Among these ORFs, a putative tail structural protein (ORF 48) had the lowest homology (less than 65%) with the related genes of the above-mentioned phages, which are homologous to the genome of bacteriophage PAJD-1 (**Table 3**). Furthermore, BLAST analysis identified no ORFs associated with drug resistance, pathogenicity or lysogenisation, such as site-specific integrases or repressors in the whole-genome of PAJD-1.

Determination of the One-Step Growth Curve and Adsorption Ability of PAJD-1

To identify the different phases of the phage infection process, a one-step growth curve of PAJD-1 was determined. The results revealed that a latent period (defined as the time interval between the absorption and the beginning of the first burst) was about 20 min, and the burst size was estimated as 223 PFU per infected cell (**Figure 4A**), which was calculated as the ratio of the final count of liberated phage particles to the initial count of infected bacterial cells. Furthermore, the adsorption rates of PAJD-1 were determined. After 5 min of phage–bacteria incubation, about 95% of the phage particles were attached to the host cells (**Figure 4B**). After 30 min, only 65% of the phage particles were adsorbed, indicating that phage PAJD-1 had begun to lyse bacteria and that progeny phages were produced (**Figure 4B**).

The Temperature and pH Stability of Phage PAJD-1

To evaluate the suitability of phage PAJD-1 for potential clinical application in the future, a series of physical and chemical stabilities of phage PAJD-1 were examined. The stability of

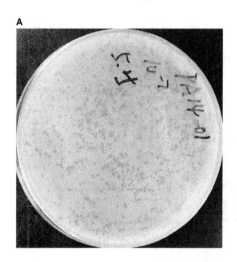
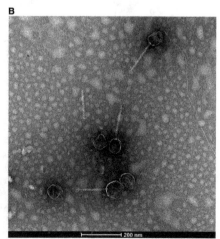

FIGURE 2 | Morphological images of PAJD-1. **(A)** Single-plaque in a double-layer agar plate. **(B)** Transmission electron microscopy image of PAJD-1.

TABLE 2 | The sequence identity of the PAJD-1 genome with other *Pseudomonas* phage.

Accession	Other phages	Phage type	Genome size (bp)	Morphology	Query cover
KX129925.1	*Pseudomonas* phage NP1	Lytic	58566	Siphoviridae	94%
MN504636.1	*Pseudomonas* phage Quinobequin-P09	Lytic	58277	Siphoviridae	93%
NC_041953.1	*Pseudomonas* phage PaMx25	Lytic	57899	Siphoviridae	93%
KX898399.1	*Pseudomonas* phage JG012	Lytic	58359	Siphoviridae	93%
KX898400.1	*Pseudomonas* phage JG054	Lytic	57839	Siphoviridae	90%

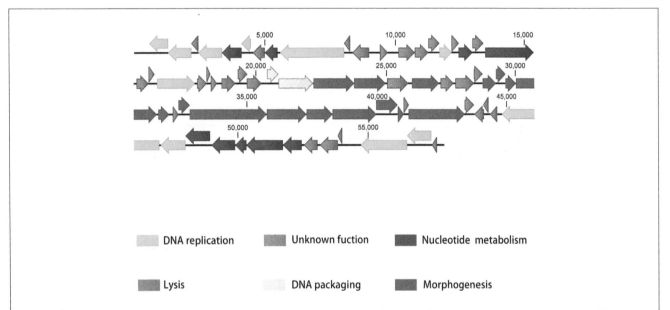

FIGURE 3 | The genome map of PAJD-1. The ORFs in the direction of transcription is shown by arrows. Groups of functional genes are indicated by different colours, including morphogenesis (purple), DNA replication (light green), nucleotide metabolism (blue), lysis (red), DNA packaging (pink), and hypothetical proteins (bottle green) modules.

TABLE 3 | The sequence identity of the PAJD-1 ORF48 with other *Pseudomonas* phage.

Accession	Description	The corresponding phage	Identity
KX129925.1	putative structural protein	*Pseudomonas* phage JG012	64.3%
MN504636.1	Putative virion structural protein	*Pseudomonas* phage NP1	63.51%
NC_041953.1	hypothetical protein	*Pseudomonas* phage Quinobequin-P09	61.86%
KX898399.1	hypothetical protein	*Pseudomonas* phage JG054	60.83%
KX898400.1	structural protein	*Pseudomonas* phage PaMx25	60.43%
YP_006561077.1	tail fiber structural protein	*Pseudomonas* phage MP1412	52.38%

phage PAJD-1 was investigated at several temperatures. We found that the activity of phage PAJD-1 remained stable over a wide range of temperatures up to 50°C. Higher temperatures resulted in progressive inactivation. Phage PAJD-1 was completely inactivated when heated to 65°C (**Figure 5A**). Moreover, **Figure 5A** shows that PAJD-1 maintained more than 80% of its bactericidal activity when stored at 4°C and -80°C for 6 months. pH stability was evaluated in SM buffers adjusted to values between pH 2 and pH 12. Phage PAJD-1 remained at a relatively high survival rate (more than 80%) in the pH range of 5 to 8. Beyond these values, the activity decreased dramatically (**Figure 5B**).

Phage Treatment in a Mouse Model of *P. aeruginosa*-Induced Mastitis

To evaluate the therapeutic potential of phage PAJD-1 *in vivo*, assays were performed on female lactating mice infected with MDR *P. aeruginosa* strain PAmas5, which was isolated from milk samples diagnosed as mastitis positive and efficiently lysed by PAJD-1 *in vitro* (**Table 1**). The results showed that the mammary glands of mice treated with PBS had the highest CFU burden (about log 5.79 CFU/gland). By contrast, mammary glands from mice treated with antibiotic had the lowest CFU burden (about log 2.41 CFU/gland). Mammary glands from the phage-treated mice had median CFU burdens

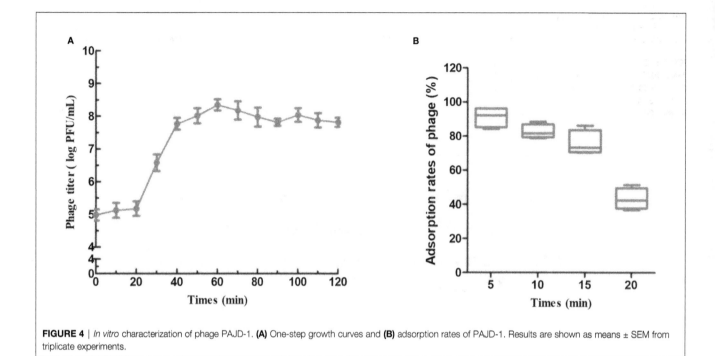

FIGURE 4 | *In vitro* characterization of phage PAJD-1. **(A)** One-step growth curves and **(B)** adsorption rates of PAJD-1. Results are shown as means ± SEM from triplicate experiments.

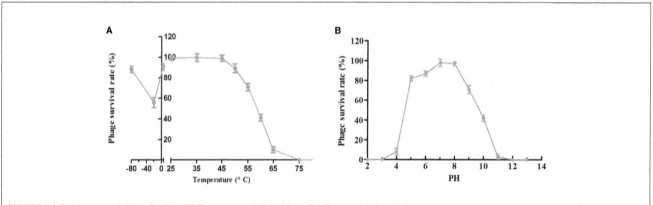

FIGURE 5 | Stability tests of phage PAJD-1. **(A)** Temperature stability: phage PAJD-1 was incubated at various temperatures as indicated. **(B)** pH stability: phage PAJD-1 was incubated at different pH conditions for 3 h. Results are shown as means ± SEM from triplicate experiments.

of about log 3.08 CFU/gland, significantly lower than the PBS control group ($p < 0.01$, **Figure 6**).

Damage to the mammary glands was observed by anatomical photograph in the mice (**Figure S1**). Representative images after histopathological examination are shown in **Figure 7**. The histopathological changes were semi-quantified as the tissue alteration score as shown in **Figure 7E**. Healthy lactating mice revealed normal healthy lactating alveoli without pathological changes (**Figure 7B**); however, the mammary glands of the PBS-treated mice with *P. aeruginosa*-induced mastitis showed obvious oedema and bleeding (**Figure S1A**). The H&E results showed an obvious intraglandular neutrophilic infiltration. The acinar epithelial cells were necrotic and detached with the acinar space infiltrated by a very large number of interstitial inflammatory cells (**Figure 7A**). By contrast, the mice treated

with antibiotics exhibited relatively normal mammary glands (slight hyperaemia), and a minimal degree of necrotic acinar epithelial cells and interstitial inflammation were identified (**Figures S1D** and **7D**). Compared with the PBS-treated mice, the mammary gland tissues of the mice from the phage-treated group showed relatively moderate oedema and bleeding (**Figure S1C**). Patchy, minimal neutrophilic inflammation and necrotic acinar epithelial cells were observed only in several glands (**Figure 7C**).

The Expression, Purification and Lytic Activity of PlyPAJD-1

To determine the bacteriolytic activity of the lysin (PlyPAJD-1) from phage PAJD-1, PlyPAJD-1 was expressed and purified. The results showed that PlyPAJD-1 was successfully expressed in

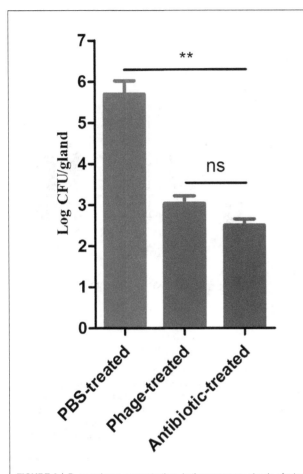

FIGURE 6 | *P. aeruginosa* concentrations in the mammary glands of mice treated with phage PAJD-1. The fourth abdominal mammary gland was infected with *P. aeruginosa* PAmas5. After 6 h, the mice were treated with the phage, an antibiotic and PBS. After 24 h, the L4 mammary glands were aseptically removed. Results are shown as means ± SEM from triplicate experiments. Significant differences ($p < 0.01$) are indicated by asterisks and ns represents no significant.

E. coli BL-21, and the size was 19.5 kDa (**Figure 8A**). The purified protein concentration was 2.1 mg/mL (data not shown). To evaluate the bacteriolytic activity of the PlyPAJD-1 protein against *P. aeruginosa*, a plate lytic assay was performed. The results showed a marked inhibition zone around the punched hole where the PlyPAJD-1 lay (**Figure 8B**). Notably, PlyPAJD-1 could not kill *P. aeruginosa* directly without pre-treatment with EDTA (**Figure 8C**). The lytic spectrum of PlyPAJD-1 against different *P. aeruginosa* is shown in **Figure 8D**. The result showed that after treatment with PlyPAJD-1, the concentrations of 90% (18/20) of the *P. aeruginosa* strains were significantly reduced compared with the strains treated with PBS.

DISCUSSION

In recent years, the incidence of clinical mastitis due to *P. aeruginosa* and the associated risk of large economic losses

have increased in large dairy herds, causing significant problems for affected farmers (Kawai et al., 2017; Klaas and Zadoks, 2018). Consistent with the previous issue, our study found that *P. aeruginosa* might become the major pathogenic bacterium that survives on the milk or udder surface of cows with mastitis (Kawai et al., 2017; Schauer et al., 2021). Notably, all five *P. aeruginosa* isolates from these cows were MDR. Therefore, there is an urgent need for novel therapies to treat and prevent bovine mastitis caused by *P. aeruginosa*.

With the rapid development of phage therapy, the use of phages against *P. aeruginosa* infections has been widely studied in experimental infections in humans and animals (Raz et al., 2019; Ng et al., 2020). In this study, we successfully isolated a lytic phage against *P. aeruginosa* from sewage in a dairy farm. The isolated PAJD-1, which was different from other *Siphoviridae* of previous reports (Amgarten et al., 2017; Jeon and Yong, 2019), showed intraspecific broad-spectrum lytic activities and good bactericidal activity against MDR *P. aeruginosa* strains (**Table 1**). It is known that the adsorption capacity, which is affected by the receptor-binding proteins (RBPs) of a phage, is the most important factor in determining its bactericidal broad-spectrum (Rios et al., 2016). Studies have found that through the exchange or insertion of RBPs (for instance, tail fibre protein) of virulent phages, such as members of the T3 or T7 families, the host range of related phages has been modified and expanded (Ando et al., 2015; Yehl et al., 2019). In this study, the hypothetical tail fibre protein of PAJD-1 (gb48) showed relatively low homology to other NP1-like phages (less than 65%), suggesting that phage PAJD-1 might have a different or relatively broad lytic spectrum than other NP1-like phages. Besides a wide host range, an optimal phage therapeutic agent necessitates certain features, such as a strictly lytic lifestyle, no toxins, and antibiotic-resistant genes (Rios et al., 2016). In addition to the intraspecific broad spectrum, the clarity of the genetic background is also a key factor for the application of bacteriophages (Rios et al., 2016). Genome sequence analysis showed that no ORFs associated with drug resistance, pathogenicity, or lysogenisations (such as site-specific integrases or repressors) were identified, which indicated that PAJD-1 has the potential for biocontrol and therapy.

Moreover, a high number of therapeutic phages (at least 1×10^8 PFU/mL) must be used to ensure sufficient contact and rapid infection of targeted cells. Selected phages should be easily propagated in liquid media with high titre (Brovko et al., 2012). Our study found that phage PAJD-1 rapidly proliferated (from 1×10^5 PFU/mL to 3×10^8 PFU/mL) within *P. aeruginosa* at 60 min after infection based on assays of one-step kinetics. Moreover, PAJD-1 showed a relatively short latent adsorption period (20 min) but a remarkable adsorption capacity (95% of adsorption rate). These findings indicate that the concentration of PAJD-1 can be achieved quickly and efficiently for application.

Among the physiological properties of phages, temperature and pH stability are considered important factors in the survival of phages during infectivity and storage (Wang et al., 2016).

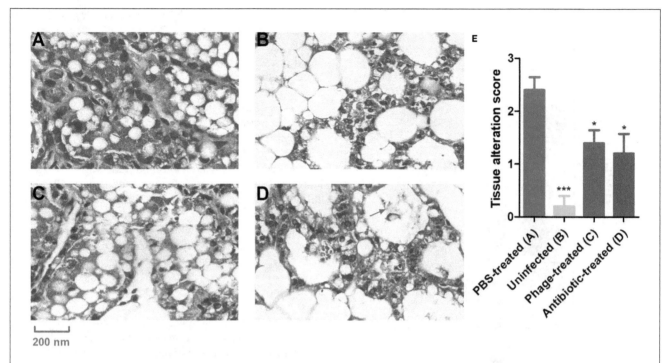

FIGURE 7 | PAJD-1 reduced *P. aeruginosa*-induced mammary gland lesions of mice. Mice were infected with *P. aeruginosa* PAmas5 strains and treated with **(C)** PAJD-1 and **(D)** ceftiofur sodium. **(A)** Mice were treated with PBS after infection as a medium-treated group. **(B)** An uninfected mouse served as a positive control. **(E)** The tissue alteration score was measured in tissue sections above. The scoring criteria were present in the materials and methods section. Mammary glands were collected 24 h after treatment and processed for H&E staining and microscopic examination. Results are shown as means ± SEM. Asterisks indicate when the tissue alteration score of uninfected mice and mice treated with PAJD-1 or ceftiofur sodium after infection were significantly lower (***$p < 0.001$ and *$p < 0.05$) than untreated mice after infection. The red arrows indicate neutrophilic infiltration. Magnification × 100, scale bars represent 200 nm.

Therefore, phages that have high stability at various temperatures and pH values are better candidates for applications, such as alternative therapeutic agents (Rios et al., 2016). Our study found that phage PAJD-1 showed a relatively broad range of temperature tolerance and pH stability. PAJD-1 stored at 4°C and -80°C for at least half a year maintained antibacterial activity. These data can be used to optimize the storage and therapeutic application of phages under various physicochemical conditions.

Scholars have reported many successful outcomes for the local and systemic application of phages in the treatment of human and animal infections with *P. aeruginosa*. For example, Jeon and Yong reported that nasal inhalation of phage significantly decreased the *P. aeruginosa* concentrations in the lungs of mice with pneumonia (Jeon and Yong, 2019). Moreover, there have been two clinical trials of *P. aeruginosa* phage therapy: one trial involving treatment of a *P. aeruginosa*-infected ear (Wright et al., 2009) and the other a treatment of burn infections (Jault et al., 2019). Nevertheless, there are no reports of *P. aeruginosa* infection nor a phage therapy model for murine mastitis. In this work, we successfully established a mouse model with mammary glands infected using *P. aeruginosa* strains isolated from cows with mastitis. In order to block adverse impact (reduced and variable disease induction) from suckling pups, we performed 'forced weaning' (removal of pups from the lactating female) before the time of mastitis induction

(Ingman et al., 2015). However, prolonged forced weaning resulted in rapid accumulation of milk in the mammary gland causing some complication (Nazemi et al., 2014), which convoluted the analysis of mastitis induction. Therefore, consistent with most studies, we completed the experiment within 48 h following mastitis induction and forced weaning (Gonen et al., 2007; Breyne et al., 2014). Importantly, phage PAJD-1 exhibited the same satisfactory curative effect as antibiotics against mastitis infection. Moreover, no adverse effects were observed due to phage treatment in this study.

Compared with phages, the application of lysins, which are derived from phages, has been widely studied in recent years (Wang et al., 2018; Raz et al., 2019); in particular, lysins of phages that overcome Gram-positive pathogens infection (Rios et al., 2016; Wang et al., 2018). However, lysins were not initially recommended against Gram-negative pathogens because their impermeable outer membrane blocked lysin contact with peptidoglycans, which is the target of lysins (Gutierrez and Briers, 2020). Phage PAJD-1 had a strong bactericidal effect against a broad spectrum of bacteria, suggesting that the lysin encoded by the phage had a strong bactericidal effect. Therefore, the PlyPAJD-1 (lysin of PAJD-1) was expressed and purified. However, PlyPAJD-1 could not penetrate the outer membrane directly to kill bacteria, but it showed synergetic bactericidal efficacy when combined with EDTA, which disrupts the outer

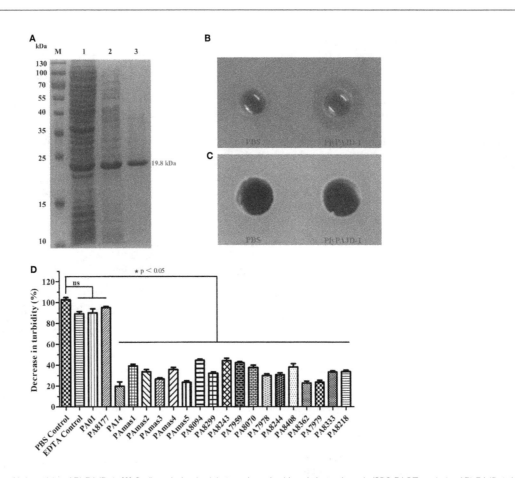

FIGURE 8 | The expression and lytic activity of PlyPAJD-1. **(A)** Sodium dodecyl sulphate–polyacrylamide gel electrophoresis (SDS-PAGE) analysis of PlyPAJD-1. M, molecular size marker; Lane 1, unpurified protein; Lane 2, flow-through sample; Lane 3, purified PlyPAJD-1 (19.8 kDa); **(B, C)** show the inhibition zone around the punched hole where the PlyPAJD-1 and PBS in bacteria pre-treated **(B)** with EDTA or **(C)** without EDTA, respectively. **(D)** The lytic spectrum of PlyPAJD-1 against different *P. aeruginosa*. Results are shown as means ± SEM from triplicate experiments. Significant differences (*p* < 0.05) are indicated by asterisks and ns represents no significant.

membrane by removing stabilizing cations and facilitating bacterial lysis by PlyPAJD-1 (Yang et al., 2018). At present, many studies have proposed different methods to transform lysin to effectively kill Gram-negative strains, including combining lysins with outer membrane permeabilizers (Oliveira et al., 2016), protein engineering (Wang et al., 2017; Yan et al., 2017) and formulating with nanocarriers (Ciepluch et al., 2019), which is the focus of our future research.

CONCLUSION

In conclusion, the results presented herein provide insight into a lytic phage PAJD-1, which exhibited a wide host range, and strong lytic activity and stability under various conditions. Clearly, our animal experiments demonstrated that phage PAJD-1 can protect mice from mastitis infection by MDR *P. aeruginosa*. Thus, phage PAJD-1 may be an alternative antimicrobial agent in the clinic.

ETHICS STATEMENT

The animal study was reviewed and approved by Ethical Committee for Animal Experiments of Shanghai Jiao Tong University.

AUTHOR CONTRIBUTIONS

YY, JS, and ZW designed the experiments. ZW, YX, and YG performed the experiments and collected the data. ZW, MG, YL, XZ, and YC collected and analyzed the data. JS, JM, and HW performed critical revision of the article. ZW wrote the manuscript. All authors contributed to the article and approved the submitted version.

ACKNOWLEDGMENTS

We appreciate Professor Xinhong Li at the Shanghai Jiao Tong University for sharing the *P. aeruginosa* PA01 and PA14. We

REFERENCES

Altschul, S. F., Madden, T. L., Schaffer, A. A., Zhang, J., Zhang, Z., Miller, W., et al (1997). Gapped BLAST and PSI-BLAST: A New Generation of Protein Database Search Programs. *Nucleic Acids Res.* 25, 3389–3402. doi: 10.1093/nar/25.17.3389

Amgarten, D., Martins, L. F., Lombardi, K. C., Antunes, L. P., De Souza, A. P. S., Nicastro, G. G., et al (2017). Three Novel *Pseudomonas* Phages Isolated From Composting Provide Insights Into the Evolution and Diversity of Tailed Phages. *BMC Genomics* 18, 346. doi: 10.1186/s12864-017-3729-z

Ando, H., Lemire, S., Pires, D. P., and Lu, T. K. (2015). Engineering Modular Viral Scaffolds for Targeted Bacterial Population Editing. *Cell Syst.* 1 (3), 187–196. doi: 10.1016/j.cels.2015.08.013

Bachta, K. E. R., Allen, J. P., Cheung, B. H., Chiu, C. H., and Hauser, A. R. (2020). Systemic Infection Facilitates Transmission of *Pseudomonas aeruginosa* in Mice. *Nat. Commun.* 11, 543. doi: 10.1038/s41467-020-14363-4

Breyne, K., Cool, S. K., Demon, D., Demeyere, K., Vandenberghe, T., Vandenabeele, P., et al (2014). Non-Classical proIL-1beta Activation During Mammary Gland Infection Is Pathogen-Dependent But Caspase-1 Independent. *PloS One* 9, e105680. doi: 10.1371/journal.pone.0105680

Brovko, L. Y., Anany, H., and Griffiths, M. W. (2012). Bacteriophages for Detection and Control of Bacterial Pathogens in Food and Food-Processing Environment. *Adv. Food Nutr. Res.* 67, 241–288. doi: 10.1016/B978-0-12-394598-3.00006-X

Camperio, C., Armas, F., Biasibetti, E., Frassanito, P., Giovannelli, C., Spuria, L., et al (2017). A Mouse Mastitis Model to Study the Effects of the Intramammary Infusion of a Food-Grade *Lactococcus Lactis* Strain. *PloS One* 12, e0184218. doi: 10.1371/journal.pone.0184218

Caporaso, J. G., Kuczynski, J., Stombaugh, J., Bittinger, K., Bushman, F. D., Costello, E. K., et al (2010). QIIME Allows Analysis of High-Throughput Community Sequencing Data. *Nat. Methods* 7 (5), 335–336. doi: 10.1038/nmeth.f.303

Caporaso, J. G., Lauber, C. L., Walters, W. A., Berg-Lyons, D., Huntley, J., Fierer, N., et al (2012). Ultra-High-Throughput Microbial Community Analysis on the Illumina HiSeq and MiSeq Platforms. *ISME J.* 6 (8), 1621–1624. doi: 10.1038/ismej.2012.8

Chegini, Z., Khoshbayan, A., Taati Moghadam, M., Farahani, I., Jazireian, P., and Shariati, A. (2020). Bacteriophage Therapy Against *Pseudomonas aeruginosa* Biofilms: A Review. *Ann. Clin. Microbiol. Antimicrob.* 19, 45. doi: 10.1186/s12941-020-00389-5

Ciepluch, K., Maciejewska, B., Galczynska, K., Kuc-Ciepluch, D., Bryszewska, M., Appelhans, D., et al (2019). The Influence of Cationic Dendrimers on Antibacterial Activity of Phage Endolysin Against *P. aeruginosa* Cells. *Bioorg. Chem.* 91, 103121. doi: 10.1016/j.bioorg.2019.103121

Desantis, T. Z., Hugenholtz, P., Larsen, N., Rojas, M., Brodie, E. L., Keller, K., et al (2006). Greengenes, a Chimera-Checked 16S rRNA Gene Database and Workbench Compatible With ARB. *Appl. Environ. Microbiol.* 72, 5069–5072. doi: 10.1128/AEM.03006-05

Dzuliashvili, M., Gabitashvili, K., Golidjashvili, A., Hoyle, N., and Gachechiladze, K. (2007). Study of Therapeutic Potential of the Experimental *Pseudomonas* Bacteriophage Preparation. *Georgian Med. News* 174, 81–88.

Edgar, R. C. (2010). Search and Clustering Orders of Magnitude Faster Than BLAST. *Bioinformatics* 26, 2460–2461. doi: 10.1093/bioinformatics/btq461

El Garch, F., Youala, M., Simjee, S., Moyaert, H., Klee, R., Truszkowska, B., et al (2020). Antimicrobial Susceptibility of Nine Udder Pathogens Recovered From Bovine Clinical Mastitis Milk in Europe 2015-2016: VetPath Results. *Vet. Microbiol.* 245, 108644. doi: 10.1016/j.vetmic.2020.108644

Fathizadeh, H., Saffari, M., Esmaeili, D., Moniri, R., and Salimian, M. (2020). Evaluation of Antibacterial Activity of Enterocin A-colicin E1 Fusion Peptide. *Iran. J. Basic Med. Sci.* 23, 1471–1479. doi: 10.22038/ijbms.2020.47826.11004

Fukuda, K., Ishida, W., Uchiyama, J., Rashel, M., Kato, S., Morita, T., et al (2012). *Pseudomonas aeruginosa* Keratitis in Mice: Effects of Topical Bacteriophage KPP12 Administration. *PloS One* 7 (10), e47742. doi: 10.1371/journal.pone.0047742

Gonen, E., Vallon-Eberhard, A., Elazar, S., Harmelin, A., Brenner, O., Rosenshine, I., et al (2007). Toll-Like Receptor 4 Is Needed to Restrict the Invasion of *Escherichia Coli* P4 Into Mammary Gland Epithelial Cells in a Murine Model of Acute Mastitis. *Cell Microbiol.* 9, 2826–2838. doi: 10.1111/j.1462-5822.2007.00999.x

Gutierrez, D., and Briers, Y. (2020). Lysins Breaking Down the Walls of Gram-Negative Bacteria, No Longer a No-Go. *Curr. Opin. Biotechnol.* 68, 15–22. doi: 10.1016/j.copbio.2020.08.014

Hesse, S., and Adhya, S. (2019). Phage Therapy in the Twenty-First Century: Facing the Decline of the Antibiotic Era; Is it Finally Time for the Age of the Phage? *Annu. Rev. Microbiol.* 73, 155–174. doi: 10.1146/annurev-micro-090817-062535

Ingman, W. V., Glynn, D. J., and Hutchinson, M. R. (2015). Mouse Models of Mastitis - How Physiological Are They? *Int. Breastfeed. J.* 10, 12. doi: 10.1186/s13006-015-0038-5

Jault, P., Leclerc, T., Jennes, S., Pirnay, J. P., Que, Y. A., Resch, G., et al (2019). Efficacy and Tolerability of a Cocktail of Bacteriophages to Treat Burn Wounds Infected by *Pseudomonas aeruginosa* (PhagoBurn): A Randomised, Controlled, Double-Blind Phase 1/2 Trial. *Lancet Infect. Dis.* 19, 35–45. doi: 10.1016/S1473-3099(18)30482-1

Javed, M., Jentzsch, B., Heinrich, M., Ueltzhoeffer, V., Peter, S., Schoppmeier, U., et al (2020). Transcriptomic Basis of Serum Resistance and Virulence Related Traits in XDR *P. aeruginosa* Evolved Under Antibiotic Pressure in a Morbidostat Device. *Front. Microbiol.* 11, 619542. doi: 10.3389/fmicb.2020.619542

Jeon, J., and Yong, D. (2019). Two Novel Bacteriophages Improve Survival in Galleria Mellonella Infection and Mouse Acute Pneumonia Models Infected With Extensively Drug-Resistant *Pseudomonas aeruginosa. Appl. Environ. Microbiol.* 85 (9), e02900–e02918. doi: 10.1128/AEM.02900-18

Kawai, K., Shinozuka, Y., Uchida, I., Hirose, K., Mitamura, T., Watanabe, A., et al (2017). Control of *Pseudomonas* Mastitis on a Large Dairy Farm by Using Slightly Acidic Electrolyzed Water. *Anim. Sci. J.* 88, 1601–1605. doi: 10.1111/asj.12815

Keane, O. M. (2019). Symposium Review: Intramammary Infections-Major Pathogens and Strain-Associated Complexity. *J. Dairy Sci.* 102, 4713–4726. doi: 10.3168/jds.2018-15326

Khalid, A., Lin, R. C. Y., and Iredell, J. R. (2020). A Phage Therapy Guide for Clinicians and Basic Scientists: Background and Highlighting Applications for Developing Countries. *Front. Microbiol.* 11, 599906. doi: 10.3389/fmicb.2020.599906

Klaas, I. C., and Zadoks, R. N. (2018). An Update on Environmental Mastitis: Challenging Perceptions. *Transbound Emerg. Dis.* 65 (Suppl1), 166–185. doi: 10.1111/tbed.12704

Maslova, E., Shi, Y., Sjoberg, F., Azevedo, H. S., Wareham, D. W., and Mccarthy, R. R. (2020). An Invertebrate Burn Wound Model That Recapitulates the Hallmarks of Burn Trauma and Infection Seen in Mammalian Models. *Front. Microbiol.* 11, 998. doi: 10.3389/fmicb.2020.00998

Morella, N. M., Gomez, A. L., Wang, G., Leung, M. S., and Koskella, B. (2018). The Impact of Bacteriophages on Phyllosphere Bacterial Abundance and Composition. *Mol. Ecol.* 27, 2025–2038. doi: 10.1111/mec.14542

Nazemi, S., Aalbaek, B., Kjelgaard-Hansen, M., Safayi, S., Klaerke, D. A., and Knight, C. H. (2014). Expression of Acute Phase Proteins and Inflammatory Cytokines in Mouse Mammary Gland Following *Staphylococcus Aureus* Challenge and in Response to Milk Accumulation. *J. Dairy Res.* 81, 445–454. doi: 10.1017/S0022029914000454

Ng, R. N., Tai, A. S., Chang, B. J., Stick, S. M., and Kicic, A. (2020). Overcoming Challenges to Make Bacteriophage Therapy Standard Clinical Treatment Practice for Cystic Fibrosis. *Front. Microbiol.* 11, 593988. doi: 10.3389/fmicb.2020.593988

Oliveira, H., Vilas Boas, D., Mesnage, S., Kluskens, L. D., Lavigne, R., Sillankorva, S., et al (2016). Structural and Enzymatic Characterization of ABgp46, a Novel Phage Endolysin With Broad Anti-Gram-Negative Bacterial Activity. *Front. Microbiol.* 7, 208. doi: 10.3389/fmicb.2016.00208

Ong, S. P., Azam, A. H., Sasahara, T., Miyanaga, K., and d Tanji, Y. (2020). Characterization of *Pseudomonas* Lytic Phages and Their Application as a Cocktail With Antibiotics in Controlling *Pseudomonas aeruginosa. J. Biosci. Bioeng.* 129, 693–699. doi: 10.1016/j.jbiosc.2020.02.001

Otto, M. (2014). Physical Stress and Bacterial Colonization. *FEMS Microbiol. Rev.* 38, 1250–1270. doi: 10.1111/1574-6976.12088

Pajunen, M., Kiljunen, S., and Skurnik, M. (2000). Bacteriophage phiYeO3-12, Specific for *Yersinia Enterocolitica* Serotype O:3, Is Related to Coliphages T3 and T7. *J. Bacteriol.* 182, 5114–5120. doi: 10.1128/JB.182.18.5114-5120.2000

Principi, N., Silvestri, E., and Esposito, S. (2019). Advantages and Limitations of Bacteriophages for the Treatment of Bacterial Infections. *Front. Pharmacol.* 10, 513. doi: 10.3389/fphar.2019.00513

Raz, A., Serrano, A., Hernandez, A., Euler, C. W., and Fischetti, V. A. (2019). Isolation of Phage Lysins That Effectively Kill *Pseudomonas aeruginosa* in Mouse Models of Lung and Skin Infection. *Antimicrob. Agents Chemother.* 63 (7), e00024–19. doi: 10.1128/AAC.00024-19

Rios, A. C., Moutinho, C. G., Pinto, F. C., Del Fiol, F. S., Jozala, A., Chaud, M. V., et al (2016). Alternatives to Overcoming Bacterial Resistances: State-of-the-Art. *Microbiol. Res.* 191, 51–80. doi: 10.1016/j.micres.2016.04.008

Schauer, B., Wald, R., Urbantke, V., Loncaric, I., and Baumgartner, M. (2021). Tracing Mastitis Pathogens-Epidemiological Investigations of a *Pseudomonas aeruginosa* Mastitis Outbreak in an Austrian Dairy Herd. *Animals (Basel)* 11 (2), 279. doi: 10.3390/ani11020279

Segata, N., Izard, J., Waldron, L., Gevers, D., Miropolsky, L., Garrett, W. S., et al (2011). Metagenomic Biomarker Discovery and Explanation. *Genome Biol.* 12, R60. doi: 10.1186/gb-2011-12-6-r60

Tummler, B. (2019). Emerging Therapies Against Infections With *Pseudomonas aeruginosa*. *F1000Res* 8, F1000 Faculty Rev-1371. doi: 10.12688/f1000research.19509.1

Wang, S., Gu, J., Lv, M., Guo, Z., Yan, G., Yu, L., et al (2017). The Antibacterial Activity of *E. Coli* Bacteriophage Lysin Lysep3 Is Enhanced by Fusing the *Bacillus Amyloliquefaciens* Bacteriophage Endolysin Binding Domain D8 to the C-Terminal Region. *J. Microbiol.* 55, 403–408. doi: 10.1007/s12275-017-6431-6

Wang, Z., Kong, L., Liu, Y., Fu, Q., Cui, Z., Wang, J., et al (2018). A Phage Lysin Fused to a Cell-Penetrating Peptide Kills Intracellular Methicillin-Resistant *Staphylococcus Aureus* in Keratinocytes and has Potential as a Treatment for Skin Infections in Mice. *Appl. Environ. Microbiol.* 84 (12), e00380–e00318. doi: 10.1128/AEM.00380-18

Wang, Z., Zheng, P., Ji, W., Fu, Q., Wang, H., Yan, Y., et al (2016). SLPW: A Virulent Bacteriophage Targeting Methicillin-Resistant *Staphylococcus Aureus In Vitro* and *In Vivo*. *Front. Microbiol.* 7, 934. doi: 10.3389/fmicb.2016.00934

Wright, A., Hawkins, C. H., Anggard, E. E., and Harper, D. R. (2009). A Controlled Clinical Trial of a Therapeutic Bacteriophage Preparation in Chronic Otitis Due to Antibiotic-Resistant *Pseudomonas aeruginosa*; A Preliminary Report of Efficacy. *Clin. Otolaryngol.* 34, 349–357. doi: 10.1111/j.1749-4486.2009.01973.x

Yang, Y., Le, S., Shen, W., Chen, Q., Huang, Y., Lu, S., et al (2018). Antibacterial Activity of a Lytic Enzyme Encoded by *Pseudomonas aeruginosa* Double Stranded RNA Bacteriophage phiYY. *Front. Microbiol.* 9, 1778. doi: 10.3389/fmicb.2018.01778

Yan, G., Liu, J., Ma, Q., Zhu, R., Guo, Z., Gao, C., et al (2017). The N-Terminal and Central Domain of Colicin A Enables Phage Lysin to Lyse *Escherichia Coli* Extracellularly. *Antonie Van Leeuwenhoek* 110, 1627–1635. doi: 10.1007/s10482-017-0912-9

Yehl, K., Lemire, S., Yang, A. C., Ando, H., Mimee, M., Torres, M. T., et al (2019). Engineering Phage Host-Range and Suppressing Bacterial Resistance Through Phage Tail Fiber Mutagenesis. *Cell* 179, 459–469.e459. doi: 10.1016/j.cell.2019.09.015

Zhang, H., Zhang, C., Wang, H., Yan, Y. X., and Sun, J. (2016). A Novel Prophage Lysin Ply5218 With Extended Lytic Activity and Stability Against *Streptococcus Suis* Infection. *FEMS Microbiol. Lett.* 363 (18), fnw186. doi: 10.1093/femsle/fnw186

Permissions

The contributors of this book come from diverse backgrounds, making this book a truly international effort. This book will bring forth new frontiers with its revolutionizing research information and detailed analysis of the nascent developments around the world.

We would like to thank all the contributing authors for lending their expertise to make the book truly unique. They have played a crucial role in the development of this book. Without their invaluable contributions this book wouldn't have been possible. They have made vital efforts to compile up to date information on the varied aspects of this subject to make this book a valuable addition to the collection of many professionals and students.

This book was conceptualized with the vision of imparting up-to-date information and advanced data in this field. To ensure the same, a matchless editorial board was set up. Every individual on the board went through rigorous rounds of assessment to prove their worth. After which they invested a large part of their time researching and compiling the most relevant data for our readers.

The editorial board has been involved in producing this book since its inception. They have spent rigorous hours researching and exploring the diverse topics which have resulted in the successful publishing of this book. They have passed on their knowledge of decades through this book. To expedite this challenging task, the publisher supported the team at every step. A small team of assistant editors was also appointed to further simplify the editing procedure and attain best results for the readers.

Apart from the editorial board, the designing team has also invested a significant amount of their time in understanding the subject and creating the most relevant covers. They scrutinized every image to scout for the most suitable representation of the subject and create an appropriate cover for the book.

The publishing team has been an ardent support to the editorial, designing and production team. Their endless efforts to recruit the best for this project, has resulted in the accomplishment of this book. They are a veteran in the field of academics and their pool of knowledge is as vast as their experience in printing. Their expertise and guidance has proved useful at every step. Their uncompromising quality standards have made this book an exceptional effort. Their encouragement from time to time has been an inspiration for everyone.

The publisher and the editorial board hope that this book will prove to be a valuable piece of knowledge for researchers, students, practitioners and scholars across the globe.

List of Contributors

Thais Arns and Eduardo A. Donadi
Department of Basic and Applied Immunology, Ribeirão Preto Medical School, University of São Paulo, Ribeirão Preto, Brazil

Dinler A. Antunes, Jayvee R. Abella, Maurício M. Rigo and Lydia E. Kavraki
Department of Computer Science, Rice University, Houston, TX, United States

Silvana Giuliatti
Department of Genetics, Ribeirão Preto Medical School, University of São Paulo, Ribeirão Preto, Brazil

Bo-Eun Kwon, Jae-Hee Ahn, Eun-Kyoung Park, Hyunjin Jeong and Hyun-Jeong Ko
Laboratory of Microbiology and Immunology, College of Pharmacy, Kangwon National University, Chuncheon, South Korea

Hyo-Ji Lee and Yu-Jin Jung
Department of Biological Sciences, Kangwon National University, Chuncheon, South Korea

Sung Jae Shin
Department of Microbiology, Institute for Immunology and Immunological Disease, Brain Korea 21 PLUS Project for Medical Science, Yonsei University College of Medicine, Seoul, South Korea

Hye-Sook Jeong, Jung Sik Yoo and EunKyoung Shin
Division of Vaccine Research, Center for Infectious Disease Research, Korea National Institute of Health (KNIH), Korea Centers for Disease Control and Prevention (KCDC), Cheongju, South Korea

Sang-Gu Yeo
Sejong Institute of Health and Environment, Sejong, South Korea

Sun-Young Chang
Laboratory of Microbiology, College of Pharmacy and Research Institute of Pharmaceutical Science and Technology (RIPST), Ajou University, Suwon, South Korea

Pei Wang, Longyu Yi, Xin Liu and Qunwei Lu
Key Laboratory of Molecular Biophysics of Ministry of Education, Department of Biomedical Engineering, College of Life Science and Technology, Center for Human Genome Research, Huazhong University of Science and Technology, Wuhan, China

Xue Zhang, Lizhan Chen and Yang Cao
Jiangsu Key Laboratory of Marine Pharmaceutical Compound Screening, Jiangsu Key Laboratory of Marine Biological Resources and Environment, Co-Innovation Center of Jiangsu Marine Bio-industry Technology, School of Pharmacy, Jiangsu Ocean University, Lianyungang, China

Chao Ma, Shihui Fan, Yu Wang, Haitao Yang, Mingsheng Lyu, Jingquan Dong and Song Gao
Jiangsu Key Laboratory of Marine Biological Resources and Environment, Jiangsu Key Laboratory of Marine Pharmaceutical Compound Screening, Co-Innovation Center of Jiangsu Marine Bio-industry Technology, School of Pharmacy, Jiangsu Ocean University, Lianyungang, China

Elliot Whittard, James Redfern, Roobinidevi Ragupathy, Sladjana Malic and Mark C. Enright
Department of Life Sciences, Manchester Metropolitan University, Manchester, United Kingdom

Guoqing Xia
Lydia Becker Institute of Immunology and Inflammation, University of Manchester, Manchester, United Kingdom

Andrew Millard
Department of Genetics and Genome Biology, University of Leicester, Leicester, United Kingdom

Mauro César da Silva, Fernanda Silva Medeiros, Neila Caroline Henrique da Silva, Fabiana Oliveira dos Santos Gomes, Thailany Thays Gomes and Christina Alves Peixoto
Laboratory of Immunogenetics, Department of Immunology, Aggeu Magalhães Institute, Oswaldo Cruz Foundation, Recife, Brazil

Larissa Albuquerque Paiva
Getúlio Vargas Hospital, Pernambuco Health Department, Recife, Brazil

Matheus Costa e Silva and Eduardo Antônio Donadi
Clinical Immunology Division, Department of Medicine, School of Medicine of Ribeirão Preto, University of São Paulo (USP), Ribeirão Preto, Brazil

Maria Carolina Valença Rygaard
Laboratory of Molecular Biology, IMIP Hospital, Pediatric Oncology Service, Recife, Brazil

Norma Lucena-Silva
Laboratory of Immunogenetics, Department of Immunology, Aggeu Magalhães Institute, Oswaldo Cruz Foundation, Recife, Brazil
Laboratory of Molecular Biology, IMIP Hospital, Pediatric Oncology Service, Recife, Brazil

Maria Luiza Bezerra Menezes
Department of Maternal and Child, Faculty of Medical Sciences, University of Pernambuco, Recife, Brazil

Stefan Welkovic
Integrated Health Center Amaury de Medeiros (CISAM), University of Pernambuco, Recife, Brazil

Maria Alice Freitas Queiroz, Ednelza da Silva Graça Amoras, Tuane Carolina Ferreira Moura, Sandra Souza Lima, Ricardo Ishak and Antonio Carlos Rosário Vallinoto
Laboratory of Virology, Institute of Biological Sciences, Federal University of Pará, Belém, Brazil

Carlos Araújo da Costa and Maisa Silva de Sousa
Laboratory of Cellular and Molecular Biology, Tropical Medicine Center, Federal University of Pará, Belém, Brazil

Xin Tan and Yingfei Ma
Shenzhen Key Laboratory of Synthetic Genomics, Guangdong Provincial Key Laboratory of Synthetic Genomics, CAS Key Laboratory of Quantitative Engineering Biology, Shenzhen Institute of Synthetic Biology, Shenzhen Institute of Advanced Technology, Chinese Academy of Sciences, Shenzhen, China

Huaisheng Chen, Yichun Jiang and Xueyan Liu
Department of Critical Care Medicine, Shenzhen People's Hospital (The Second Clinical Medical College of Jinan University, The First Affiliated Hospital of South University of Science and Technology), Shenzhen, China

Min Zhang and Wei Huang
Shenzhen People's Hospital, Shenzhen Institute of Respiratory Diseases, Shenzhen, China
Bacteriology and Antibacterial Resistance Surveillance Laboratory, Shenzhen People's Hospital (The Second Clinical Medical College, Jinan University, The First Affiliated Hospital, Southern University of Science and Technology), Shenzhen, China

Ying Zhao
Department of Geriatrics, Shenzhen People's Hospital (The Second Clinical Medical College of Jinan University, The First Affiliated Hospital of South University of Science and Technology), Shenzhen, China

Min Song, Dongmei Wu, Yang Hu, Haiyan Luo and Gongbo Li
Department of Neurology, The Second Affiliated Hospital of Chongqing Medical University, Chongqing, China

Michelle Seif, Hermann Einsele and Jürgen Löffler
Department of Internal Medicine II, University Hospital Wuerzburg, Würzburg, Germany

Yi Qiao, Ge Jiang and Hui Shen
Jiangsu Institute of Oceanology and Marine Fisheries, Nantong, China

George Blundell-Hunter, Gemma E. Beecham and Peter W. Taylor
School of Pharmacy, University College London, London, United Kingdom

David Negus
School of Science & Technology, Nottingham Trent University, Nottingham, United Kingdom

Matthew J. Dorman
Parasites and Microbes Programme, Wellcome Sanger Institute, Hinxton, United Kingdom

Derek J. Pickard
Department of Medicine, University of Cambridge, Addenbrooke's Hospital, Cambridge, United Kingdom

Phitchayapak Wintachai and Supayang P. Voravuthikunchai
Faculty of Science, Prince of Songkla University, Songkhla, Thailand

Nicholas R. Thomson
Parasites and Microbes Programme, Wellcome Sanger Institute, Hinxton, United Kingdom
Department of Infectious and Tropical Diseases, London School of Hygiene & Tropical Medicine, London, United Kingdom

Antonio J. Martín-Galiano and Michael J. McConnell
Intrahospital Infections Laboratory, National Centre for Microbiology, Instituto de Salud Carlos III, Majadahonda, Spain

Junrong Liang, Shuai Qin, Ran Duan, Haoran Zhang, Deming Tang, Dongyue Lv, Zhaokai He, Hui Mu, Meng Xiao, Jinchuan Yang, Huaiqi Jing and Xin Wang
State Key Laboratory of Infectious Disease Prevention and Control, National Institute for Communicable Disease Control and Prevention, Chinese Center for Disease Control and Prevention, Beijing, China

Weiwei Wu
State Key Laboratory of Infectious Disease Prevention and Control, National Institute for Communicable Disease Control and Prevention, Chinese Center for Disease Control and Prevention, Beijing, China
Sanitary Inspection Center, Xuzhou Municipal Centre for Disease Control and Prevention, Xuzhou, China

Xu Li
School of Light Industry, Beijing Technology and Business University, Beijing, China

Guoming Fu
Sanitary Inspection Center, Subei Mongolian Autonomous County Center for Disease Control and Prevention, Jiuquan, China

Xinmin Lu
Sanitary Inspection Center, Akesai Kazakh Autonomous County Center for Disease Control and Prevention, Jiuquan, China

Vijay Singh Gondil, Mengwei Jiang and Junhua Li
CAS Key Laboratory of Special Pathogens and Biosafety, Center for Biosafety Mega-Science, Wuhan Institute of Virology, Chinese Academy of Sciences, Wuhan, China

Fazal Mehmood Khan, Changchang Li, Junping Yu, Hongping Wei and Hang Yang
CAS Key Laboratory of Special Pathogens and Biosafety, Center for Biosafety Mega-Science, Wuhan Institute of Virology, Chinese Academy of Sciences, Wuhan, China
International College, University of Chinese Academy of Sciences, Beijing, China

Gunaraj Dhungana, Madhav Regmi and Rajani Malla
Central Department of Biotechnology, Tribhuvan University, Kirtipur, Nepal

Roshan Nepal
Central Department of Biotechnology, Tribhuvan University, Kirtipur, Nepal
Adelaide Medical School, Faculty of Health and Medical Sciences, The University of Adelaide, Adelaide, SA, Australia

Ming Liu, Fenxia Fan, Zhe Li, Yufeng Fan, Jingyun Zhang, Yuanming Huang, Zhenpeng Li, Jie Li and Biao Kan
State Key Laboratory for Infectious Disease Prevention and Control, National Institute for Communicable Disease Control and Prevention, Chinese Center for Disease Control and Prevention, Beijing, China

Huihui Sun
State Key Laboratory for Infectious Disease Prevention and Control, National Institute for Communicable Disease Control and Prevention, Chinese Center for Disease Control and Prevention, Beijing, China
National Institute of Environment Health, Chinese Center for Disease Control and Prevention, Beijing, China

Jialiang Xu
School of Light Industry, Beijing Technology and Business University, Beijing, China

Thomas Sécher, Alexie Mayor and Nathalie Heuzé-Vourc'h
INSERM U1100, Centre d'Etude des Pathologies Respiratoires, Tours, France
Centre d'Etude des Pathologies Respiratoires, Université de Tours, Tours, France

Yifei Lu
Institute of Burn Research, Southwest Hospital, State Key Lab of Trauma, Burn and Combined Injury, Army Medical University, Chongqing, China

Yingran Wang
Department of Clinical Laboratory Medicine, Southwest Hospital, Army Medical University, Chongqing, China

Jing Wang, Yan Zhao, Gang Li and Shuguang Lu
Department of Microbiology, College of Basic Medical Science, Army Medical University, Chongqing, China

Qiu Zhong
Department of Clinical Laboratory Medicine, Daping Hospital, Army Medical University, Chongqing, China

Zhifeng Fu
College of Pharmaceutical Sciences, Southwest University, Chongqing, China

Jiachen Huang, Darren Diaz and Jarrod J. Mousa
Department of Infectious Diseases, College of Veterinary Medicine, University of Georgia, Athens, GA, United States
Center for Vaccines and Immunology, College of Veterinary Medicine, University of Georgia, Athens, GA, United States

Xiang Wang, Zuozhou Xie, Jinhong Zhao, Zhenghua Zhu, Chen Yang and Yi Liu
Department of Pulmonary and Critical Care Medicine, The Second People's Hospital of Kunming, Kunming, China

Xinwei Zou
School of Agriculture and Biology, Shanghai Jiao Tong University, Shanghai Key Laboratory of Veterinary Biotechnology, Shanghai, China

Mengting Guo, Ya Gao, Yibing Xue, Yuanping Liu, Xiaoyan Zeng, Yuqiang Cheng, Jingjiao Ma, Hengan Wang, Jianhe Sun, Zhaofei Wang and Yaxian Yan
School of Agriculture and Biology, Shanghai Jiao Tong University, Shanghai Key Laboratory of Veterinary Biotechnology, Shanghai, ChinaW

Index